Psoriasis and Psoriatic Arthritis

Psoriasis and Psoriatic Arthritis

Editor: Cooper Ginger

AMERICAN
MEDICAL PUBLISHERS
www.americanmedicalpublishers.com

AMERICAN
MEDICAL PUBLISHERS
www.americanmedicalpublishers.com

Cataloging-in-Publication Data

Psoriasis and psoriatic arthritis / edited by Cooper Ginger.
p. cm.
Includes bibliographical references and index.
ISBN 979-8-88740-403-5
1. Psoriasis. 2. Psoriatic arthritis. 3. Skin--Diseases. 4. Arthritis.
5. Dermatology. I. Ginger, Cooper.
RL321 .P76 2023
616.526--dc23

American Medical Publishers,
41 Flatbush Avenue,
1st Floor, New York,
NY 11217, USA

ISBN 979-8-88740-403-5 (Hardback)

Contents

Preface IX

Chapter 1 **Potential Role of Cytochrome c and Tryptase in Psoriasis and Psoriatic Arthritis Pathogenesis: Focus on Resistance to Apoptosis and Oxidative Stress** 1
Maria Sole Chimenti, Flavia Sunzini, Laura Fiorucci, Elisabetta Botti, Giulia Lavinia Fonti, Paola Conigliaro, Paola Triggianese, Luisa Costa, Francesco Caso, Alessandro Giunta, Maria Esposito, Luca Bianchi, Roberto Santucci and Roberto Perricone

Chapter 2 **IL-36γ is a Strong Inducer of IL-23 in Psoriatic Cells and Activates Angiogenesis** 12
Charlie Bridgewood, Gareth W. Fearnley, Anna Berekmeri, Philip Laws, Tom Macleod, Sreenivasan Ponnambalam, Martin Stacey, Anne Graham and Miriam Wittmann

Chapter 3 **The Role of Helper T Cells in Psoriasis** 26
Peng Hu, Mengyao Wang, Hu Gao, Ai Zheng, Jinhui Li, Dezhi Mu and Jiyu Tong

Chapter 4 **Psoriasis: Classical vs. Paradoxical: The Yin-Yang of TNF and Type I Interferon** 36
Alessio Mylonas and Curdin Conrad

Chapter 5 **Potential Immunological Links Between Psoriasis and Cardiovascular Disease** 46
Aparna P. Sajja, Aditya A. Joshi, Heather L. Teague, Amit K. Dey and Nehal N. Mehta

Chapter 6 **Long Non-Coding RNAs Play a Role in the Pathogenesis of Psoriatic Arthritis by Regulating MicroRNAs and Genes Involved in Inflammation and Metabolic Syndrome** 56
Marzia Dolcino, Andrea Pelosi, Piera Filomena Fiore, Giuseppe Patuzzo, Elisa Tinazzi, Claudio Lunardi and Antonio Puccetti

Chapter 7 **Epidermal mTORC1 Signaling Contributes to the Pathogenesis of Psoriasis and Could Serve as a Therapeutic Target** 72
Claudia Buerger

Chapter 8 **Human Leukocyte Antigen-Class I Alleles and the Autoreactive T Cell Response in Psoriasis Pathogenesis** 79
Jörg Christoph Prinz

Chapter 9 **Psoriasis, Cardiovascular Events and Biologics: Lights and Shadows** 86
Giuseppina Caiazzo, Gabriella Fabbrocini, Roberta Di Caprio, Annunziata Raimondo, Emanuele Scala, Nicola Balato and Anna Balato

Chapter 10 **The Interplay Between Keratinocytes and Immune Cells in the Pathogenesis of Psoriasis** 98
Cristina Albanesi, Stefania Madonna, Paolo Gisondi and Giampiero Girolomoni

Chapter 11 **PSORI-CM02 Formula Increases CD4+ Foxp3+ Regulatory T Cell Frequency and Ameliorates Imiquimod-Induced Psoriasis in Mice** 105
Haiming Chen, Huazhen Liu, Chuanjian Lu, Maojie Wang, Xiong Li, Hui Zhao, Yuhong Yan, Wanling Yu, Ling Han and Zhenhua Dai

Chapter 12 **The Interleukin-23/Interleukin-17 Axis Links Adaptive and Innate Immunity in Psoriasis** 117
Michael P. Schön and Luise Erpenbeck

Chapter 13 **Thrombosis in Psoriasis: Cutaneous Cytokine Production as a Potential Driving Force of Haemostatic Dysregulation and Subsequent Cardiovascular Risk** 130
Maria J. E. Visser, Gareth Tarr and Etheresia Pretorius

Chapter 14 **Transcription Factor Retinoid-Related Orphan Receptor γt: A Promising Target for the Treatment of Psoriasis** 147
Lipeng Tang, Xiaozhi Yang, Yongxin Liang, Hesong Xie, Zhenhua Dai and Guangjuan Zheng

Chapter 15 **Anti-LL37 Antibodies are Present in Psoriatic Arthritis (PsA) Patients: New Biomarkers in PsA** 155
Loredana Frasca, Raffaella Palazzo, Maria S. Chimenti, Stefano Alivernini, Barbara Tolusso, Laura Bui, Elisabetta Botti, Alessandro Giunta, Luca Bianchi, Luca Petricca, Simone E. Auteri, Francesca Spadaro, Giulia L. Fonti, Mario Falchi, Antonella Evangelista, Barbara Marinari, Immacolata Pietraforte, Francesca R. Spinelli, Tania Colasanti, Cristiano Alessandri, Fabrizio Conti, Elisa Gremese, Antonio Costanzo, Guido Valesini, Roberto Perricone and Roberto Lande

Chapter 16 **Gamma Delta T Cells and their Pathogenic Role in Psoriasis** 171
Cong Qi, Yazhuo Wang, Ping Li and Jingxia Zhao

Chapter 17 **CLA^+ T Cell Response to Microbes in Psoriasis** 183
Carmen De Jesús-Gil, Ester Ruiz-Romeu, Marta Ferran, Anca Chiriac, Gustavo Deza, Péter Hóllo, Antonio Celada, Ramon M. Pujol and Luis F. Santamaria-Babí

Chapter 18 **The IL-17 Family of Cytokines in Psoriasis: IL-17A and Beyond** 188
Nicolo Costantino Brembilla, Luisa Senra and Wolf-Henning Boehncke

Chapter 19 **Systemic Inflammation and Cardiovascular Comorbidity in Psoriasis Patients: Causes and Consequences** 201
Wolf-Henning Boehncke

Chapter 20 **Neutrophils in Psoriasis** 214
Chih-Chao Chiang, Wei-Jen Cheng, Michal Korinek, Cheng-Yu Lin and Tsong-Long Hwang

Chapter 21 **T Cell Hierarchy in the Pathogenesis of Psoriasis and Associated Cardiovascular Comorbidities......226**
Fabio Casciano, Paolo D. Pigatto, Paola Secchiero, Roberto Gambari and Eva Reali

Permissions

List of Contributors

Index

Preface

Psoriasis is a non-communicable and chronic autoimmune disease. It is characterized by red, itchy scaly patches mostly on the knees, elbows, back and scalp. There are five main forms of psoriasis. It includes plaque psoriasis, guttate psoriasis, inverse psoriasis, pustular psoriasis, and erythrodermic psoriasis. It is a genetic disease, which is stimulated by environmental factors. Stress, obesity, smoking, alcohol consumption, skin dryness, HIV infection, and certain drugs are some key factors that prompt this condition. It leads to several complications such as conjunctivitis, metabolic syndrome, Crohn's disease, Parkinson's disease, etc. Diagnosis varies according to the appearance of the skin. It includes differential diagnosis and in certain cases a skin biopsy. Psoriatic arthritis is a type of inflammatory arthritis which affects people who have psoriasis The most common treatments for mild to moderate psoriasis include topical treatments (application of creams or ointments), phototherapy, and systemic treatment (oral and injected medications). Treatment of psoriatic arthritis involves biological therapies, non-steroidal anti-inflammatory drugs and steroid injections. From theories to research to practical applications, case studies related to various topics of relevance to psoriasis and psoriatic arthritis have been included in this book. Students, immunologists, doctors, researchers, and all interested in this medical condition will find it beneficial.

This book is a comprehensive compilation of works of different researchers from varied parts of the world. It includes valuable experiences of the researchers with the sole objective of providing the readers (learners) with a proper knowledge of the concerned field. This book will be beneficial in evoking inspiration and enhancing the knowledge of the interested readers.

In the end, I would like to extend my heartiest thanks to the authors who worked with great determination on their chapters. I also appreciate the publisher's support in the course of the book. I would also like to deeply acknowledge my family who stood by me as a source of inspiration during the project.

Editor

1

Potential Role of Cytochrome c and Tryptase in Psoriasis and Psoriatic Arthritis Pathogenesis: Focus on Resistance to Apoptosis and Oxidative Stress

Maria Sole Chimenti[1], Flavia Sunzini[1], Laura Fiorucci[2], Elisabetta Botti[3], Giulia Lavinia Fonti[1], Paola Conigliaro[1], Paola Triggianese[1], Luisa Costa[4], Francesco Caso[4], Alessandro Giunta[3], Maria Esposito[3], Luca Bianchi[3], Roberto Santucci[2] and Roberto Perricone[1]*

[1] Rheumatology, Allergology and Clinical Immunology, University of Rome Tor Vergata, Rome, Italy, [2] Department of Clinical Sciences and Translational Medicine, University of Rome Tor Vergata, Rome, Italy, [3] Dermatology, University of Rome Tor Vergata, Rome, Italy, [4] Rheumatology Unit, Department of Clinical Medicine and Surgery, University of Naples Federico II, Naples, Italy

***Correspondence:**
Maria Sole Chimenti
maria.sole.chimenti@unroma2.it

Psoriasis (PsO) is an autoimmune disease characterized by keratinocyte proliferation, chronic inflammation and mast cell activation. Up to 42% of patients with PsO may present psoriatic arthritis (PsA). PsO and PsA share common pathophysiological mechanisms: keratinocytes and fibroblast-like synoviocytes are resistant to apoptosis: this is one of the mechanism facilitating their hyperplasic growth, and at joint level, the destruction of articular cartilage, and bone erosion and/or proliferation. Several clinical studies regarding diseases characterized by impairment of cell death, either due to apoptosis or necrosis, reported cytochrome c release from the mitochondria into the extracellular space and finally into the circulation. The presence of elevated cytochrome c levels in serum has been demonstrated in diseases as inflammatory arthritis, myocardial infarction and stroke, and liver diseases. Cytochrome c is a signaling molecule essential for apoptotic cell death released from mitochondria to the cytosol allowing the interaction with protease, as the apoptosis protease activation factor, which lead to the activation of factor-1 and procaspase 9. It has been demonstrated that this efflux from the mitochondria is crucial to start the intracellular signaling responsible for apoptosis, then to the activation of the inflammatory process. Another inflammatory marker, the tryptase, a trypsin-like serine protease produced by mast cells, is released during inflammation, leading to the activation of several immune cells through proteinase-activated receptor-2. In this review, we aimed at discussing the role played by cytochrome c and tryptase in PsO and PsA pathogenesis. To this purpose, we searched pathogenetic mechanisms in PUBMED database and review on oxidative stress, cytochrome c and tryptase and their potential role during inflammation in PsO and PsA. To this regard, the cytochrome c release into the extracellular space and tryptase may have a role in skin and joint inflammation.

Keywords: psoriatic arthritis, psoriatic disease, autoimmunity, oxidative stress, apoptosis, cytochrome c and tryptase

INTRODUCTION

Psoriasis (PsO) is an inflammatory skin disease characterized by plaques of thickened and scaling skin due to keratinocyte proliferation, chronic inflammation linked to the presence of several innate and acquired immune cells, and mast cells activation (1). Psoriatic arthritis (PsA) is a chronic inflammatory arthritis that may be present in up to 42% of individuals affected by PsO (2). PsA is clinically characterized by inflammation of periarticular (e.g., enthesis) and articular structures. PsO and PsA share common pathophysiological mechanisms: the marked tortuosity of blood vessels and infiltration of plasma cell and mononuclear cells are observed in both the psoriatic plaque and PsA articular space (3). For both diseases, the pathogenesis is multi-factorial with underlying autoimmune mechanism (4). Genetic predisposition, as human leukocyte antigens (HLA)-Cw0602 and the HLAB27 allele, and an altered immune response can induce inflammation of skin and joints (5). Cytokines, as Tumor Necrosis Factor-alpha (TNF-α), interleukin (IL)-1β, IL-6, IL-17, and IL-18, are over-expressed in skin lesions, in peripheral blood, synovial membrane, and synovial fluid of PsA patients (6). Moreover, keratinocytes and fibroblast-like synoviocytes (FLS) exhibit similar resistance to apoptosis, one of the key mechanism that may facilitate psoriatic plaque growth and the hyperplasic progression of FLS in the synovium, destruction of articular cartilage and bone damage. PsA pathogenesis is only partially understood and the interest in the pathophysiological role of the synovium is recently growing (7). Pro-inflammatory mediators, responsible for joint inflammation, may be secreted at skin level and blocking this pathological communication may represent a new fascinating therapeutic objective. The primum movens seems to be the activation of the innate immunity. Several markers have been studied, among them, elevated S100A8 and S100A9 levels were observed in fluid samples from inflamed tissues in PsA synovium and in skin psoriasis in patients affected by both PsA and PsO (8). To this regard, inflammatory mediators, at an early stage, may predict articular involvement helping in preventing joint damage. Recently, the involvement of oxidative stress in PsO and PsA pathogenesis has been considered (9). Disruption of redox signaling, caused by oxidative stress, brings molecular damage which inevitably impacts on angiogenesis, inflammation, and function/activation of dendritic cells, lymphocytes, and keratinocytes (10). Cytochrome c, whose structure is shown in **Figure 1A**, is floating into the peripheral mitochondrial membrane and mediates the electron transfer (eT) throughout the respiratory chain (11–14). Reactive oxygen species (ROS) formation induces the release of cytochrome c into the cytosol (15, 16), where it binds to the apoptosis protease activation factor (APAf-1) forming with ATP or dATP, the apoptosome; this complex activates procaspase 9, which triggers an enzymatic cascade that brings to cell apoptosis (17–19). Several clinical studies regarding diseases characterized by cell death, either due to apoptosis or necrosis, reported cytochrome c release from the mitochondria into the extracellular space and finally into the circulation. Elevated cytochrome c levels in serum were found in chronic and acute diseases, including inflammatory arthritis, myocardial infarction and stroke, and liver diseases (20–22). Its role as an inducer of skin and joint inflammation has been proposed. In particular, a link between cytochrome c, skin inflammation, and keratinocytes proliferation was demonstrated during ROS production (23). ROS dysregulation and cytochrome c release have been associated with PsO, and were reported to be the cause of associated skin inflammation (24). During inflammation, another relevant pathway involves tryptase, a trypsin-like serine protease produced by mast cells and stored in intracellular vesicles. It is a catalytically active tetramer made of identical subunits, each having the catalytic triad residues (25) (shown in **Figures 1B,C**) and represents the major protein present in mast cells granules (26, 27). The tetrameric structure and the presence of heparin are necessary *in vivo* for the tryptase function (28). Tryptase activates, both *in vivo* and *in vitro*, a number of cells involved during innate and adaptive immune response, through proteinase-activated receptor-2 (PAR-2), thus contributing to the perpetuation of inflammation (29). The activation of PAR-2 brings about, in some circumstances, apoptosis inhibition (30). Several new interesting pathogenetic ways have been recently assumed in Psoriatic disease pathogenesis (23, 25). This review aims at discussing the role played by two new inflammatory mediators, as cytochrome c and as tryptase, in regulating extrinsic and intrinsic apoptotic pathways in PsO and PsA pathogenesis (as described in **Figures 2, 3**). The role of oxidative stress, linked to psoriatic disease pathogenesis, will be highlightened. Moreover, the review will focus on the relationship of these two molecules with oxidative stress and their potential role as inflammatory markers in PsO and PsA.

POTENTIAL ROLE OF CYTOCHROME C AND TRYPTASE IN PSORIASIS AND PSORIATIC ARTHRITIS

Cytochrome c, Apoptosis and Chronic Inflammation

Cytochrome c was found to be one of the key signaling molecules during programmed cell death-apoptosis. As explained above, its translocation into the cytoplasm leads to its interaction with APAf-1 and, in presence of ATP/dATP, to the final activation of procaspase 9. These stages are crucial for the completion of the apoptosis (16). In normal conditions, the apoptosis leads to cells death in dysfunctional cells owing to the strictly regulated pathways which are vital to maintain the homeostasis. A disequilibrium in the regulation of the apoptotic way may lead to defective immune responses and, consequently, to infections, tumor growth and autoimmune diseases. There are two intracellular pathways leading to apoptosis: the extrinsic, mediated by death-receptors, and the intrinsic or mitochondrial pathway (32). ROS are known to cause mitochondrial damage and dysfunction, which can cause the rise of cytochrome c release into the cytoplasm, as part of the intrinsic pathway, and the activation of the apoptotic pathway (33). In this context, it has been demonstrated that an increase in the release of cytochrome c from the mitochondria into the cytosol, is regulated by B-cells follicular lymphoma (Bcl)-2 family proteins (33). Therefore, the regulatory effect of the Bcl-2 family is essential for

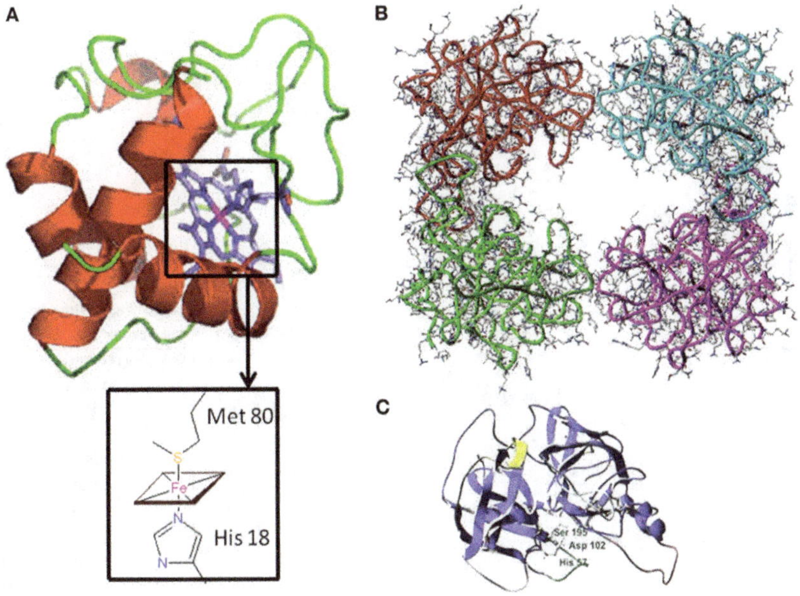

FIGURE 1 | Three-dimensional structure of Cytochrome c and Tryptase **(A)** Horse heart cytochrome c structure characterized by X-ray crystallography (6). In the inset, the fifth and sixth ligands (His 18 and Met 80, respectively) to the Fe-Heme are shown. **(B)** Human β-tryptase tetramer structure as determined by X-ray crystallography (11). **(C)** Tryptase monomer structure: the catalytic triad residues (Ser 195, His 57, and Asp 102) are highlighted.

the control of apoptosis and can determine the cell's fate (33). Schultz and colleagues described how deregulation of apoptosis, linked to the intrinsic pathway, may contribute to autoimmunity (34). They observed that mainly Fas ligand (FasL) contributes in the pathogenesis of autoimmune diseases. FasL and other (TNF) ligands bind death receptors and induce: the release of cytochrome c and the expression of both flavoprotein apoptosis-inducing factor and the second mitochondria-derived activator of caspases, known as DIABLO (inhibitor of anti-apoptotic factors and activator of procaspase) (34). The consequence is the activation of caspases with the induction of cell death through DNA and protein cleavage. Cellular damage may release potential autoantigens and may be the basis for autoimmunity and inflammation.

During autoimmune diseases, the regulation of self-reactive B cells, in order to inhibit autoantibody production, may be critical. B cells' tolerance consists in the inhibition of completely or partially autoreactive B cells by using different mechanisms. Cell death pathways are the most reliable system to eliminate autoreactive B cells and to prevent autoimmunity (35). The presence of autoreactive cells and mitochondrial markers, as cytochrome c, may be relevant also in PsO and PsA pathogenesis (22, 36). In PsO, a dysregulation of cytochrome c has been demonstrated. Indeed, a higher serum and mitochondrial levels were observed compared to healthy skin; this contributes to epidermal hyperplasia (37). Concerning PsA, the result is synovial inflammation and joint destruction (38). PsA is microscopically characterized by lining layer hyperplasia, infiltration of B and T lymphocytes, and activation of the innate immune response that lead to vascular remodeling and angiogenesis into the joint (39). The characteristic PsA synovitis has inflammatory infiltration of macrophages, lymphocytes, and plasma cells that cause FLS hyperplasia and chronically, joint and bone damage (40). A cytochrome c dysregulation may also result in an inadequate apoptosis. To this regard, both the FLS and keratinocytes display a resistance to apoptosis leading to synovial and epidermal hyperplasia which are the hallmark of synovitis and psoriatic plaques genesis (41, 42). In this context, impaired apoptosis may contribute to the perpetuation of the inflammatory process (43). For this apoptotic resistant state, Mitomycin C (MMC), which is a bacteric anti-tumor antibiotic, has been investigated as potential treatment in inflammatory arthritis. This agent has shown an inhibitory effect on fibroblast proliferation by inducing apoptosis (39). Furthermore, Yan and coll. have demonstrated that MMC can decrease cell liability and provoke apoptosis in FLS obtained from patients affected by inflammatory arthritis, as rheumatoid arthritis (RA). A possible mechanism involved in the MMC inhibitory effect on FLS may regard the intrinsic mitochondrial pathway. To this regard, MMC stimulates the production of ROS and induces the release of cytochrome c, and consequently it may activate the caspases' cascade (33).

Tryptase and Chronic Inflammation

Among cells that participate to the inflammatory status, the role of mast cells during inflammation was well demonstrated in the literature (44). Mast cells activation into joints and skin can cause the release of vasoactive mediators, such as histamine, prostanoids, and cytokines which contribute to inflammation (44, 45). Moreover, tryptase, released by mast cells, play an important role in the pathogenesis of inflammatory arthritis (46). Different pathogenetic mechanisms are linked to tryptase

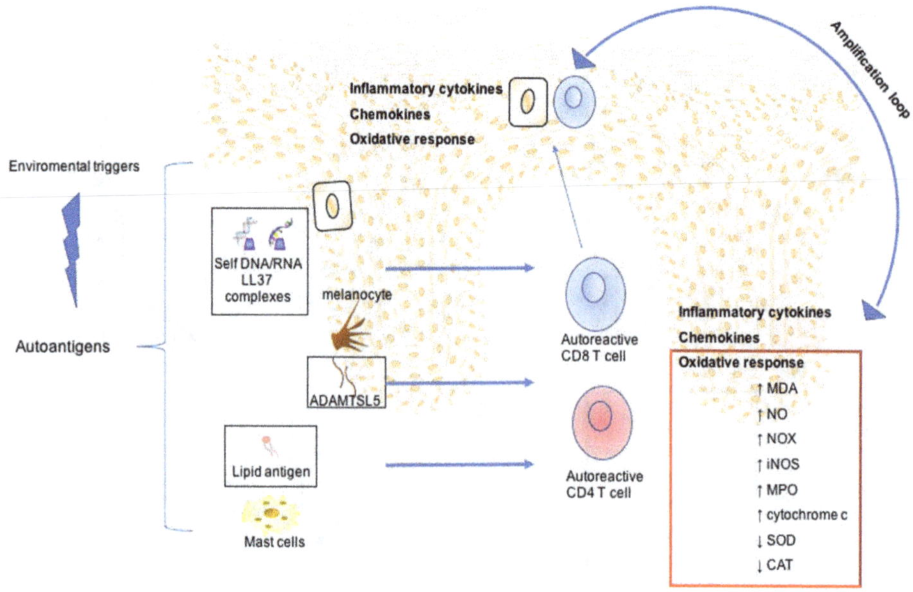

FIGURE 2 | Mechanisms involved in Psoriasis arthritis pathogenesis. In a summary view, environmental triggers induce the expression of autoantigens, such as LL37 by keratinocytes, ADAMTSL5 by melanocytes, and lipid antigen by mast cells. This leads to expansion and activation of autoreactive CD8 and CD4 T cells. Although CD4 T cells remain within the dermis producing a large plethora of inflammatory cytokines, activated CD8 T cells migrate into the epidermis. Subsequently, potentially upon recognition of autoantigens in the epidermis CD8 T cells release other inflammatory mediators, which in turn mediate skin cell homing and remain as resident memory T cells in the epidermis. All this inflammatory process is maintained and amplified by oxidative stress sustained by production of NADPH-oxidase (NOX), inducible nitric oxide synthase (iNOS) myeloperoxidase (MPO), malondialdehyde (MDA), nitric oxide (NO), and serum cytochrome c and decreased of antioxidant status such as superoxide dismutase (SOD), catalase (CAT).

release: it is expressed in high concentration in synovial fluids from patients affected by RA, PsA, and reactive arthritis (47). The link between PsA and tryptase is supported also by the presence of corticotropin releasing hormone receptor 1 in PsA synovial biopsy. This hormone and its receptor have been demonstrated in the joints of patients affected by PsA and not in the control group. This hormone can enhance the intercellular matrix degradation by inducing tryptase release by mast cells (48). Intriguingly, a mast cell subset able to produce IL-17 was detected in rheumatoid synovium (49) and in psoriasis plaques, resulting to be the prevalent IL-17 producing cells (50, 51). The relevant role of IL-17 in the pathogenesis of PsO and PsA is pointed out also by the efficacy of biological drugs as IL-17 inhibitors for both skin and joint involvement in these diseases (52–55). To note, tryptase showed to have several pathogenic roles in PsO and PsA patients: (1) it can induce the production and release of several pro-inflammatory cytokines, such as IL-1β, IL-8, TNFα, and IL-6 (56, 57); (2) it stimulates leukocytes migration into the joints by PAR-2, ICAM-1, CXCR2, and IL-8, directly causing and amplifying the inflammatory process (58–60); (3) it activates, by cleavage, proteolytic enzymes, such as prostromelysin, procollagenase, and MMP-3 which contributes to matrix degradation (61, 62). Furthermore, it has been demonstrated that mast cells proteinases, as tryptase, secreted in excess under the influence of inflammatory stimuli of specific cytokines, degrade the joint matrix *in vitro*. Tryptase damages various matrix components by the activation of matrix metalloproteinases (62). Mast cells can express several cytokines, as TNF-α and IL-1β, and various profibrotic cytokines such as TGF-α and IL-4, suggesting numerous functional roles for Mast cells during chronic inflammation (63). In particular, synovial mast cells *in vitro* release tryptase and activate latent collagenase (64), participating to the development of the typical PsA synovial hypertrophy (65).

EVIDENCE FOR AUTOIMMUNE PATHWAYS AND OXIDATIVE STRESS IN PSORIASIS

The Autoimmune Side of Psoriasis Pathogenesis

PsO is immune-mediated inflammatory cutaneous disease characterized by keratinocyte proliferation and chronic inflammation (58). Recently, evidence has supported that PsO has an autoimmune pathogenesis and three different autoantigens have been identified so far: cathelicidin LL37, a domain thrombospondin type 1 motif-like 5 (ADAMTSL5) present in metalloproteases, and lipid antigens generated by phospholipase called PLA2G4D (66, 67). LL37 is a peptide upregulated in psoriatic skin with antimicrobial properties, LL37 can bind self RNA and DNA in complexes which are able to activate plasmacytoid and myeloid dendritic cells (68). This leads to an expansion of LL37-specific T cells producing pathogenic cytokines such as INF-γ, IL17, and IL-22. LL37 presentation to CD8 and CD4 T cells is mediated by HLA-Class I, in particular (HLA)-Cw0602 and HLA-Class II molecules respectively (69). ADAMTSL5 is an autoantigen presented by (HLA)-Cw0602 in

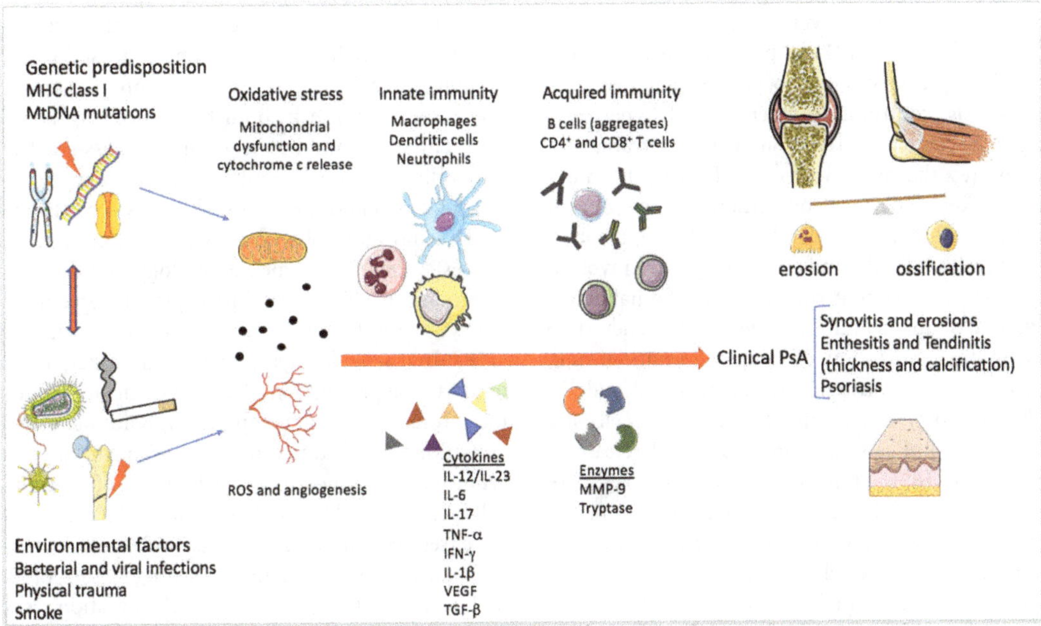

FIGURE 3 | Mechanisms involved in Psoriatic arthritis pathogenesis. The figure summarizes the pathogenesis of Psoriatic arthritis (PsA). The enthesitis seems to be the primum movens of the disease, even if the heterogeneity of systemic involvement and clinical manifestations is extremely wide (31). Genetic and environmental factors predispose a healthy individual and contribute to the development of the disease. Mitochondrial dysfunction, angiogenesis and increased production of reactive oxygen species (ROS) seem to be present since the early disease onset. The role of the innate immunity in the tolerance disruption and in the production of a pro-inflammatory milieu is very early and essential in the pathogenesis of both PsA and Psoriasis. Adaptive immunity participates later by perpetuating and further increasing the inflammation. Several soluble mediators, such as pro-inflammatory cytokines and proteases, can be found in the synovial fluid and sera of PsA patients.

PsO, the derived peptide can stimulate psoriatic T cells but not T cells from healthy individuals, resulting in IL17 production (68). Moreover, ADAMTSL5 and LL37 are increased in psoriatic lesions and are co-expressed by many immune cells, dendritic cells, neutrophils, macrophages, and T cells within skin. Both ADAMTSL5 and LL37 can be decreased by treatment with IL-17 or TNF-α inhibitors (70). Lastly, there is evidence for non-peptide autoantigen in PsO. T cells from PsA patients can recognize also lipid antigens generated in mast cells by PLA2G4D which are presented by CD1a. PLA2G4D is expressed in psoriatic skin lesions, but not in skin of healthy individuals (71). PsO pathogenesis is multifactorial, resulting from a combination of genetic, epigenetic, and environmental factors which lead to activation of an abnormal immune response. Working models for PsO suggest that several immune cells may present these antigens to autoreactive T cells with following activation and clonal expansion (60). This mechanism induces cytokines production, immune cells activation, and cell recruitment which in turn contributes to the amplification of inflammatory response and keratinocytes proliferation in PsO.

The Role of Oxidative Stress in Psoriasis Pathogenesis

In this complex pathogenesis, oxidative stress and free radical production play a role in skin inflammation (23). It was demonstrated that a reduction of antioxidant and augmented oxidant activities in psoriasis exists (72, 73). Moreover, a reciprocal amplification loop may exist between inflammation and oxidative stress in PsO. It is known that ROS production during oxidative stress activates cellular proinflammatory signaling mostly the JAK–STAT, MAPK/AP-1, and NF-κB pathways, leading to the production of cytokines, chemokines, and growth factors which are involved in the pathogenesis of psoriasis (74–77). Interestingly, activator protein-1 (AP-1) activates peroxisome proliferator-activated receptor δ (PPARδ) which is up-regulated in PsO, inducing proliferation and preventing apoptosis of keratinocytes, via the activation of heparin-binding EGF-like growth factor (HB-EGF) and activation of Protein Kinase Ba/Akt1 pathway, respectively (78, 79).

On the other hand, oxidative stress may originate by endogenous stimuli such as Th1 and Th17 cytokines, which are able to induce the production of NADPH-oxidase (NOX), inducible nitric oxide synthase (iNOS) and myeloperoxidase (MPO) and from environmental agents that may be also the cause of inflammation (80). Moreover, it has been recently demonstrated that MPO can be considered as a marker of systemic inflammation in Psoriatic disease (81).

Gabr and colleagues demonstrated a positive correlation between serum malondialdehyde, nitric oxide and serum cytochrome c levels and disease severity (measured by PASI score). On the contrary, a negative correlation with superoxide dismutase (SOD), catalase, and total antioxidant status was reported (36). Increased levels of mitochondria cytochrome c were also observed in lesional psoriatic skin compared to non-affected skin, and this increase is reversed by methotrexate

(MTX) treatment (37). Indeed, during MTX therapy, an increased cytosolic cytochrome c level and consequent cleaved caspase-9 were also observed (37). Apoptotic dysregulation has been reported in psoriatic keratinocytes, which display a resistance to apoptosis, contributing to epidermal hyperplasia (42). Accordingly, in a recent article, after UVB irradiation, psoriatic keratinocytes showed a less cytosolic cytochrome c level compared to keratinocytes from healthy skin (82). A wide type of cells, such as T cells, dendritic cells, neutrophils, keratinocytes, mast cells, NK cells and macrophages are involved in PsO pathogenesis with different roles and specific hallmarks (83). The activation of innate immune system is believed to play a key role in the initial step of plaque formation, and, in this context, mast cells contribute producing IL-22 and IL-17 (52, 84). Furthermore, a high number of mast cells are present in the affected skin as well as the associated release of tryptase and histamine (85). Tryptase positive mast cells are increased in psoriatic lesional skin compared to normal skin, and tryptase mainly is localized in the dermis, at dermis-epidermal junction and around blood vessels, as showed by Steinhoff and collaborators through immunohistochemistry experiments (45). Tryptase participates to PsO inflammation through specific cytokines and neuropeptides production. Indeed, Tryptase acts by PAR2 cleavage, which is highly expressed in mast cells and in keratinocytes of PsO skin lesions (86–88). PAR2 exerts its inflammatory effects inducing the production of proinflammatory cytokines such as TNFα, IL-1ß, IL-6, IL-8, and granulocytes macrophage-colony stimulation factor (GM-CSF) (57, 87, 89). In details, TNFα is a landmark inflammatory mediator in PsO, being one of the first target of monoclonal antibody therapy (90) and GM-CSF is a mediator for maturation of Langerhans cells and stimulates keratinocytes proliferation (91, 92). On the other hand IL-6, which is also highly expressed in PsO, is able to stimulate keratinocytes proliferation (93) and contributes to the differentiation of Th17 cells which play a key role in PsO pathogenesis (94). Interestingly, PAR2 is also able to induce skin inflammation also through neurogenic mechanism, stimulating sensory C-fibers to produce some neuropeptides such as calcitonin gene-related peptide and substance P (95).

ROLE OF AUTOIMMUNITY AND OXIDATIVE STRESS IN PSORIATIC ARTHRITIS

The Autoimmune Side of Psoriatic Arthritis Pathogenesis

The autoimmune side of PsA pathogenesis has been demonstrated by the presence of autoreactive T cells in synovium from PsA patients, which were activated by a homologous protein antigen, expressed in the synovium (4). Furthermore, the association with major histocompatibility complex class I molecules, the loci HLA-Cw6 or HLA-B27 in particular, leads to the presentation by those molecules of an autoantigen with the consequent production of antibodies against autoantigens. Additionally, the good response to immunosuppressive agents and cytokines blockers supports the involvement of autoreactive cells participating at the autoimmune process (96). Histologically, the PsA synovium presented both clonal and non-clonal T cells (97), and the link between skin and synovium T cells-clones (98) has been demonstrated. This indicates that a common antigen might drive the T cell response in both the target organs. Concerning the joint-enthesal complex, a group of cross-reactive PsA-specific antibodies, directed against peptides expressed in both the psoriatic skin and the inflamed enthesis, has been demonstrated by Dolcino and collaborators (99). Moreover, recent evidence suggests that PsA synovial biology involves several type of immune cells. The same histological heterogeneity observed in RA synovium has also been detected in psoriatic synovial tissue (100). In particular, lymphocytes infiltrates, in PsA synovium, tend to aggregate in lymphoid agglomerates, supporting the presence of an ectopic lymphoid neogenesis (LN), and autoantibody production (100). Conigliaro et al. previously reported an abnormal distribution of peripheral blood B cells in both RA and PsA patients (101). Peripheral B cells were reduced in PsA patients and their level were restored after anti-TNF treatment suggesting a role of B cells in PsA pathogenesis (101). During inflammation, several protein modifications may occur supporting the strong link between autoimmunity and inflammation. Among them, the effects of carbamylation on proteins and its effect in inflammatory arthritis has been recently investigated. Carbamylation is a post transcriptional modification on lysine, the effect on protein function and biochemical properties includes a change of the ability in polymerization, sensitivity to proteinases, and binding avidity to antibodies (102). To date, it is well known that carbamylation happens during inflammation, after the release of MPO by neutrophils, generating a pro-inflammatory loop. Carbamylated proteins are recognized by circulating antibodies, the anti-carbamylated protein (anti-CarP) antibodies that have been identified in patients with RA, also before the clinical onset of the disease (38). The presence of anti-CarP antibodies in sera from PsA patients with active disease, in the absence of rheumatoid factor and/or other known autoantibodies specificities, was demonstrated (96, 102). Interestingly, the circulating anti-CarP antibodies levels showed to be a good diagnostic test for PsA patients in comparison to healthy subject. A further support of an autoimmune origin is the discovery of a peptide antigen, called the PsA antigen, recognized by IgG derived from PsA patients' sera. This peptide shows homologies with peptides expressed both in skin and enthesis, as a further demonstration that an immunologic disequilibrium has a role in the pathogenesis of PsA (99).

The Role of Oxidative Stress in Psoriatic Arthritis Pathogenesis

The activation of innate immunity is believed to have a role in PsA pathogenesis (96). In particular, the monocyte/macrophages population has a relevant role during inflammation at the enthesal level: it participates to the tolerance disruption in PsA patients and activates the release of mediators linked to the oxidative stress (103, 104). The oxidative damage in PsA is mainly due to a dramatic production of ROS that saturate the compensatory antioxidant enzymes and molecules, such as glutathione and SOD (105). The substantial producers of ROS are present in the mitochondrial membrane, NADPH oxidase and eT chain. The consequence of the unbalanced production of ROS is the leakage of cytochrome c from mitochondria, which activates the caspases cascade leading to apoptotic cell death (105). This reaction occurs also in cells populating inflamed joints, like synoviocytes, chondrocytes, lymphocytes and monocytes. To note, oxidative stress can lead to cyclooxygenase-2 and MMP9/13 expression and modulates apoptotic pathways and NF-κB. All of them are relevant mediators during inflammatory arthritis pathogenesis (106–109). Recent studies have highlighted the possible role of oxidative stress in PsA. Altered levels of oxidative metabolites, for example carbonyl groups, F2-isoprostanes, hydroperoxides, and sulfhydryl groups, were detected in PsA patients when compared to healthy donors (110–112). A similar study, showed a higher serum peroxide concentration and a lower antioxidant capacity in sera from patients affected by RA, PsA, and PsO in comparison with healthy individuals (113). The connection between circulating ROS and inflammation was investigated in RA, PsA, and ankylosing spondylitis patients in whom ROS in sera were higher when compared to controls (113, 114). Interestingly, after anti-TNFα treatment, a reduced value of circulating ROS was detected (114). Furthermore, the circulating peripheral blood mononuclear cells in patients with inflammatory arthritis have high levels of peroxidated lipid and altered polarization of the mitochondria membrane; these alterations correlate with patients disease activity (115). Furthermore, oxidative stress takes part also in the pathogenesis of comorbidities that may affect PsA patients. Patients with PsA have an accelerated atherosclerosis, and so a higher cardiovascular risk compared to healthy subjects (116). In this context, oxidative stress plays a relevant role in the pathogenesis of atherosclerosis: it induces the oxidative modification of LDL. The oxidized LDL takes part in many phases of atherogenesis and are strictly related to the inflammatory process (117). Moreover, oxidative modifications of LDL have been linked to the presence of TNFα and HDL may be altered during inflammation. Modified HDL lose their capacity to remove cholesterol from atherosclerotic lesions and have a reduced antioxidant activity (118). During inflammation, the release of TNFα is one of the main contributor of increased ROS production, and this is strongly related to disease activity (119). Then, the presence of ROS supports oxidative stress, further stimulating in this way cell damage and atherogenesis (113). Recent findings demonstrated that ROS were found not only into the blood stream and in circulating cells, but also into the joint. In synovial fluid of PsA patients, a higher ROS production, angiogenesis, and, DNA damage was found when compared to an osteoarthritis group (120–122); this is a further demonstration that oxidative stress has a role in the pathogenesis. Interestingly, a role of hypoxia was proven during inflammatory arthritis pathogenesis. A negative correlation between pO2 in synovial fluid of RA and PsA patients and level of macroscopic synovitis, disease activity, sublining layer thickness, and cells infiltration were demonstrated. In addition, hypoxic intra-articular environment and oxidative stress induce the production of pro-inflammatory cytokines (106). Ng and coll. confirmed this link by demonstrating a high expression of NOX in RA and PsA synovial tissue, which correlates with intra-articular pO2 and angiogenesis. A reduction of NOX expression was observed after 3 months of anti-TNFα treatment, in association with raised pO2 and a lower disease activity (123). The oxidative stress, measured as rate of mitochondrial DNA (mtDNA) mutations, is increased in RA and PsA synoviocytes; and it is correlated to high reactive ROS, reduced expression of cytochrome c oxidase, and low level of intra-articular pO2 (8). As a further evidence of the link between inflammation and oxidative stress, Harty et al demonstrated that the levels of mitochondrial DNA (mtDNA) point mutations in synovial tissue from patients with inflammatory arthritis was related to *in vivo* hypoxia and oxidative stress levels (124). The authors described a correlation between mtDNA mutation rate, the expression of TNFα and macroscopic arthroscopic signs of inflammation in RA and PsA patients. Patients were then treated with anti-TNFα, and only in anti-TNFα-responders the mtDNA mutations frequency was reduced. Moreover, the addition of recombinant TNFα in RA and PsA synoviocytes culture induces mtDNA mutations (124). These data suggest that antioxidant agents may be potentially useful as an add-on treatment to conventional therapies in the management of inflammatory arthritis and in autoimmune diseases (125, 126).

CONCLUSIONS

All studies converge to establish that in autoimmune diseases as PsO and PsA, oxidative stress, cell apoptosis and inflammation may lead to cytochrome c released from the mitochondria into the extracellular space. The future perspective given by data from the literature is that serum cytochrome c can be measured and used for diagnosing and assessing cell death during systemic diseases. The role of cytochrome c has been associated with autoimmune diseases and its release from mitochondria into the cytoplasm may be considered as a marker of inflammation and autoimmunity. Besides, several evidence suggests that mast cells activation is implicated in PsO and PsA pathogenesis. Those cells and the release of tryptase support the relevant role of innate immunity in PsO and PsA development. In this context, both cytochrome c and tryptase are detected during the inflammatory process. They may act as potential triggers in the perpetuation of the pro-inflammatory loop. In this context, mediators released from mast cells or mitochondrial activity may be used as marker of disease or as target in the treatment of autoimmune diseases. However, further studies are needed to better understand the potential contribution of cytochrome c and tryptase in autoimmune disease pathogenesis during oxidative stress and their potential correlation with disease activity and as markers of treatment efficacy.

AUTHOR CONTRIBUTIONS

MC, FS, and LF conceived the review and wrote the introduction and the paragraph concerning psoriatic arthritis. GF, ME, AG, and RS helped in writing the part concerning cytochrome c and tryptase. EB and LB wrote the paragraph concerning psoriasis. PC, PT, FC, and LC supervised the paper. RP conceived and revised the manuscript.

ACKNOWLEDGMENTS

The authors would like to thank Mrs. Laura Mathew, native English speaker, for her assistance in editing the English version of this manuscript.

REFERENCES

1. Fitzgerald O, Dougados M. Psoriatic arthritis: one or more diseases? *Best Pract Res Clin Rheumatol.* (2006) 20:435–50. doi: 10.1016/j.berh.2006.02.002
2. Gladman DD, Antoni C, Mease P, Clegg DO, Nash P. Psoriatic arthritis: epidemiology, clinical features, course, and outcome. *Ann Rheum Dis.* (2005) 64:14–7. doi: 10.1136/ard.2004.032482
3. Haroon M, Winchester R, Giles JT, Heffernan E, FitzGerald O. Certain class I HLA alleles and haplotypes implicated in susceptibility play a role in determining specific features of the psoriatic arthritis phenotype. *Ann Rheum Dis.* (2016) 75:155–62. doi: 10.1136/annrheumdis-2014-205461
4. Chimenti MS, Ballanti E, Perricone C, Cipriani P, Giacomelli R, Perricone R. Immunomodulation in psoriatic arthritis: focus on cellular and molecular pathways. *Autoimmun Rev.* (2013) 12:599–606. doi: 10.1016/j.autrev.2012.10.002
5. Fiocco U, Stramare R, Martini V, Coran A, Caso F, Dalla Costa L, et al. Quantitative imaging by pixelbased contrast-enhanced ultrasound reveals a linear relationship between synovial vascular perfusion and the recruitment of pathogenic IL-17A-F(+)IL-23(+) CD161(+) CD4(+) T helper cells in psoriatic arthritis joints. *Clin Rheumatol.* (2017) 36:391–9. doi: 10.1007/s10067-016-3500-x
6. McGonagle D, Conaghan PG, Emery P. Psoriatic arthritis: a unified concept twenty years on. *Arthritis Rheum.* (1999) 42:1080–6. doi: 10.1002/1529-0131(199906)42:6<1080::AID-ANR2>3.0.CO;2-7
7. Chimenti MS, Triggianese P, Botti E, Narcisi A, Conigliaro P, Giunta A, et al. S100A8/A9 in psoriatic plaques from patients with psoriatic arthritis. *J Int Med Res.* (2016) 44:33–7. doi: 10.1177/0300060515598900
8. Biniecka M, Connolly M, Gao W, Ng CT, Balogh E, Gogarty M, et al. Redox-mediated angiogenesis in the hypoxic joint of inflammatory arthritis. *Arthritis Rheumatol.* (2014) 66:3300–10. doi: 10.1002/art.38822
9. Lin X, Huang T. Oxidative stress in psoriasis and potential therapeutic use of antioxidants. *Free Radic Res.* (2016) 50:585–95. doi: 10.3109/10715762.2016.1162301
10. Bushnell GW, Louie GV, Brayer GD. High-resolution three-dimensional structure of horse heart cytochrome c. *J Mol Biol.* (1990) 214:585–95. doi: 10.1016/0022-2836(90)90200-6
11. Pettigrew GW, Moore GR. *Cytochromes c. Biological aspects.* Heidelberg: Springer-Verlag (1987)
12. Tognaccini L, Ciaccio C, D'Oria V, Cervelli M, Howes BD, Coletta M, et al. Structure-function relationships in human cytochrome c: the role of tyrosine 67. *J Inorg Biochem.* (2016) 155:56–66. doi: 10.1016/j.jinorgbio.2015.11.011
13. Hannibal L, Tomasina F, Capdevila DA, Demicheli V, Tórtora V, Alvarez-Paggi D, et al. Alternative conformations of cytochrome c: structure, function, and detection. *Biochemistry* (2016) 55:407–28. doi: 10.1021/acs.biochem.5b01385
14. Patriarca A, Eliseo T, Sinibaldi F, Piro MC, Melis R, Paci M, et al. ATP acts as a regulatory effector in modulating structural transitions of cytochrome c: implications for apoptotic activity. *Biochemistry* (2009) 48:3279–87. doi: 10.1021/bi801837e
15. Santucci R, Sinibaldi F, Polticelli F, Fiorucci L. Role of cardiolipin in mitochondrial diseases and apoptosis. *Curr Med Chem.* (2014) 21:2702–14.
16. Lamkanfi M, Declercq W, Depuydt B, Kalai M, Saelens X, Vandenabeele P. *In Caspases: Their Role in Cell Death and Cell Survival.* Dordrecht: Kluwer Academic Publishers (2002) pp.1–40.
17. Antonsson B. Mitochondria and the Bcl-2 family proteins in apoptosis signalling pathways. *Mol Cell Biochem.* (2004) 256–257:141–55.
18. Patriarca A, Polticelli F, Piro MC, Sinibaldi F, Mei G, Bari M et al. Conversion of cytochrome c into a peroxidase: inhibitory mechanisms and implication for neurodegenerative diseases. *Arch Biochem Biophys.* (2012) 522:62–9. doi: 10.1016/j.abb.2012.03.028
19. Radhakrishnan J, Wang S, Ayoub IM, Kolarova JD, Levine RF, Gazmuri RJ. Circulating levels of cytochrome c after resuscitation from cardiac arrest: a marker of mitochondrial injury and predictor of survival. *Am. J. Physiol. Heart Care Circ. Physiol.* (2007) 292:H767–75. doi: 10.1152/ajpheart.00468.2006
20. Shi Q, Yang X, Mattes WB, Mendrick DL, Harrill AH, Beger RD. Circulating mitochondrial biomarkers for drug-induced liver injury. *Biomark Med.* (2015) 9:1215–23. doi: 10.2217/bmm.15.59
21. Kretz-Rommel A, Rubin RL. Early cellular events in systemic autoimmunity driven by chromatin-reactive T cells. *Cell. Immunol.* (2001) 208:125–36. doi: 10.1006/cimm.2001.1774
22. Omori E, Morioka S, Matsumoto K, Ninomiya-Tsuji J. TAK1 regulates reactive oxygen species and cell death in keratinocytes, which is essential for skin integrity. *J Biol Chem.* (2008) 283:26161–8. doi: 10.1074/jbc.M804513200
23. Rashmi R, Rao KSJ, Basavaraj KH. A comprehensive review of biomarkers in psoriasis. *Clin Exp Dermatol.* (2009) 34:658–63. doi: 10.1111/j.1365-2230.2009.03410.x
24. Sommerhoff CP, Bode W, Pereira PJB, Stubbs MT, Stürzebecher J, Piechottka GP, et al. The structure of the human βII-tryptase tetramer: Fo(u)r better or worse. *Proc Natl Acad Sci USA.* (1999) 96:10984–91.
25. Atiakshin D, Buchwalow I, Samoilova V, Tiemann M. Tryptase as a polyfunctional component of mast cells. *Histochem Cell Biol.* (2018) 149:461–77. doi: 10.1007/s00418-018-1659-8
26. Fiorucci L, Ascoli F. Mast cell tryptase, a still enigmatic enzyme. *Cell Mol Life Sci.* (2004) 61:1278–95. doi: 10.1007/s00018-004-3400-0
27. Gambacurta A, Fiorucci L, Basili P, Erba F, Amoresano A, Ascoli F. Bovine tryptases. cDNA cloning, tissue specific expression and characterization of the lung isoform. *Eur J Biochem.* (2003) 270:507–17.
28. Fiorucci L, Erba F, Coletta M, Ascoli F. Evidence for multiple interacting binding sites in bovine tryptase. *FEBS Lett.* (1995) 363:81–4.
29. Olivera A, Beaven MA, Metcalfe DD. Mast cells signal their importance in health and disease. *J Allergy Clin Immunol.* (2018) 142:381–93. doi: 10.1016/j.jaci.2018.01.034
30. Rothmeier AS, Ruf W. Protease-activated receptor 2 signalling in inflammation. *Semin Immunopathol.* (2012) 34:133-49. doi: 10.1007/s00281-011-0289-1
31. Kaeley GS, Eder L, Aydin SZ, Gutierrez M, Bakewell C. Enthesitis: a hallmark of psoriatic arthritis. *Semin Arthritis Rheum.* (2018) 48:34–43. doi: 10.1016/j.semarthrit.2017.12.008
32. Wang J, Yuan L, Xiao H, Xiao C, Wang Y, Liu X. Momordin Ic induces HepG2 cell apoptosis through MAPK and PI3K/Akt-mediated mitochondrial pathways. *Apoptosis* (2013) 18:751–65. doi: 10.1007/s10495-013-0820-z

33. Yan C, Kong D, Ge D, Zhang Y, Zhang X, Su C, et al. Mitomycin C induces apoptosis in rheumatoid arthritis fibroblast-like synoviocytes via a mitochondrial-mediated pathway. *Cell Physiol Biochem.* (2015) 35:1125–36. doi: 10.1159/000373938
34. Schultz DR, Harrington WJ Jr. Apoptosis: programmed cell death at a molecular level. *Semin Arthritis Rheum.* (2003) 32:345–69. doi: 10.1053/sarh.2003.50005
35. Deming PB, Rathmell JC. Mitochondria, cell death, and B cell tolerance. *Curr Dir Autoimmun.* (2006) 9:95–119. doi: 10.1159/000090774
36. Gabr SA, Al-Ghadir AH. Role of cellular oxidative stress and cytochrome c in the pathogenesis of psoriasis. *Arch Dermatol Res.* (2012) 304:451–7. doi: 10.1007/s00403-012-1230-8
37. Elango T, Thirupathi A, Subramanian S, Ethiraj P, Dayalan H, Gnanaraj P. Methotrexate treatment provokes apoptosis of proliferating keratinocyte in psoriasis patients. *Clin Exp Med.* (2017) 17:371–81. doi: 10.1007/s10238-016-0431-4
38. Conigliaro P, Chimenti MS, Triggianese P, Sunzini F, Novelli L, Perricone C, et al. Autoantibodies in inflammatory arthritis. *Autoimmun Rev.* (2016) 15:673–83. doi: 10.1016/j.autrev.2016.03.003
39. Seong GJ, Park C, Kim CY, Hong YJ, So HS, Kim SD, et al. Mitomycin-C induces the apoptosis of human Tenon's capsule fibroblast by activation of c-Jun N-terminal kinase 1 and caspase-3 protease. *Invest Ophthalmol Vis Sci.* (2005) 46:3545–52. doi: 10.1167/iovs.04-1358
40. Alivernini S, Tolusso B, Petricca L, Bui L, Di Sante G, Peluso G, et al. Synovial features of patients with rheumatoid arthritis and psoriatic arthritis in clinical and ultrasound remission differ under anti-TNF therapy: a clue to interpret different chances of relapse after clinical remission? *Ann Rheum Dis.* (2017) 76:1228–36. doi: 10.1136/annrheumdis-2016-210424
41. Bartok B, Firestein GS. Fibroblast-like synoviocytes: key effector cells in rheumatoid arthritis. *Immunol Rev.* (2010) 233:233–55. doi: 10.1111/j.0105-2896.2009.00859.x
42. Kastelan M, Prpic-Massari L, Brajac I. Apoptosis in psoriasis. *Acta Dermatovenereol Croat* (2009) 17:182–6.
43. Gao W, McGarry T, Orr C, McCormick J, Veale DJ, Fearon U. Tofacitinib regulates synovial inflammation in psoriatic arthritis, inhibiting STAT activation and induction of negative feedback inhibitors. *Ann Rheum Dis.* (2016) 75:311–5. doi: 10.1136/annrheumdis-2014-207201
44. Woolley DE, Tetlow LC. Mast cell activation and its relation to proinflammatory cytokine production in the rheumatoid lesion. *Arthritis Res.* (1999) 2:65–74. doi: 10.1186/ar70
45. Steinhoff M, Corvera CU, Thoma MS, Kong W, McAlpine BE, Caughey GH, et al. Proteinase-activated receptor-2 in human skin: tissue distribution and activation of keratinocytes by mast cell tryptase. *Exp Dermatol.* (1999) 8: 282–94.
46. Denadai-Souza A, Ribeiro CM, Rolland C, Thouard A, Deraison C, Scavone C, et al. Effect of tryptase inhibition on joint inflammation: a pharmacological and lentivirus-mediated gene transfer study. *Arthritis Res Ther.* (2017) 19:124. doi: 10.1186/s13075-017-1326-9
47. Lavery JP, Lisse JR. Preliminary study of the tryptase levels in the synovial fluid of patients with inflammatory arthritis. *Ann Allergy* (1994) 72:425–7.
48. McEvoy AN, Bresnihan B, FitzGerald O, Murphy EP. Corticotropin-releasing hormone signaling in synovial tissue from patients with early inflammatory arthritis is mediated by the type 1 alpha corticotropin-releasing hormone receptor. *Arthritis Rheum.* (2001) 44:1761–7. doi: 10. 1002/1529-0131(200108)44:8<1761::AID-ART311>3.0.CO;2-D45
49. Cua DJ, Tato CM. Innate IL-17-producing cells: the sentinels of the immune system. *Nat Rev Immunol.* (2010) 10:479–89. doi: 10.1038/nri2800
50. Hueber AJ, Asquith DL, Miller AM, Reilly J, Kerr S, Leipe J, et al. Mast cells express IL-17A in rheumatoid arthritis synovium. *J Immunol.* (2010) 184:3336–40. doi: 10.4049/jimmunol.0903566
51. Res PC, Piskin G, de Boer OJ, van der Loos CM, Teeling P, Bos JD, et al. Overrepresentation of IL-17A and IL-22 producing CD8 T cells in lesional skin suggests their involvement in the pathogenesis of psoriasis. *PLoS ONE* (2010) 5:e14108. doi: 10.1371/journal.pone.0014108
52. Lin AM, Rubin CJ, Khandpur R, Wang JY, Riblett M, Yalavarthi S, et al. Mast cells and neutrophils release IL-17 through extracellular trap formation in psoriasis. *J Immunol.* (2011) 187:490–500. doi: 10.4049/jimmunol.1100123
53. McInnes IB, Sieper J, Braun J, Emery P, van der Heijde D, Isaacs JD, et al. Efficacy and safety of secukinumab, a fully human anti-interleukin-17A monoclonal antibody, in patients with moderate-to-severe psoriatic arthritis: a 24-week, randomised, double-blind, placebo-controlled, phase II proof-of-concept trial. *Ann Rheum Dis.* (2014) 73:349–56. doi: 10.1136/annrheumdis-2012-202646
54. Leonardi C, Matheson R, Zachariae C, Cameron G, Li L, Edson-Heredia E, et al. Anti-interleukin-17 monoclonal antibody ixekizumab in chronic plaque psoriasis. *N Engl J Med.* (2010) 366:1190–9. doi: 10.1056/NEJMoa1109997
55. Patel DD, Lee DM, Kolbinger F, Antoni C. Effect of IL-17A blockade with secukinumab in autoimmune diseases. *Ann Rheum Dis.* (2013) 72:116–23. doi: 10.1136/annrheumdis-2012-202371
56. Compten SJ, Cairns JA, Holgate ST, Walls AF. The role of mast cell tryptase in regulating endothelial cell proliferation, cytokine release, and adhesion molecule expression: Tryptase induces expression of mRNA for IL-1b and IL-8 and stimulates the selective release of IL-8 from human umbilical vein endothelial cells. *J Immunol.* (1998) 161:1939–46.
57. Malamud V, Vaaknin A, Abramsky O, Mor M, Burgess LE, Ben-Yehudah A. Tryptase activates peripheral blood mononuclear cells causing the synthesis and release of TNF-alpha, IL-6, and IL-1 beta: Possible relevance to multiple sclerosis. *J Neuroimmunol.* (2013) 138:115–22. doi: 10.1016/S0165-5728(03)00090-0
58. Sawamukai N, Yukawa S, Saito K, Nakayamada S, Kambayashi T, Tanaka Y. Mast cell-derived tryptase inhibits apoptosis of human rheumatoid synovial fibroblasts via rho-mediated signaling. *Arthritis Rheum.* (2010) 62:952–9. doi: 10.1002/art.27331
59. Botti E, Spallone G, Caruso R, Monteleone G, Chimenti S, Costanzo A. Psoriasis, from pathogenesis to therapeutic strategies: IL-21 as a novel potential therapeutic target. *Curr Pharm Biotechnol.* (2012) 13:1861–7. doi: 10.2174/138920112802273281
60. Lande R, Botti E, Jandus C, Dojcinovic D, Fanelli G, Conrad C, et al. The antimicrobial peptide LL37 is a T-cell autoantigen in psoriasis. *Nat Commun.* (2014) 5:5621. doi: 10.1038/ncomms6621
61. Lees M, Taylor DJ, Wolley DE. Mast cell proteinase activates precursor forms of collegenase and stromelysin, but not of gelatinase A and B. *Eur J Biochem.* (1994) 223:171–77.
62. Shin K, Nigrovic PA, Crish J, Boilard E, McNeil HP, Larabee KS, et al. Mast cells contribute to autoimmune inflammatory arthritis via their tryptase/heparin complexes. *J Immunol.* (2009) 182:647–56. doi: 10.4049/jimmunol.182.1.647
63. Gotis-Graham I, Smith M, Parker A, McNeil HP. Synovial mast cell responses during clinical improvement in early rheumatoid arthritis. *Ann Rheum Dis.* (1998) 57:664–71.
64. Gruber BL, Schwartz LB, Ramamurthy NS, Irani AM, Marches MJ. Activation of latent rheumatoid synovial collagenasebyhumanmastcelltryptase. *J Immunol.* (1998) 140:3936–42.
65. Gruber BL, Marchese MJ, Suzuki K, Schwartz LB, Ckada Y, Nagase H. Synovial procollagenase activation by human mast cells tryptase: dependence upon matrix metalloproteinase 3 activation. *J Clin Investig.* (1989) 84:1657–62. doi: 10.1172/JCI114344
66. Lande R, Gregorio J, Facchinetti V, Chatterjee B, Wang YH, Homey B, et al. Plasmacytoid dendritic cells sense self-DNA coupled with antimicrobial peptide. *Nature* (2007) 449:564–9. doi: 10.1038/nature06116
67. Albanesi C, Madonna S, Gisondi P, Girolomoni G. The interplay between keratinocytes and immune cells in the pathogenesis of psoriasis. *Front Immunol.* (2018) 9:1549. doi: 10.3389/fimmu.2018.01549.47-4863
68. Cheung KL, Jarrett R, Subramaniam S, Salimi M, Gutowska-Owsiak D, Chen YL, et al. Psoriatic T cells recognize neolipid antigens generated by mast cell phospholipase delivered by exosomes and presented by CD1a. *J Exp Med.* (2016) 213:2399–412. doi: 10.1084/jem.201 60258
69. Arakawa A, Siewert K, Stöhr J, Besgen P, Kim SM, Rühl G, et al. Melanocyte antigen triggers autoimmunity in human psoriasis. *J Exp Med.* (2015) 212:2203–12. doi: 10.1084/jem.20151093
70. Gilliet M, Lande R. Antimicrobial peptides and self-DNA in autoimmune skin inflammation. *Curr Opin Immunol.* (2008) 20:401–7. doi: 10.1016/j.coi.2008.06.008

71. Fuentes-Duculan J, Bonifacio KM, Hawkes JE, Kunjravia N, Cueto I, Li X, et al. Autoantigens ADAMTSL5 and LL37 are significantly upregulated in active Psoriasis and localized with keratinocytes, dendritic cells and other leukocytes. *Exp Dermatol.* (2017) 26:1075–82. doi: 10.1111/exd.1337
72. Yildirim M, Inaloz HS, Baysal V, Delibas N. The role of oxidants and antioxidants in psoriasis. *J Eur Acad Dermatol Venereol.* (2003) 17:34–36. doi: 10.1046/j.1468-3083.2003.00641.x
73. Baz K, Cimen MY, Kokturk A, Yazici AC, Eskandari G, Ikizoglu G, et al. Oxidant / antioxidant status in patients with psoriasis. *Yonsei Med J.* (2003) 44:987–90. doi: 10.3349/ymj.2003.44.6.987
74. Simon AR, Rai U, Fanburg BL, Cochran BH. Activation of the JAK-STAT pathway by reactive oxygen species. *Am J Physiol.* (1998) 275:C1640–52.
75. Dhar A, Young MR, Colburn NH. The role of AP-1, NF-kappaB and ROS/NOS in skin carcinogenesis: the JB6 model is predictive. *Mol Cell Biochem.* (2002) 234–235:185–93. doi: 10.1023/A:1015948505117
76. Shim JS, Kwon YY, Han YS, Hwang JK. Inhibitory effect of panduratin A on UV-induced activation of mitogen-activated protein kinases (MAPKs) in dermal fibroblast cells. *Planta Med.* (2008) 74:1446–50. doi: 10.1055/s-2008-1081352
77. Zhou Q, Mrowietz U, Rostami-Yazdi M. Oxidative stress in the pathogenesis of psoriasis. *Free Radic Biol Med.* (2009) 47:891–905. doi: 10.1016/j.freeradbiomed.2009.06.033
78. Romanowska M, al Yacoub N, Seidel H, Donandt S, Gerken H, Phillip S, et al. PPARdelta enhances keratinocyte proliferation in psoriasis and induces heparin-binding EGF-like growth factor. *J Invest Dermatol.* (2008) 128:110–24. doi: 10.1038/sj.jid.5700943
79. Westergaard M, Henningsen J, Johansen C, Rasmussen S, Svendsen ML, Jensen UB, et al. Expression and localization of peroxisome proliferator-activated receptors and nuclear factor kappaB in normal and lesional psoriatic skin. *J Invest Dermatol.* (2003) 121:1104–17. doi: 10.1046/j.1523-1747.2003.12536.x
80. Peluso I, Morabito G, Urban L, Ioannone F, Serafini M. Oxidative stress in atherosclerosis development: the central role of LDL and oxidative burst. *Endocr Metab Immune Disord Drug Targets* (2012) 12:351–60. doi: 10.2174/187153012803832602
81. Cretu D, Gao L, Liang K, Soosaipillai A, Diamandis EP, Chandran V. Differentiating psoriatic arthritis from psoriasis without psoriatic arthritis using novel serum biomarkers. *Arthritis Care Res.* (2018) 70:454–61. doi: 10.1002/acr.23298
82. Eding CB, Enerbäck C. Involved and uninvolved psoriatic keratinocytes display a resistance to apoptosis that may contribute to epidermal thickness. *Acta Derm Venereol.* (2017) 97:788–96. doi: 10.2340/00015555-2656
83. Chiricozzi A, Romanelli M, Panduri S, Donetti E, Prignano F. Relevance of *in vitro* 3-D skin models in dissecting cytokine contribution to psoriasis pathogenesis. *Histol Histopathol.* (2017) 32:893–8. doi: 10.14670/HH-11-877
84. Mashiko S, Bouguermouh S, Rubio M, Baba N, Bissonnette R, Sarfati M. Human mast cells are major IL-22 producers in patients with psoriasis and atopic dermatitis. *J Allergy Clin Immunol.* (2015) 136:351–9. doi: 10.1016/j.jaci.2015.01.033
85. Harvima IT, Naukkarinen A, Paukkonen K, Harvima RJ, Aalto ML, Schwartz LB, et al. Mast cell tryptase and chymase in developing and mature psoriatic lesions. *Arch Dermatol Res.* (1993) 285:184–92.
86. Moormann C, Artuc M, Pohl E, Varga G, Buddenkotte J, Vergnolle N, et al. Functional characterization and expression analysis of the proteinase-activated receptor-2 in human cutaneous mast cells. *J Invest Dermatol.* (2006) 126:746–55. doi: 10.1038/sj.jid.570016
87. Carvalho RF, Nilsson G, Harvima IT. Increased mast cell expression of PAR-2 in skin inflammatory diseases and release of IL-8 upon PAR-2 activation. *Exp Dermatol.* (2010) 19:117–22. doi: 10.1111/j.1600-0625.2009.00998.x
88. Santulli RJ, Derian CK, Darrow AL, Tomko KA, Eckardt AJ, Seiberg M, et al. Evidence for the presence of a protease-activated receptor distinct from the thrombin receptor in human keratinocytes. *Proc Natl Acad Sci USA.* (1995) 92:9151–5.
89. Wakita H, Furukawa F, Takigawa M. Thrombin and trypsin stimulate granulocyte-macrophage colony-stimulating factor and interleukin-6 gene expression in cultured normal human keratinocytes. *Proc Assoc Am Phys.* (1997) 109:190–207.
90. Oh CJ, Das KM, Gottlieb AB. Treatment with anti-tumor necrosis factor alpha (TNF-alpha) monoclonal antibody dramatically decreases the clinical activity of psoriasis lesions. *J Am Acad Dermatol.* (2000) 42:829–30. doi: 10.1067/mjd.2000.105948
91. Heufler C, Koch F, Schuler G. Granulocyte/macrophage colony-stimulating factor and interleukin-1 mediate the maturation of murine epidermal Langerhans cells into potent immunostimulatory dendritic cells. *J Exp Med.* (1988) 167:700–8.
92. Braunstein S, Kaplan G, Gottlieb AB, Schwartz M, Walsh G, Abalos RM, et al. GM-CSF activates regenerative epidermal growth and stimulates keratinocyte proliferation in human skin *in vivo*. *J Invest Dermatol.* (1994) 103:601–4.
93. Grossman RM, Krueger J, Yourish D, Granelli-Piperno A, Murphy DP, May LT, et al. Interleukin 6 is expressed in high levels in psoriatic skin and stimulates proliferation of cultured human keratinocytes. *Proc Nati Acad Sci USA.* (1989) 86:6367–71.
94. Zhou LI, Ivanov I, Spolski R, Min R, Shenderov K, Egawa T, et al. IL-6 programs TH-17 cell differentiation by promoting sequential engagement of the IL-21 and IL-23 pathways. *Nat Immunol.* (2007) 8:967–74. doi: 10.1038/ni1488
95. Harvima IT, Nilsson G. Stress, the neuroendocrine system and mast cells: current understanding of their role in psoriasis. *Expert Rev Clin Immunol.* (2012) 8:235–41. doi: 10.1586/eci.12.1
96. Chimenti MS, Triggianese P, Nuccetelli M, Terracciano C, Crisanti A, Guarino MD, et al. Auto-reactions, autoimmunity and psoriatic arthritis. *Autoimmun Rev.* (2015) 14:1142–6. doi: 10.1016/j.autrev.2015.08.003
97. Fitzgerald O, Winchester R. Psoriatic arthritis: from pathogenesis to therapy. *Arthritis Res Ther.* (2009) 11:214. doi: 10.1186/ar2580
98. Tassiulas I, Duncan SR, Centola M, Theofilopoulos AN, Boumpas DT. Clonal characteristics of T cell infiltrates in skin and synovium of patients with psoriatic arthritis. *Hum Immunol.* (1999) 60:479–91.
99. Dolcino M, Lunardi C, Ottria A, Tinazzi E, Patuzzo G, Puccetti A. Crossreactive autoantibodies directed against cutaneous and joint antigens are present in psoriatic arthritis. *PLoS ONE* (2014) 16:e115424. doi: 10.1371/journal.pone.0115424
100. Cañete JD, Santiago B, Cantaert T, Sanmartí R, Palacin A, Celis R, et al. Ectopic lymphoid neogenesis in psoriatic arthritis. *Ann Rheum Dis.* (2007) 66:720–6. doi: 10.1136/ard.2006.062042
101. Conigliaro P, Triggianese P, Perricone C, Chimenti MS, Di Muzio G, Ballanti E, et al. Restoration of peripheral blood natural killer and B cell levels in patients affected by rheumatoid and psoriatic arthritis during etanercept treatment. *Clin Exp Immunol.* (2014) 177:234–43. doi: 10.1111/cei.12335
102. Jaisson S, Larreta-Garde V, Bellon G, Hornebeck W, Garnotel R, Gillery P. Carbamylation differentially alters type I collagen sensitivity to various collagenases. *Matrix Biol.* (2007) 26:190–6. doi: 10.1016/j.matbio.2006.10.008
103. Wang H, Peters T, Kess D, Sindrilaru A, Oreshkova T, Van Rooijen N, et al. Activated macrophages are essential in a murine model for T cell-mediated chronic psoriasiform skin inflammation. *J Clin Invest.* (2006) 116:2105–14. doi: 10.1172/JCI27180
104. McGonagle D, Marzo-Ortega H, O'Connor P, Gibbon W, Hawkey P, Henshaw K, et al. Histological assessment of the early enthesitis lesion in spondyloarthropathy. *Ann Rheum Dis.* (2002) 61:534–7. doi: 10.1136/ard.61.6.534
105. Hamanaka RB, Chandel NS. Mitochondrial reactive oxygen species regulate hypoxic signaling. *Curr Opin Cell Biol.* (2009) 21:894–9. doi: 10.1016/j.ceb.2009.08.005
106. Kumagai T, Matsukawa N, Kaneko Y, Kusumi Y, Mitsumata M, Uchida K. A lipid peroxidation-derived inflammatory mediator: identification of 4-hydroxy-2-nonenal as a potential inducer of cyclooxygenase-2 in macrophages. *J Biol Chem.* (2004) 279:48389–96. doi: 10.1074/jbc.M409935200
107. Page S, Fischer C, Baumgartner B, Haas M, Kreusel U, Loidl G, et al. 4-Hydroxynonenal prevents NF-kappaB activation and tumor necrosis factor expression by inhibiting IkappaB phosphorylation and subsequent proteolysis. *J Biol Chem.* (1999) 274:11611–8.

108. Distler JH, Wenger RH, Gassmann M, Kurowska M, Hirth A, Gay S, et al. Physiologic responses to hypoxia and implications for hypoxia-inducible factors in the pathogenesis of rheumatoid arthritis. *Arthritis Rheum.* (2004) 50:10–23. doi: 10.1002/art.11425
109. Radisky DC, Levy DD, Littlepage LE, Liu H, Nelson CM, Fata JE, et al. Rac1b and reactive oxygen species mediate MMP-3-induced EMT and genomic instability. *Nature* (2005) 436:123–7. doi: 10.1038/nature03688
110. Korzon M, Renke J, Popadiuk S, Wozniak M. Carbonyl content in plasma proteins of children with connective tissue inflammatory diseases. *Pol J Environ Stud.* (1998) 7:376–7.
111. Basu S, Whiteman M, Mattey DL, Halliwell B. Raised levels of F(2)-isoprostanes and prostaglandin F(2alpha) in different rheumatic diseases. *Ann Rheum Dis.* (2001) 60:627–31. doi: 10.1136/ard.60.6.627
112. Firuzi O, Fuksa L, Spadaro C, Bousová I, Riccieri V, Spadaro A, et al. Oxidative stress parameters in different systemic rheumatic diseases. *J Pharm Pharmacol.* (2006) 58:951–7. doi: 10.1211/jpp.58.7.0010
113. Coaccioli S, Panaccione A, Biondi R, Sabatini C, Landucci P, Del Giorno R, et al. Evaluation of oxidative stress in rheumatoid and psoriatic arthritis and psoriasis. *Clin Ter.* (2009) 160:467–72.
114. Túnez I, Feijóo M, Huerta G, Montilla P, Muñoz E, Ruíz A, et al. The effect of infliximab on oxidative stress in chronic inflammatory joint disease. *Curr Med Res Opin.* (2007) 23:1259–67. doi: 10.1185/030079907X187955
115. Moodley D, Mody G, Patel N, Chuturgoon AA. Mitochondrial depolarisation and oxidative stress in rheumatoid arthritis patients. *Clin Biochem.* (2008) 41:1396–401. doi: 10.1016/j.clinbiochem.2008.08.072
116. Puig L. Cardiometabolic comorbidities in psoriasis and psoriatic arthritis.*Int J Mol Sci.* (2017) 19:E58. doi: 10.3390/ijms19010058
117. Yang X, Li Y, Li Y, Ren X, Zhang X, Hu D, Gao Y, et al. Oxidative stress-mediated atherosclerosis: mechanisms and therapies. *Front Physiol.* (2017) 8:600. doi: 10.3389/fphys.2017.00600
118. Nuttall SL, Heaton S, Piper MK, Martin U, Gordon C. Cardiovascular risk in systemic lupus erythematosus–evidence of increased oxidative stress and dyslipidaemia. *Rheumatology (Oxford)* (2003) 42:758–62. doi: 10.1093/rheumatology/keg212
119. Chimenti MS, Triggianese P, Conigliaro P, Candi E, Melino G, Perricone R. The interplay between inflammation and metabolism in rheumatoid arthritis. *Cell Death Dis.* (2015) 6:e1887. doi: 10.1038/cddis.2015.24
120. Firuzi O, Spadaro A, Spadaro C, Riccieri V, Petrucci R, Marrosu G, et al. Protein oxidation markers in the serum and synovial fluid of psoriatic arthritis patients. *J Clin Lab Anal.* (2008) 22:210–5. doi: 10.1002/jcla.20243
121. Kennedy A, Ng CT, Biniecka M, Saber T, Taylor C, O'Sullivan J, et al. Angiogenesis and blood vessel stability in inflammatory arthritis. *Arthritis Rheum.* (2010) 62:711–21. doi: 10.1002/art.27287
122. Biniecka M, Kennedy A, Fearon U, Ng CT, Veale DJ, O'Sullivan JN. Oxidative damage in synovial tissue is associated with *in vivo* hypoxic status in the arthritic joint. *Ann Rheum Dis.* (2010) 69:1172–8. doi: 10.1136/ard.2009.111211
123. Ng CT, Biniecka M, Kennedy A, McCormick J, Fitzgerald O, Bresnihan B, et al. Synovial tissue hypoxia and inflammation *in vivo. Ann Rheum Dis.* (2010) 69:1389–95. doi: 10.1136/ard.2009.119776
124. Biniecka M, Fox E, Gao W, Ng CT, Veale DJ, Fearon U, et al. Hypoxia induces mitochondrial mutagenesis and dysfunction in inflammatory arthritis. *Arthritis Rheum.* (2011) 63:2172–82. doi: 10.1002/art.30395
125. Harty LC, Biniecka M, O'Sullivan J, Fox E, Mulhall K, Veale DJ, et al. Mitochondrial mutagenesis correlates with the local inflammatory environment in arthritis. *Ann Rheum Dis.* (2012) 71:582–8. doi: 10.1136/annrheumdis-2011-200245
126. Chimenti MS, Perricone C, Novelli L, Caso F, Costa L, Bogdanos D, et al. Interaction between microbiome and host genetics in psoriatic arthritis. *Autoimmun Rev.* (2018) 17:276–83. doi: 10.1016/j.autrev.2018.01.002

2

IL-36γ is a Strong Inducer of IL-23 in Psoriatic Cells and Activates Angiogenesis

Charlie Bridgewood[1], Gareth W. Fearnley[2], Anna Berekmeri[3,4], Philip Laws[3,5], Tom Macleod[4], Sreenivasan Ponnambalam[2], Martin Stacey[4], Anne Graham[6] and Miriam Wittmann[1,5,7]**

[1] Centre of Skin Sciences, School of Chemistry and Biosciences, University of Bradford, Bradford, United Kingdom, [2] Endothelial Cell Biology Unit, School of Molecular and Cellular Biology, University of Leeds, Leeds, United Kingdom, [3] Department of Dermatology, Chapel Allerton Hospital, Leeds, United Kingdom, [4] Faculty of Biological Sciences, School of Molecular and Cellular Biology, University of Leeds, Leeds, United Kingdom, [5] National Institute of Health Research (NIHR), Leeds Biomedical Research Centre (BRC), Chapel Allerton Hospital, Leeds, United Kingdom, [6] Biomedical Sciences, School of Chemistry and Biosciences, University of Bradford, Bradford, United Kingdom, [7] Leeds Institute of Rheumatic and Musculoskeletal Medicine (LIRMM), University of Leeds, Leeds, United Kingdom

***Correspondence:**
Anne Graham
a.graham@bradford.ac.uk;
Miriam Wittmann
m.wittmann@leeds.ac.uk

The IL-1 family member cytokine IL-36γ is recognised as key mediator in the immunopathology of psoriasis, hallmarks of which involve the activation of both resident and infiltrating inflammatory myeloid cells and aberrant angiogenesis. This research demonstrates a role for IL-36γ in both myeloid activation and angiogenesis. We show that IL-36γ induces the production of psoriasis-associated cytokines from macrophages (IL-23 and TNFα) and that this response is enhanced in macrophages from psoriasis patients. This effect is specific for IL-36γ and could not be mimicked by other IL-1 family cytokines such as IL-1α. IL-36γ was also demonstrated to induce endothelial tube formation and branching, in a VEGF-A-dependent manner. Furthermore, IL-36γ-stimulated macrophages potently activated endothelial cells and led to increased adherence of monocytes, effects that were markedly more pronounced for psoriatic macrophages. Interestingly, regardless of stimulus, psoriasis monocytes showed increased adherence to both the stimulated and unstimulated endothelium when compared with monocytes from healthy individuals. Collectively, these findings show that IL-36γ has the potential to enhance endothelium directed leucocyte infiltration into the skin and strengthen the IL-23/IL-17 pathway adding to the growing evidence of pathogenetic roles for IL-36γ in psoriatic responses. Our findings also point to a cellular response, which could potentially explain cardiovascular comorbidities in psoriasis in the form of endothelial activation and increased monocyte adherence.

Keywords: psoriasis, IL-36γ, IL-23, macrophages, monocytes, angiogenesis, endothelial, inflammation

INTRODUCTION

Psoriasis is an immune mediated inflammatory disease which affects 2–3% of the world's population (1). Psoriatic lesions manifest as hyperkeratotic plaques, dermo-epidermal inflammation, and aberrant blood vessel formation caused by the complex interplay between tissue resident cells, dendritic cells, macrophages, and T cells and resultant enhanced expression of the IL-23–Th17/Th22 and IL-12–IFNγ/TNFα pathways (2).

IL-36α, IL-36β, and IL-36γ are members of the IL-1 family of cytokines that signal through a common receptor composed of IL-36 receptor (IL-36R) and IL-1R/AcP to activate NF-κB and MAPKs, such as p38 and JNK, and promote inflammatory responses.

IL-36α, IL-36β, and IL-36γ are members of the wider IL-1 family of cytokines. These cytokines mediate inflammatory events through the IL-36R and activate NF-κB and MAPKs, such as p38 and JNK in susceptible cells. The significance of IL-36γ for psoriatic inflammation is increasingly being recognised (3–6). IL-36 cytokines, in particular IL-36γ is dramatically upregulated in lesional psoriasis when compared with healthy controls (5). As well as acting as a psoriatic biomarker, loss-of-function mutations in the IL-36R antagonist (IL-36RA) in multiple cohorts of generalised pustular psoriasis (GPP) patients provide evidence that IL-36 plays a causative role in the pathology of psoriasis (7–9). IL-36 has recently also been implicated in other skin inflammatory diseases including acne and hidradenitis suppurativa, and allergic contact dermatitis (10, 11). IL-36γ, which is highly expressed by epithelial cells, is thought to be released in the context of cell damage or *via* non-conventional secretory pathways (12–14). Following release, it has been shown that IL-36γ is processed into its bioactive form by cathepsin S and results in the subsequent stimulation of surrounding tissues (15). IL-36R-mediated signal transduction has been shown to induce the release of pro-inflammatory cytokines (e.g., IL-8, TNFα, and IL-6), upregulate antimicrobial peptides and proliferative mediators such as defensins and HB-EGF, as well as T cell attracting or polarising cytokines such as CCL20 and IL-12, respectively (16–19).

Angiogenesis is the formation of new blood vessels from the preexisting vasculature and is a hallmark of psoriasis lesions (20). Microvascular changes within psoriasis lesions include pronounced dilation, increased permeability and endothelial cell proliferation. Immature permeable blood vessels may enhance dermal inflammation through immune cell recruitment (21, 22). A recent study confirmed a positive correlation between hypervascularisation and disease severity (23). Excessive capillary-venular dilatation precedes development of psoriatic inflammation, and resolution of these vascular changes is associated with remission of psoriasis lesions (24). VEGF-A is thought to be the driving force behind angiogenesis observed in psoriatic lesions. Mice that overexpress VEGF-A show an inflammatory response that histologically resembles psoriasis (25, 26). The *VEGFA* gene is located on chromosome 6 at 6p21, close to PSORS 1, which is a known chromosomal locus for psoriasis susceptibility (27, 28). The +405 CC *VEGFA* genotype, also known as the "high VEGF-A-producing genotype," is associated with early onset psoriasis, whereas the "low VEGF-A-producing genotype" has no association with psoriasis (29–31). This suggests that the pro-angiogenic potential of an individual may influence disease progression.

Treatment of human psoriasis with biologics has unequivocally shown that activation of the IL-23/IL-17 pathway is key for clinical symptom development (32). IL-23 induces and maintains the differentiation of IL-17- and IL-22-producing lymphocytes, which serve as the primary source of IL-17 and IL-22, both of which orchestrate epidermal hyperplasia and tissue inflammation in psoriasis (2). In murine induced psoriasis models, infiltrating macrophages, monocytes, and monocyte-derived dendritic cells and their subsequent T cell activating cytokines such as IL-23 have been shown to drive inflammation (33–37). A mechanistic link between IL-36 and the IL-23/IL-17 axis is becoming increasingly clear (6, 38–40). Work on other inflammatory skin diseases has also highlighted a correlation between IL-36 and IL-17 (41, 42).

Whilst previous reports have shown that IL-36γ induces inflammatory mediators from macrophages, little is known about its ability to induce psoriasis relevant cytokines such as TNFα and IL-23 (16). The ability of IL-36γ to induce such inflammatory mediators from infiltrating macrophages could escalate the inflammatory cascade by activating surrounding fibroblasts, endothelial cells (18), and keratinocytes and ultimately lead to further immune cell recruitment. In recent studies, GPP patients with DITRA (Deficiency of IL-36R Antagonist) showed significant disease improvement after receiving monocyte apheresis therapy, highlighting the potential importance of an IL-36-macrophage axis in the pathology of psoriasis (43, 44).

In this study, we highlight the role of IL-36γ in both macrophage and vascular activation in the context of psoriatic lesions. Our data demonstrate that IL-36γ induces the secretion of a key driver of psoriasis, IL-23, by macrophages and that this induction is enhanced in macrophages of psoriasis patients. IL-36γ also induces angiogenesis and branching of endothelial cells in a VEGF-A-dependent manner. Supernatant from IL-36γ treated macrophages potently activate endothelial cells and increased ICAM-1 expression. Psoriasis monocytes show an increased adhesion to both stimulated and untreated endothelial cells. Overall, the presented findings add to the growing body of evidence for IL-36γ as highly relevant molecule in psoriasis immunopathology.

MATERIALS AND METHODS

Cell Isolations and Cell Culture

Blood was collected in sodium citrate tubes. PBMCs were separated using Lymphoprep density gradient centrifugation. Monocytes were isolated from PBMCs using magnetic separation CD14+ beads (Miltenyi Biotech) using the Dynal MPC column (Invitrogen, CA, USA). Monocytes were resuspended in RPMI (ThermoFisher Scientific, MA, USA) containing 10% FCS and penicillin/streptomycin (100 U/100 mg/ml; both Life Technologies, Carlsbad, CA, USA). CD14+ purity was tested by FACs analysis with mouse antihuman CD14 FITC conjugated or mouse IgG isotype control (both 1:100; both ImmunoTools, Friesoythe, Germany). Purity for healthy patients was >90% (Figure S2 in Supplementary Material). Umbilical cords were supplied by Bradford Royal Infirmary under the approval and processing of Ethical Tissue Bradford. Human umbilical vein endothelial cells (HUVECs) were isolated from umbilical cords in a previously described method (45). Monocytes were seeded onto plates (dependent on application) in RPMI overnight to generate day 1 macrophages.

Macrophage Purity and IL-36R Confirmation

Isolated macrophages were seeded onto coverslips overnight. Cells were washed in PBS and fixed in 4% formaldehyde for 20 min. Cells were then blocked for 1 h in 5% BSA in PBS. Cells were incubated overnight with rabbit anti-human IL-36R 1:500 (Novus Biologics, Littleton, CO, USA) or rabbit IgG isotype control (1:500; Abcam, Cambridge, UK). Cells were then washed with PBS and incubated with donkey anti-rabbit Alexa 594 conjugated and mouse anti-human CD14 FITC conjugated or mouse IgG isotype control (both 1:100; both ImmunoTools, Friesoythe, Germany). Cells were visualised using the EVOS XL microscope (Thermo Fisher Scientific).

Patient Demographics

Details on patients who gave blood for the study are listed below in (**Table 1**). All patients included are under care in the dermatology department and have a diagnosis of plaque psoriasis; one patient presented mainly with palmoplantar pustular psoriasis at the time point blood was taken. Patients receiving conventional systemic treatment known to change the biological response of leucocytes, in particular methotrexate, cyclosporine A, or leflunomide were excluded from the study. For this experimental setup, where cells were isolated involving multiple washing steps, cell culture and *ex vivo* stimulation, biologics treatment was not an exclusion criteria. We carefully checked the dataset, and there was no tendency for a difference in our outcome measured between cells derived from patients with or without biologics treatment.

As for the healthy controls, none were known to suffer from psoriasis, eczema or any active inflammatory disease under systemic treatment. Healthy controls were matched regarding gender distribution; the age range was between 28 and 52.

Macrophage Cytokine Stimulation

Monocytes were seeded at 1×10^5 in 96-well plates (Greiner Bio-One, Stonehouse, UK) in RPMI overnight to generate day 1 macrophages. Where relevant, macrophages were primed for 24 h with IFNγ 20 ng/ml. Macrophages were stimulated with IL-36γ protein, which was generated as previously described (15, 46), IL-17, TNFα, and IL-1α (PeproTech, Rocky Hill, NJ, USA). Following 48 h stimulation, supernatant was stored at −80°C. Concentrations of IL-23 and TNFα were measured using ELISA kits from eBioscience/ThermoFisher (Waltham, MA, USA). ELISAs were carried out according to the manufacturer's protocols. Reproducibility of the supernatants was confirmed by triplicate testing, with <10% error.

Tubulogenesis Assay

Primary human foreskin fibroblasts (PromoCell, Heidelberg, Germany) were cultured in 48-well plates in complete DMEM [containing 10% (v/v) FCS, 1% (v/v) non-essential amino acids and 1% (v/v) sodium pyruvate] until confluent. 6,500 HUVECs were seeded onto the fibroblasts monolayer in a 1 ml 1:1 mixture of complete DMEM and ECGM (PromoCell). Cells were left to acclimatise for 24 h. Media were aspirated and replaced with fresh ECGM ± growth factors (VEGF-A, 10 ng/ml) or IL-36 (50 ng/ml) or inhibitors (IL-36RA, 50 ng/ml), Sutent (Sigma, 1 nM) or anti-VEGF-A neutralising antibody (R&D Systems, 50 or 100 ng/ml) as indicated; media were replaced every 2–3 days for 9 days. Cocultures were fixed in 200 µl 10% (v/v) formalin for 20 min and blocked in 5% (w/v) BSA for 30 min at RT. Cocultures were then incubated with 1 µg/ml mouse anti-human PECAM-1 (CD31) (Santa Cruz, Dallas, TX, USA) overnight at 4°C. Cells were washed three times with PBS before incubation with anti-mouse Alexa Fluor 594 conjugate (Invitrogen) for 3 h at RT. Wells were washed three times with PBS. Endothelial tubules were visualised *via* immunofluorescence microscopy using an EVOS-fl inverted digital microscope (Thermo Fisher Scientific). Three random fields were imaged per well. Total tubule length and number of branch points were quantified from each photographic field using the open source software AngioQuant (www.cs.tut.fi/sgn/csb/angioquant) and values were averaged. For a more detailed method, see Ref. (47).

VEGF-A Induction Quantification by Immunoblot and ELISA

Endothelial or fibroblast cells were seeded into 6-well plates and cultured in ECGM or complete DMEM until ~80%

TABLE 1 | Patient demographics.

Diagnosis	Age	Gender	Disease duration (years)	PsA	PASI	Current systemic treatment
Plaque psoriasis	48	Female	42	Yes	Minimal disease activity	Secukinumab
Plaque psoriasis	38	Male	10	No	14.4	None
Plaque psoriasis	43	Female	Unknown	No	Minimal disease activity	Ustekinumab
Plaque psoriasis	55	Male	10	No	Minimal disease activity	None
Plaque psoriasis	41	Male	10	Yes	Minimal disease activity	Adalimumab
Plaque psoriasis	24	Female	13	No	5.1	None
Plaque psoriasis	52	Male	13	No	6	Ustekinumab
Plaque psoriasis	48	Male	10	No	8.1	None
Plaque psoriasis	29	Female	22	No	7.7	None
Plaque psoriasis	41	Female	28	Yes	1.2	Ustekinumab
Plaque psoriasis	35	Male	15	No	4	Ustekinumab
Plaque psoriasis	37	Male	10	No	8	None
Plaque psoriasis	48	Female	30	Yes	13	None
Pustular palmoplantar and plaque psoriasis	70	Female	Unknown	No	Minimal disease activity	Ustekinumab

PsA, psoriatic arthritis; PASI, Psoriasis Area and Severity Index.

confluent. Cells were then washed twice with PBS and starved in MCDB131 + 0.2% (w/v) BSA for 2 h before stimulation with IL-36 (50 ng/ml) for 24 h. Cells were then washed twice with ice-cold PBS and lysed in 2% (w/v) SDS, TBS, 1 mM PMSF and protease inhibitor cocktail (Sigma-Aldrich). Protein concentration was determined using the bicinchoninic acid assay (ThermoFisher). 20 µg of protein lysate was subjected to SDS-PAGE before transfer onto nitrocellulose membrane and analysis *via* immunoblotting using antibodies against VEGF-A, VEGFR1, and VEGFR2 (R&D Systems). For a detailed immunoblot protocol, see Ref. (48). The relative expression of the non-stimulated control was set to 1, and all other results expressed as a ratio of this. To measure VEGF-A secretion from both cell types, the supernatant was tested using VEGF-A ELISA kit (eBioscience/ThermoFisher).

Macrophage Supernatant-Endothelial Activation Assay

Following 48 h stimulation, supernatant was removed and stored at −80°C. HUVEC was cultured on black TC grade fluorescence plates (PerkinElmer, Waltham, MA, USA), in PromoCell endothelial cell media containing penicillin/streptomycin (100 U/100 mg/ml) (Life Technologies, Carlsbad, CA, USA). Supernatant was cultured with HUVEC at ratio of 1:10 for 24 h. Recombinant IL-36γ was added to control wells to serve as a blank. After 24 h, the cells were fixed for 15 min with 4% formaldehyde in PBS. Mouse anti-human ICAM-1 FITC or mouse IgG isotype control was added (1:500) (BioLegend, San Diego, CA, USA). The fluorescence intensity of each well was measured using the Promega GloMax plate reader (Madison, WI, USA). For immunocytochemistry, the cells were visualised using the EVOS XL microscope.

Monocyte Adherence Assays

Monolayers of HUVEC were grown to confluence in 24-well plates (Greiner Bio-One). HUVECs were stimulated with macrophage supernatant as above, or with TNFα (10 ng/ml) for 24 h and then suspended in fresh media before experiments. 1×10^5 monocytes were added per chamber for 30 min. After 30 min, non-adherent cells were washed away, and the cells were fixed using 4% formaldehyde in PBS and blocked in 5% BSA in PBS for 1 h. The cells were the stained with mouse anti-human CD14 FITC conjugated or mouse IgG isotype control (both 1:100) (both ImmunoTools). The cells were visualised using the EVOS XL microscope, and the number of adhered cells counted using ImageJ software.

Statistical Analysis

This was performed using a one-way analysis of variance (ANOVA) followed by Tukey's *post hoc* test, two-way ANOVA followed by Bonferroni multiple comparison or single unpaired *t*-test using GraphPad Prism software (La Jolla, CA, USA). Significant differences between control and test groups were evaluated with p values less than $^{*}p < 0.05$, $^{**}p < 0.01$, $^{***}p < 0.001$, and $^{****}p < 0.0001$ indicated on the graphs. Error bars represent the SEM.

RESULTS

IL-36γ Induces Increased IL-23 and TNFα from Psoriasis Macrophages

Psoriasis is driven by aberrant type-3 immune responses, characterised by high levels of IL-17 and IL-22 (32, 49). A key inducer of type-3 responses is IL-23, which is expressed by antigen-presenting cells including macrophages upon stimulation with TLRs agonists such as LPS and flagellin (50, 51). IL-36γ is an abundant and prominent mediator in skin psoriasis, and we were interested in its ability to induce IL-23 expression by macrophages.

In support of previous mRNA data (52) IL-36R protein was found to be expressed by blood derived CD14+ monocyte/macrophages (**Figure 1A**) ($n = 3$, healthy). To assess the functional significance of IL-36γ interactions with macrophages, IL-36γ stimulation was performed for 48 h before analysis of TNFα and IL-23 secretion *via* ELISA (**Figure 1B**). As macrophages are known to be sensitive to LPS stimulation, boiled IL-36γ was included as a control for potential endotoxin contamination of the protein preparation. TNFα induction was measured at 24 and 48 h (Figure S1 in Supplementary Material). Differences between treatment groups became more apparent when more time was allowed for the secreted mediator to accumulate. Both 10 and 50 ng/ml IL-36γ induced a significant increase in IL-23 secretion when compared with unstimulated cells, which was further amplified when the macrophages were primed with IFNγ 20 ng/ml. For both doses of IL-36γ, macrophages from psoriatic donors secreted significantly more IL-23 compared with cells from healthy individuals. Other psoriasis relevant mediators such as IL-17, TNFα, and IL-1 did not induce a significant increase in IL-23 secretion, regardless of IFNγ priming. IL-36γ also induced significant TNFα secretion from macrophages, as did both IL-1 and IL-17 when compared with untreated controls. However, following IFNγ priming, IL-36γ induced secretion exceeded both IL-1 and IL-17.

IL-36-Stimulated Endothelial Cell Tubulogenesis

IL-36's relationship with angiogenesis in the context of inflammation is presently unknown. To close this knowledge gap, we investigated the role of IL-36 in blood vessel formation. Endothelial cell tubulogenesis was assessed using an endothelial-fibroblast coculture assay. Here, human endothelial cells were cocultured on a monolayer of primary human fibroblasts, before IL-36 or VEGF-A (positive control) stimulation, fixation, and visualisation of PECAM-1 positive endothelial cells (**Figure 2A**). Quantification revealed that both IL-36γ and IL-36α (50 ng/ml) stimulation produced a significant increase in both tubule length (**Figure 2B**) and branch point number (**Figure 2C**). Such effects were dependent on IL-36/IL-36R interactions, as treatment with an IL-36RA impaired IL-36-stimulated tubulogenesis (**Figures 2A–C**). Endothelial cell tubulogenesis was also enhanced in response to VEGF-A (10 ng/ml; **Figures 2A,D,E**); however, as expected, this was unaffected by co-treatment with IL-36RA (**Figures 2A,D,E**). Thus, these data show that IL-36R-mediated signal transduction promotes endothelial cell tubulogenesis.

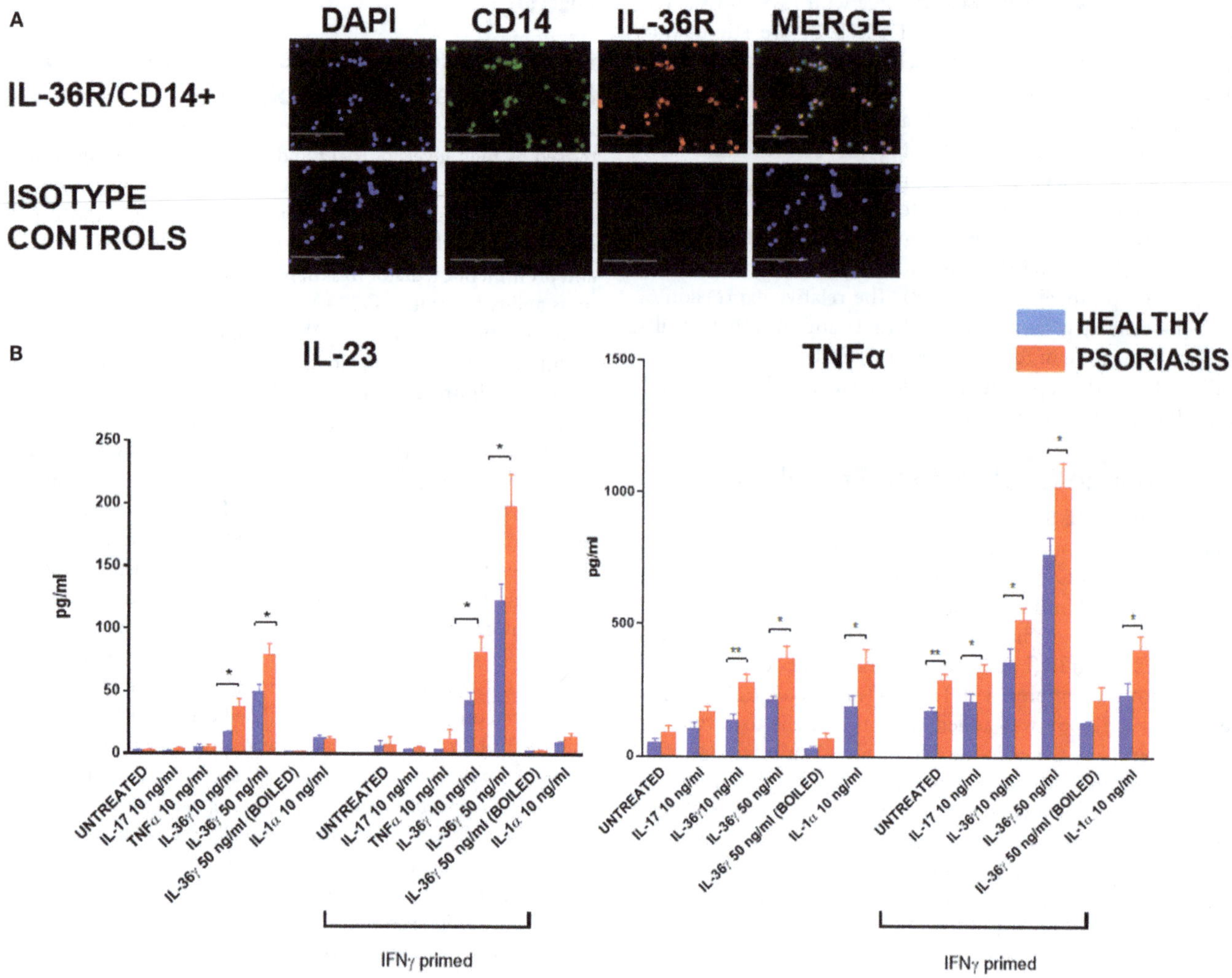

FIGURE 1 | **(A)** IL-36 receptor (IL-36R) (red) on macrophages; CD14+ (green) (magnification 20x). **(B)** Following 48 h stimulation with IL-36γ, IL-1α, IL-17A, TNFα, and IFNγ (24 h priming), supernatant was analysed by ELISA for TNFα and IL-23. Unpaired *t*-test $^{*}p < 0.05$, $^{**}p < 0.01$ psoriasis versus healthy (sample size: psoriasis = 9, healthy = 9, and boiled control $n = 3$).

IL-36-Stimulated Endothelial Cell Tubulogenesis Is VEGF-A Dependent

VEGF-A is a strong promoter of angiogenesis (53) and endothelial cell tube formation (**Figure 2**). Pro-angiogenic molecules such as IL-6 have been shown to induce the expression and secretion of VEGF-A; therefore, one possibility was that IL-36-mediated endothelial cell tube formation could be dependent on increased VEGF-A signalling. To test this, human endothelial cells were cocultured on a bed of primary human fibroblasts and stimulated with IL-36 or VEGF-A (positive control) in the presence or absence of an anti-VEGF-A neutralising antibody or the VEGFR inhibitor, Sutent (**Figure 3A**). Here, quantification revealed that IL-36-stimulated (50 ng/ml) endothelial cell tubulogenesis was significantly impaired in response to either the anti-VEGF-A neutralising antibody (50 and 100 ng/μl) or Sutent (1 nM; **Figures 3A–C**). As expected, VEGF-A-stimulated endothelial cell tubulogeneis was also impaired in response to either the anti-VEGF-A neutralising antibody or Sutent (**Figures 3A,D,E**). Therefore, these data show that IL-36-stimulated endothelial cell tube formation is dependent on VEGF-A-mediated signal transduction.

IL-36 Stimulation Upregulates VEGF-A Protein Levels in Fibroblast Cells

After concluding IL-36-induced angiogenesis is dependent on VEGF-A-mediated signal transduction (**Figure 3**), we assessed the effect of IL-36 stimulation on the protein levels of VEGF-A and its receptors VEGFR1 and VEGFR2. Here, endothelial or fibroblast cells were serum-starved before IL-36 stimulation (50 ng/ml; 24 h); cells were then lysed and subjected to immunoblotting (**Figure 3A**). Here, IL-36 stimulation significantly increased VEGF-A protein levels (~2-fold) in primary fibroblasts (**Figures 4A,B**), but not in endothelial cells (**Figures 4A,B**). IL-36 also induced significant VEGF secretion by fibroblasts, but not endothelial cells, as detected by ELISA (**Figure 4C**). However, IL-36

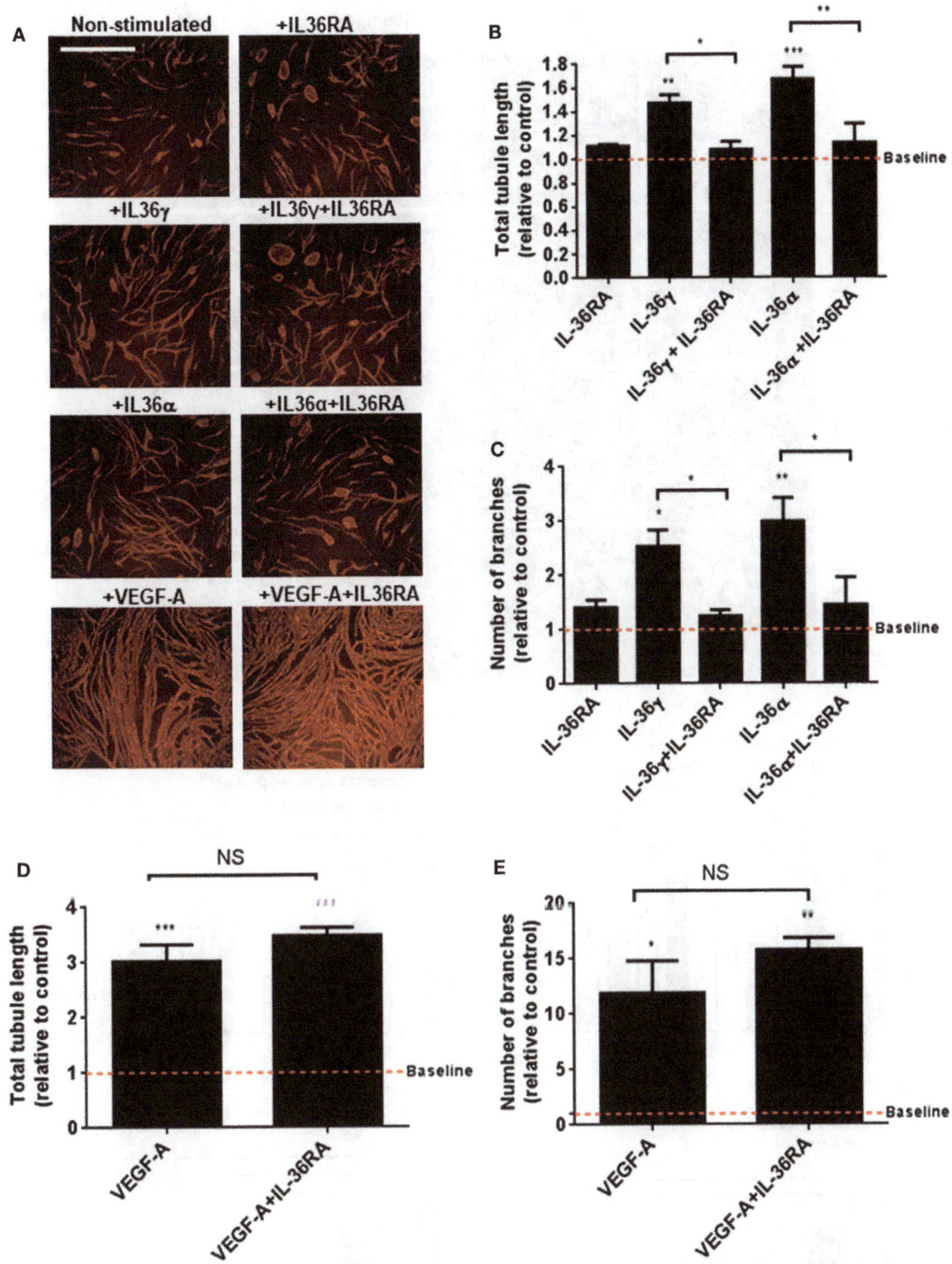

FIGURE 2 | IL-36 stimulates endothelial cell tubulogenesis. **(A)** Human umbilical vein endothelial cells were cocultured on a bed of primary human fibroblasts for 9 days and stimulated with either IL-36 (50 ng/ml) or VEGF-A (10 ng/ml). Cocultures were then fixed and stained for PECAM-1, before visualisation using immunofluorescence microscopy. **(B,C)** Quantification of **(B)** total tubule length or **(C)** number of branches upon IL-36 stimulation. **(D,E)** Quantification of **(D)** total tubule length or **(E)** number of branches upon VEGF-A stimulation. Scale bar represents 1,000 μm ($n = 3$). One-way analysis of variance was performed ($^{*}p < 0.05$, $^{**}p < 0.01$, and $^{***}p < 0.001$).

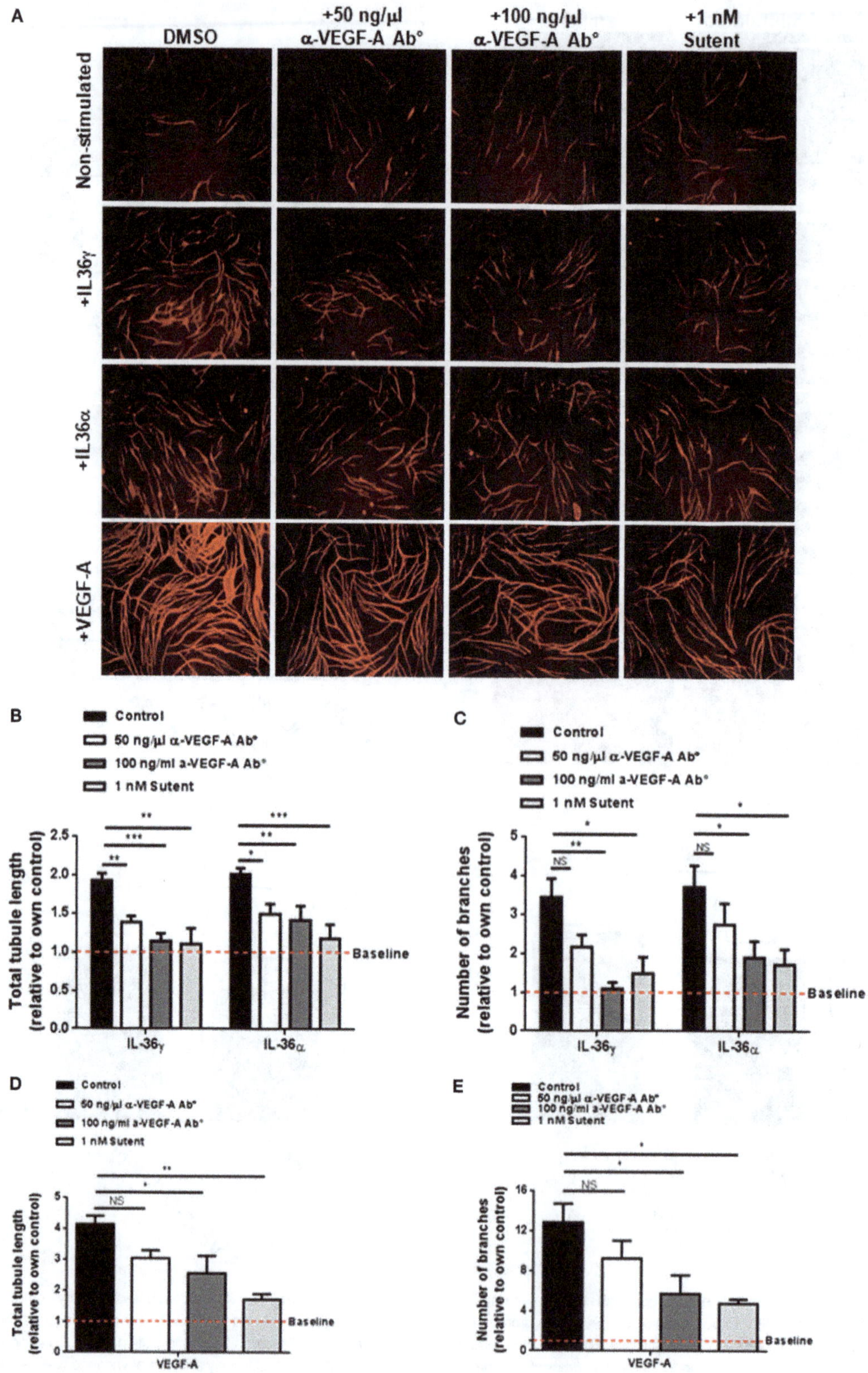

FIGURE 3 | IL-36-stimulated endothelial cell tubulogenesis is VEGF-A dependent. **(A)** Human umbilical vein endothelial cells were cocultured on a bed of primary human fibroblasts for 9 days and stimulated with either IL-36 (50 ng/ml) or VEGF-A (10 ng/ml) ± 50 ng/ml anti-VEGF-A antibody, 100 ng/ml anti-VEGF-A antibody, or 1 nM Sutent. Cocultures were then fixed and stained for PECAM-1, before visualisation using immunofluorescence microscopy. **(B,C)** Quantification of **(B)** total tubule length or **(C)** number of branches upon IL-36 stimulation. **(D,E)** Quantification of **(D)** total tubule length or **(E)** number of branches upon VEGF-A stimulation. Scale bar represents 1,000 μm ($n = 3$). Two-way analysis of variance (ANOVA) **(C,D)** and one-way ANOVA **(D,E)** were applied (*$p < 0.05$, **$p < 0.01$, and ***$p < 0.001$).

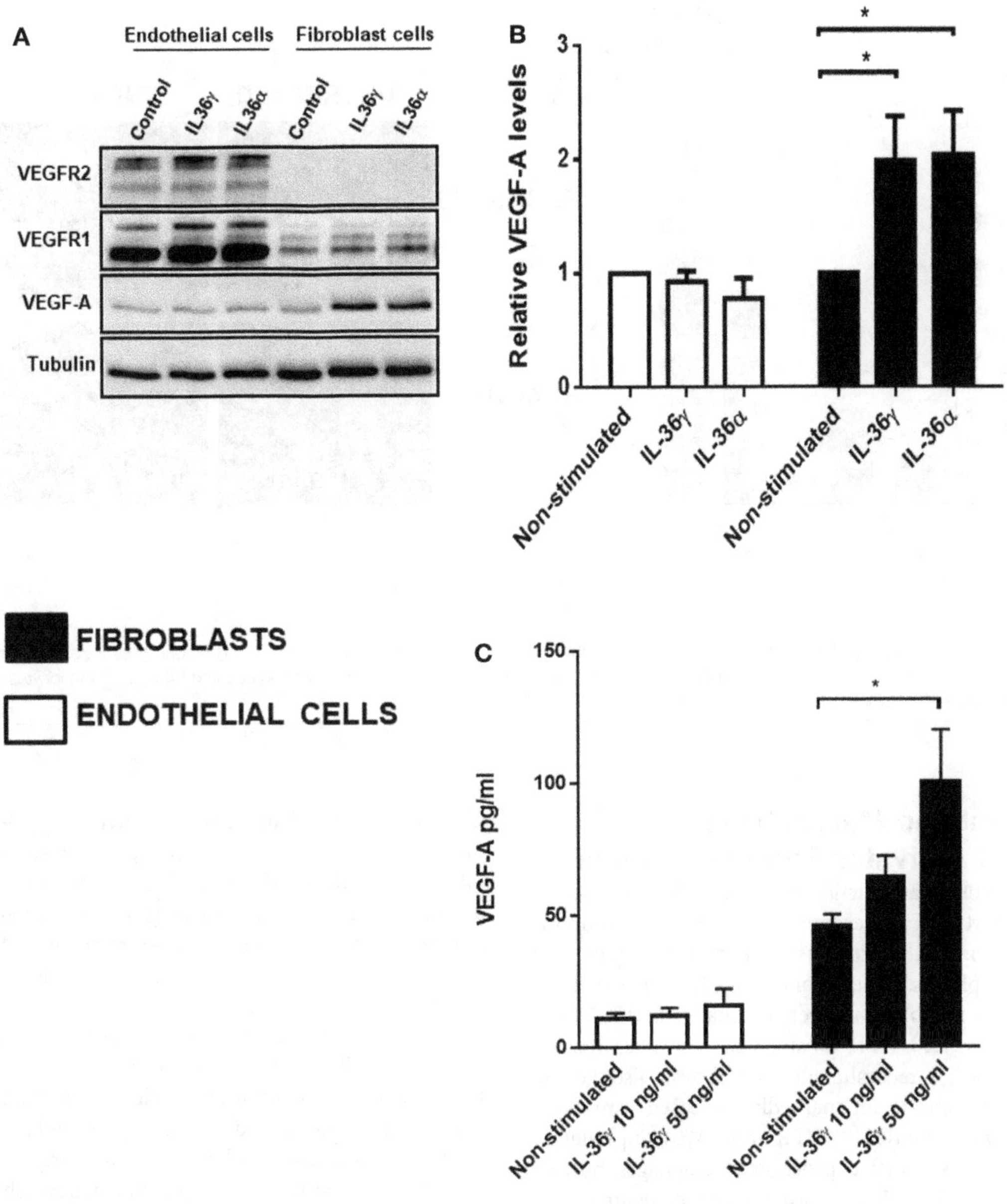

FIGURE 4 | IL-36 stimulates VEGF-A expression and secretion by primary human fibroblasts. **(A)** Human umbilical vein endothelial cells or foreskin-derived fibroblasts were stimulated with IL-36 (50 ng/ml) for 24 h, before cell lysis. Endothelial cell or fibroblast lysates were processed for detection of VEGF-A protein levels *via* immunoblot analysis. **(B)** Quantification of VEGF-A protein levels upon IL-36 stimulation by 2D-densitometry ($n = 3$). **(C)** The supernatant from both the stimulated cell types was also tested for VEGF-A protein concentration. Two-way analysis of variance was performed (*$p < 0.05$).

stimulation had no significant effect on VEGFR1 or VEGFR2 protein levels in either cell type (**Figure 4A**). These data suggest that IL-36-induced VEGF-A secretion from surrounding fibroblasts cell is capable of stimulating endothelial cell tubulogenesis.

Psoriasis Monocytes Show Increased Adhesion

As monocyte recruitment is crucial for psoriasis lesion development, but also comorbidities associated with psoriasis such as atherosclerosis, we decided to investigate the adhesive properties of psoriasis patients' monocytes to HUVECs. To fully visualise potential differences in monocyte adhesion we worked with non-stimulated HUVEC monolayers but also used the best described stimulus, TNFα, to reliably upregulate adhesion molecules on endothelial cells (54). Psoriasis and healthy monocytes (healthy $n = 8$, psoriasis $n = 8$) were allowed to adhere for 30 min to HUVECs. Psoriasis patients' monocytes showed increased adherence to both untreated and TNFα activated HUVECs (**Figures 5A,B**).

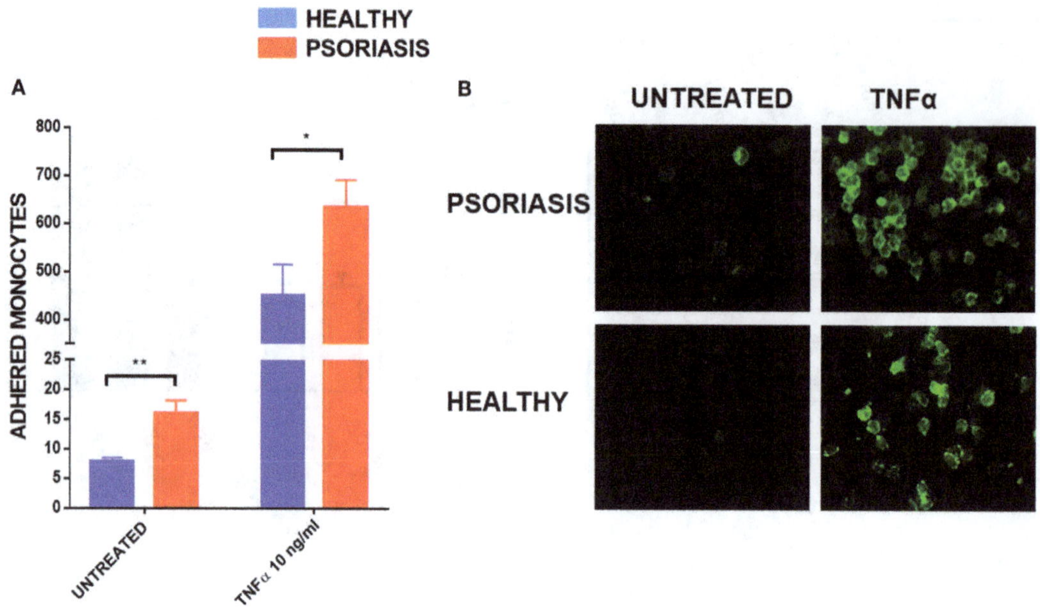

FIGURE 5 | Human umbilical vein endothelial cell monolayer was stimulated with or without TNFα 10 ng for 24 h. 1 × 10^5 monocytes were allowed to adhere to the monolayer for 30 min. Cells were visualised by immunofluorescence microscopy following CD14+ staining **(B)** and counted **(A)** (patient monocytes: psoriasis = 8; healthy = 8). Magnification 40×. Unpaired *t*-test *$p < 0.05$ and **$p < 0.01$.

IL-36γ-Stimulated Macrophage Supernatant Activates Endothelial Cells

To further understand the functional role of IL-36γ beyond the epidermal compartment we examined the aspect of immune cell recruitment into the skin using endothelial cells and monocytes/macrophages. Supernatants from IL-36γ-stimulated macrophages were incubated with endothelial cells (HUVECs) for 24 h at a ratio of 1:10. As IL-36 alone has pro-inflammatory effects on HUVEC, a recombinant control was also added. IL-36γ-stimulated supernatant markedly increased expression of the adhesion molecule ICAM-1 (**Figures 6A,B**). Supernatant derived from IL-36γ-stimulated, psoriasis macrophages induced significantly more ICAM-1 expression when compared with healthy macrophages (**Figures 6A,B**). Stimulation of HUVECs with psoriasis macrophage supernatant resulted in increased adhesion of both healthy and psoriasis monocytes (**Figure 6C**) (healthy $n = 8$, psoriasis $n = 8$). However, regardless of HUVEC stimulation (untreated or treated, supernatant from healthy or psoriasis macrophages), psoriasis monocytes showed increased endothelial adhesion.

DISCUSSION

IL-36γ is an IL-1 family cytokine with an increasingly recognised importance in the pathology of psoriasis (5). Various myeloid cells are thought to contribute to the pathology of psoriasis, including macrophages (33). Myeloid cells are capable of secreting IL-23 and thus contributing to the IL-23/IL-17 axis, prominent in psoriasis (36). The central role of a type-3 immune response shift in psoriatic inflammation is convincingly demonstrated by the overwhelmingly positive therapeutic response of biologics interfering with the IL-23/IL-17 axis, which leads to complete or almost complete clearing of psoriatic symptoms in a large number of patients receiving these treatments. Within psoriasis lesions, monocytes, macrophages and dendritic cells all show positive staining for IL-23 (55).

With IL-36γ being released by keratinocytes, probably in the context of cellular stress/environmental challenges, its downstream actions on dermal cells including fibroblasts, endothelial cells but also resident and infiltrating myeloid cells such as macrophages could represent a key step in both early and chronic lesion pathology. While IL-36γ has previously been shown to induce IL-23 mRNA in murine bone marrow derived dendritic cells, we here report secretion of IL-23 protein by human macrophages (56). Interestingly, other inflammatory cytokines prominent in psoriatic lesions, TNFα, IL-17, and IL-1, had little or no ability to induce IL-23 when compared with IL-36γ. Psoriasis macrophages secreted significantly more IL-23 following IL-36γ stimulation than healthy macrophages. Our findings also complement findings from an imiquimod-induced mouse model of psoriasis which has shown to be dependent on MyD88 signalling in macrophages (57). Whilst macrophage derived IL-23 is thought to be crucial to the immunopathological development of psoriasis lesions, we are the first to report a viable cytokine agonist for this induction, in IL-36γ. Clinical case reports also support our findings and the idea of a potential IL-36-macrophage pathway within psoriasis pathology. Two case reports show patients with DITRA, who suffer from a lack of function mutation in the endogenous IL-36RA, benefit from monocyte apheresis treatment (44, 58).

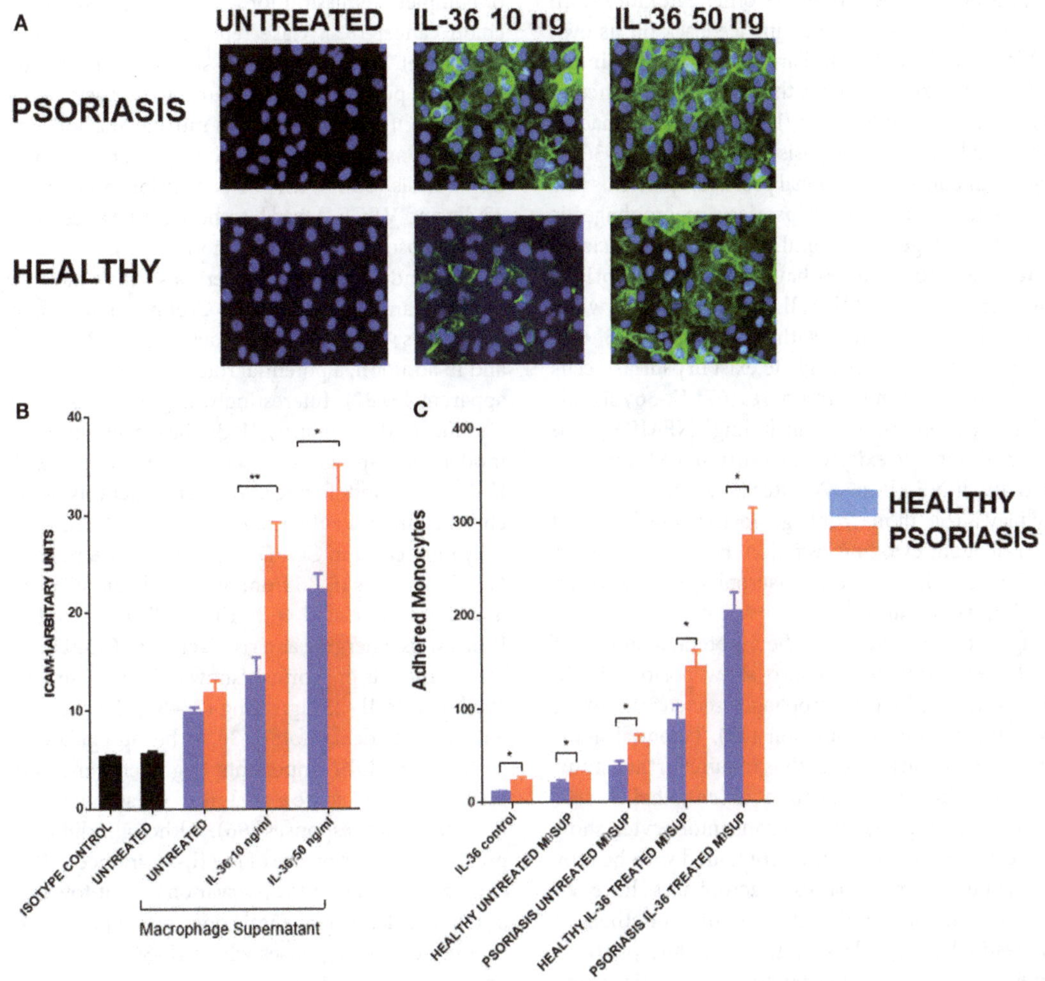

FIGURE 6 | **(A,B)** Supernatants from IL-36γ stimulated psoriasis or healthy macrophages were used to stimulate human umbilical vein endothelial cell (HUVECs) for 24 h, and ICAM-1 (green) and DAPI (blue) expression as visualised by immunofluorescence microscopy is depicted in panel **(A)** and intensity of staining measured by fluorescence absorbance summarised in panel [**(B)**; psoriasis $n = 8$, healthy $n = 8$]. **(C)** Healthy and psoriasis monocytes (1×10^5) were allowed to adhere to a HUVEC monolayer for 30 min. The monolayer was stimulated with supernatant derived from IL-36-stimulated/non-stimulated psoriasis or healthy derived macrophage supernatant. Patient monocytes: psoriasis $n = 8$, healthy $n = 8$. Unpaired *t*-test $^*p < 0.05$ and $^{**}p < 0.01$.

IL-36γ induced secretion of IL-23 was enhanced when macrophages were primed and activated with IFNγ. IFNγ enhancement of/priming for IL-23 secretion from macrophages has previously also been shown with other TIR agonists such as TLRs (50, 59). IFNγ has also been shown to induce an inflammatory phenotype characteristic of psoriasis when injected into the skin and serum levels correlate with disease severity (60, 61). In this context it is noteworthy that IL-36, similar to other IL-1 family members has been shown to enhance IFNγ production in CD4+ T cells (62, 63). We found in our experimental setting that synergy with IFNγ is a prominent feature for IL-36 induced responses but not for IL-17, TNFα, or the IL-1 family member and TIR agonist IL-1. Previous reports have also shown that IL-1 induced TNFα secretion from macrophages is not enhanced by IFNγ (64).

TNFα was prominently induced in macrophages by IL-36γ. Similar to IL-23, psoriasis macrophages had higher basal expression levels and secreted significantly more TNFα when stimulated with IL-36γ. Consequently, IL-36γ induced TNFα from infiltrating macrophages would be well placed to potently stimulate the surrounding tissues to further orchestrate the immune response, activate the endothelium, and increase leucocyte migration.

TNFα is known to be a prominent inflammatory activator of the endothelium and we show that IL-36 induced macrophage supernatant is a potent activator of the endothelium, with the adhesion molecule ICAM-1 showing upregulation (65). In accordance with enhanced cytokine secretion seen from psoriasis macrophages, their supernatant was able to achieve increased endothelial activation when compared with healthy supernatant. Deciphering the most important activator of the endothelium within the supernatant will require further study. Whilst, TNFα is a known activator of the endothelium and several biologic treatments targeting TNFα have proved successful in psoriasis conditions (66), IL-36γ is known to induce other cytokines from macrophages (including a positive autocrine feedback on its own production) which could induce similar effects. The key information from this set of experiments is the striking difference in the endothelium activating potential of IL-36-stimulated macrophages between healthy and psoriasis individuals. IL-36 is expressed in high abundance in all lesional psoriasis epidermis (5).

Enhanced cytokine secretion from psoriasis macrophages is characteristic of the exaggerated immune response associated with psoriasis (67). Previous studies have also shown psoriasis macrophages to secrete increased IL-8, IL-1α/β, and TNFα when untreated and this is in agreement with our findings (68, 69). Numerous genetic variations are thought to exist in psoriasis cells which lead to dysregulated immune responses (67). IL-36γ signals through NF-κB, and various variants—including TNFAIP3 (A20) and CARD14—are thought to exist within psoriasis cells that lead to increased activity of NF-κB (67, 70). Recent studies also suggest IL-36 may play a role in macrophage polarisation (40), and thereby affect subsequent cytokine secretion. However, whether IL-36 has a direct or indirect role in macrophage polarisation within psoriasis is as yet unknown.

Whilst damaged keratinocytes may be a potential source of IL-36γ, macrophages within lesions also show positive IL-36 staining (6). Interestingly, lung macrophages secrete IL-36γ in microparticles following LPS stimulation (71). Potential autocrine actions of IL-36 on macrophages thus require further study.

We report that following stimulation of endothelial cells with IL-36 induced macrophage supernatant, monocytes show significantly increased adherence. When compared with healthy controls, supernatants from psoriasis macrophages have an increased ability to stimulate and adhere to the endothelium (ICAM-1). Interestingly, regardless of the stimulus, psoriasis monocytes showed increased adhesion to both unstimulated and stimulated endothelial cells. A previous study has also found monocytes from psoriasis patients to show increased activation and integrin expression (72).

We report here that IL-36γ induced angiogenesis is dependent on VEGF-A induction. VEGF-A is perhaps the best documented inducer of angiogenesis, and its presence in psoriasis lesions is long established (73). VEGF-A and both VEGFRs are overexpressed in psoriasis lesions and serum levels of VEGF-A correlate with PASI (74–76). A genetic variant in *VEGFA* is also associated with more severe psoriasis (+405 CC) and is thought to result in increased VEGF-A production (29, 31). Interestingly, the same SNP is also associated with poor prognosis in patients with chronic heart failure (77). Importantly, it is thought that angiogenesis precedes symptomatic lesion formation; so it could be hypothesised that IL-36γ released from damaged keratinocytes would be well placed to stimulate VEGF-A synthesis and thus angiogenesis when compared with other cytokines that would have importance in a chronic lesion (78).

Angiogenesis has even been muted as a potential therapeutic target for psoriasis (20, 79, 80). Case reports have demonstrated improvements in PASI through targeting pro-angiogenic factors such as VEGF-A. Bevacizumab, a monoclonal antibody against VEGF-A used in the treatment for solid cancers, has also been shown to be effective in treating psoriasis, including one case of complete remission for a patient being treated for metastatic colon cancer (81). Case reports for tyrosine kinase inhibitors that target VEGFRs such as sunitinib and sorafenib also have produced positive results regarding psoriasis symptom reduction (82–84). Of interest, G6-31, a murine antibody against VEGF-A has demonstrated therapeutic improvement, in a mouse model of psoriasis (85). VALPHA is a fusion protein that targets both TNFα and VEGF-A and has shown to be effective in treating TPA induced psoriasis in mouse models (86).

The findings presented here also may have implications for other inflammatory diseases. Crohn's shares some immunological aspects with psoriasis, namely the IL-23/IL-17 axis activation, and in addition, a potential role for IL-36 in Crohn's is becoming apparent (6, 87). Interestingly, angiogenesis is also a feature of Crohn's (88). Similarly, IL-36 has been implicated in mouse models of respiratory infection and again linked to the IL-23/IL-17 axis, and furthermore, angiogenesis is associated with chronic lung inflammation (40, 89, 90). Whilst IL-36 is yet to be fully implicated in COPD, cigarette smoke, the causative agent of COPD, induces IL-36 from bronchial epithelial cells (91). COPD is heavily associated with Th17 cell driven inflammation (92). Psoriasis is emerging as a risk factor for COPD, and furthermore, mouse models of psoriasis show enhanced airway inflammation attributed to IL-23 signalling (93–95). For skin diseases there is emerging evidence for IL-36 to be upregulated in pathologies with neutrophil components (e.g., acne and hidradenitis suppurativa) and to some extent in all inflammatory diseases involving epidermal responses (96). Although, difficult to dissect the precise *in vivo* relevance of the IL-36-induced VEGF-A mediated angiogenesis, multiple observations point towards an important potential role. Angiogenesis does play a physiological important role in healing responses where IL-36 could have an important impact (97). In a mouse model of psoriasis, systemic anti-VEGF-A treatment has also reduced skin inflammation (85). However, VEGF-A is also induced by other skin inflammatory mediators such as TNFα, and the net effect of IL-36 remains to be shown in future *in vivo* studies.

Our data greatly support previous data suggesting a role for IL-36 in the pathology of psoriasis. IL-36 has been shown to be intimately involved in the epidermal changes characterising psoriatic lesions. This study provides further evidence of a direct relationship between the development of a Th17 psoriatic phenotype and IL-36. IL-36 acts on tissue infiltrating macrophage and actively promotes recruitment of monocytes which cumulatively amplify IL-23 expression, thus promoting polarisation of lymphocytes for increased IL-17/IL-22 expression. In addition, IL-36 directed angiogenesis is dependent on VEGF, a recognised precursor to the development of a psoriatic plaque. We therefore demonstrate a central, pivotal role of IL-36 in the development and propagation of psoriatic disease. This builds on current understanding of psoriasis pathogenesis and provides a further potential therapeutic target in managing disease. Given its potential role in establishing a psoriatic plaque this may offer an opportunity to affect the disease course through preventing a chronic disease signature being established. Thus, deciphering the exact significance of IL-36 in the psoriatic disease continuum remains an important issue for further translational and clinical studies.

ETHICS STATEMENT

This study was approved by Yorkshire and the Humber—Leeds West Research Ethics Committee with written informed consent from all subjects (PDAR study: REC 16/YH/0086).

AUTHOR CONTRIBUTIONS

CB wrote manuscript and conducted macrophage experiments. GF performed angiogenesis experiments and help write the manuscript. AB, PL, and MW delivered the clinical ethical and patient-related aspects of the projects and obtained clinical samples. PL and SP contributed to critical appraisal of results. TM generated and provided IL-36 molecules. MS, MW, and AG contributed to experimental planning, critical discussion of results obtained, as well as manuscript correction.

ACKNOWLEDGMENTS

The authors thank Ethical Tissue Bradford, for providing HUVEC cells. They thank patients and healthy volunteers who supported the research project. This article presents independent research supported by the National Institute for Health Research (NIHR) Leeds Biomedical Research Centre (BRC). The views expressed are those of the authors and not necessarily those of the NHS, the NIHR, or the Department of Health.

REFERENCES

1. Nestle FO, Kaplan DH, Barker J. Psoriasis. *N Engl J Med* (2009) 361(5):496–509. doi:10.1056/NEJMra0804595
2. Lowes MA, Suárez-Fariñas M, Krueger JG. Immunology of psoriasis. *Annu Rev Immunol* (2014) 32:227–55. doi:10.1146/annurev-immunol-032713-120225
3. Towne JE, Sims JE. IL-36 in psoriasis. *Curr Opin Pharmacol* (2012) 12(4):486–90. doi:10.1016/j.coph.2012.02.009
4. He Q, Chen H.-x, Li W, Wu Y, Chen S.-j, Yue Q, et al. IL-36 cytokine expression and its relationship with p38 MAPK and NF-κB pathways in psoriasis vulgaris skin lesions. *J Huazhong Univ Sci Technol Med Sci* (2013) 33(4):594–9. doi:10.1007/s11596-013-1164-1
5. D'Erme AM, Wilsmann-Theis D, Wagenpfeil J, Holzel M, Ferring-Schmitt S, Sternberg S, et al. IL-36[gamma] (IL-1F9) is a biomarker for psoriasis skin lesions. *J Invest Dermatol* (2015) 135(4):1025–32. doi:10.1038/jid.2014.532
6. Boutet MA, Bart G, Penhoat M, Amiaud J, Brulin B, Charrier C, et al. Distinct expression of interleukin (IL)-36alpha, beta and gamma, their antagonist IL-36Ra and IL-38 in psoriasis, rheumatoid arthritis and Crohn's disease. *Clin Exp Immunol* (2016) 184(2):159–73. doi:10.1111/cei.12761
7. Marrakchi S, Guigue P, Renshaw BR, Puel A, Pei X-Y, Fraitag S, et al. Interleukin-36-receptor antagonist deficiency and generalized pustular psoriasis. *N Engl J Med* (2011) 365(7):620–8. doi:10.1056/NEJMoa1013068
8. Kanazawa N, Nakamura T, Mikita N, Furukawa F. Novel IL36RN mutation in a Japanese case of early onset generalized pustular psoriasis. *J Dermatol* (2013) 40(9):749–51. doi:10.1111/1346-8138.12227
9. Sugiura K, Takemoto A, Yamaguchi M, Takahashi H, Shoda Y, Mitsuma T, et al. The majority of generalized pustular psoriasis without psoriasis vulgaris is caused by deficiency of interleukin-36 receptor antagonist. *J Invest Dermatol* (2013) 133(11):2514–21. doi:10.1038/jid.2013.230
10. Balato A, Mattii M, Caiazzo G, Raimondo A, Patruno C, Balato N, et al. IL-36gamma is involved in psoriasis and allergic contact dermatitis. *J Invest Dermatol* (2016) 136(7):1520–3. doi:10.1016/j.jid.2016.03.020
11. Di Caprio R, Balato A, Caiazzo G, Lembo S, Raimondo A, Fabbrocini G, et al. IL-36 cytokines are increased in acne and hidradenitis suppurativa. *Arch Dermatol Res* (2017) 309(8):673–8. doi:10.1007/s00403-017-1769-5
12. Carrier Y, Ma HL, Ramon HE, Napierata L, Small C, O'Toole M, et al. Inter-regulation of Th17 cytokines and the IL-36 cytokines in vitro and in vivo: implications in psoriasis pathogenesis. *J Invest Dermatol* (2011) 131(12):2428–37. doi:10.1038/jid.2011.234
13. Tortola L, Rosenwald E, Abel B, Blumberg H, Schafer M, Coyle AJ, et al. Psoriasiform dermatitis is driven by IL-36-mediated DC-keratinocyte cross-talk. *J Clin Invest* (2012) 122(11):3965–76. doi:10.1172/jci63451
14. Medina-Contreras O, Harusato A, Nishio H, Flannigan KL, Ngo V, Leoni G, et al. Cutting edge: IL-36 receptor promotes resolution of intestinal damage. *J Immunol* (2016) 196(1):34–8. doi:10.4049/jimmunol.1501312
15. Ainscough JS, Macleod T, McGonagle D, Brakefield R, Baron JM, Alase A, et al. Cathepsin S is the major activator of the psoriasis-associated proinflammatory cytokine IL-36γ. *Proc Natl Acad Sci U S A* (2017) 114(13):E2748–57. doi:10.1073/pnas.1620954114
16. Foster AM, Baliwag J, Chen CS, Guzman AM, Stoll SW, Gudjonsson JE, et al. IL-36 promotes myeloid cell infiltration, activation, and inflammatory activity in skin. *J Immunol* (2014) 192(12):6053–61. doi:10.4049/jimmunol.1301481
17. Li N, Yamasaki K, Saito R, Fukushi-Takahashi S, Shimada-Omori R, Asano M, et al. Alarmin function of cathelicidin antimicrobial peptide LL37 through IL-36gamma induction in human epidermal keratinocytes. *J Immunol* (2014) 193(10):5140–8. doi:10.4049/jimmunol.1302574
18. Bridgewood C, Stacey M, Alase A, Lagos D, Graham A, Wittmann M. IL-36gamma has proinflammatory effects on human endothelial cells. *Exp Dermatol* (2017) 26(5):402–8. doi:10.1111/exd.13228
19. Scheibe K, Backert I, Wirtz S, Hueber A, Schett G, Vieth M, et al. IL-36R signalling activates intestinal epithelial cells and fibroblasts and promotes mucosal healing in vivo. *Gut* (2017) 66(5):823–38. doi:10.1136/gutjnl-2015-310374
20. Heidenreich R, Röcken M, Ghoreschi K. Angiogenesis drives psoriasis pathogenesis. *Int J Exp Pathol* (2009) 90(3):232–48. doi:10.1111/j.1365-2613.2009.00669.x
21. Braverman IM, Yen A. Ultrastructure of the capillary loops in the dermal papillae of psoriasis. *J Invest Dermatol* (1977) 68(1):53–60. doi:10.1111/1523-1747.ep12485169
22. Braverman IM, Sibley J. Role of the microcirculation in the treatment and pathogenesis of psoriasis. *J Invest Dermatol* (1982) 78(1):12–7. doi:10.1111/1523-1747.ep12497850
23. Rosina P, Giovannini A, Gisondi P, Girolomoni G. Microcirculatory modifications of psoriatic lesions during topical therapy. *Skin Res Technol* (2009) 15(2):135–8. doi:10.1111/j.1600-0846.2008.00336.x
24. Kulka JP. Microcirculatory impairment as a factor in inflammatory tissue damage. *Ann N Y Acad Sci* (1964) 116:1018–44. doi:10.1111/j.1749-6632.1964.tb52565.x
25. Detmar M, Brown LF, Schon MP, Elicker BM, Velasco P, Richard L, et al. Increased microvascular density and enhanced leukocyte rolling and adhesion in the skin of VEGF transgenic mice. *J Invest Dermatol* (1998) 111(1):1–6. doi:10.1046/j.1523-1747.1998.00262.x
26. Xia YP, Li B, Hylton D, Detmar M, Yancopoulos GD, Rudge JS. Transgenic delivery of VEGF to mouse skin leads to an inflammatory condition resembling human psoriasis. *Blood* (2003) 102(1):161–8. doi:10.1182/blood-2002-12-3793
27. Trembath RC, Clough RL, Rosbotham JL, Jones AB, Camp RD, Frodsham A, et al. Identification of a major susceptibility locus on chromosome 6p and evidence for further disease loci revealed by a two stage genome-wide search in psoriasis. *Hum Mol Genet* (1997) 6(5):813–20. doi:10.1093/hmg/6.5.813
28. Brogan IJ, Khan N, Isaac K, Hutchinson JA, Pravica V, Hutchinson IV.

Novel polymorphisms in the promoter and 5' UTR regions of the human vascular endothelial growth factor gene. *Hum Immunol* (1999) 60(12):1245–9. doi:10.1016/S0198-8859(99)00132-9

29. Diaz BV, Lenoir MC, Ladoux A, Frelin C, Demarchez M, Michel S. Regulation of vascular endothelial growth factor expression in human keratinocytes by retinoids. *J Biol Chem* (2000) 275(1):642–50. doi:10.1074/jbc.275.1.642
30. Detmar M. Evidence for vascular endothelial growth factor (VEGF) as a modifier gene in psoriasis. *J Invest Dermatol* (2004) 122(1):xiv–xv. doi:10.1046/j.0022-202X.2003.22140.x
31. Young HS, Summers AM, Read IR, Fairhurst DA, Plant DJ, Campalani E, et al. Interaction between genetic control of vascular endothelial growth factor production and retinoid responsiveness in psoriasis. *J Invest Dermatol* (2006) 126(2):453–9. doi:10.1038/sj.jid.5700096
32. Puig L. The role of IL 23 in the treatment of psoriasis. *Expert Rev Clin Immunol* (2017) 13(6):525–34. doi:10.1080/1744666x.2017.1292137
33. Clark RA, Kupper TS. Misbehaving macrophages in the pathogenesis of psoriasis. *J Clin Invest* (2006) 116(8):2084–7. doi:10.1172/jci29441
34. Stratis A, Pasparakis M, Rupec RA, Markur D, Hartmann K, Scharffetter-Kochanek K, et al. Pathogenic role for skin macrophages in a mouse model of keratinocyte-induced psoriasis-like skin inflammation. *J Clin Invest* (2006) 116(8):2094–104. doi:10.1172/jci27179
35. Wang H, Peters T, Kess D, Sindrilaru A, Oreshkova T, Van Rooijen N, et al. Activated macrophages are essential in a murine model for T cell-mediated chronic psoriasiform skin inflammation. *J Clin Invest* (2006) 116(8):2105–14. doi:10.1172/JCI27180
36. Zaba LC, Fuentes-Duculan J, Eungdamrong NJ, Abello MV, Novitskaya I, Pierson KC, et al. Psoriasis is characterized by accumulation of immunostimulatory and Th1/Th17 cell-polarizing myeloid dendritic cells. *J Invest Dermatol* (2009) 129(1):79–88. doi:10.1038/jid.2008.194
37. Fuentes-Duculan J, Suarez-Farinas M, Zaba LC, Nograles KE, Pierson KC, Mitsui H, et al. A subpopulation of CD163-positive macrophages is classically activated in psoriasis. *J Invest Dermatol* (2010) 130(10):2412–22. doi:10.1038/jid.2010.165
38. Blumberg H, Dinh H, Dean C Jr, Trueblood ES, Bailey K, Shows D, et al. IL-1RL2 and its ligands contribute to the cytokine network in psoriasis. *J Immunol* (2010) 185(7):4354–62. doi:10.4049/jimmunol.1000313
39. Chi HH, Hua KF, Lin YC, Chu CL, Hsieh CY, Hsu YJ, et al. IL-36 signaling facilitates activation of the NLRP3 inflammasome and IL-23/IL-17 axis in renal inflammation and fibrosis. *J Am Soc Nephrol* (2017) 28(7):2022–37. doi:10.1681/asn.2016080840
40. Kovach MA, Singer B, Martinez-Colon G, Newstead MW, Zeng X, Mancuso P, et al. IL-36gamma is a crucial proximal component of protective type-1-mediated lung mucosal immunity in Gram-positive and -negative bacterial pneumonia. *Mucosal Immunol* (2017) 10(5):1320–34. doi:10.1038/mi.2016.130
41. Thomi R, Kakeda M, Yawalkar N, Schlapbach C, Hunger RE. Increased expression of the interleukin-36 cytokines in lesions of hidradenitis suppurativa. *J Eur Acad Dermatol Venereol* (2017) 31(12):2091–6. doi:10.1111/jdv.14389
42. Zebrowska A, Wozniacka A, Juczynska K, Ociepa K, Waszczykowska E, Szymczak I, et al. Correlation between IL36alpha and IL17 and activity of the disease in selected autoimmune blistering diseases. *Mediators Inflamm* (2017) 2017:8980534. doi:10.1155/2017/8980534
43. Sugiura K, Haruna K, Suga Y, Akiyama M. Generalized pustular psoriasis caused by deficiency of interleukin-36 receptor antagonist successfully treated with granulocyte and monocyte adsorption apheresis. *J Eur Acad Dermatol Venereol* (2014) 28(12):1835–6. doi:10.1111/jdv.12383
44. Koike Y, Okubo M, Kiyohara T, Fukuchi R, Sato Y, Kuwatsuka S, et al. Granulocyte and monocyte apheresis can control juvenile generalized pustular psoriasis with mutation of IL36RN. *Br J Dermatol* (2017) 177(6):1732–6. doi:10.1111/bjd.15509
45. Eccles KA, Sowden H, Porter KE, Parkin SM, Homer-Vanniasinkam S, Graham AM. Simvastatin alters human endothelial cell adhesion molecule expression and inhibits leukocyte adhesion under flow. *Atherosclerosis* (2008) 200(1):69–79. doi:10.1016/j.atherosclerosis.2007.12.018
46. Macleod T, Doble R, McGonagle D, Wasson CW, Alase A, Stacey M, et al. Neutrophil elastase-mediated proteolysis activates the anti-inflammatory cytokine IL-36 receptor antagonist. *Sci Rep* (2016) 6:24880. doi:10.1038/srep24880
47. Fearnley GW, Smith GA, Odell AF, Latham AM, Wheatcroft SB, Harrison MA, et al. Vascular endothelial growth factor A-stimulated signaling from endosomes in primary endothelial cells. *Methods Enzymol* (2014) 535:265–92. doi:10.1016/b978-0-12-397925-4.00016-x
48. Fearnley GW, Wheatcroft SB, Ponnambalam S. Detection and quantification of vascular endothelial growth factor receptor tyrosine kinases in primary human endothelial cells. *Methods Mol Biol* (2015) 1332:49–65. doi:10.1007/978-1-4939-2917-7_4
49. Hao JQ. Targeting interleukin-22 in psoriasis. *Inflammation* (2014) 37(1):94–9. doi:10.1007/s10753-013-9715-y
50. van de Wetering D, de Paus RA, van Dissel JT, van de Vosse E. Salmonella induced IL-23 and IL-1β allow for IL-12 production by monocytes and Mϕ1 through induction of IFN-γ in CD56(+) NK/NK-like T cells. *PLoS One* (2009) 4(12):e8396. doi:10.1371/journal.pone.0008396
51. Peral de Castro C, Jones SA, Ni Cheallaigh C, Hearnden CA, Williams L, Winter J, et al. Autophagy regulates IL-23 secretion and innate T cell responses through effects on IL-1 secretion. *J Immunol* (2012) 189(8):4144–53. doi:10.4049/jimmunol.1201946
52. Dietrich D, Martin P, Flacher V, Sun Y, Jarrossay D, Brembilla N, et al. Interleukin-36 potently stimulates human M2 macrophages, Langerhans cells and keratinocytes to produce pro-inflammatory cytokines. *Cytokine* (2016) 84:88–98. doi:10.1016/j.cyto.2016.05.012
53. Hoeben A, Landuyt B, Highley MS, Wildiers H, Van Oosterom AT, De Bruijn EA. Vascular endothelial growth factor and angiogenesis. *Pharmacol Rev* (2004) 56(4):549–80. doi:10.1124/pr.56.4.3
54. Mattila P, Majuri ML, Mattila PS, Renkonen R. TNF alpha-induced expression of endothelial adhesion molecules, ICAM-1 and VCAM-1, is linked to protein kinase C activation. *Scand J Immunol* (1992) 36(2):159–65. doi:10.1111/j.1365-3083.1992.tb03087.x
55. Yawalkar N, Tscharner GG, Hunger RE, Hassan AS. Increased expression of IL-12p70 and IL-23 by multiple dendritic cell and macrophage subsets in plaque psoriasis. *J Dermatol Sci* (2009) 54(2):99–105. doi:10.1016/j.jdermsci.2009.01.003
56. Vigne S, Palmer G, Lamacchia C, Martin P, Talabot-Ayer D, Rodriguez E, et al. IL-36R ligands are potent regulators of dendritic and T cells. *Blood* (2011) 118(22):5813–23. doi:10.1182/blood-2011-05-356873
57. Costa S, Marini O, Bevilacqua D, DeFranco AL, Hou B, Lonardi S, et al. Role of MyD88 signaling in the imiquimod-induced mouse model of psoriasis: focus on innate myeloid cells. *J Leukoc Biol* (2017) 102(3):791–803. doi:10.1189/jlb.3MA0217-054RR
58. Tominaga C, Yamamoto M, Imai Y, Yamanishi K. A case of old age-onset generalized pustular psoriasis with a deficiency of IL-36RN (DITRA) treated by granulocyte and monocyte apheresis. *Case Rep Dermatol* (2015) 7(1):29–35. doi:10.1159/000380876
59. Butchar JP, Parsa KVL, Marsh CB, Tridandapani S. IFNγ enhances IL-23 production during *Francisella* infection of human monocytes. *FEBS Lett* (2008) 582(7):1044–8. doi:10.1016/j.febslet.2008.02.058
60. Abdallah MA, Abdel-Hamid MF, Kotb AM, Mabrouk EA. Serum interferon-gamma is a psoriasis severity and prognostic marker. *Cutis* (2009) 84(3):163–8.
61. Johnson-Huang LM, Suárez-Fariñas M, Pierson KC, Fuentes-Duculan J, Cueto I, Lentini T, et al. A single intradermal injection of IFN-γ induces an inflammatory state in both non-lesional psoriatic and healthy skin. *J Invest Dermatol* (2012) 132(4):1177–87. doi:10.1038/jid.2011.458
62. Renne J, Schäfer V, Werfel T, Wittmann M. Interleukin-1 from epithelial cells fosters T cell-dependent skin inflammation. *Br J Dermatol* (2010) 162(6):1198–205. doi:10.1111/j.1365-2133.2010.09662.x
63. Vigne S, Palmer G, Martin P, Lamacchia C, Strebel D, Rodriguez E, et al. IL-36 signaling amplifies Th1 responses by enhancing proliferation and Th1 polarization of naive CD4+ T cells. *Blood* (2012) 120(17):3478–87. doi:10.1182/blood-2012-06-439026
64. Ikejima T, Okusawa S, Ghezzi P, van der Meer JW, Dinarello CA. Interleukin-1 induces tumor necrosis factor (TNF) in human peripheral blood mononuclear cells in vitro and a circulating TNF-like activity in rabbits. *J Infect Dis* (1990) 162(1):215–23. doi:10.1093/infdis/162.1.215
65. Meekins JW, McLaughlin PJ, West DC, McFadyen IR, Johnson PM. Endothelial cell activation by tumour necrosis factor-alpha (TNF-alpha) and the development of pre-eclampsia. *Clin Exp Immunol* (1994) 98(1):110–4. doi:10.1111/j.1365-2249.1994.tb06615.x

66. Yost J, Gudjonsson JE. The role of TNF inhibitors in psoriasis therapy: new implications for associated comorbidities. *F1000 Med Rep* (2009) 1:30. doi:10.3410/M1-30
67. Harden JL, Krueger JG, Bowcock AM. The immunogenetics of psoriasis: a comprehensive review. *J Autoimmun* (2015) 64:66–73. doi:10.1016/j.jaut.2015.07.008
68. Okubo Y, Koga M. Peripheral blood monocytes in psoriatic patients overproduce cytokines. *J Dermatol Sci* (1998) 17(3):223–32. doi:10.1016/S0923-1811(98)00019-X
69. Nishibu A, Han GW, Iwatsuki K, Matsui T, Inoue M, Akiba H, et al. Overexpression of monocyte-derived cytokines in active psoriasis: a relation to coexistent arthropathy. *J Dermatol Sci* (1999) 21(1):63–70. doi:10.1016/S0923-1811(99)00031-6
70. Sun Y, Mozaffarian A, Arnett HA, Dinh H, Trueblood ES, Towne JE. 253. *Cytokine* (2013) 63(3):303. doi:10.1016/j.cyto.2013.06.256
71. Kovach MA, Singer BH, Newstead MW, Zeng X, Moore TA, White ES, et al. IL-36gamma is secreted in microparticles and exosomes by lung macrophages in response to bacteria and bacterial components. *J Leukoc Biol* (2016) 100(2):413–21. doi:10.1189/jlb.4A0315-087R
72. Golden JB, Groft SG, Squeri MV, Debanne SM, Ward NL, McCormick TS, et al. Chronic psoriatic skin inflammation leads to increased monocyte adhesion and aggregation. *J Immunol* (2015) 195(5):2006–18. doi:10.4049/jimmunol.1402307
73. Marina ME, Roman II, Constantin A-M, Mihu CM, TĂTaru AD. VEGF involvement in psoriasis. *Clujul Med* (2015) 88(3):247–52. doi:10.15386/cjmed-494
74. Detmar M, Brown LF, Claffey KP, Yeo KT, Kocher O, Jackman RW, et al. Overexpression of vascular permeability factor/vascular endothelial growth factor and its receptors in psoriasis. *J Exp Med* (1994) 180(3):1141–6. doi:10.1084/jem.180.3.1141
75. Young HS, Summers AM, Bhushan M, Brenchley PE, Griffiths CE. Single-nucleotide polymorphisms of vascular endothelial growth factor in psoriasis of early onset. *J Invest Dermatol* (2004) 122(1):209–15. doi:10.1046/j.0022-202X.2003.22107.x
76. Nofal A, Al-Makhzangy I, Attwa E, Nassar A, Abdalmoati A. Vascular endothelial growth factor in psoriasis: an indicator of disease severity and control. *J Eur Acad Dermatol Venereol* (2009) 23(7):803–6. doi:10.1111/j.1468-3083.2009.03181.x
77. van der Meer P, de Boer RA, White HL, van der Steege G, Hall AS, Voors AA, et al. The VEGF +405 CC promoter polymorphism is associated with an impaired prognosis in patients with chronic heart failure: a MERIT-HF substudy. *J Card Fail* (2005) 11(4):279–84. doi:10.1016/j.cardfail.2004.11.006
78. Telner P, Fekete Z. The capillary responses in psoriatic skin. *J Invest Dermatol* (1961) 36:225–30. doi:10.1038/jid.1961.36
79. Guérard S, Pouliot R. The role of angiogenesis in the pathogenesis of psoriasis: mechanisms and clinical implications. *J Clin Exp Dermatol Res* (2012) S2:7. doi:10.4172/2155-9554.S2-007
80. Weidemann AK, Crawshaw AA, Byrne E, Young HS. Vascular endothelial growth factor inhibitors: investigational therapies for the treatment of psoriasis. *Clin Cosmet Investig Dermatol* (2013) 6:233–44. doi:10.2147/CCID.S35312
81. Akman A, Yilmaz E, Mutlu H, Ozdogan M. Complete remission of psoriasis following bevacizumab therapy for colon cancer. *Clin Exp Dermatol* (2009) 34(5):e202–4. doi:10.1111/j.1365-2230.2008.02991.x
82. Fournier C, Tisman G. Sorafenib-associated remission of psoriasis in hypernephroma: case report. *Dermatol Online J* (2010) 16(2):17.
83. Narayanan S, Callis-Duffin K, Batten J, Agarwal N. Improvement of psoriasis during sunitinib therapy for renal cell carcinoma. *Am J Med Sci* (2010) 339(6):580–1. doi:10.1097/MAJ.0b013e3181dd1aa5
84. Antoniou EA, Koutsounas I, Damaskos C, Koutsounas S. Remission of psoriasis in a patient with hepatocellular carcinoma treated with sorafenib. *In Vivo* (2016) 30(5):677–80.
85. Schonthaler HB, Huggenberger R, Wculek SK, Detmar M, Wagner EF. Systemic anti-VEGF treatment strongly reduces skin inflammation in a mouse model of psoriasis. *Proc Natl Acad Sci U S A* (2009) 106(50):21264–9. doi:10.1073/pnas.0907550106
86. Jung K, Lee D, Lim HS, Lee SI, Kim YJ, Lee GM, et al. Double anti-angiogenic and anti-inflammatory protein Valpha targeting VEGF-A and TNF-alpha in retinopathy and psoriasis. *J Biol Chem* (2011) 286(16):14410–8. doi:10.1074/jbc.M111.228130
87. Siakavellas SI, Bamias G. Role of the IL-23/IL-17 axis in Crohn's disease. *Discov Med* (2012) 14(77):253–62.
88. Alkim C, Alkim H, Koksal AR, Boga S, Sen I. Angiogenesis in inflammatory bowel disease. *Int J Inflam* (2015) 2015:970890. doi:10.1155/2015/970890
89. Matarese A, Santulli G. Angiogenesis in chronic obstructive pulmonary disease: a translational appraisal. *Transl Med UniSa* (2012) 3:49–56.
90. Kovach MA, Newstead MW, Zeng X, Peters-Golden M, Standiford TJ. IL-36γ is a potent inducer of type I and IL-17 cytokine induction during lung infection. *Am J Respir Care Med* (2015) 191: A6148.
91. Parsanejad R, Fields WR, Steichen TJ, Bombick BR, Doolittle DJ. Distinct regulatory profiles of interleukins and chemokines in response to cigarette smoke condensate in normal human bronchial epithelial (NHBE) cells. *J Interferon Cytokine Res* (2008) 28(12):703–12. doi:10.1089/jir.2008.0139
92. Alcorn JF, Crowe CR, Kolls JK. TH17 cells in asthma and COPD. *Annu Rev Physiol* (2010) 72:495–516. doi:10.1146/annurev-physiol-021909-135926
93. Dreiher J, Weitzman D, Shapiro J, Davidovici B, Cohen AD. Psoriasis and chronic obstructive pulmonary disease: a case-control study. *Br J Dermatol* (2008) 159(4):956–60. doi:10.1111/j.1365-2133.2008.08749.x
94. Li X, Kong L, Li F, Chen C, Xu R, Wang H, et al. Association between psoriasis and chronic obstructive pulmonary disease: a systematic review and meta-analysis. *PLoS One* (2015) 10(12):e0145221. doi:10.1371/journal.pone.0145221
95. Nadeem A, Al Harbi NO, Ansari MA, Al-Harbi MM, El-Sherbeeny AM, Zoheir KM, et al. Psoriatic inflammation enhances allergic airway inflammation through IL-23/STAT3 signaling in a murine model. *Biochem Pharmacol* (2017) 124:69–82. doi:10.1016/j.bcp.2016.10.012
96. Walsh PT, Fallon PG. The emergence of the IL-36 cytokine family as novel targets for inflammatory diseases. *Ann N Y Acad Sci* (2016). doi:10.1111/nyas.13280
97. Tonnesen MG, Feng X, Clark RA. Angiogenesis in wound healing. *J Investig Dermatol Symp Proc* (2000) 5(1):40–6. doi:10.1046/j.1087-0024.2000.00014.x

3

The Role of Helper T Cells in Psoriasis

Peng Hu[1,2,3†], Mengyao Wang[1,4†], Hu Gao[1,4,5†], Ai Zheng[1,4], Jinhui Li[1,2,3], Dezhi Mu[1,2,3*] and Jiyu Tong[1,4,6*]*

[1] West China Second University Hospital, Sichuan University, Chengdu, China, [2] Department of Pediatrics, West China Second University Hospital, Sichuan University, Chengdu, China, [3] Key Laboratory of Obstetrics & Gynecologic and Pediatric Diseases and Birth Defects of the Ministry of Education, Sichuan University, Chengdu, China, [4] Key Laboratory of Birth Defects and Related Diseases of Women and Children, Sichuan University, Ministry of Education, Chengdu, China, [5] Department of Emergency, West China Second University Hospital, Sichuan University, Chengdu, China, [6] Department of Immunology, West China School of Basic Medical Sciences and Forensic Medicine, Sichuan University, Chengdu, China

***Correspondence:**
Jinhui Li
yoyolee824@163.com
Dezhi Mu
mudz@scu.edu.cn
Jiyu Tong
jiyu.tong@scu.edu.cn

†These authors have contributed equally to this work and share first authorship

Psoriasis is a complex, chronic relapsing and inflammatory skin disorder with a prevalence of approximately 2% in the general population worldwide. Psoriasis can be triggered by infections, physical injury and certain drugs. The most common type of psoriasis is psoriasis vulgaris, which primarily features dry, well-demarcated, raised red lesions with adherent silvery scales on the skin and joints. Over the past few decades, scientific research has helped us reveal that innate and adaptive immune cells contribute to the chronic inflammatory pathological process of psoriasis. In particular, dysfunctional helper T cells (Th1, Th17, Th22, and Treg cells) are indispensable factors in psoriasis development. When stimulated by certain triggers, antigen-presenting cells (APCs) can release pro-inflammatory factors (IL-23, IFN-α and IL-12), which further activate naive T cells and polarize them into distinct helper T cell subsets that produce numerous cytokines, such as TNF, IFN-γ, IL-17 and IL-22, which act on keratinocytes to amplify psoriatic inflammation. In this review, we describe the function of helper T cells in psoriasis and summarize currently targeted anti-psoriatic therapies.

Keywords: Th17, Tregs, psoriasis, cytokines, biologics

INTRODUCTION

Psoriasis is a complex, chronic relapsing and inflammatory skin disorder with an overall prevalence of 2% in the general population worldwide (1). The most common type of psoriasis is psoriasis vulgaris, which primarily manifests as dry, well-demarcated, raised red lesions with adherent silvery scales on the skin and joints and accounts for nearly 90% of all psoriasis cases. Psoriasis is also associated with multiple comorbidities, such as arthritis, obesity, diabetes mellitus, depression, hypertension, cardiovascular disease, and reduced quality of life (2).

Although the exact mechanism that triggers psoriasis remains unclear, it is currently accepted that psoriasis is induced or exacerbated by either nonspecific triggers, such as infections [such as Streptococcus (3)], physical injury [such as scratching and tattoos (4)], drugs [such as β blockers, lithium and antimalarials (5, 6)] or some specific autoantigens [such as cathelicidin LL-37, melanocytic ADAMTSL5, lipid antigen PLA2G4D and keratin 17 (7)]. Pathologically, psoriasis is characterized by epidermal acanthosis (thickening of the viable layers), hyperkeratosis (thickened cornified layer), and parakeratosis (cell nuclei present in the cornified layer) (8). Over the past 50 years, researchers have performed substantial work to explore the underlying mechanism of the link between skin injury and keratinocyte dysfunction, which drives the development and progression of psoriasis. A series of basic and clinical studies has shown that psoriasis is mediated by components of both the innate and adaptive immune systems. It was reported that innate immune cells such as natural killer (NK) cells, NKT cells, neutrophils, mast cells, γδ T cells, and dendritic cells (DCs) were significantly increased in psoriatic lesions and could frequently release pathogenic mediators such as TNF-α and interleukin 23 (IL-23) (9–13). As another important source of cytokines, adaptive immune cells have been the subject of academic interest since 1979. A variety of studies showed that several related cytokines, such as tumor necrosis factor-α (TNF-α), interferon γ (IFN-γ), interleukin 23 (IL-23), interleukin 17 (IL-17), and interleukin 22 (IL-22), were highly correlated with psoriasis. Recently, autoreactive T cells against specific autoantigens were also found to produce related pathogenic cytokines, especially IFN-γ and IL-17. Lande et al. demonstrated specific CD4 and CD8 T-cell responses and increased IFN-γ and IL-17 production to LL37 in psoriatic patients (14), while Arakwa et al. identified ADAMTSL5 as an autoantigen recognized by specific CD8 T-cells (15). Specially, for CD8 T cells, both autoantigens were showed to be presented in the peptide-binding groove of the human leukocyte antigen (HLA)-class I molecule encoded by the major psoriasis risk gene, HLA-Cw*06:02 (14, 15). Consistently, keratin peptides that share sequences with Streptococcal M-protein can be recognized by T cells from psoriatic patients (16–18). Subsequent evidences showed that full-length keratin 17 and its peptide fragments induce T cell proliferation and IFN-γ production, particularly in patients with the HLA-Cw*06:02 allele (19, 20). Furthermore, clinic studies showed that matched biological agents against these cytokines could also induce effective therapeutic results. Moreover, among them, IL-17, which is mainly produced by γδ T cells, CD4+ helper T cells (Th17 cells), and CD8+ cytotoxic T cells (Tc17 cells), seems to be most strongly implicated in psoriasis; thus, T cells, especially helper T (Th) cells, have become a hot topic in psoriasis pathogenesis. Here, we reviewed the biogenesis and function of helper T cells in psoriasis and briefly summarized currently targeted therapies.

ROLE OF HELPER T CELLS IN PSORIASIS

When Mueller et al. used cyclosporine A, an immunosuppressive agent that inhibits T cell proliferation and cytokine production, to treat psoriasis and then observed surprising therapeutic efficacy, researchers realized the potential role of T cells in psoriasis pathogenesis (21). Later, Prinz et al. isolated 10 T cell lines and 105 T cell clones from the dermis and epidermis of psoriatic skin specimens and subsequently found that T cells and their secreted products, such as IFN-γ, could contribute to keratinocyte proliferation (22). Then, Baker et al. showed that the initial phase of psoriasis was dominated by epidermal infiltration of activated CD4+ T cells, indicating a primary immune trigger for the inflammatory and hyper-proliferative processes (23). In the current model, the crosstalk between keratinocytes and various immune cells, especially helper T cells, plays a central role in the progression of psoriasis (**Figure 1**).

Th1/Th17/Th22 Cells in Psoriasis

A study from the University of Mainz investigated cytokines secreted by T cells obtained from epidermal specimens of psoriatic patients and showed that nearly all T cells tested produced Th1-related cytokines (IFN-γ, TNF-α, and IL-2), whereas only a minority of cells secreted Th2-related cytokines (IL-4 and IL-10) (24). In the same year, another study suggested that IFN-γ, which is produced mainly by Th1 cells, is capable of enhancing keratinocyte proliferation *in vitro* (22). These results defined psoriasis as a Th1 cell-mediated disease. However, the administration of humanized monoclonal antibodies against IFN-γ and TNF-α does not significantly improve psoriasis, suggesting that Th1 cells or their related cytokines may not be critical in the pathogenesis of psoriasis (25).

While assessing the involvement of IL-23 in the induction and maintenance of chronic inflammatory diseases, Harrington et al. first recognized the distinct CD4+ T cells - known as Th17 cells (26, 27). IL-23, a heterodimeric cytokine composed of a unique p19 chain and a p40 chain that is shared with IL-12, is essential for the survival and development of Th17 cells (28). There is growing evidence to suggest that the IL-23/Th17 axis and the related cytokines have critical roles in psoriasis. Enhanced expression of IL-23 at the mRNA and protein levels could be detected in psoriatic skin compared with healthy skin. Moreover, intradermal injection of IL-23 in murine models can stimulate keratinocyte proliferation and cause epidermal hyperplasia, and anti-IL-12/IL-23 and anti-IL-23 agents have shown highly effective therapeutic effects in clinical trials (29–32). In 2007, Wilson et al. found that Th17 cells may participate in the pathological processes of psoriasis through the coordinated expression of IL-17A, IL-17F, IL-22, IL-21 and IL-26 (33). Both IL-17A and IL-17F are subtypes of IL-17, and they have been shown to be elevated in psoriatic lesions and the peripheral blood of psoriatic patients (34). Clinical randomized trials have shown beneficial effects of IL-17A and IL-17F antibodies, validating IL-17A and IL-17F as potential therapeutic targets (35–38). Further studies demonstrated that IL-22 also mediates IL-23/Th17 axis-induced psoriasis-like skin inflammation (39). Zheng et al. suggested that IL-22, which acts in synergy with IL-17, might play an essential role in the pathogenesis of autoimmune diseases such as psoriasis (39). Subsequently, scientific research highlighted that IL-17 and IL-22 may mediate distinct downstream pathways that contribute to the psoriatic phenotype: IL-17 is more pro-inflammatory than IL-22, while IL-22 impairs keratinocyte differentiation (40). In addition, Van Belle et al. showed that IL-22 played major roles not only in the development of pustules and acanthosis but also in

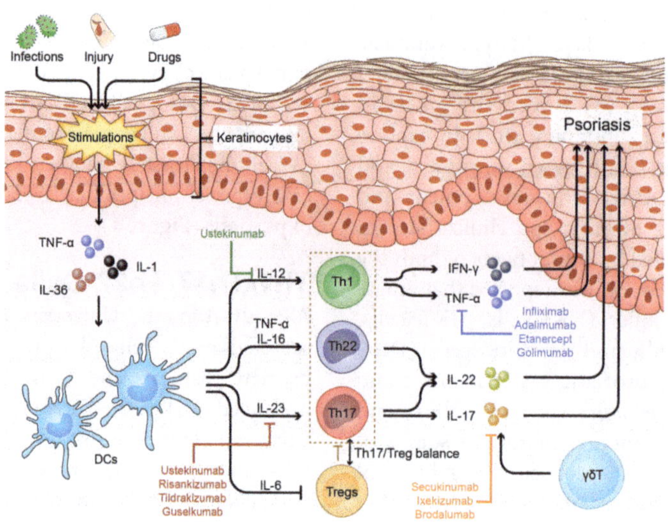

FIGURE 1 | Immune dysfunction of psoriasis. Psoriasis is driven by many nonspecific triggers. Triggers such as infections and physical injury stimulate DCs to release pro-inflammatory factors (IL-23, TNF-α and IL-12). These cytokines in turn activate the IL-23 and/or IL-22 pathway to induce Th17 and/or Th22 cell differentiation, resulting in the production of numerous psoriatic cytokines, such as TNF-α, IFN-γ, IL-17 and IL-22, which act on keratinocytes to amplify psoriatic inflammation. In addition, skin infiltrating cells, such as γδT cells, contribute to the disease development *via* producing IL-17, and Treg cells and the Th17/Treg balance also play important roles in the pathogenesis of psoriasis.

neutrophil infiltration in a mouse model triggered by the Toll-like receptor (TLR) 7/8 agonist imiquimod (41). The IL-23/Th17 axis and the related cytokines could further amplify keratinocyte proliferation and cause epidermal hyperplasia (42).

Later, Nograles et al. discovered a new subtype of T cells by analyzing the T cell subsets in skin biopsies and peripheral blood collected from psoriatic patients by intracellular cytokine staining and flow cytometry, and these cells were called Th22 cells (43). Moreover, research from Trifari et al. solidified this view. The researchers identified another population of human helper T cells that produced abundant IL-22 and IL-13 but no IFN-γ, IL-4 or IL-17. IL-22, as we described above, is required for the pathogenesis and development of many autoimmune diseases (44). Kagami et al. analyzed T cell numbers in the circulation of psoriatic patients and showed that in addition to Th1 and Th17 cells, Th22 cells were also increased in psoriatic patients (45). Notably, IL-22 deficiency caused a significant decrease in epidermal acanthosis and dermal inflammation induced by IL-23 (39). These studies established the crucial role of the IL-23/Th17 axis and the IL-22/Th22 pathway in the pathogenesis and development of psoriasis. However, it has been reported that Th1 and Th17 cells may contribute to the pathogenesis and development of psoriasis. Researchers argued that IFN-γ secreted mainly by Th1 cells could induce Th17 cells *via* IL-1 and IL-23. Furthermore, IFN-γ can also stimulate antigen-presenting cells (APCs) to produce CCL20, which is responsible for the migration of IL-17+ T cells (46). Considering the role of IL-22, it can no longer be denied that psoriasis is a Th1/Th17/Th22-mediated autoimmune disease.

Treg Cells in Psoriasis

Treg cells are a special subset of helper T cells that are characterized by high expression of the CD25, alpha-chain of IL-2 receptor. Then Foxp3 (Forkhead Box P3), a transcription factor of the fork head/winged-helix family, was found as the most important transcription factor for controlling the development and function of Treg cells. Treg cells can suppress the activities of other effector immune cells mainly by direct contact and/or the secretion of suppressive cytokines, such as IL-10 and transforming growth factor (TGF)-β (47). Hence, Treg cells are prominently associated with peripheral tolerance, autoimmune diseases and chronic inflammatory diseases, including psoriasis (48).

Studies investigating the percentage of Treg cells in lesional skin or peripheral blood have contradictory evidence, which varied in different psoriasis subtypes, disease states, Treg definition, and types of samples (49–55). Interestingly, the function of Treg cells was consistently demonstrated to be impaired (56). Both Sugiyama et al. and Li B et al. observed that circulating CD4+CD25+ Treg cells in psoriatic patients failed to suppress the proliferation of normal CD4+CD25- responder T cells during co-culture (56, 57). Similar results were reported in pediatric patients (58).

The unstable expression (downregulation) of Foxp3 reflects the dysfunction of Treg cells in psoriasis, and numerous upstream regulators have been reported. One of these regulators is the pro-inflammatory cytokine milieu, especially high levels of IL-6. Indeed, IL-6 was highly expressed in the plasma and lesional skin of psoriatic patients (59). In an *in vitro* model, Goodman et al. reported that human Treg cell-mediated suppression of responder T cell proliferation could be reversed by culture with rhIL6 (recombinant human IL-6) or activated DCs, which highly express IL-6 (59). Furthermore, under IL-6 stimulation, elevated phosphorylation of the transcription factor Stat3 was noted in dysfunctional Treg cells (60). Stat3 acts as a downstream molecule of IL-6R and can bind to a silencing element within the Foxp3 locus, leading to a reduction in the expression of Foxp3. Furthermore, Zhao et al. reported that increased expression of microRNA-210 in CD4+ T cells from patients with psoriasis vulgaris repressed Foxp3 expression and subsequently inhibited the production of IL-10 and TGF-β (61). In addition, in a CD18-knockout mouse model, a spontaneous psoriasiform phenotype was observed, accompanied by Treg cell dysfunction. Adoptive transfer of wild-type Treg cells into CD18-knockout mice markedly reduced the psoriasis area and severity index (PASI) scores. Wang et al. revealed that reduced CD18 expression on CD4+CD25+CD127− Tregs resulted in deceased expression of TGF-β1 by disrupting their cell-cell contact with DCs (62).

Because the differentiation of Th17 and Treg cells is reciprocally regulated by shared and different cytokines, it is not surprising that the cytokine milieu of the psoriatic skin microenvironment may cause an imbalance. Zhang et al. and Wang et al. independently reported a positive association between the ratio of Th17 cells to Treg cells in peripheral blood and PASI scores (51, 61). As mentioned previously, IL-6, which is a critical cytokine for Th17 differentiation, inhibits Treg cells by inhibiting the expression of Foxp3 in psoriasis pathogenesis (63). Furthermore, a group of IL-17A+/Foxp3 +/CD4+ triple-positive cells were identified in the lesional skin of psoriasis patients (64). These cells maintain a high RORγt/ Foxp3 ratio to promote the production of IL-17A. This evidence suggests important plasticity between Th17 and Treg cells in psoriasis (64). Specifically, Singh et al. reported a mechanism by which reduced CD18 levels could promote the conversion of Treg cells to Th17 cells in a CD18-knockout mouse model of psoriasis (65). In addition, Ma et al. showed that the Th17/Treg imbalance was also regulated by the Notch1 signaling pathway, which is known to be a conserved signaling pathway involved in cell development and differentiation of multiple organisms and tissues (66). In their experiments, the expression of Notch1 and its target gene Hes-1 were positively correlated with PASI scores and the ratios of Th17/Treg cells. Correspondingly, Notch receptor inhibitors reduced the percentage of Th17 cells and the Th17/Treg ratio (66).

Currently, it is relatively clear that Treg cells and the Th17/ Treg balance play important roles in the pathogenesis of psoriasis; however, the underlying mechanisms that drive Treg cell dysfunction and the imbalance in Th17/Treg cells still need to be further investigated.

T Follicular Helper Cells

T follicular helper (Tfh) cells, characterized by the high expression of chemokine CXC receptor 5 (CXCR5), are another specialized subset of CD4+ T cells. With expression of IL-21, CXCL13 and PD-1, they exert B helper activities in a manner primarily dependent on IL-21 (67). Tfh cells can be further classified as three subpopulations, including Type 17 (CXCR3-CCR6+), Type 1 (CXCR3 + CCR6-), and Type 2 (CXCR3-CCR6-) cells. Recently, Tfh cells have been shown to be involved in the pathogenesis of psoriasis. Niu et al. and Wang et al. demonstrated that the frequency of circulating Tfh were elevated in psoriasis and positively correlated with serum IL-21 levels and PASI scores (68, 69), suggesting Tfh cells as potential contributors to psoriasis pathogenesis. Moreover, Caruso et al. reported that increased IL-21 was produced primarily by CD4+ T cells in psoriatic lesions (70). Although other markers, like CXCR5, were not analyzed to define CD4+ T cell subsets, a part of the IL-21-producing CD4 T cells were co-producing IFN-γ or IL-17. Consistently, Wang et al. observed that CXCR3−CCR6+ Tfh type 17 subset, which secrete the Th17 cytokines IL-17A and IL-22, increased and correlated with PASI score in psoriasis (71).

TARGETED PSORIASIS THERAPIES

Recognition of the IL-23/Th17 axis and IL-22/Th22 pathway vigorously promoted the development of targeted therapies. To date, targeted therapies that have been approved by the Food and Drug Administration (FDA) for psoriasis treatment have shown promising effects (72, 73). There are also various new biologic agents that exhibit promising therapeutic efficacy in clinical trials (72, 73). **Table 1** shows the targeted agents for psoriasis treatment, and we briefly discuss the agents targeting the IL-23/Th17 axis and IL-22/Th22 pathway in the treatment of psoriasis.

Targeting IL-23

IL-23 is a heterodimeric cytokine composed of a unique p19 chain and a p40 chain shared with IL-12. Targeted drugs include antibodies that inhibit the p19 subunit of IL-23 and the p40 subunit of both IL-12 and IL-23. Ustekinumab and Briakinumab, which are human interleukin-12/23 monoclonal antibodies, have been approved by the FDA and have shown significant efficacy in patients with moderate to severe plaque psoriasis (29, 32). Risankizumab and Tildrakizumab are agents that target the unique IL-23 subunit p19. The results of randomized controlled, phase 3 trials showed that these agents have superior efficacy to placebo or Ustekinumab in the treatment of moderate-to-severe plaque psoriasis (30, 31). Data from clinical trials have shown that IL-23 inhibitors have convincing safety profiles; however, long-term observations indicate that adverse events still occur during the treatment. A multicentre, randomized, double-blind, placebo-controlled clinical trial of Ustekinumab showed that adverse events were observed in 217 (53·1%) patients in the 45 mg group, 197 (47·9%) in the 90 mg group and 204 (49·8%) in the placebo group (80). The most common adverse effects included infections, headache and injection-site reactions (98).

Targeting IL-17

Additional categories of biologic agents include fully human interleukin-17A/F monoclonal antibodies. Secukinumab and Ixekizumab can directly neutralize IL-17A and have excellent and sustained efficacy for psoriatic patients with or without PsA and nail psoriasis (37, 38, 90, 99–101). Bimekizumab, a human anti-IL-17 drug that inhibits both IL-17A and IL-17F, induced convincing clinical improvements in psoriatic patients with or

TABLE 1 | US food and drug administration–approved biologic treatments for psoriasis.

Biologics	Drug	Main Trials (Reference)	N	Control Intervention	Efficacy (VS Control Intervention)	
					PASI 75	PASI 90
Anti-TNF	Etanercept	Papp et al. (74)	583	PBO	49% at week 12 (VS 3%)	21% at week 12 (VS 1%)
	Infliximab	Reich et al. (75)	378	PBO	80% at week 10 (VS 3%)	57% at week 10 (VS 1%)
					82% at week 24 (VS 4%)	58% at week 24 (VS 1%)
					61% at week 50 (VS N/A)	45% at week 50 (VS N/A)
		Barker et al. (76)	868	MTX	78% at week 16 (VS 42%)	54.5% at week 16 (VS 19.1%)
					76.9% at week 26 (VS 30.7%)	51.0% at week 26 (VS 14.9%)
	Adalimumab	Menter et al. (77)	1212	PBO	71% at week 16 (VS 7%)	N/A
	Certolizumab pegol	Gottlieb et al. (78)	461	PBO	82% at week 16 (VS 9.9%)	52.2% at week 16 (VS 2.5%)
					83.6% at week 48 (VS N/A)	
		Lebwohl et al. (79)	224	Etanercept	66.7% at week 12 (VS 53.3%)	N/A
Anti-IL-23	Ustekinumab	Leonardi et al. (32)	511	PBO	66.4% at week 12 (VS 3.1%)	36.7% at week 12 (VS 2.0%)
					78.6% at week 28 (VS N/A)	55.6% at week 28 (VS N/A)
		Papp et al. (80)	821	PBO	75.7% at week 12 (VS 3.7%)	50.9% at week 12 (VS 0.7%)
					78.5% at week 28 (VS N/A)	54.3% at week 28 (VS N/A)
	Briakinumab	Gottlieb et al. (81)	347	Etanercept/PBO	81.9% at week 12 (VS 56.0%/7.4%)	N/A
		Strober et al. (29)	350	Etanercept/PBO	80.6% at week 12 (VS 39.6%/6.9%)	55.4% at week 12 (VS 13.7%/4.2%)
	Tildrakizumab	Reich et al. (31)	463	PBO	62% at week 12 (VS 6%)	35% at week 12 (VS 3%)
			783	Etanercept/PBO	66% at week 12 (VS 48%/6%)	37% at week 12 (VS 21%/1%)
	Guselkumab	Blauvelt et al. (82)	663	Adalimumab	91.2% at week 16 (VS 73.1%)	73.3% at week 16 (VS 49.7%)
					91.2% at week 24 (VS 72.2%)	80.2% at week 24 (VS 53.0%)
					87.8% at week 48 (VS 62.6%)	76.3% at week 48 (VS 47.9%)
		Reich et al. (83)	1048	Secukinumab	85% at week 48 (VS 80%)	84% at week 48 (VS 70%)
		Thaçi et al. (84)	119	FAE	90.0% at week 24 (VS 27.1%)	81.7% at week 24 (VS 13.6%)
	Risankizumab	Gordon et al. (30)	506	Ustekinumab/PBO	N/A	75.3% at week 16 (VS 42%/4.9%)
			491	Ustekinumab/PBO	N/A	74.8% at week 16 (VS 47.5%/2.0%)
		Reich et al. (85)	605	Adalimumab	91% at week 16 (VS 72%)	72% at week 16 (VS 47%)
		Warren et al. (86)	327	Secukinumab	92% at week 16 (VS 80%)	74% at week 16 (VS 66%)
					90% at week 52 (VS 70%)	87% at week 52 (VS 57%)
Anti-IL-17	Secukinumab	Langley et al. (38)	493	PBO	81.6% at week 12 (VS 4.5%)	59.2% at week 12 (VS 1.2%)
			979	Etanercept/PBO	77.1% at week 12 (VS 44%/4.9%)	54.2% at week 12 (VS 20.7%/1.5%)
		Thaçi et al. (87)	676	Ustekinumab	93.1% at week 16 (VS 82.7%)	79.0% at week 16 (VS 57.6%)
		Blauvelt 2017 (88)	676	Ustekinumab	92.5% at week 24 (VS 83.6%)	80.8% at week 24 (VS 66.3%)
					91.6% at week 52 (VS 78.2%)	74.9% at week 52 (VS 60.6%)
		Bagel et al. (89)	1102	Ustekinumab	89.0% at week 52 (VS 82.1%)	73.2% at week 52 (VS 59.8%)
	Ixekizumab	Griffiths et al. (90)	877	Etanercept/PBO	89.7% at week 12 (VS 41.6%/2.4%)	70.7% at week 12 (VS 18.7%/0.6%)
			960	Etanercept/PBO	87.3% at week 12 (VS 53.4%/7.3%)	68.1% at week 12 (VS 25.7%/3.1%)
		Gordon et al. (91)	864	PBO	89.1% at week 12 (VS 3.9%)	70.9% at week 12 (VS 0.5%)
			385	N/A	83% at week 60	73% at week 60
		Blauvelt et al. (92)	385	N/A	83.6% at week 108	70.3% at week 108
		Lebwohl et al. (93)	385	N/A	82.8% at week 204	48.3% at week 204
		Reich et al. (94)	162	MTX/FAE	91% at week 24 (VS 70%/22%)	80% at week 24 (VS 39%/9%)
		Blauvelt et al. (95)	1027	Guselkumab	23% at week 2 (VS 5%)	58% at week 8 (VS 36%)
					No statistically difference at week 24	No statistically difference at week 24
	Brodalumab	Lebwohl et al. (96)	1221	Ustekinumab/PBO	86% at week 12 (VS 70%/8%)	N/A
		Papp et al. (36)	1252	Ustekinumab/PBO	85% at week 12 (VS 69%/6%)	N/A
			441	PBO	83.3% at week 12 (VS 2.7%)	70.3% at week 12 (VS 0.9%)
		Pinter et al. (97)	149	FAE	81.0% at week 24 (VS 38.1%)	65.7% at week 12 (VS 21.9%)

TNF, tumor necrosis factor; N, Number of participants; PASI 75/90, a 75%/90% reduction in Psoriasis Area Severity Index (PASI) score compared with baseline; N/A, Not Applicable; MTX, Methotrexate; FAE, fumaric acid esters; PBO, Placebo.

without psoriatic arthritis (35, 102). Brodalumab is a human anti-IL-17 receptor antagonist (IL-17RA) (36). The feature that broadly blocks IL-17A, IL-17F, IL-17C and IL-17E enables IL-17RA to rapidly improve the clinical and histological features of psoriasis (103). It was shown that Brodalumab may even be effective in those who failed to respond to Secukinumab and Ixekizumab (103, 104). Although all these antagonists showed robust efficacy, unexpected side effects have also been reported. The most common adverse effects are infections, such as bacterial infection and tuberculosis; others, such as headache and diarrhea, are less common (73).

Targeting IL-22

IL-22 is an essential cytokine for psoriasis development. ILV-095, an IL-22 receptor antagonist that was developed to treat psoriasis, failed in a phase I clinical trial because the expected endpoints could not be met (105). Another humanized monoclonal antibody against the IL-22 receptor, IL-094, was suspended for similar reasons (105). Thus far, biological therapies against the IL-22 receptor need to be further investigated in the future.

Targeting JAK/STAT Pathway

The Janus kinase (JAK) signal transducer and activator of transcription (STAT) signaling pathway (JAK/STAT pathway) transduce signals from multitudes of cytokines and growth factors and plays a major role in the pathogenesis of many inflammatory and autoimmune diseases. Due to the essential role in forwarding the IL-23/Th17 axis and IL-22/Th22 pathway signals into cell, JAK/STAT pathway has received increasing attention recently in psoriasis (106). Furthermore, it is an attractive idea that to blockade multiple psoriasis related cytokines rather than specific to one signaling pathway by inhibiting of JAKs. Indeed, there are already several biologic agents that target JAK/STAT pathway in clinical trials: Tofacitinib (NCT01241591) for JAK1 and JAK3 (107); Baricitinib (NCT01490632) for JAK1 and JAK2 (108); Itacitinib (NCT01634087) and Solcitinib (NCT01782664) for JAK1 (109, 110); PF-06700841 (NCT02969018) for JAK1 and TYK2 (111); and PF-06826647 (NCT03895372) and Deucravacitinib (NCT03924427) for TYK2 (112, 113). Many of them have shown promising efficacy, especially selective TYK2 inhibitors, whereas the adverse effect and long-term safety still need to be emphasized.

CONCLUSIONS

Over the past 50 years, substantial scientific research has suggested that T cells are closely associated with the pathogenesis of psoriasis. These cells serve as a link connecting nonspecific triggers and keratinocyte dysfunction. Triggers such as infections and physical injury stimulate antigen-presenting cells (APCs) to release pro-inflammatory factors (IL-23, IFN-α and IL-12). These cytokines in turn activate the IL-23 and/or IL-22 pathway to induce Th17 and/or Th22 cell differentiation, resulting in the production of numerous psoriatic cytokines, such as TNF, IFN-γ, IL-17 and IL-22, which act on keratinocytes to amplify psoriatic inflammation. Nowadays, on the one hand, the observation that Treg and/or Th17/Treg balance is frequently dysregulated in psoriatic patients hints at the critical role of Treg cells in controlling psoriatic inflammation. One possible mechanism by which the Th17/Treg balance is disturbed in psoriatic lesions attributes to the high levels of IL-6. And Tfh cells, which has been proved to be one of the major sources of IL-21, are also involve in the pathogenesis of psoriasis. Additionally, it has been reported that γδT cells, which are the major IL-17-producing cells in the skin, also play critical roles in psoriasis pathogenesis. On the other hand, biological agents targeting TNF, IL-23 and IL-17 have shown promising efficacy during the clinical treatment of psoriasis, while IL-6 inhibitors, IL-21 inhibitors and recombinant human IL-10 treatment didn't attain the results as expected. Moreover, many clinical trials are ongoing to uncover new targets in psoriasis. For example, JAK inhibitors paved the way of inhibiting multiple pro-inflammatory cytokines together and have shown clinical efficacy in both phase II and III trials. All these advancements are ascribed to the continuous exploration of the pathogenesis of psoriasis. However, there are still some issues that need to be addressed. First, adverse events cannot be ignored during treatment, which may be feasibly due to the broad biological effects of these cytokines. In addition, several limitations, such as the difficulty of effecting a cure, the need for long-term medication and ease of recurrence after drug withdrawal, still exist. All this evidence highlights that our understanding of psoriasis is insufficient, especially the crosstalk of multiple immune cells and cytokines in psoriasis, which still needs to be studied in depth. Further studies should focus on identifying current therapeutic approaches and novel, efficient targets to help overcome the adverse effects and limitations.

AUTHOR CONTRIBUTIONS

JL, DM and JT conceived of the presented idea. PH, and MW summarized the reference and draft the manuscript. HG organized the figure and table. JL, DM and JT supervised the project and contributed equally to the final version of the manuscript. All authors contributed to the article and approved the submitted version.

REFERENCES

1. Lowes MA, Suarez-Farinas M, Krueger JG. Immunology of Psoriasis. *Annu Rev Immunol* (2014) 32:227–55. doi: 10.1146/annurev-immunol-032713-120225
2. Griffiths CE, Barker JN. Pathogenesis and Clinical Features of Psoriasis. *Lancet (London England)* (2007) 370(9583):263–71. doi: 10.1016/s0140-6736(07)61128-3
3. Groot J, Blegvad C, Nybo Andersen AM, Zachariae C, Skov L. Tonsillitis and Pediatric Psoriasis: Cohort and Cross-Sectional Analyses of Offspring From the Danish National Birth Cohort. *J Am Acad Dermatol* (2020) 82(3):666–74. doi: 10.1016/j.jaad.2019.08.010
4. Kluger N, Estève E, Fouéré S, Dupuis-Fourdan F, Jegou MH, Lévy-Rameau C. Tattooing and Psoriasis: A Case Series and Review of the Literature. *Int J Dermatol* (2017) 56(8):822–7. doi: 10.1111/ijd.13646
5. Awad VM, Sakhamuru S, Kambampati S, Wasim S, Malik BH. Mechanisms of Beta-Blocker Induced Psoriasis, and Psoriasis *De Novo* at the Cellular Level. *Cureus* (2020) 12(7):e8964. doi: 10.7759/cureus.8964
6. Balak DM, Hajdarbegovic E. Drug-Induced Psoriasis: Clinical Perspectives. *Psoriasis (Auckland NZ)* (2017) 7:87–94. doi: 10.2147/ptt.S126727

7. Ten Bergen LL, Petrovic A, Aarebrot AK, Appel S. Current Knowledge on Autoantigens and Autoantibodies in Psoriasis. *Scand J Immunol* (2020) 92 (4):e12945. doi: 10.1111/sji.12945
8. Boehncke WH, Schön MP. Psoriasis. *Lancet (London England)* (2015) 386 (9997):983–94. doi: 10.1016/s0140-6736(14)61909-7
9. Kastelan M, Prpic Massari L, Gruber F, Zamolo G, Zauhar G, Coklo M, et al. Perforin Expression Is Upregulated in the Epidermis of Psoriatic Lesions. *Br J Dermatol* (2004) 151(4):831–6. doi: 10.1111/j.1365-2133.2004.06168.x
10. Ottaviani C, Nasorri F, Bedini C, de Pita O, Girolomoni G, Cavani A. CD56brightCD16(-) NK Cells Accumulate in Psoriatic Skin in Response to CXCL10 and CCL5 and Exacerbate Skin Inflammation. *Eur J Immunol* (2006) 36(1):118–28. doi: 10.1002/eji.200535243
11. Lin AM, Rubin CJ, Khandpur R, Wang JY, Riblett M, Yalavarthi S, et al. Mast Cells and Neutrophils Release IL-17 Through Extracellular Trap Formation in Psoriasis. *J Immunol (Baltimore Md 1950)* (2011) 187(1):490–500. doi: 10.4049/jimmunol.1100123
12. Martin B, Hirota K, Cua DJ, Stockinger B, Veldhoen M. Interleukin-17-Producing Gammadelta T Cells Selectively Expand in Response to Pathogen Products and Environmental Signals. *Immunity* (2009) 31(2):321–30. doi: 10.1016/j.immuni.2009.06.020
13. Deng YX, Chang C, Lu QJ. The Inflammatory Response in Psoriasis: A Comprehensive Review. *Clin Rev Allergy Immunol* (2016) 50(3):377–89. doi: 10.1007/s12016-016-8535-x
14. Lande R, Botti E, Jandus C, Dojcinovic D, Fanelli G, Conrad C, et al. The Antimicrobial Peptide LL37 Is a T-Cell Autoantigen in Psoriasis. *Nat Commun* (2014) 5:5621. doi: 10.1038/ncomms6621
15. Arakawa A, Siewert K, Stohr J, Besgen P, Kim SM, Ruhl G, et al. Melanocyte Antigen Triggers Autoimmunity in Human Psoriasis. *J Exp Med* (2015) 212 (13):2203–12. doi: 10.1084/jem.20151093
16. Valdimarsson H, Sigmundsdóttir H, Jónsdóttir I. Is Psoriasis Induced by Streptococcal Superantigens and Maintained by M-Protein-Specific T Cells That Cross-React With Keratin? *Clin Exp Immunol* (1997) 107 Suppl 1:21–4. doi: 10.3389/fimmu.2018.01390
17. Gudmundsdottir AS, Sigmundsdottir H, Sigurgeirsson B, Good MF, Valdimarsson H, Jonsdottir I. Is an Epitope on Keratin 17 a Major Target for Autoreactive T Lymphocytes in Psoriasis? *Clin Exp Immunol* (1999) 117 (3):580–6. doi: 10.1046/j.1365-2249.1999.01013.x
18. Johnston A, Gudjonsson JE, Sigmundsdottir H, Love TJ, Valdimarsson H. Peripheral Blood T Cell Responses to Keratin Peptides That Share Sequences With Streptococcal M Proteins Are Largely Restricted to Skin-Homing CD8(+) T Cells. *Clin Exp Immunol* (2004) 138(1):83–93. doi: 10.1111/j.1365-2249.2004.00600.x
19. Valdimarsson H, Thorleifsdottir RH, Sigurdardottir SL, Gudjonsson JE, Johnston A. Psoriasis–as an Autoimmune Disease Caused by Molecular Mimicry. *Trends Immunol* (2009) 30(10):494–501. doi: 10.1016/j.it.2009.07.008
20. Yunusbaeva M, Valiev R, Bilalov F, Sultanova Z, Sharipova L, Yunusbayev B. Psoriasis Patients Demonstrate HLA-Cw*06:02 Allele Dosage-Dependent T Cell Proliferation When Treated With Hair Follicle-Derived Keratin 17 Protein. *Sci Rep* (2018) 8(1):6098. doi: 10.1038/s41598-018-24491-z
21. Mueller W, Herrmann B. Cyclosporin A for Psoriasis. *New Engl J Med* (1979) 301(10):555. doi: 10.1056/NEJM197909063011016
22. Prinz JC, Gross B, Vollmer S, Trommler P, Strobel I, Meurer R, et al. T-Cell Clones From Psoriasis Skin-Lesions Can Promote Keratinocyte Proliferation In-Vitro via Secreted Products. *Eur J Immunol* (1994) 24(3):593–8. doi: 10.1002/eji.1830240315
23. Baker BS, Swain AF, Fry L, Valdimarsson H. Epidermal Lymphocytes-T and Hla-Dr Expression in Psoriasis. *Br J Dermatol* (1984) 110(5):555–64. doi: 10.1016/B978-0-407-00338-5.50047-8
24. Schlaak JF, Buslau M, Jochum W, Hermann E, Girndt M, Gallati H, et al. T-Cells Involved in Psoriasis Vulgaris Belong to the Th1 Subset. *J Invest Dermatol* (1994) 102(2):145–9. doi: 10.1111/1523-1747.ep12371752
25. Harden JL, Johnson-Huang LM, Chamian MF, Lee E, Pearce T, Leonardi CL, et al. Humanized Anti-IFN-Gamma (HuZAF) in the Treatment of Psoriasis. *J Allergy Clin Immunol* (2015) 135(2):553–6. doi: 10.1016/j.jaci.2014.05.046
26. Aggarwal S, Ghilardi N, Xie MH, de Sauvage FJ, Gurney AL. Interleukin-23 Promotes a Distinct CD4 T Cell Activation State Characterized by the Production of Interleukin-17. *J Biol Chem* (2003) 278(3):1910–4. doi: 10.1074/jbc.M207577200
27. Harrington LE, Hatton RD, Mangan PR, Turner H, Murphy TL, Murphy KM, et al. Interleukin 17-Producing CD4+ Effector T Cells Develop *via* a Lineage Distinct From the T Helper Type 1 and 2 Lineages. *Nat Immunol* (2005) 6(11):1123–32. doi: 10.1038/ni1254
28. Piskin G, Sylva-Steenland RM, Bos JD, Teunissen MB. *In Vitro* and *In Situ* Expression of IL-23 by Keratinocytes in Healthy Skin and Psoriasis Lesions: Enhanced Expression in Psoriatic Skin. *J Immunol (Baltimore Md 1950)* (2006) 176(3):1908–15. doi: 10.4049/jimmunol.176.3.1908
29. Strober BE, Crowley JJ, Yamauchi PS, Olds M, Williams DA. Efficacy and Safety Results From a Phase III, Randomized Controlled Trial Comparing the Safety and Efficacy of Briakinumab With Etanercept and Placebo in Patients With Moderate to Severe Chronic Plaque Psoriasis. *Br J Dermatol* (2011) 165(3):661–8. doi: 10.1111/j.1365-2133.2011.10419.x
30. Gordon KB, Strober B, Lebwohl M, Augustin M, Blauvelt A, Poulin Y, et al. Efficacy and Safety of Risankizumab in Moderate-to-Severe Plaque Psoriasis (UltIMMa-1 and UltIMMa-2): Results From Two Double-Blind, Randomised, Placebo-Controlled and Ustekinumab-Controlled Phase 3 Trials. *Lancet (London England)* (2018) 392(10148):650–61. doi: 10.1016/s0140-6736(18)31713-6
31. Reich K, Papp KA, Blauvelt A, Tyring SK, Sinclair R, Thaçi D, et al. Tildrakizumab Versus Placebo or Etanercept for Chronic Plaque Psoriasis (reSURFACE 1 and reSURFACE 2): Results From Two Randomised Controlled, Phase 3 Trials. *Lancet (London England)* (2017) 390 (10091):276–88. doi: 10.1016/s0140-6736(17)31279-5
32. Leonardi CL, Kimball AB, Papp KA, Yeilding N, Guzzo C, Wang Y, et al. Efficacy and Safety of Ustekinumab, a Human Interleukin-12/23 Monoclonal Antibody, in Patients With Psoriasis: 76-Week Results From a Randomised, Double-Blind, Placebo-Controlled Trial (PHOENIX 1). *Lancet (London England)* (2008) 371(9625):1665–74. doi: 10.1016/S0140-6736(08)60725-4
33. Wilson NJ, Boniface K, Chan JR, McKenzie BS, Blumenschein WM, Mattson JD, et al. Development, Cytokine Profile and Function of Human Interleukin 17-Producing Helper T Cells. *Nat Immunol* (2007) 8(9):950–7. doi: 10.1038/ni1497
34. Lowes MA, Kikuchi T, Fuentes-Duculan J, Cardinale I, Zaba LC, Haider AS, et al. Psoriasis Vulgaris Lesions Contain Discrete Populations of Th1 and Th17 T Cells. *J Invest Dermatol* (2008) 128(5):1207–11. doi: 10.1038/sj.jid.5701213
35. Papp KA, Merola JF, Gottlieb AB, Griffiths CEM, Cross N, Peterson L, et al. Dual Neutralization of Both Interleukin 17A and Interleukin 17F With Bimekizumab in Patients With Psoriasis: Results From BE ABLE 1, a 12-Week Randomized, Double-Blinded, Placebo-Controlled Phase 2b Trial. *J Am Acad Dermatol* (2018) 79(2):277–+. doi: 10.1016/j.jaad.2018.03.037
36. Papp KA, Reich K, Paul C, Blauvelt A, Baran W, Bolduc C, et al. A Prospective Phase III, Randomized, Double-Blind, Placebo-Controlled Study of Brodalumab in Patients With Moderate-to-Severe Plaque Psoriasis. *Br J Dermatol* (2016) 175(2):273–86. doi: 10.1111/bjd.14493
37. Leonardi C, Maari C, Philipp S, Goldblum O, Zhang L, Burkhardt N, et al. Maintenance of Skin Clearance With Ixekizumab Treatment of Psoriasis: Three-Year Results From the UNCOVER-3 Study. *J Am Acad Dermatol* (2018) 79(5):824–30 e2. doi: 10.1016/j.jaad.2018.05.032
38. Langley RG, Elewski BE, Lebwohl M, Reich K, Griffiths CE, Papp K, et al. Secukinumab in Plaque Psoriasis–Results of Two Phase 3 Trials. *New Engl J Med* (2014) 371(4):326–38. doi: 10.1056/NEJMoa1314258
39. Zheng Y, Danilenko DM, Valdez P, Kasman I, Eastham-Anderson J, Wu JF, et al. Interleukin-22, a T(H)17 Cytokine, Mediates IL-23-Induced Dermal Inflammation and Acanthosis. *Nature* (2007) 445(7128):648–51. doi: 10.1038/nature05505
40. Nograles KE, Zaba LC, Guttman-Yassky E, Fuentes-Duculan J, Suarez-Farinas M, Cardinale I, et al. Th17 Cytokines Interleukin (IL)-17 and IL-22 Modulate Distinct Inflammatory and Keratinocyte-Response Pathways. *Br J Dermatol* (2008) 159(5):1092–102. doi: 10.1111/j.1365-2133.2008.08769.x
41. Van Belle AB, de Heusch M, Lemaire MM, Hendrickx E, Warnier G, Dunussi-Joannopoulos K, et al. IL-22 Is Required for Imiquimod-Induced

Psoriasiform Skin Inflammation in Mice. *J Immunol* (2012) 188(1):462–9. doi: 10.4049/jimmunol.1102224

42. Schon MP, Erpenbeck L. The Interleukin-23/Interleukin-17 Axis Links Adaptive and Innate Immunity in Psoriasis. *Front Immunol* (2018) 9:1323. doi: 10.3389/fimmu.2018.01323
43. Nograles KE, Zaba LC, Shemer A, Fuentes-Duculan J, Cardinale I, Kikuchi T, et al. IL-22-Producing "T22" T Cells Account for Upregulated IL-22 in Atopic Dermatitis Despite Reduced IL-17-Producing T(H)17 T Cells. *J Allergy Clin Immunol* (2009) 123(6):1244–52. doi: 10.1016/j.jaci.2009.03.041
44. Trifari S, Kaplan CD, Tran EH, Crellin NK, Spits H. Identification of a Human Helper T Cell Population That has Abundant Production of Interleukin 22 and Is Distinct From T-H-17, T(H)1 and T(H)2 Cells. *Nat Immunol* (2009) 10(8):864–U73. doi: 10.1038/ni.1770
45. Kagami S, Rizzo HL, Lee JJ, Koguchi Y, Blauvelt A. Circulating Th17, Th22, and Th1 Cells Are Increased in Psoriasis. *J Invest Dermatol* (2010) 130 (5):1373–83. doi: 10.1038/jid.2009.399
46. Kryczek I, Bruce AT, Gudjonsson JE, Johnston A, Aphale A, Vatan L, et al. Induction of IL-17(+) T Cell Trafficking and Development by IFN-Gamma: Mechanism and Pathological Relevance in Psoriasis. *J Immunol* (2008) 181 (7):4733–41. doi: 10.4049/jimmunol.181.7.4733
47. Sakaguchi S, Yamaguchi T, Nomura T, Ono M. Regulatory T Cells and Immune Tolerance. *Cell* (2008) 133(5):775–87. doi: 10.1016/j.cell.2008.05.009
48. Nussbaum L, Chen YL, Ogg GS. Role of Regulatory T Cells in Psoriasis Pathogenesis and Treatment. *Br J Dermatol* (2021) 184(1):14–24. doi: 10.1111/bjd.19380
49. Priyadarssini M, Divya Priya D, Indhumathi S, Rajappa M, Chandrashekar L, Thappa DM. Immunophenotyping of T Cells in the Peripheral Circulation in Psoriasis. *Br J Biomed Sci* (2016) 73(4):174–9. doi: 10.1080/09674845.2016.1207869
50. Richetta AG, Mattozzi C, Salvi M, Giancristoforo S, D'Epiro S, Milana B, et al. CD4+ CD25+ T-Regulatory Cells in Psoriasis. Correlation Between Their Numbers and Biologics-Induced Clinical Improvement. *Eur J Dermatol EJD* (2011) 21(3):344–8. doi: 10.1684/ejd.2011.1362
51. Zhang L, Yang XQ, Cheng J, Hui RS, Gao TW. Increased Th17 Cells are Accompanied by FoxP3(+) Treg Cell Accumulation and Correlated With Psoriasis Disease Severity. *Clin Immunol (Orlando Fla)* (2010) 135(1):108–17. doi: 10.1016/j.clim.2009.11.008
52. Yun WJ, Lee DW, Chang SE, Yoon GS, Huh JR, Won CH, et al. Role of CD4CD25FOXP3 Regulatory T Cells in Psoriasis. *Ann Dermatol* (2010) 22 (4):397–403. doi: 10.5021/ad.2010.22.4.397
53. Yan KX, Fang X, Han L, Zhang ZH, Kang KF, Zheng ZZ, et al. Foxp3+ Regulatory T Cells and Related Cytokines Differentially Expressed in Plaque vs. Guttate Psoriasis Vulgaris. *Br J Dermatol* (2010) 163(1):48–56. doi: 10.1111/j.1365-2133.2010.09742.x
54. Fujimura T, Okuyama R, Ito Y, Aiba S. Profiles of Foxp3+ Regulatory T Cells in Eczematous Dermatitis, Psoriasis Vulgaris and Mycosis Fungoides. *Br J Dermatol* (2008) 158(6):1256–63. doi: 10.1111/j.1365-2133.2008.08504.x
55. Bovenschen HJ, van Vlijmen-Willems IM, van de Kerkhof PC, van Erp PE. Identification of Lesional CD4+ CD25+ Foxp3+ Regulatory T Cells in Psoriasis. *Dermatol (Basel Switzerland)* (2006) 213(2):111–7. doi: 10.1159/000093849
56. Li B, Lei J, Yang L, Gao C, Dang E, Cao T, et al. Dysregulation of Akt-FOXO1 Pathway Leads to Dysfunction of Regulatory T Cells in Patients With Psoriasis. *J Invest Dermatol* (2019) 139(10):2098–107. doi: 10.1016/j.jid.2018.12.035
57. Sugiyama H, Gyulai R, Toichi E, Garaczi E, Shimada S, Stevens SR, et al. Dysfunctional Blood and Target Tissue CD4+CD25high Regulatory T Cells in Psoriasis: Mechanism Underlying Unrestrained Pathogenic Effector T Cell Proliferation. *J Immunol (Baltimore Md 1950)* (2005) 174(1):164–73. doi: 10.4049/jimmunol.174.1.164
58. Zhang L, Li Y, Yang X, Wei J, Zhou S, Zhao Z, et al. Characterization of Th17 and FoxP3(+) Treg Cells in Paediatric Psoriasis Patients. *Scand J Immunol* (2016) 83(3):174–80. doi: 10.1111/sji.12404
59. Goodman WA, Levine AD, Massari JV, Sugiyama H, McCormick TS, Cooper KD. IL-6 Signaling in Psoriasis Prevents Immune Suppression by Regulatory T Cells. *J Immunol (Baltimore Md 1950)* (2009) 183(5):3170–6. doi: 10.4049/jimmunol.0803721
60. Goodman WA, Young AB, McCormick TS, Cooper KD, Levine AD. Stat3 Phosphorylation Mediates Resistance of Primary Human T Cells to Regulatory T Cell Suppression. *J Immunol (Baltimore Md 1950)* (2011) 186(6):3336–45. doi: 10.4049/jimmunol.1001455
61. Wang XY, Chen XY, Li J, Zhang HY, Liu J, Sun LD. MiR-200a Expression in CD4+ T Cells Correlates With the Expression of Th17/Treg Cells and Relevant Cytokines in Psoriasis Vulgaris: A Case Control Study. *Biomed Pharmacother = Biomed Pharmacother* (2017) 93:1158–64. doi: 10.1016/j.biopha.2017.06.055
62. Wang H, Peters T, Sindrilaru A, Kess D, Oreshkova T, Yu XZ, et al. TGF-Beta-Dependent Suppressive Function of Tregs Requires Wild-Type Levels of CD18 in a Mouse Model of Psoriasis. *J Clin Invest* (2008) 118(7):2629–39. doi: 10.1172/jci34916
63. Kimura A, Kishimoto T. IL-6: Regulator of Treg/Th17 Balance. *Eur J Immunol* (2010) 40(7):1830–5. doi: 10.1002/eji.201040391
64. Bovenschen HJ, van de Kerkhof PC, van Erp PE, Woestenenk R, Joosten I, Koenen HJ. Foxp3+ Regulatory T Cells of Psoriasis Patients Easily Differentiate Into IL-17A-Producing Cells and Are Found in Lesional Skin. *J Invest Dermatol* (2011) 131(9):1853–60. doi: 10.1038/jid.2011.139
65. Singh K, Gatzka M, Peters T, Borkner L, Hainzl A, Wang H, et al. Reduced CD18 Levels Drive Regulatory T Cell Conversion Into Th17 Cells in the CD18hypo Pl/J Mouse Model of Psoriasis. *J Immunol (Baltimore Md 1950)* (2013) 190(6):2544–53. doi: 10.4049/jimmunol.1202399
66. Ma L, Xue H, Gao T, Gao M, Zhang Y. Notch1 Signaling Regulates the Th17/Treg Immune Imbalance in Patients With Psoriasis Vulgaris. *Mediators Inflammation* (2018) 2018:3069521. doi: 10.1155/2018/3069521
67. Long D, Chen Y, Wu H, Zhao M, Lu Q. Clinical Significance and Immunobiology of IL-21 in Autoimmunity. *J Autoimmun* (2019) 99:1–14. doi: 10.1016/j.jaut.2019.01.013
68. Niu J, Song Z, Yang X, Zhai Z, Zhong H, Hao F. Increased Circulating Follicular Helper T Cells and Activated B Cells Correlate With Disease Severity in Patients With Psoriasis. *J Eur Acad Dermatol Venereol JEADV* (2015) 29(9):1791–6. doi: 10.1111/jdv.13027
69. Wang Y, Wang L, Yang H, Yuan W, Ren J, Bai Y. Activated Circulating T Follicular Helper Cells Are Associated With Disease Severity in Patients With Psoriasis. *J Immunol Res* (2016) 2016:7346030. doi: 10.1155/2016/7346030
70. Caruso R, Botti E, Sarra M, Esposito M, Stolfi C, Diluvio L, et al. Involvement of Interleukin-21 in the Epidermal Hyperplasia of Psoriasis. *Nat Med* (2009) 15(9):1013–5. doi: 10.1038/nm.1995
71. Wang Y, Wang L, Shi Y, Wang F, Yang H, Han S, et al. Altered Circulating T Follicular Helper Cell Subsets in Patients With Psoriasis Vulgaris. *Immunol Lett* (2017) 181:101–8. doi: 10.1016/j.imlet.2016.09.008
72. Cai YH, Fleming C, Yan J. New Insights of T Cells in the Pathogenesis of Psoriasis. *Cell Mol Immunol* (2012) 9(4):302–9. doi: 10.1038/cmi.2012.15
73. Liu T, Li S, Ying S, Tang S, Ding Y, Li Y, et al. The IL-23/IL-17 Pathway in Inflammatory Skin Diseases: From Bench to Bedside. *Front Immunol* (2020) 11:594735. doi: 10.3389/fimmu.2020.594735
74. Papp KA, Tyring S, Lahfa M, Prinz J, Griffiths CE, Nakanishi AM, et al. A Global Phase III Randomized Controlled Trial of Etanercept in Psoriasis: Safety, Efficacy, and Effect of Dose Reduction. *Br J Dermatol* (2005) 152 (6):1304–12. doi: 10.1111/j.1365-2133.2005.06688.x
75. Reich K, Nestle FO, Papp K, Ortonne JP, Evans R, Guzzo C, et al. Infliximab Induction and Maintenance Therapy for Moderate-to-Severe Psoriasis: A Phase III, Multicentre, Double-Blind Trial. *Lancet (London England)* (2005) 366(9494):1367–74. doi: 10.1016/s0140-6736(05)67566-6
76. Barker J, Hoffmann M, Wozel G, Ortonne JP, Zheng H, van Hoogstraten H, et al. Efficacy and Safety of Infliximab vs. Methotrexate in Patients With Moderate-to-Severe Plaque Psoriasis: Results of an Open-Label, Active-Controlled, Randomized Trial (RESTORE1). *Br J Dermatol* (2011) 165 (5):1109–17. doi: 10.1111/j.1365-2133.2011.10615.x
77. Menter A, Tyring SK, Gordon K, Kimball AB, Leonardi CL, Langley RG, et al. Adalimumab Therapy for Moderate to Severe Psoriasis: A Randomized, Controlled Phase III Trial. *J Am Acad Dermatol* (2008) 58(1):106–15. doi: 10.1016/j.jaad.2007.09.010
78. Gottlieb AB, Blauvelt A, Thaçi D, Leonardi CL, Poulin Y, Drew J, et al. Certolizumab Pegol for the Treatment of Chronic Plaque Psoriasis: Results Through 48 Weeks From 2 Phase 3, Multicenter, Randomized, Double-

Blinded, Placebo-Controlled Studies (CIMPASI-1 and CIMPASI-2). *J Am Acad Dermatol* (2018) 79(2):302–14.e6. doi: 10.1016/j.jaad.2018.04.012

79. Lebwohl M, Blauvelt A, Paul C, Sofen H, Węgłowska J, Piguet V, et al. Certolizumab Pegol for the Treatment of Chronic Plaque Psoriasis: Results Through 48 Weeks of a Phase 3, Multicenter, Randomized, Double-Blind, Etanercept- and Placebo-Controlled Study (CIMPACT). *J Am Acad Dermatol* (2018) 79(2):266–76.e5. doi: 10.1016/j.jaad.2018.04.013
80. Papp KA, Langley RG, Lebwohl M, Krueger GG, Szapary P, Yeilding N, et al. Efficacy and Safety of Ustekinumab, a Human Interleukin-12/23 Monoclonal Antibody, in Patients With Psoriasis: 52-Week Results From a Randomised, Double-Blind, Placebo-Controlled Trial (PHOENIX 2). *Lancet (London England)* (2008) 371(9625):1675–84. doi: 10.1016/S0140-6736(08)60726-6
81. Gottlieb AB, Leonardi C, Kerdel F, Mehlis S, Olds M, Williams DA. Efficacy and Safety of Briakinumab vs. Etanercept and Placebo in Patients With Moderate to Severe Chronic Plaque Psoriasis. *Br J Dermatol* (2011) 165 (3):652–60. doi: 10.1111/j.1365-2133.2011.10418.x
82. Blauvelt A, Papp KA, Griffiths CE, Randazzo B, Wasfi Y, Shen YK, et al. Efficacy and Safety of Guselkumab, an Anti-Interleukin-23 Monoclonal Antibody, Compared With Adalimumab for the Continuous Treatment of Patients With Moderate to Severe Psoriasis: Results From the Phase III, Double-Blinded, Placebo- and Active Comparator-Controlled VOYAGE 1 Trial. *J Am Acad Dermatol* (2017) 76(3):405–17. doi: 10.1016/j.jaad.2016.11.041
83. Reich K, Armstrong AW, Langley RG, Flavin S, Randazzo B, Li S, et al. Guselkumab Versus Secukinumab for the Treatment of Moderate-to-Severe Psoriasis (ECLIPSE): Results From a Phase 3, Randomised Controlled Trial. *Lancet (London England)* (2019) 394(10201):831–9. doi: 10.1016/s0140-6736(19)31773-8
84. Thaçi D, Pinter A, Sebastian M, Termeer C, Sticherling M, Gerdes S, et al. Guselkumab Is Superior to Fumaric Acid Esters in Patients With Moderate-to-Severe Plaque Psoriasis Who Are Naive to Systemic Treatment: Results From a Randomized, Active-Comparator-Controlled Phase IIIb Trial (POLARIS). *Br J Dermatol* (2020) 183(2):265–75. doi: 10.1111/bjd.18696
85. Reich K, Gooderham M, Thaçi D, Crowley JJ, Ryan C, Krueger JG, et al. Risankizumab Compared With Adalimumab in Patients With Moderate-to-Severe Plaque Psoriasis (IMMvent): A Randomised, Double-Blind, Active-Comparator-Controlled Phase 3 Trial. *Lancet (London England)* (2019) 394 (10198):576–86. doi: 10.1016/s0140-6736(19)30952-3
86. Warren RB, Blauvelt A, Poulin Y, Beeck S, Kelly M, Wu T, et al. Efficacy and Safety of Risankizumab vs. Secukinumab in Patients With Moderate-to-Severe Plaque Psoriasis (IMMerge): Results From a Phase III, Randomized, Open-Label, Efficacy-Assessor-Blinded Clinical Trial. *Br J Dermatol* (2021) 184(1):50–9. doi: 10.1111/bjd.19341
87. Thaçi D, Blauvelt A, Reich K, Tsai TF, Vanaclocha F, Kingo K, et al. Secukinumab is Superior to Ustekinumab in Clearing Skin of Subjects With Moderate to Severe Plaque Psoriasis: CLEAR, A Randomized Controlled Trial. *J Am Acad Dermatol* (2015) 73(3):400–9. doi: 10.1016/j.jaad.2015.05.013
88. Blauvelt A, Reich K, Tsai TF, Tyring S, Vanaclocha F, Kingo K, et al. Secukinumab Is Superior to Ustekinumab in Clearing Skin of Subjects With Moderate-to-Severe Plaque Psoriasis Up to 1 Year: Results From the CLEAR Study. *J Am Acad Dermatol* (2017) 76(1):60–9.e9. doi: 10.1016/j.jaad.2016.08.008
89. Bagel J, Blauvelt A, Nia J, Hashim P, Patekar M, de Vera A, et al. Secukinumab Maintains Superiority Over Ustekinumab in Clearing Skin and Improving Quality of Life in Patients With Moderate to Severe Plaque Psoriasis: 52-Week Results From a Double-Blind Phase 3b Trial (CLARITY). *J Eur Acad Dermatol Venereol JEADV* (2021) 35(1):135–42. doi: 10.1111/jdv.16558
90. Griffiths CE, Reich K, Lebwohl M, van de Kerkhof P, Paul C, Menter A, et al. Comparison of Ixekizumab With Etanercept or Placebo in Moderate-to-Severe Psoriasis (UNCOVER-2 and UNCOVER-3): Results From Two Phase 3 Randomised Trials. *Lancet (London England)* (2015) 386 (9993):541–51. doi: 10.1016/S0140-6736(15)60125-8
91. Gordon KB, Blauvelt A, Papp KA, Langley RG, Luger T, Ohtsuki M, et al. Phase 3 Trials of Ixekizumab in Moderate-To-Severe Plaque Psoriasis. *New Engl J Med* (2016) 375(4):345–56. doi: 10.1056/NEJMoa1512711
92. Blauvelt A, Gooderham M, Iversen L, Ball S, Zhang L, Agada NO, et al. Efficacy and Safety of Ixekizumab for the Treatment of Moderate-to-Severe Plaque Psoriasis: Results Through 108 Weeks of a Randomized, Controlled Phase 3 Clinical Trial (UNCOVER-3). *J Am Acad Dermatol* (2017) 77 (5):855–62. doi: 10.1016/j.jaad.2017.06.153
93. Lebwohl MG, Gordon KB, Gallo G, Zhang L, Paul C. Ixekizumab Sustains High Level of Efficacy and Favourable Safety Profile Over 4 Years in Patients With Moderate Psoriasis: Results From UNCOVER-3 Study. *J Eur Acad Dermatol Venereol JEADV* (2020) 34(2):301–9. doi: 10.1111/jdv.15921
94. Reich K, Augustin M, Thaçi D, Pinter A, Leutz A, Henneges C, et al. A 24-Week Multicentre, Randomized, Open-Label, Parallel-Group Study Comparing the Efficacy and Safety of Ixekizumab vs. Fumaric Acid Esters and Methotrexate in Patients With Moderate-to-Severe Plaque Psoriasis Naive to Systemic Treatment. *Br J Dermatol* (2020) 182(4):869–79. doi: 10.1111/bjd.18384
95. Blauvelt A, Leonardi C, Elewski B, Crowley JJ, Guenther LC, Gooderham M, et al. A Head-to-Head Comparison of Ixekizumab vs. Guselkumab in Patients With Moderate-to-Severe Plaque Psoriasis: 24-Week Efficacy and Safety Results From a Randomized, Double-Blinded Trial. *Br J Dermatol* (2021) 184(6):1047–58. doi: 10.1111/bjd.19509
96. Lebwohl M, Strober B, Menter A, Gordon K, Weglowska J, Puig L, et al. Phase 3 Studies Comparing Brodalumab With Ustekinumab in Psoriasis. *New Engl J Med* (2015) 373(14):1318–28. doi: 10.1056/NEJMoa1503824
97. Pinter A, Hoffmann M, Reich K, Augustin M, Kaplan K, Gudjónsdóttir SD, et al. A Phase 4, Randomized, Head-to-Head Trial Comparing the Efficacy of Subcutaneous Injections of Brodalumab to Oral Administrations of Fumaric Acid Esters in Adults With Moderate-to-Severe Plaque Psoriasis (CHANGE). *J Eur Acad Dermatol Venereol JEADV* (2021) 35(3):701–11. doi: 10.1111/jdv.16932
98. Ghoreschi K, Balato A, Enerback C, Sabat R. Therapeutics Targeting the IL-23 and IL-17 Pathway in Psoriasis. *Lancet (London England)* (2021) 397 (10275):754–66. doi: 10.1016/S0140-6736(21)00184-7
99. Nash P, Kirkham B, Okada M, Rahman P, Combe B, Burmester GR, et al. Ixekizumab for the Treatment of Patients With Active Psoriatic Arthritis and an Inadequate Response to Tumour Necrosis Factor Inhibitors: Results From the 24-Week Randomised, Double-Blind, Placebo-Controlled Period of the SPIRIT-P2 Phase 3 Trial. *Lancet (London England)* (2017) 389 (10086):2317–27. doi: 10.1016/S0140-6736(17)31429-0
100. Mease PJ, van der Heijde D, Ritchlin CT, Okada M, Cuchacovich RS, Shuler CL, et al. Ixekizumab, an Interleukin-17A Specific Monoclonal Antibody, for the Treatment of Biologic-Naive Patients With Active Psoriatic Arthritis: Results From the 24-Week Randomised, Double-Blind, Placebo-Controlled and Active (Adalimumab)-Controlled Period of the Phase III Trial SPIRIT-P1. *Ann Rheum Dis* (2017) 76(1):79–87. doi: 10.1136/annrheumdis-2016-209709
101. McInnes IB, Mease PJ, Kirkham B, Kavanaugh A, Ritchlin CT, Rahman P, et al. Secukinumab, a Human Anti-Interleukin-17A Monoclonal Antibody, in Patients With Psoriatic Arthritis (FUTURE 2): A Randomised, Double-Blind, Placebo-Controlled, Phase 3 Trial. *Lancet (London England)* (2015) 386(9999):1137–46. doi: 10.1016/S0140-6736(15)61134-5
102. Ritchlin CT, Kavanaugh A, Merola JF, Schett G, Scher JU, Warren RB, et al. Bimekizumab in Patients With Active Psoriatic Arthritis: Results From a 48-Week, Randomised, Double-Blind, Placebo-Controlled, Dose-Ranging Phase 2b Trial. *Lancet (London England)* (2020) 395(10222):427–40. doi: 10.1016/S0140-6736(19)33161-7
103. Langley RG, Armstrong AW, Lebwohl MG, Blauvelt A, Hsu S, Tyring S, et al. Efficacy and Safety of Brodalumab in Patients With Psoriasis Who had Inadequate Responses to Ustekinumab: Subgroup Analysis of Two Randomized Phase III Trials. *Br J Dermatol* (2019) 180(2):306–14. doi: 10.1111/bjd.17318
104. Kimmel G, Chima M, Kim HJ, Bares J, Yao CJ, Singer G, et al. Brodalumab in the Treatment of Moderate to Severe Psoriasis in Patients When Previous Anti-Interleukin 17A Therapies Have Failed. *J Am Acad Dermatol* (2019) 81 (3):857–9. doi: 10.1016/j.jaad.2019.05.007
105. Antoniu SA. Discontinued Drugs 2011: Pulmonary, Allergy, Gastrointestinal and Arthritis. *Expert Opin Invest Drugs* (2012) 21(11):1607–18. doi: 10.1517/13543784.2012.712112
106. Raychaudhuri SK, Abria C, Raychaudhuri SP. Regulatory Role of the JAK STAT Kinase Signalling System on the IL-23/IL-17 Cytokine Axis in

Psoriatic Arthritis. *Ann Rheum Dis* (2017) 76(10):e36. doi: 10.1136/annrheumdis-2016-211046

107. Valenzuela F, Paul C, Mallbris L, Tan H, Papacharalambous J, Valdez H, et al. Tofacitinib Versus Etanercept or Placebo in Patients With Moderate to Severe Chronic Plaque Psoriasis: Patient-Reported Outcomes From a Phase 3 Study. *J Eur Acad Dermatol Venereol JEADV* (2016) 30(10):1753–9. doi: 10.1111/jdv.13702
108. Clinical Trails. Available at: https://clinicaltrials.gov/ct2/show/NCT01490632?cond=NCT01490632&draw=2&rank=1.
109. Clinical Trails. Available at: https://clinicaltrials.gov/ct2/show/NCT01634087?cond=NCT01634087&draw=1&rank=1.
110. Clinical Trails. Available at: https://clinicaltrials.gov/ct2/show/NCT02969018?cond=NCT02969018&draw=2&rank=1.
111. Forman SB, Pariser DM, Poulin Y, Vincent MS, Gilbert SA, Kieras EM, et al. TYK2/JAK1 Inhibitor PF-06700841 in Patients With Plaque Psoriasis: Phase IIa, Randomized, Double-Blind, Placebo-Controlled Trial. *J Invest Dermatol* (2020) 140(12):2359–70 e5. doi: 10.1016/j.jid.2020.03.962
112. Clinical Trails. Available at: https://clinicaltrials.gov/ct2/show/NCT03895372?cond=NCT03895372&draw=1&rank=1.
113. Clinical Trails. Available at: https://clinicaltrials.gov/ct2/show/NCT03924427?cond=NCT03924427&draw=2&rank=1.

4

Psoriasis: Classical vs. Paradoxical: The Yin-Yang of TNF and Type I Interferon

*Alessio Mylonas and Curdin Conrad**

Department of Dermatology, University Hospital CHUV, Lausanne, Switzerland

***Correspondence:**
Curdin Conrad
curdin.conrad@chuv.ch

Chronic plaque psoriasis is a common debilitating skin disease. The identification of the pathogenic role of the TNF/IL-23/T_H17 pathway has enabled the development of targeted therapies used in the clinic today. Particularly, TNF inhibitors have become a benchmark for the treatment of numerous chronic inflammatory diseases such as psoriasis. Although being highly effective in psoriasis treatment, anti-TNFs can themselves induce psoriasis-like skin lesions, a side effect called paradoxical psoriasis. In this review, we provide a comprehensive look at the different cellular and molecular players involved in classical plaque psoriasis and contrast its pathogenesis to paradoxical psoriasis, which is clinically similar but immunologically distinct. Classical psoriasis is a T-cell mediated autoimmune disease driven by TNF, characterised by T-cells memory, and a relapsing disease course. In contrast, paradoxical psoriasis is caused by the absence of TNF and represents an ongoing type-I interferon-driven innate inflammation that fails to elicit T-cell autoimmunity and lacks memory T cell-mediated relapses.

Keywords: plaque psoriasis, paradoxical psoriasis, TNF, IL-23, T_H17, type I-interferon

INTRODUCTION

Psoriasis is a distinctly human, chronic, inflammatory skin disease, affecting 2–3% of the population worldwide, with prevalence varying considerably according to race and geographic location (1). Clinically, plaque type psoriasis, the most common form of psoriasis, is characterised by well-demarcated erythematous lesions covered with silvery-white scales. These lesions are histologically reflected by keratinocyte hyperproliferation leading to epidermal hyperplasia (acanthosis), characteristic elongation of the rete ridges (papillomatosis), thickening of the cornified layer (hyperkeratosis), and incomplete keratinocyte differentiation resulting in retention of nuclei in the stratum corneum (parakeratosis). Leukocytes, including T-cells, dendritic cells, neutrophils, and macrophages make up a considerable dermal and epidermal immune cell infiltrate. Psoriasis is caused by the interaction of predisposing genetic factors and environmental triggers leading to dysregulated innate and adaptive immune responses. Today, psoriasis is widely regarded as a T-cell-mediated autoimmune disease and skin infiltrating T lymphocytes play key effector roles by driving disease development and maintenance. Dendritic cells producing TNF and IL-23 stimulate activation of both $CD4^+$ and $CD8^+$ T-cells, which in turn migrate into the epidermis. Upon recognition of autoantigens, T-cells produce T_H17-cytokines such as IL-17A, IL-17F, and IL-22, which drive the psoriatic phenotype by inducing keratinocyte hyperproliferation. In support of this, several single nucleotide polymorphisms cluster throughout this pathway including genes in the TNF/dendritic cell activation pathway (*TNFAIP3, REL, TN1P1, NFKBIA*) as well as in the T-cell activation (*HLA-Cw6, ERAP1/ZAP70, ETS1, SOCS1, TNFRSF9*), and T_H17/T_C17-differentiation pathways (*IL23A, IL23R*) (2, 3). Consequently, antibodies targeting the pathogenic TNF/IL-23/IL-17 pathway have revolutionised psoriasis treatment over the past 15 years and are widely used in the clinic today.

In particular, TNF blockade has become the benchmark in management of numerous chronic inflammatory diseases, such as rheumatoid arthritis, Crohn's disease, and psoriasis (4–7). As such, more than two million patients have already been treated with anti-TNFs and, with the advent of biosimilars, these figures are expected to grow further over the coming years. Yet, targeting TNF is not without consequence, as TNF is a potent pro-inflammatory cytokine known to coordinate immune responses and play an important role in limiting the spread of infectious pathogens. Thus, TNF blockade leads to an increased risk of infections and slightly increased risk for certain malignancies. However, more surprisingly, anti-TNF treatment can also induce new psoriasis-like skin lesions in about 2–5% of treated patients (8).

As anti-TNFs are amongst the most potent anti-inflammatory drugs used in the treatment of psoriasis, developing psoriasis-like skin lesions due to TNF blockade was somewhat paradoxical—hence the designation "paradoxical psoriasis."

This review aims to provide a focussed overview of the latest developments in the T-cell and cytokine networks in classical psoriasis, and contrast them to paradoxical psoriasis induced by anti-TNFs, which is clinically similar to psoriasis but immunologically distinct. Finally, these findings will be put into perspective with future avenues of research and possible clinical interventions.

CLASSICAL PSORIASIS

The Established Role of T-Helper and the Revisited Cytotoxic T-Cells

The pathogenic role for T-cells in psoriasis is well-established and stems from the following clinical observations and experimental findings: Immunosuppressive agents, such as cyclosporine, or therapies specifically targeting T-cells are efficacious in psoriasis treatment (9–12). *HLA-Cw6* represents the strongest genetic risk variant associated with psoriasis (13). Molecular analysis of psoriasis tissue showed that lesional T-cells are oligoclonal (14) and recognise epidermal autoantigens (15–18). Finally, clinically relevant xenotransplant models of psoriasis have demonstrated an essential functional role for T-cells (19–21).

T-cells migrate into inflamed skin through expression of the skin-homing Cutaneous Lymphocyte-associated Antigen (CLA) (22), LFA-1 and $\alpha_4\beta_1$ (23), and the chemokine receptors CCR8 and CCR10 (24). More specifically T_H1 cells use CXCR3 and CCR4 (25), whereas T_H17 cells use CCR4 and CCR6 (26). Among the most well-described chemokines involved in T-cell migration to the skin are CCL27 (27, 28), and CCL20 (29) produced by keratinocytes upon an inflammatory trigger. While circulating T-cells certainly play an important role in skin immunopathology, there are twice as many T-cells residing in normal healthy skin than are present in the circulation (22). Moreover, pathogenic oligoclonal T-cells remain resident in resolved psoriatic skin lesions suggesting that disease recurrence might be initiated through reactivation of skin-resident T-cells (30). Indeed, these skin-resident memory T-cells were found to be sufficient to drive psoriasis development without further recruitment of circulating cells (19, 20). Activation within the skin led to proliferation of T-cells in the dermal compartment, which preceded keratinocyte hyperproliferation. In fact, the psoriatic phenotype was only induced by migration of T-cells into the epidermis and blockade of the epidermal infiltration by T-cells prevented the development of a psoriatic lesion (20). These findings suggest that intraepidermal T-cells reflect key effector cells in psoriasis.

Traditionally, much attention has been given to differentiated $CD4^+$ T-cell subsets across chronic inflammatory diseases (31–34), including psoriasis (35). However, $CD8^+$ T-cells, which are present in healthy skin as tissue resident memory T-cells (36), have been shown to produce a similar cytokine profile (37). In psoriasis, dermal T-cell infiltrates are mostly comprised of $CD4^+$ cells, whereas the majority of T-cells in the epidermis—which represent key effector cells—are $CD8^+$ (19). Indeed, we could recently show that intraepidermal $CD8^+$ T-cells are functionally essential for psoriasis (38).

Psoriasis has been studied extensively from a genetics perspective, with HLA class I alleles known for more than 40 years to be heavily implicated (39). The *HLA-Cw6* variant is the strongest psoriasis susceptibility allele and has 10-fold higher association with early-onset severe psoriasis. As to how exactly class I HLA molecules might contribute to the pathogenesis of psoriasis is not entirely clear. But in light of the fundamental role of epidermal $CD8^+$ T-cells in psoriasis, the fact that lesional T-cells are of oligoclonal origin and $CD8^+$ T-cells recognise peptide antigens presented on MHC class I molecules suggest a role for epidermal (auto-)antigens in psoriasis. As mentioned above, epidermal $CD8^+$ T-cells in psoriasis are key effectors in psoriasis (20), and they are of oligoclonal origin (14, 30)—thus potentially recognising common antigens. Taken together with *HLA-Cw6* representing the strongest genetic risk variant associated with psoriasis, this suggests that recognition of epidermal (auto-)antigens by $CD8^+$ T-cells is pathogenic in psoriasis.

Indeed, the streptococcal M protein from *Streptococcus pyogenes* has been identified as an antigen target of primarily $CD8^+$ T-cells (40). T-cells directed against the streptococcal M-protein had the ability to react to keratin 14, which is overexpressed in psoriatic skin, due to sequence homology and antigenic similarity (molecular mimicry). Thus, the immune response to a streptococcal infection could divert T-cells toward skin antigens and cause skin pathology. Intriguingly, streptococcal throat infections are a well-known trigger factor for onset and exacerbation of psoriasis.

Other recently identified epidermal autoantigens include keratin 7 (41) and the antimicrobial peptide LL37 expressed by keratinocytes (17) as well as the melanocyte antigen ADAMTSL5 (18). Finally, CD1a-restricted lipids were also found to elicit T-cell responses in psoriatic patients (42). Interestingly, CD1a-autoreactive T-cells isolated from skin were identified as T_H22 cells producing IL-22 (43), a cytokine overexpressed in psoriasis and known to drive keratinocyte hyperproliferation.

Antigen-recognition by T-cells is thought to play a pivotal role in psoriasis, but an all-encompassing consensus on the nature of autoreactivity has yet to be reached. Despite this, all of the identified auto-antigens to date are significantly upregulated in psoriatic skin as compared to uninvolved or healthy skin. Because the majority can be induced locally upon injury, the prevailing model postulates that skin trauma could lead to upregulation of putative auto-antigens and their recognition by tissue-resident antigen-experienced T-cells in psoriasis patients.

Cytokine Networks: The TNF/IL-23/IL-17 Axis

Nowadays, the pathogenic role of the TNF/IL-23/T_H17 axis in psoriasis is well-known and numerous biologics targeting the different cytokines of this pro-inflammatory pathway are widely used in the clinic. Yet, the arrival of TNF blockers in the early 2000s completely revolutionised the management of psoriasis and other chronic inflammatory diseases. Despite underwhelming results of anti-TNF in sepsis (44), the successful use in rheumatoid arthritis (RA) spurred trials in other chronic inflammatory diseases such as Crohn's disease, psoriasis and psoriatic arthritis (45).

TNF is known to be potently produced by immune and non-immune cells including macrophages, T-cells, dendritic cells (DC), neutrophils, and fibroblasts. One of its major roles is to mount appropriate adaptive immune responses to tumors and pathogens. This is achieved through several mechanisms. Induction of DC-maturation leads to upregulation of CD40, CD80, CD83, and CD86 thereby potentiating T-cell receptor (TCR)-mediated responses and amplifying weak antigen affinity interactions (46). It also serves to limit the immune-suppressive effects of regulatory T-cells (47) and to enhance proliferation and survival of committed effector memory T-cells. In line with these findings, TNF is critically required to mount effective $CD8^+$ T-cell responses against tumors and for the recruitment of T-cells into tumor sites (48). These pro-inflammatory effects of TNF are corroborated in psoriasis, where TNF is found to dictate the inflammatory environment in several ways (49–52). In detailed histological and molecular investigations, it was found to be mostly produced by mature conventional DCs. Blockade of TNF leads to an initial reduction of the chemokine CCL20, which preferentially recruits T_H17 cells into inflamed tissue, coinciding with loss of IL-17 and diminution of dermal and epidermal T-cells. In addition, it leads to normalisation of DC numbers and reduction of IL-23 cytokine expression, followed by normalised keratinocyte differentiation, and eventually to histological improvement and clinical response. Taken together, TNF maintains a pro-inflammatory environment that primes pathogenic T_H17 T-cells through induction of IL-23, maintaining them at the site of inflammation, and sustaining T_H17 cytokine production (53, 54).

Though TNF might contribute to increased IL-17 production by T_H17 cells (55), IL-23 directly governs T_H17 cytokine production both by critically participating in T_H17 cell polarisation as well as by stimulating production of IL-17 by differentiated T_H17 cells (56, 57). Initial supportive evidence for a functional role of IL-23 in psoriasis included the clinical efficacy of an anti-p40 monoclonal antibody (blocking both IL-12 and IL-23) in psoriasis (58) and the association of a single nucleotide polymorphism in the *IL23R* gene in psoriasis patients (55, 59). Confirmation soon followed by the successful use of IL-23-specific antibodies in clinically relevant mouse models and then in patients (60, 61). In addition, IL-4 abrogated T_H17 cell-mediated inflammation by selectively silencing IL-23 in antigen-presenting cells while sparing IL-12/T_H1 immunity (62) and resulting in therapeutic outcome. In psoriasis, IL-23 is mainly produced by activated DCs but keratinocytes and other non-immune cells probably contribute to its production. In fact, it has been shown recently that TNF-dependent epigenetic control of IL-23 expression in keratinocytes plays a role in chronic skin inflammation (63).

T_H17 cytokines, such as IL-17A, IL-17F, and IL-22, represent the key effector cytokines in psoriasis pathogenesis as they directly drive the development of a psoriatic phenotype. They induce epidermal hyperproliferation, attract neutrophils to the skin, and activate keratinocytes to produce chemokines and antimicrobial peptides, which sustain the inflammatory process (64). There are six homologous IL-17 cytokines (A through F) which are produced by either haematopoietic or non-haematopoietic cells, can signal through different combinations of receptors, and mediate distinct biological activities. The individual members are reviewed in this issue by Brembilla et al. (65). Besides the aforementioned effects in the pathogenesis of psoriasis, IL-17 can act in synergy with TNF to further potentiate expression of multiple pro-inflammatory mediators known to play a role in psoriasis, such as IL-8, beta-defensins, S100A proteins, IL-19, and CCL20 (29, 66–68). As such, concurrent inhibition of TNF and IL17 might result in more effective therapy. Though, a bi-specific dual variable domain immunoglobulin targeting both cytokines did not demonstrate increased efficacy compared to anti-TNF in RA (69), this remains to be tested in psoriasis.

While antibodies targeting IL-17 have shown great efficacy in psoriasis (53, 70), blockade of IL-22 failed to meet primary end points in clinical trials indicating distinct role for IL-17 and IL-22 in psoriasis. IL-22, which is produced by T_H17 cells (71) and exclusively by a distinct T_H22 subpopulation (72, 73), had previously been regarded as a very promising target. In psoriasis, IL-22 is found to be produced by dermal $CD4^+$ but also by epidermal $CD8^+$ T_C17 and $CD4^+$ T_H22 cells (38, 74, 75), as well as Innate Lymphoid Cells (76, 77), and mast cells (78). Interestingly, skin-resident T-cells mediating disease memory in clinically resolved psoriasis plaques were found to be epidermal T_C17 and T_H22 cells producing mainly IL-22 (75). Upon binding to its heterodimeric receptor consisting of IL-22RA1 and IL10Rβ (79), which is expressed on keratinocytes (80), IL-22 induces proliferation of keratinocytes and inhibits terminal maturation (81, 82). While transient expression of IL-22 upon skin injury promotes epidermal remodelling with re-epithelisation of skin wounds (74), its chronic expression by psoriatic T-cells drives keratinocyte hyperproliferation and epidermal hyperplasia. In line with this, in transgenic mice, IL-22 was sufficient to induce a skin phenotype that resembles psoriasis (82), and the psoriatic phenotype induced by skin injection of IL-23 was abrogated in IL-22-deficient mice (83). However, the pathogenic function of IL-22 shows redundancy with other members of the IL-20 subfamily of cytokines such as IL-19 and IL-20, potentially rendering its blockade clinically ineffective in humans.

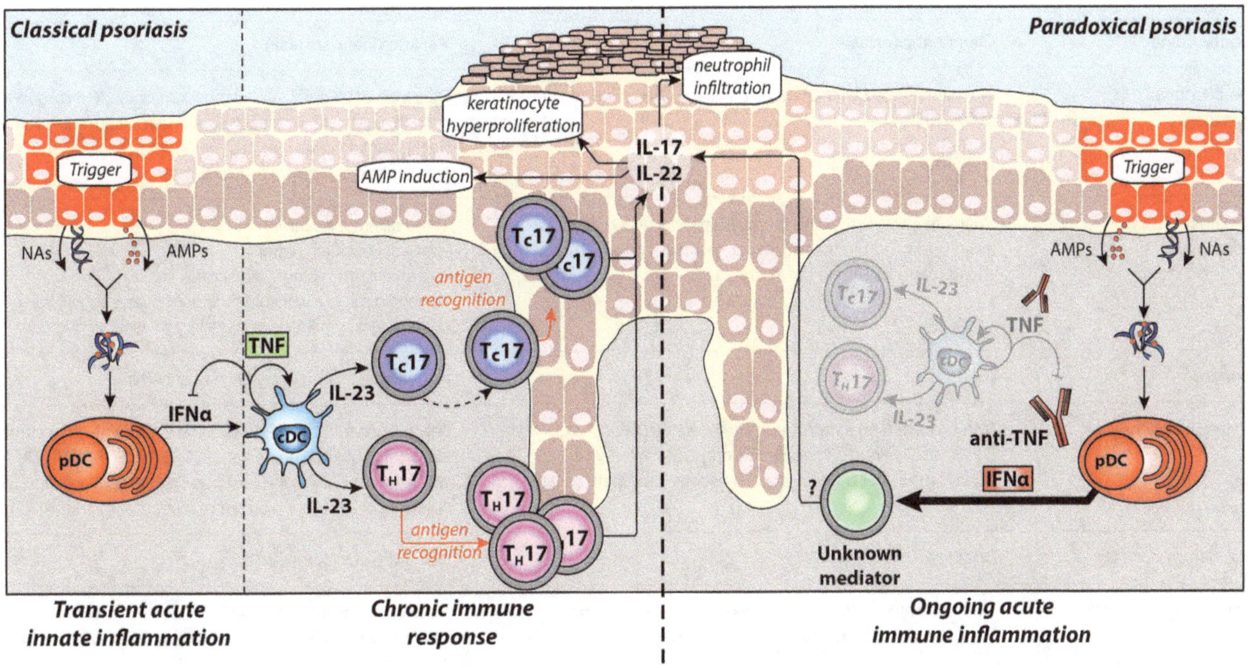

FIGURE 1 | Pathogenesis of classical plaque psoriasis and paradoxical psoriasis. Antimicrobial peptides (AMPs), which are produced by keratinocytes upon skin injury or released by neutrophils, form complexes with nucleic acids (NAs) released by dying cells. These complexes activate plasmacytoid dendritic cells (pDC) to produce large amounts IFNα during the acute/early phase of psoriasis pathogenesis. IFNα activates conventional dendritic cells (cDCs), which in turn produce TNF and IL-23. TNF induces the maturation of cDCs and pDCs, which lose their ability to produce IFNα. Thus, in classical psoriasis, early IFNα production gets relayed by TNF that controls and limits the IFNα production by pDCs via a negative feedback loop (through induction of pDC maturation). Subsequently, IL-23 and other pro-inflammatory cytokines produced by cDCs drive the activation of potentially autoreactive T-cells, which proliferate and, particularly CD8$^+$ T_C cells, migrate into the epidermis. Upon antigen recognition they produce the T_H17 cytokines IL-17 and IL-22 that induce keratinocyte hyperproliferation, attract neutrophils to the skin, and upregulate AMP production providing a positive feedback loop eventually resulting in the psoriatic phenotype (chronic/late phase). Normally, during anti-TNF therapy, the absence of TNF and consequently of downstream cytokines suppresses pathogenic T-cells thereby alleviating classical psoriasis. However, in patients developing paradoxical psoriasis, TNF blockade inhibits pDC maturation and leads to sustained IFNα production. In addition, as cDC cannot mature in absence of TNF, paradoxical psoriasis fails to elicit a T cell mediated autoimmune response. Thus, paradoxical psoriasis remains in an ongoing IFNα-driven acute immune inflammation independent of T-cells. The exact pathogenic downstream mechanism of IFNα-driven paradoxical psoriasis skin lesions remains to be fully elucidated.

Detailed knowledge about the pathogenesis of chronic plaque psoriasis and the central role for the TNF/IL-23/T_H17 pathway has led to the development of therapies targeting the pathogenic cytokines, including anti-TNFs, anti-p40 (IL-12/IL-23), anti-p19 (IL-23 specific), anti-IL-17A, and anti-IL-17 receptor antibodies. This pathway and its pathogenic mechanisms in classical plaque psoriasis are illustrated in **Figure 1**. However, less is known about instigators of psoriasis and pathogenic upstream triggers of acute cutaneous inflammation.

Type I Interferons, Setting the Tone for Autoimmunity?

Type I IFNs are key cytokines in antiviral host defence due to their ability to limit viral replication and to induce an effective antiviral immune response (84, 85). They promote maturation of myeloid DCs and priming of CD8$^+$ T-cells (86), induce T-cell proliferation (87), and sustain their survival (88). In addition, type-I IFNs stimulate differentiation of B-cells into antibody-secreting plasma cells (89). Thus, type-I IFNs are essential for the induction of an effective immune response against viruses. Although produced by all nucleated cells, they are preferentially expressed by a rare type of circulating cells called plasmacytoid dendritic cells (pDCs) (90). Upon viral recognition through endosomal Toll-like receptors (TLR) 7 and 9, pDCs produce extraordinary amounts of type-I IFN, and, therefore, have also been called professional IFN producing cells (90, 91). Under normal conditions, pDCs are not present in peripheral tissues, but they get recruited to the skin in case of infection, injury, autoimmunity, and cancer (64). Skin wounding induces rapid skin infiltration of pDCs and transient expression of type-I IFNs, which accelerate re-epithelialisation (92).

As self-nucleic acids are abundantly released into the extracellular environment during apoptotic and necrotic cell death, it is essential that pDCs avoid inappropriate activation by host-derived nucleic acid, but retain the ability to quickly respond to viral DNA and RNA. To achieve this, TLRs that sense nucleic acids are located intracellularly within endosomes, which prevents activation by extracellular self-DNA/RNA but allows immune response to viruses that actively invade the cells. Moreover, extracellular nucleases rapidly degrade nucleic acid released by dying cells without affecting DNA or RNA contained within viruses (93). Thus, under normal circumstances

TABLE 1 | Classical vs. Paradoxical psoriasis- differences, similarities, and treatment strategies.

Characteristics	Classical psoriasis	Paradoxical psoriasis
Clinico-phenotypic presentation	Well-demarcated erythematous plaques covered with silvery-white scales.	Presence of different psoriatic patterns including plaque-type, guttate, pustular forms as well as eczematiform presentation. Palmoplantar zones affected more often. Non-cicatricial alopecia regularly noted.
Histo-pathological appearance	Characteristic psoriatic histology: Epidermal hyperplasia (acanthosis), papillomatosis, hyper-/parakeratosis, dermal, and epidermal immune cell infiltrates.	Three different patterns: -classical psoriatic pattern -eczematiform pattern with spongiosis -lichenoid pattern with interface dermatitis often all these patterns are simultaneously present at variable degrees.
Recurrence	Relapsing.	Non-relapsing (upon cessation of anti-TNF).
Genetic associations	Many known (and established): *HLA-Cw6*, *IL12B*, *IL23A*, *IL23R*, and various components along type-I interferon signalling, NF-KB signalling, and other signalling pathways.	Few proposed: *IL23R* (an allele that is protective concerning classical psoriasis), and *FBXL19*, *CTLA4*, *SCL12A8*, *TAPI* which have an unclear role in paradoxical psoriasis and the outcome of the allele is undetermined.
Role of TNF	Driven by TNF.	Induced by blockade of TNF.
Role of adaptive immunity	T-cell mediated. Intraepidermal and dermal (autoimmune) T_H/T_C17-cells found throughout skin lesions.	T-cell independent. Significant reduced numbers of intraepidermal $CD8^+$ T_C-cells as compared to classical psoriasis.
Role of innate immunity	Transiently driven by pDC derived type-I IFN during the early phase of psoriasis development. Mature cDCs and neutrophils present in large numbers in skin lesions of chronic/late phase of classical psoriasis.	Driven by unabated type-I IFN produced by non-maturing pDCs. Immature dendritic cells, and neutrophils often present in lesions. Role for other cell types not known (particularly in mediating the psoriatic phenotype).
Pathogenic mechanism	Chronic (autoimmune) T_H/T_C17-mediated inflammation	Unabated, ongoing type-I IFN-driven innate inflammation, absence of T-cell autoimmunity.
Treatment avenues	-targeting TNF highly effective	-switch to different class of biologics (other than anti-TNF) often needed in severe cases of paradoxical psoriasis
	Various other treatment strategies validated:	In the absence of detailed knowledge about the pathogenic pathways, proposition of:
	-targeting of IL-12/IL-23 highly effective -targeting of IL-23 highly effective -targeting IL-17A and its receptor highly effective -targeting type-I interferon is ineffective in established classical chronic plaque-type psoriasis.	-use of anti-IL12/IL23 (successful in case reports) -unknown efficacy of IL-23 specific biologics -unknown efficacy of targeting IL-17A and its receptor -targeting type-I interferons and/or pDCs potentially effective

host-derived self-DNA/RNA released by apoptotic or damaged cells cannot activate TLR9 and 7. However, they can become potent triggers of pDC activation and type-I IFN production in the presence of endogenous antimicrobial peptides (AMP) such as LL37 and beta-defensins (94–96). AMPs are typically not expressed in healthy skin under steady-state conditions, but are transiently produced by keratinocytes or released by infiltrating neutrophils in response to skin wounding or infections (97–99). Their cationic and amphipathic structure allows AMPs to interact with and disrupt microbial membranes, which typically contain a high degree of negative charges (100). Besides their role as direct effector molecules against microorganisms, AMPs are also involved in the initiation of inflammation by breaking innate tolerance to otherwise inert extracellular self-DNA and self-RNA. Cationic AMPs bind to negatively charged fragments of nucleic acid to form aggregated and condensed structures that are resistant to extracellular degradation. Translocation of these complexes into endosomes and activation of TLR7 and 8 (RNA), or TLR9 (DNA) lead to sustained production of IFNα and IFNβ by pDCs (94–96).

Under physiological conditions, AMP-expression with activation of pDCs by AMP-nucleic acid complexes is transient, controlled by the damaging or infectious stimulus. By contrast, in psoriasis, the expression of AMPs is persistent and leads to sustained production of type-I IFNs by pDCs, which accumulate in the dermis of early developing psoriatic lesions (101). Subsequently, these trigger activation of myeloid DCs and autoreactive T-cells. Recent work has demonstrated that IFNα particularly drives the activation and skin infiltration of pathogenic $CD8^+$ T-cells in psoriasis (102). Moreover, IFNα conditioned DCs produce large amounts of IL-23 (103, 104) indicating an important role for type-I IFNs in driving T_H/T_C17-mediated (auto)immunity in psoriasis. Indeed, depletion of pDCs or blocking type-I IFN signalling both inhibited psoriasis development confirming that its overexpression by pDCs reflects a critical early/acute event in the pathogenesis of psoriasis (101). This is further supported by the observations that *de novo* psoriasis or pre-existing psoriasis can be triggered and/or aggravated by IFNα therapy (105–108) and the TLR7 agonist imiquimod (109, 110). Interestingly, epidermal trauma, which induces AMP expression by keratinocytes and attracts pDCs into the skin, is also a typical trigger of psoriasis known as Koebner phenomenon.

Taken together, type-I IFNs play a critical role in the acute/early phase of psoriasis pathogenesis by (1) activating dermal myeloid DC, (2) inducing their maturation by upregulating co-stimulatory molecules and HLA molecules, and (3) participating in T_H/T_C17 polarisation of autoimmune T-cells through induction of IL-23 production by myeloid DCs (**Figure 1**).

PARADOXICAL PSORIASIS

Almost two decades of clinical experience with anti-TNFs have provided considerable advances in our understanding of the biology of TNF. More than 2 million patients have been treated with anti-TNFs so far.

Expected side effects such as increased susceptibility to infection and a slightly increased risk for malignancies have been confirmed (111–113), though the cancer risk still remains a matter of debate (114, 115). However, the observation that anti-TNFs, which are normally extremely effective in the treatment of chronic inflammatory diseases, could lead to aggravation of pre-existing autoimmune diseases and onset of new inflammatory diseases, was unexpected and a paradox. In fact, lupus-like syndrome can be observed in 0.5–1% of anti-TNF treated patients and 2–5% of patients develop psoriasis-like skin lesions, called paradoxical psoriasis (8, 116, 117). They represent important side effects in the treatment of major chronic autoimmune diseases as they potentially necessitate treatment cessation. Since the first description of paradoxical psoriasis (117, 118), numerous cases have been reported (119–121). Paradoxical psoriasis appears independently of the underlying disease or the type of anti-TNF agent used and regresses upon discontinuation of therapy, which suggests that paradoxical psoriasis does represent a side effect of TNF blockade and not *de novo* psoriasis. Though the side effect is a well-established phenomenon, its pathogenesis had remained elusive and only recently, the dysbalance of TNF and type-I IFN (yin-yang of TNF and IFNα) has been confirmed as a pathogenic mechanism underlying paradoxical psoriasis (8).

The first clues for a link between anti-TNF therapy and increased type-I IFN expression came from the observation that anti-TNF therapy induces an IFN signature in blood of juvenile arthritis patients (122). Likewise, anti-TNF treatments promote formation of anti-nuclear antibodies (123), which are associated with increased type-I IFN levels in SLE patients (124). Furthermore, anti-TNFs can induce or aggravate lupus, a well-known type-I IFN-driven autoimmune disease (125, 126). Indeed, patients with anti-TNF induced paradoxical psoriasis showed an increased IFN signature in lesional skin (127). Recently, we could confirm that TNF controls the production of type I-IFN by pDCs and that anti-TNF induces its unabated overexpression driving paradoxical psoriasis (8).

Upon activation, pDCs produce type-I IFNs first, which is relayed by their production of TNF. TNF induces maturation of pDCs, which upregulate costimulatory molecules and lose their ability to produce interferons (8, 128). Thereby, TNF limits the duration of type-I IFN production by pDCs, while conversely, TNF blockade decreases pDC maturation and extends their ability to produce type-I IFN. This supports a yin-yang model of TNF and type-I IFN. In classical plaque psoriasis, early transient overexpression of type-I IFN is replaced by a dominant TNF-driven chronic inflammation. In contrast, TNF blockade leads to an ongoing type-I IFN mediated acute inflammation in paradoxical psoriasis (**Figure 1**).

Another important distinction between the two entities is that in paradoxical psoriasis, unlike classical psoriasis, T-cells play a redundant role (8). Hence, both classical and paradoxical psoriasis are induced by pDC-derived type-I IFN. But while classical psoriasis develops into a T-cell mediated autoimmune disease, paradoxical psoriasis represents an ongoing type-I IFN-driven innate immune response that fails to elicit T cell autoimmunity. In line with this, there are no relapses of paradoxical psoriasis upon discontinuation of anti-TNF therapy, which supports lack of T-cell mediated disease memory in paradoxical psoriasis.

It remains unclear what triggers the activation of pDCs and eventually drives paradoxical psoriasis. Potentially certain environmental factors such as microbes could trigger development of paradoxical psoriasis, as a considerable number of patients have been found to have concurrent superinfections (129). Furthermore, the yin yang of TNF and type-I IFN, the pathogenic mechanism underlying paradoxical psoriasis, is inherently true for healthy individuals as much as patients. But only 2–5% of anti-TNF treated patients develop paradoxical psoriasis indicating that there is another key determining factor such as genetic predisposition for paradoxical psoriasis. Among polymorphisms associated with psoriasis, five have been identified to also be associated to paradoxical psoriasis, and these include *IL23R*, *FBXL19*, *CTLA4*, *SLC12A8*, and *TAP1* (130) though it remains to be determined exactly how they would fit in the pathological mechanism.

Though classical and paradoxical psoriasis have similarities in their clinical presentation, many distinctions have been identified in recent years as to the pathogenic mechanism. **Table 1** summarises key similarities and differences between the two entities, and highlights potential treatment strategies.

OUTLOOK

Detailed knowledge on classical plaque psoriasis, particularly by identifying the relevant role of the TNF/IL-23/T_H17 axis in its pathogenesis, has allowed for novel, more targeted therapies.

Though newer treatments targeting IL-23 and IL-17 show better efficacy, today, anti-TNFs remain a gold-standard in psoriasis management. Yet important immunological side effects of TNF blockade, such as paradoxical psoriasis and lupus-like syndrome, may require premature discontinuation of an otherwise effective treatment option for patients. These side effects are caused by an unabated type-I IFN-driven immune response making it an intriguing target in these patients. While, anti-IFNs have not shown efficacy in chronic plaque psoriasis confirming the distinct inflammatory pathways in chronic and acute forms of classical psoriasis (131), they provided promising results in SLE. Therefore, type-I IFN blockade might be a valuable treatment option in acute forms of psoriasis such as erythrodermic or guttate psoriasis as well as in paradoxical psoriasis. However, simultaneous inhibition of the interferon pathway together with the ongoing TNF blockade might increase the infectious risk too considerably. Therefore, targeting IFN-producing pDCs (i.e., *via* anti-ILT-7, anti-BDCA2) or inhibiting TLR 7 and 9, thereby blocking pDC activation, could provide more suitable therapeutic options in patients that need continuation of their anti-TNF treatment. In this way, production of type-I IFNs by monocytes and stromal cells would remain intact and might allow sufficient immune responses toward infectious agents.

Despite considerable advances in the understanding of paradoxical psoriasis and its pathogenesis, several questions are still unanswered. Downstream mechanisms that mediate the interferon-driven psoriatic phenotype of paradoxical psoriasis remain unknown as IFNα does not directly induce keratinocyte hyperproliferation. The identification of cytokines involved and their cellular source might provide additional novel targets for therapeutic intervention. In addition, biomarkers to predict side effects such as paradoxical psoriasis and lupus-like syndrome could help optimising the management of patients with chronic inflammatory diseases.

AUTHOR CONTRIBUTIONS

AM and CC wrote and edited the manuscript and figures.

ACKNOWLEDGMENTS

We acknowledge funding from the Gottfried & Julia Bangerter-Rhyner Foundation, the University Hospital of Lausanne (CHUV), and the Faculty of Biology and Medicine of the University of Lausanne (FBM-UNIL).

REFERENCES

1. Parisi R, Symmons DP, Griffiths CE, Ashcroft DM, et al. Global epidemiology of psoriasis: a systematic review of incidence and prevalence. *J Invest Dermatol.* (2013) 133:377–85. doi: 10.1038/jid.2012.339
2. Tsoi LC, Spain SL, Knight J, Ellinghaus E, Stuart PE, Capon F, et al. Identification of 15 new psoriasis susceptibility loci highlights the role of innate immunity. *Nat Genet.* (2012) 44:1341–8. doi: 10.1038/ng.2467
3. Tsoi LC, Spain SL, Ellinghaus E, Stuart PE, Capon F, Knight J, et al. Enhanced meta-analysis and replication studies identify five new psoriasis susceptibility loci. *Nat Commun.* (2015) 6:7001. doi: 10.1038/ncomms8001
4. Moreland LW, Baumgartner SW, Schiff MH, Tindall EA, Fleischmann RM, Weaver AL, et al. Treatment of rheumatoid arthritis with a recombinant human Tumour Necrosis Factor Receptor (p75)-Fc fusion protein. *N Engl J Med.* (1997) 337:141–8.
5. Leonardi CL, Powers JL, Matheson RT, Goffe BS, Zitnik R, Wang A, et al. Etanercept as monotherapy in patients with psoriasis. *N Engl J Med.* (2003) 349:2014–2023. doi: 10.1056/NEJMoa030409
6. Rutgeerts P, Sandborn WJ, Feagan BG, Reinisch W, Olson A, Johanns J, et al. Infliximab for induction and maintenance therapy for ulcerative colitis. *N Engl J Med.* (2005) 353:2462–76. doi: 10.1056/NEJMoa050516
7. Taylor PC, Feldmann M. Anti-TNF biologic agents: still the therapy of choice for rheumatoid arthritis. *Nat Rev Rheumatol.* (2009) 5:578–82. doi: 10.1038/nrrheum.2009.181
8. Conrad C, Di Domizio J, Mylonas A, Belkhodja C, Demaria O, Navarini AA, et al. TNF blockade induces a dysregulated type I interferon response without autoimmunity in paradoxical psoriasis. *Nat Commun.* (2018) 9:25. doi: 10.1038/s41467-017-02466-4
9. Weinshenker BG, Bass BH, Ebers GC, Rice GP. Remission of psoriatic lesions with muromonab-CD3 (Orthoclone OKT3) treatment. *J Am Acad Dermatol.* (1989) 20:1132–3.
10. Bachelez H, Flageul B, Dubertret L, Fraitag S, Grossman R, Brousse N, et al. Treatment of recalcitrant plaque psoriasis with a humanized non-depleting antibody to CD4. *J Autoimmun* (1998) 11:53–62.
11. Gottlieb SL, Gilleaudeau P, Johnson R, Estes L, Woodworth TG, Gottlieb AB, et al. Response of psoriasis to a lymphocyte-selective toxin (DAB389IL-2) suggests primary immune, but not keratinocyte, pathogenic basis. *Nat Med.* (1995) 1:442–8.
12. Krueger GG, Ellis CN. Alefacept therapy produces remission for patients with chronic plaque psoriasis. *Br J Dermatol.* (2003) 148:784–8. doi: 10.1046/j.1365-2133.2003.05239.x
13. Nair RP, Stuart PE, Nistor I, Hiremagalore R, Chia NVC, Jenisch S, et al. Sequence and haplotype analysis supports HLA-C as the psoriasis susceptibility 1 gene. *Am J Hum Genet.* (2006) 78:827–51. doi: 10.1086/503821
14. Prinz JC, Vollmer S, Boehncke WH, Menssen A, Laisney I, Trommler P. Selection of conserved TCR VDJ rearrangements in chronic psoriatic plaques indicates a common antigen in psoriasis vulgaris. *Eur J Dermatol.* (1999) 29:3360–8.
15. Vollmer S, Menssen A, Prinz JC. Dominant lesional T cell receptor rearrangements persist in relapsing psoriasis but are absent from nonlesional skin: evidence for a stable antigen-specific pathogenic T cell response in psoriasis vulgaris. *J Invest Dermatol.* (2001) 117:1296–301. doi: 10.1046/j.0022-202x.2001.01494.x
16. Sigmundsdottir H, Sigurgeirsson B, Troye-Blomberg M, Good MF, Valdimarsson H, Jonsdottir I. Circulating T cells of patients with active psoriasis respond to streptococcal M-peptides sharing sequences with human epidermal keratins. *Scand J Immunol.* (1997) 45:688–97.
17. Lande R, Botti E, Jandus C, Dojcinovic D, Fanelli G, Conrad C, et al. The antimicrobial peptide LL37 is a T-cell autoantigen in psoriasis. *Nat Commun.* (2014) 5:5621. doi: 10.1038/ncomms6621
18. Arakawa A, Siewert K, Stöhr J, Besgen P, Kim SM, Rühl G, et al. Melanocyte antigen triggers autoimmunity in human psoriasis. *J Exp Med.* (2015) 212:2203–12. doi: 10.1084/jem.20151093
19. Boyman O, Hefti HP, Conrad C, Nickoloff BJ, Suter M, Nestle FO. Spontaneous development of psoriasis in a new animal model shows an essential role for resident T cells and tumor necrosis factor-alpha. *J Exp Med.* (2004) 199:731–6. doi: 10.1084/jem.20031482
20. Conrad C, Boyman O, Tonel G, Tun-Kyi A, Laggner U, de Fougerolles A, et al. Alpha1beta1 integrin is crucial for accumulation of epidermal T cells and the development of psoriasis. *Nat Med.* (2007) 13:836–42. doi: 10.1038/nm1605

21. Wrone-Smith T, Nickoloff BJ. Dermal injection of immunocytes induces psoriasis. *J Clin Invest.* (1996) 98:1878–87. doi: 10.1172/JCI118989
22. Clark RA, Chong B, Mirchandani N, Brinster NK, Yamanaka K, Dowgiert RK, et al. The vast majority of CLA+ T cells are resident in normal skin. *J Immunol.* (2006) 176:4431–9. doi: 10.4049/jimmunol.176.7.4431
23. Teraki Y, Miyake A, Takebayashi R, Shiohara T. Homing receptor and chemokine receptor on intraepidermal T cells in psoriasis vulgaris. *Exp Dermatol.* (2004) 29: 658–63. doi: 10.1111/j.1365-2230.2004.01638.x
24. Schaerli P, Ebert L, Willimann K, Blaser A, Roos RS, Loetscher P, et al. A skin-selective homing mechanism for human immune surveillance T cells. *J Exp Med.* (2004) 199:1265–75. doi: 10.1084/jem.20032177
25. Al-Banna NA, Vaci M, Slauenwhite D, Johnston B, Issekutz TB. CCR4 and CXCR3 play different roles in the migration of T cells to inflammation in skin, arthritic joints, and lymph nodes. *Eur J Immunol.* (2014) 44:1633–43. doi: 10.1002/eji.201343995
26. Pène J, Chevalier S, Preisser L, Vénéreau E, Guilleux MH, Ghannam S, et al. Chronically inflamed human tissues are infiltrated by highly differentiated Th17 Lymphocytes. *J Immunol.* (2008) 180:7423–30. doi: 10.4049/jimmunol.180.11.7423
27. Homey B, Alenius H, Müller A, Soto H, Bowman EP, Yuan W, et al. CCL27–CCR10 interactions regulate T cell–mediated skin inflammation. *Nat Med.* (2002) 8:157–66. doi: 10.1038/nm0202-157
28. Sigmundsdottir H, Pan J, Debes GF, Alt C, Habtezion A, Soler D, et al. DCs metabolize sunlight-induced vitamin D3 to 'program' T cell attraction to the epidermal chemokine CCL27. *Nat Immunol.* (2007) 8:285–93. doi: 10.1038/ni1433
29. Homey B, Dieu-Nosjean MC, Wiesenborn A, Massacrier C, Pin JJ, Oldham E, et al. Up-regulation of macrophage inflammatory protein-3 /CCL20 and CC chemokine receptor 6 in psoriasis. *J Immunol.* (2000) 164:6621–32. doi: 10.4049/jimmunol.164.12.6621
30. Matos TR, O'Malley JT, Lowry EL, Hamm D, Kirsch IR, Robins HS, et al. Clinically resolved psoriatic lesions contain psoriasis-specific IL-17-producing alphabeta T cell clones. *J Clin Invest.* (2017) 127:4031–41. doi: 10.1172/JCI93396
31. Matos TR, O'Malley JT, Lowry EL, Hamm D, Kirsch IR, Robins HS, et al. Diversification of T-helper-cell lineages: finding the family root of IL-17-producing cells. *Nat Rev Immunol.* (2006) 6:329–33. doi: 10.1038/nri1807
32. Raphael I, Nalawade S, Eagar TN, Forsthuber TG, T cell subsets and their signature cytokines in autoimmune and inflammatory diseases. *Cytokine* (2015) 74:5–17. doi: 10.1016/j.cyto.2014.09.011
33. Walker JA, McKenzie ANJ. TH2 cell development and function. *Nat Rev Immunol.* (2018) 18:121–33. doi: 10.1038/nri.2017.118
34. Stockinger B, Omenetti S. The dichotomous nature of T helper 17 cells. *Nat Rev Immunol.* (2017) 17:535–44. doi: 10.1038/nri.2017.50
35. Diani M, Altomare G, Reali E. T helper cell subsets in clinical manifestations of psoriasis. *J Immunol Res.* (2016) 2016:7692024. doi: 10.1155/2016/7692024
36. Watanabe R, Gehad A, Yang C, Scott LL, Teague JE, Schlapbach C, et al. Human skin is protected by four functionally and phenotypically discrete populations of resident and recirculating memory T cells. *Sci Transl Med.* (2015) 7:279ra39. doi: 10.1126/scitranslmed.3010302
37. Hijnen D, Knol EF, Gent YY, Giovannone B, Beijn SJ, Kupper TS, et al. CD8(+) T cells in the lesional skin of atopic dermatitis and psoriasis patients are an important source of IFN-gamma, IL-13, IL-17, and IL-22. *J Invest Dermatol.* (2013) 133:973–9. doi: 10.1038/jid.2012.456
38. Di Meglio P, Villanova F, Navarini AA, Mylonas A, Tosi I, Nestle FO, et al. Targeting CD8(+) T cells prevents psoriasis development. *J Allergy Clin Immunol.* (2016) 138:274–276.e276. doi: 10.1016/j.jaci.2015.10.046
39. Tiilikainen A, Lassus A, Karvonen J, Vartiainen P, Julin M. Psoriasis and HLA-Cw6. *Br J Dermatol.* (1980) 102:179–84.
40. Johnston A, Gudjonsson JE, Sigmundsdottir H, Love TJ, Valdimarsson H. Peripheral blood T cell responses to keratin peptides that share sequences with streptococcal M proteins are largely restricted to skin-homing CD8+ T-cells. *Clin Exp Dermatol.* (2004) 138:83–93. doi: 10.1111/j.1365-2249.2004.02600.x
41. Yunusbaeva M, Valiev R, Bilalov F, Sultanova Z, Sharipova L, Yunusbayev B. Psoriasis patients demonstrate HLA-Cw*06:02 allele dosage-dependent T cell proliferation when treated with hair follicle-derived keratin 17 protein. *Sci Rep.* (2018) 8:6098. doi: 10.1038/s41598-018-24491-z
42. Cheung KL, Jarrett R, Subramaniam S, Salimi M, Gutowska-Owsiak D, Chen YL, et al. Psoriatic T cells recognize neolipid antigens generated by mast cell phospholipase delivered by exosomes and presented by CD1a. *J Exp Med.* (2016) 213:2399–412. doi: 10.1084/jem.20160258
43. de Jong A, Peña-Cruz V, Cheng TY, Clark RA, Van Rhijn I, Moody DB. CD1a-autoreactive T cells are a normal component of the human alphabeta T cell repertoire. *Nat Immunol.* (2010) 11:1102–9. doi: 10.1038/ni.1956
44. Fisher CJ, Agosti JM, Opal SM, Lowry SF, Balk RA, Sadoff JC, et al. Treatment of septic shock with the tumor necrosis factor receptor:Fc fusion protein. *New Engl J Med.* (1996) 334:1697–702. doi: 10.1056/Nejm199606273342603
45. Monaco C, Nanchahal J, Taylor P, Feldmann M. Anti-TNF therapy: past, present and future. *Int Immunol.* (2015) 27:55–62. doi: 10.1093/intimm/dxu102
46. Maney NJ, Reynolds G, Krippner-Heidenreich A, Hilkens CMU. Dendritic cell maturation and survival are differentially regulated by TNFR1 and TNFR2. *J Immunol.* (2014) 193:4914–23. doi: 10.4049/jimmunol.1302929
47. Chen X, Hamano R, Subleski JJ, Hurwitz AA, Howard OM, Oppenheim JJ. Expression of costimulatory TNFR2 induces resistance of CD4+FoxP3-conventional T cells to suppression by CD4+FoxP3+ regulatory T cells. *J Immunol.* (2010) 185:174–82. doi: 10.4049/jimmunol.0903548
48. Calzascia T, Pellegrini M, Hall H, Sabbagh L, Ono N, Elford AR, et al. TNF-alpha is critical for antitumor but not antiviral T cell immunity in mice. *J Clin Invest.* (2007) 117:3833–45. doi: 10.1172/JCI32567
49. Gottlieb AB. Tumor necrosis factor blockade: mechanism of action. *J Investig Dermatol Symp Proc.* (2007) 12:1–4. doi: 10.1038/sj.jidsymp.5650029
50. Tan JK, Aphale A, Malaviya R, Sun Y, Gottlieb AB. Mechanisms of action of etanercept in psoriasis. *J Investig Dermatol Symp Proc.* (2007) 12:38–45. doi: 10.1038/sj.jidsymp.5650037
51. Zaba LC, Cardinale I, Gilleaudeau P, Sullivan-Whalen M, Suárez-Fariñas M, Fuentes-Duculan J, et al. Amelioration of epidermal hyperplasia by TNF inhibition is associated with reduced Th17 responses. *J Exp Med.* (2007) 204:3183–94. doi: 10.1084/jem.20071094
52. Zaba LC, Suárez-Fariñas M, Fuentes-Duculan J, Nograles KE, Guttman-Yassky E, Cardinale I, et al. Effective treatment of psoriasis with etanercept is linked to suppression of IL-17 signaling, not immediate response TNF genes. *J Allergy Clin Immunol.* (2009) 124:1022–10.e1-395. doi: 10.1016/j.jaci.2009.08.046
53. Langley RG, Elewski BE, Lebwohl M, Reich K, Griffiths CE, Papp K, et al. Secukinumab in plaque psoriasis–results of two phase 3 trials. *N Engl J Med.* (2014) 371:326–38. doi: 10.1056/NEJMoa1314258
54. Gordon KB, Colombel JF, Hardin DS. Phase 3 Trials of Ixekizumab in moderate to severe plaque psoriasis. *N Engl J Med.* (2016) 375:2102. doi: 10.1056/NEJMc1610828
55. Cargill M, Schrodi SJ, Chang M, Garcia VE, Brandon R, Callis KP, et al. A large-scale genetic association study confirms IL12B and leads to the identification of IL23R as psoriasis-risk genes. *Am J Hum Genet.* (2007) 80:273–90. doi: 10.1086/511051
56. Wilson NJ, Boniface K, Chan JR, McKenzie BS, Blumenschein WM, Mattson JD, et al. Development, cytokine profile and function of human interleukin 17-producing helper T cells. *Nat Immunol.* (2007) 8:950–7. doi: 10.1038/ni1497
57. Gaffen SL, Jain R, Garg AV, Cua DJ, The IL-23-IL-17 immune axis: from mechanisms to therapeutic testing. *Nat Rev Immunol.* (2014) 14:585–600. doi: 10.1038/nri3707
58. Lowes MA, Bowcock AM, Krueger JG. Pathogenesis and therapy of psoriasis. *Nature* (2007) 445:866–73. doi: 10.1038/nature05663
59. Capon F, Di Meglio P, Szaub J, Prescott NJ, Dunster C, Baumber L, et al. Sequence variants in the genes for the interleukin-23 receptor (IL23R) and its ligand (IL12B) confer protection against psoriasis. *Hum Genet.* (2007) 122:201–6. doi: 10.1007/s00439-007-0397-0
60. Tonel G, Conrad C, Laggner U, Di Meglio P, Grys K, McClanahan TK, et al. Cutting edge: a critical functional role for IL-23 in psoriasis. *J Immunol.* (2010) 185:5688–91. doi: 10.4049/jimmunol.1001538
61. Kopp T, Riedl E, Bangert C, Bowman EP, Greisenegger E, Horowitz A, et al. Clinical improvement in psoriasis with specific targeting of interleukin-23. *Nature* (2015) 521:222–6. doi: 10.1038/nature14175
62. Guenova E, Skabytska Y, Hoetzenecker W, Weindl G, Sauer K, Tham M, et al. IL-4 abrogates T(H)17 cell-mediated inflammation by selective silencing of

IL-23 in antigen-presenting cells. *Proc Natl Acad Sci USA.* (2015) 112:2163–8. doi: 10.1073/pnas.1416922112
63. Li H, Yao Q, Mariscal AG, Wu X, Hülse J, Pedersen E, et al. Epigenetic control of IL-23 expression in keratinocytes is important for chronic skin inflammation. *Nat Commun.* (2018) 9:1420. doi: 10.1038/s41467-018-03704-z
64. Conrad C, Meller S, Gilliet M. Plasmacytoid dendritic cells in the skin: to sense or not to sense nucleic acids. *Semin Immunol.* (2009) 21:101–9. doi: 10.1016/j.smim.2009.01.004
65. Brembilla NC, Senra L, Boehncke WH. The IL-17 family of cytokines in psoriasis: IL-17A and beyond. *Front Immunol.* (2018) 9:1682. doi: 10.3389/fimmu.2018.01682
66. Wang CQF, Akalu YT, Suarez-Farinas M, Gonzalez J, Mitsui H, Lowes MA, et al. IL-17 and TNF synergistically modulate cytokine expression while suppressing melanogenesis: potential relevance to psoriasis. *J Invest Dermatol.* (2013) 133:2741–52. doi: 10.1038/jid.2013.237
67. Albanesi C, Cavani A, Girolomoni G. IL-17 is produced by nickel-specific T lymphocytes and regulates ICAM-1 expression and chemokine production in human keratinocytes: synergistic or antagonist effects with IFN-g and TNF-a. *J Immunol.* (1998) 162:494–502.
68. Chiricozzi A, Guttman-Yassky E, Suárez-Fariñas M, Nograles KE, Tian S, Cardinale I, et al. Integrative responses to IL-17 and TNF-alpha in human keratinocytes account for key inflammatory pathogenic circuits in psoriasis. *J Invest Dermatol.* (2011) 131:677–87. doi: 10.1038/jid.2010.340
69. Genovese MC, Weinblatt ME, Aelion JA, Mansikka HT, Peloso PM, Chen K, et al. ABT-122, a bispecific DVD-immunoglobulin targeting TNF- and IL-17A, in RA with inadequate response to methotrexate: a randomized, double-blind study. *Arthritis Rheumatol.* (2018) 70:1710–20. doi: 10.1002/art.40580
70. Leonardi C, Matheson R, Zachariae C, Cameron G, Li L, Edson-Heredia E, et al. Anti-interleukin-17 monoclonal antibody ixekizumab in chronic plaque psoriasis. *N Engl J Med.* (2012) 366:1190–9. doi: 10.1056/NEJMoa1109997
71. Liang SC, Tan XY, Luxenberg DP, Karim R, Dunussi-Joannopoulos K, Collins M, et al. Interleukin (IL)-22 and IL-17 are coexpressed by Th17 cells and cooperatively enhance expression of antimicrobial peptides. *J Exp Med.* (2006) 203:2271–9. doi: 10.1084/jem.20061308
72. Duhen T, Geiger R, Jarrossay D, Lanzavecchia A, Sallusto F. Production of interleukin 22 but not interleukin 17 by a subset of human skin-homing memory T cells. *Nat Immunol.* (2009) 10:857–63. doi: 10.1038/ni.1767
73. Trifari S, Kaplan CD, Tran EH, Crellin NK, Spits H. Identification of a human helper T cell population that has abundant production of interleukin 22 and is distinct from T(H)-17, T(H)1 and T(H)2 cells. *Nat Immunol.* (2009) 10:864–71. doi: 10.1038/ni.1770
74. Eyerich S, Eyerich K, Pennino D, Carbone T, Nasorri F, Pallotta S, et al. Th22 cells represent a distinct human T cell subset involved in epidermal immunity and remodeling. *J Clin Invest.* (2009) 119:3573–85. doi: 10.1172/JCI40202
75. Cheuk S, Wikén M, Blomqvist L, Nylén S, Talme T, Ståhle M, et al. Epidermal Th22 and Tc17 cells form a localized disease memory in clinically healed psoriasis. *J Immunol.* (2014) 192:3111–20. doi: 10.4049/jimmunol.1302313
76. Teunissen MBM, Munneke JM, Bernink JH, Spuls PI, Res PCM, Te Velde A, et al. Composition of innate lymphoid cell subsets in the human skin: enrichment of NCR(+) ILC3 in lesional skin and blood of psoriasis patients. *J Invest Dermatol.* (2014) 134:2351–60. doi: 10.1038/jid.2014.146
77. Villanova F, Flutter B, Tosi I, Grys K, Sreeneebus H, Perera GK, et al. Characterization of innate lymphoid cells in human skin and blood demonstrates increase of NKp44+ ILC3 in psoriasis. *J Invest Dermatol.* (2014) 134:984–91. doi: 10.1038/jid.2013.477
78. Mashiko S, Bouguermouh S, Rubio M, Baba N, Bissonnette R, Sarfati M. Human mast cells are major IL-22 producers in patients with psoriasis and atopic dermatitis. *J Allergy Clin Immunol.* (2015) 136:351–359.e351. doi: 10.1016/j.jaci.2015.01.033
79. Xie MH, Aggarwal S, Ho WH, Foster J, Zhang Z, Stinson J, et al. Interleukin (IL)-22, a novel human cytokine that signals through the interferon receptor-related proteins CRF2-4 and IL-22R. *J Biol Chem.* (2000) 275:31335–9. doi: 10.1074/jbc.M005304200
80. Wolk K, Kunz S, Witte E, Friedrich M, Asadullah K, Sabat R. IL-22 increases the innate immunity of tissues. *Immunity* (2004) 21:241–54. doi: 10.1016/j.immuni.2004.07.007
81. Boniface K, Bernard FX, Garcia M, Gurney AL, Lecron JC, Morel F. IL-22 inhibits epidermal differentiation and induces proinflammatory gene expression and migration of human keratinocytes. *J Immunol.* (2005) 174:3695–702. doi: 10.4049/jimmunol.174.6.3695
82. Wolk K, Haugen HS, Xu W, Witte E, Waggie K, Anderson M, et al. IL-22 and IL-20 are key mediators of the epidermal alterations in psoriasis while IL-17 and IFN-gamma are not. *J Mol Med.* (2009) 87:523–36. doi: 10.1007/s00109-009-0457-0
83. Zheng Y, Danilenko DM, Valdez P, Kasman I, Eastham-Anderson J, Wu J, et al. Interleukin-22, a T(H)17 cytokine, mediates IL-23-induced dermal inflammation and acanthosis. *Nature* (2007) 445:648–51. doi: 10.1038/nature05505
84. Theofilopoulos AN, Baccala R, Beutler B, Kono DH. Type I interferons (alpha/beta) in immunity and autoimmunity. *Annu Rev Immunol.* (2005) 23:307–36. doi: 10.1146/annurev.immunol.23.021704.115843
85. McNab F, Mayer-Barber K, Sher A, Wack A, O'Garra A. Type I interferons in infectious disease. *Nat Rev Immunol.* (2015) 15:87–103. doi: 10.1038/nri3787
86. Le Bon A, Etchart N, Rossmann C, Ashton M, Hou S, Gewert D, et al. Cross-priming of CD8+ T cells stimulated by virus-induced type I interferon. *Nat Immunol.* (2003) 4:1009–15. doi: 10.1038/ni978
87. Tough DF, Borrow P, Sprent J. Induction of bystander T cell proliferation by viruses and type I interferon *in vivo*. *Science* (1996) 272:1947–50.
88. Marrack P, Kappler J, Mitchell T. Type I interferons keep activated T cells alive. *J Exp Med.* (1999) 189:521–30.
89. Jego G, Palucka AK, Blanck JP, Chalouni C, Pascual V, Banchereau J. Plasmacytoid dendritic cells induce plasma cell differentiation through type I interferon and interleukin 6. *Immunity* (2003) 19:225–34. doi: 10.1016/s1074-7613(03)00208-5
90. Siegal FP, Kadowaki N, Shodell M, Fitzgerald-Bocarsly PA, Shah K, Ho S, et al. The nature of the principal type 1 interferon-producing cells in human blood. *Science* (1999) 284:1835–7.
91. Cella M, Jarrossay D, Facchetti F, Alebardi O, Nakajima H, Lanzavecchia A, et al. Plasmacytoid monocytes migrate to inflamed lymph nodes and produce large amounts of type I interferon. *Nat Med.* (1999) 5:919–23. doi: 10.1038/11360
92. Gregorio J, Meller S, Conrad C, Di Nardo A, Homey B, Lauerma A, et al. Plasmacytoid dendritic cells sense skin injury and promote wound healing through type I interferons. *J Exp Med.* (2010) 207:2921–30. doi: 10.1084/jem.20101102
93. Gilliet M, Lande R. Antimicrobial peptides and self-DNA in autoimmune skin inflammation. *Curr Opin Immunol.* (2008) 20:401–7. doi: 10.1016/j.coi.2008.06.008
94. Lande R, Gregorio J, Facchinetti V, Chatterjee B, Wang YH, Homey B, et al. Plasmacytoid dendritic cells sense self-DNA coupled with antimicrobial peptide. *Nature* (2007) 449:564–9. doi: 10.1038/nature06116
95. Ganguly D, Chamilos G, Lande R, Gregorio J, Meller S, Facchinetti V, et al. Self-RNA-antimicrobial peptide complexes activate human dendritic cells through TLR7 and TLR8. *J Exp Med.* (2009) 206:1983–94. doi: 10.1084/jem.20090480
96. Lande R, Chamilos G, Ganguly D, Demaria O, Frasca L, Durr S, et al. Cationic antimicrobial peptides in psoriatic skin cooperate to break innate tolerance to self-DNA. *Eur J Immunol.* (2015) 45:203–13. doi: 10.1002/eji.201344277
97. Dorschner RA, Pestonjamasp VK, Tamakuwala S, Ohtake T, Rudisill J, Nizet V, et al. Cutaneous injury induces the release of cathelicidin anti-microbial peptides active against group A Streptococcus. *J Invest Dermatol.* (2001) 117:91–7. doi: 10.1046/j.1523-1747.2001.01340.x
98. Schauber J, Dorschner RA, Coda AB, Büchau AS, Liu PT, Kiken D, et al. Injury enhances TLR2 function and antimicrobial peptide expression through a vitamin D-dependent mechanism. *J Clin Invest.* (2007) 117:803–11. doi: 10.1172/JCI30142
99. Sorensen O, Arnljots K, Cowland JB, Bainton DF, Borregaard N. The human antibacterial cathelicidin, hCAP-18, is synthesized in myelocytes and metamyelocytes and localized to specific granules in neutrophils. *Blood* (1997) 90:2796–803.
100. Zasloff M. Antimicrobial peptides of multicellular organisms. *Nature* (2002) 415:389–95. doi: 10.1038/415389a
101. Nestle FO, Conrad C, Tun-Kyi A, Homey B, Gombert M, Boyman O, et al. Plasmacytoid predendritic cells initiate psoriasis through interferon-alpha

production. *J Exp Med.* (2005) 202:135–43. doi: 10.1084/jem.20050500

102. Stockenhuber K, Hegazy AN, West NR, Ilott NE, Stockenhuber A, Bullers SJ, et al. Foxp3(+) T reg cells control psoriasiform inflammation by restraining an IFN-I-driven CD8(+) T cell response. *J Exp Med.* (2018) 215:1987–98. doi: 10.1084/jem.20172094
103. Lapenta C, Santini SM, Spada M, Donati S, Urbani F, Accapezzato D, et al. IFN-alpha-conditioned dendritic cells are highly efficient in inducing cross-priming CD8(+) T cells against exogenous viral antigens. *Eur J Immunol.* (2006) 36:2046–60. doi: 10.1002/eji.200535579
104. Santini SM, Lapenta C, Donati S, Spadaro F, Belardelli F, Ferrantini M. Interferon-alpha-conditioned human monocytes combine a Th1-orienting attitude with the induction of autologous Th17 responses: role of IL-23 and IL-12. *PLoS ONE* (2011) 6:e17364. doi: 10.1371/journal.pone.0017364
105. Funk J, Langeland T, Schrumpf E, Hanssen LE. Psoriasis induced by interferon-a. *Br J Dermatol.* (1991) 125:463–5.
106. Lemmenmeier E, Gaus B, Schmid P, Hoffmann M. A case of erythrodermia from exacerbated psoriasis vulgaris due to treatment of acute hepatitis C. *BMC Dermatol.* (2016) 16:5. doi: 10.1186/s12895-016-0042-5
107. Damiani G, Franchi C, Pigatto P, Altomare A, Pacifico A, Petrou S, et al. Outcomes assessment of hepatitis C virus-positive psoriatic patients treated using pegylated interferon in combination with ribavirin compared to new Direct-Acting Antiviral agents. *World J Hepatol.* (2018) 10:329–36. doi: 10.4254/wjh.v10.i2.329
108. Pauluzzi P, Kokelj F, Perkan V, Pozzato G, Moretti M. Psoriasis exacerbation induced by interferon-alpha. Report of two cases. *Acta Derm Venereol.* (1993) 73:395.
109. Gilliet M, Conrad C, Geiges M, Cozzio A, Thürlimann W, Burg G, et al. Psoriasis triggered by toll-like receptor 7 agonist imiquimod in the presence of dermal plasmacytoid dendritic cell precursors. *Arch Dermatol.* (2004) 140:1490–5. doi: 10.1001/archderm.140.12.1490
110. Eyerich K, Eyerich S. Immune response patterns in non-communicable inflammatory skin diseases. *J Eur Acad Dermatol Venereol.* (2018) 32:692–703. doi: 10.1111/jdv.14673
111. Burmester GR, Panaccione R, Gordon KB, McIlraith MJ, Lacerda AP. Adalimumab: long-term safety in 23 458 patients from global clinical trials in rheumatoid arthritis, juvenile idiopathic arthritis, ankylosing spondylitis, psoriatic arthritis, psoriasis and Crohn's disease. *Ann Rheum Dis.* (2013) 72:517–24. doi: 10.1136/annrheumdis-2011-201244
112. Ali T, Kaitha S, Mahmood S, Ftesi A, Stone J, Bronze MS. Clinical use of anti-TNF therapy and increased risk of infections. *Drug Healthc Patient Saf.* (2013) 5:79–99. doi: 10.2147/DHPS.S28801
113. Bongartz T, Sutton AJ, Sweeting MJ, Buchan I, Matteson EL, Montori V. Anti-TNF antibody therapy in rheumatoid arthritis and the risk of serious infections and malignancies: systematic review and meta-analysis of rare harmful effects in randomized controlled trials. *JAMA* (2006) 295:2275–85. doi: 10.1001/jama.295.19.2275
114. Wu CY, Chen DY, Shen JL, Ho HJ, Chen CC, Kuo KN, et al. The risk of cancer in patients with rheumatoid arthritis taking tumor necrosis factor antagonists: a nationwide cohort study. *Arthritis Res Ther.* (2014) 16:449. doi: 10.1186/s13075-014-0449-5
115. Costenbader KH, Glass R, Cui J, Shadick N. Risk of serious infections and malignancies with anti-TNF antibody therapy in rheumatoid arthritis. *JAMA* (2006) 296:2201; author reply: 2203–4. doi: 10.1001/jama.296.18.2201-a
116. Aringer M, Smolen JS. The role of tumor necrosis factor-alpha in systemic lupus erythematosus. *Arthritis Res Ther.* (2008) 10:202. doi: 10.1186/ar2341
117. Sfikakis PP, Iliopoulos A, Elezoglou A, Kittas C, Stratigos A. Psoriasis induced by anti-tumor necrosis factor therapy: a paradoxical adverse reaction. *Arthritis Rheum.* (2005) 52:2513–8. doi: 10.1002/art.21233
118. Baeten D, Kruithof E, Van den Bosch F, Van den Bossche N, Herssens A, Mielants H, et al. Systematic safety follow up in a cohort of 107 patients with spondyloarthropathy treated with infliximab: a new perspective on the role of host defence in the pathogenesis of the disease? *Ann Rheum Dis.* (2003) 62:829–34. doi: 10.1136/ard.62.9.829
119. Cohen JD, Bournerias I, Buffard V, Paufler A, Chevalier X, Bagot M, et al. Psoriasis induced by tumor necrosis factor-alpha antagonist therapy: a case series. *J Rheumatol.* (2007) 34:380–5.
120. de Gannes GC, Ghoreishi M, Pope J, Russell A, Bell D, Adams S, et al. Psoriasis and pustular dermatitis triggered by TNF-{alpha} inhibitors in patients with rheumatologic conditions. *Arch Dermatol.* (2007) 143:223–31. doi: 10.1001/archderm.143.2.223
121. Brown G, Wang E, Leon A, Huynh M, Wehner M, Matro R, et al. Tumor necrosis factor-alpha inhibitor-induced psoriasis: Systematic review of clinical features, histopathological findings, and management experience. *J Am Acad Dermatol.* (2017) 76:334–41. doi: 10.1016/j.jaad.2016.08.012
122. Palucka AK, Blanck JP, Bennett L, Pascual V, Banchereau J. Cross-regulation of TNF and IFNa in autoimmune diseases. *Proc Natl Acad Sci USA.* (2005) 102:3372–7. doi: 10.1073/pnas.0408506102
123. Ivashkiv LB. Type I interferon modulation of cellular responses to cytokines and infectious pathogens: potential role in SLE pathogenesis. *Autoimmunity* (2003) 36:473–9. doi: 10.1080/08916930310001605882
124. Ytterberg SR, Schnitzer TJ. Serum interferon levels in patients with systemic lupus erythematosous. *Arthritis Rheum.* (1982) 25:401–7.
125. Bengtsson AA, Sturfelt G, Truedsson L, Blomberg J, Alm G, Vallin H, et al. Activation of type I interferon system in systemic lupus erythematosus correlates with disease activity but not with antiretroviral antibodies. *Lupus* (2000) 9:664–71. doi: 10.1191/096120300674499064
126. Blanco P, Palucka AK, Gill M, Pascual V, Banchereau J. Induction of dendritic cell differentiation by IFN-alpha in systemic lupus erythematosus. *Science* (2001) 294:1540–3. doi: 10.1126/science.1064890
127. Seneschal J, Milpied B, Vergier B, Lepreux S, Schaeverbeke T, Taïeb A. Cytokine imbalance with increased production of interferon-alpha in psoriasiform eruptions associated with antitumour necrosis factor-alpha treatments. *Br J Dermatol.* (2009) 161:1081–8. doi: 10.1111/j.1365-2133.2009.09329.x
128. Soumelis V, Liu YJ. From plasmacytoid to dendritic cell: morphological and functional switches during plasmacytoid pre-dendritic cell differentiation. *Eur J Immunol.* (2006) 36:2286–92. doi: 10.1002/eji.200636026
129. Cleynen I, Vermeire S. Paradoxical inflammation induced by anti-TNF agents in patients with IBD. *Nat Rev Gastroenterol Hepatol.* (2012) 9:496–503. doi: 10.1038/nrgastro.2012.125
130. Cabaleiro T, Prieto-Pérez R, Navarro R, Solano G, Román M, Ochoa D, et al. Paradoxical psoriasiform reactions to anti-TNFalpha drugs are associated with genetic polymorphisms in patients with psoriasis. *Pharmacogenomics J* (2016) 16:336–40. doi: 10.1038/tpj.2015.53
131. Bissonnette R, Papp K, Maari C, Yao Y, Robbie G, White WI, et al. A randomized, double-blind, placebo-controlled, phase I study of MEDI-545, an anti-interferon-alfa monoclonal antibody, in subjects with chronic psoriasis. *J Am Acad Dermatol.* (2010) 62:427–36. doi: 10.1016/j.jaad.2009.05.042

5

Potential Immunological Links Between Psoriasis and Cardiovascular Disease

*Aparna P. Sajja, Aditya A. Joshi, Heather L. Teague, Amit K. Dey and Nehal N. Mehta**

National Heart, Lung, and Blood Institute, National Institutes of Health, Bethesda, MD, United States

Correspondence:
Nehal N. Mehta
nehal.mehta@nih.gov

Preclinical and clinical research provide strong evidence that chronic, systemic inflammation plays a key role in development and progression of atherosclerosis. Indeed, chronic inflammatory diseases, such as psoriasis, are associated with accelerated atherosclerosis and increased risk of cardiovascular events. Contemporary research has demonstrated plausible mechanistic links between immune cell dysfunction and cardiometabolic disease in psoriasis. In this review, we describe the role of potential common immunological mechanisms underlying both psoriasis and atherogenesis. We primarily discuss innate and adaptive immune cell subsets and their contributions to psoriatic disease and cardiovascular morbidity. Emerging efforts should focus on understanding the interplay among immune cells, adipose tissue, and various biomarkers of immune dysfunction to provide direction for future targeted therapy.

Keywords: psoriasis, cardiovascular disease, inflammation, atherosclerosis, vascular inflammation, inflammatory cytokines

INTRODUCTION

Inflammation is the hallmark of atherosclerosis (1). Preclinical and clinical research provide strong evidence that chronic inflammation is critical to the process of atherogenesis. Chronic inflammatory diseases, such as psoriasis, are associated with accelerated atherosclerosis and increased risk of cardiovascular events (2–6). Atherosclerosis is increasingly recognized as an inflammatory process, thus similarities between atherosclerosis and chronic, systemic inflammatory diseases have become an emerging focus of interest. Almost 20% patients with coronary heart disease lack conventional risk factors (7), supporting the importance of evaluating residual inflammatory risk (8). Chronic inflammatory diseases such as psoriasis have been shown to add 6% additional risk (9, 10) to the Framingham Risk Score (8, 9) highlighting the need to understand the role of immunological processes in cardiovascular disease (CVD) for better risk stratification and treatment strategies.

CHRONIC INFLAMMATION AND CARDIOVASCULAR CO-MORBIDITIES

Patients with chronic inflammatory diseases are predisposed to cardiometabolic diseases including obesity, hypertension, and dyslipidemia (11–16)—chronic inflammatory conditions common in the general population (17–19). Obesity, particularly visceral, is strongly associated with dysregulated expression of inflammatory cytokines such as tumor necrosis factor-alpha (TNF-α), interleukin-1 beta (IL-1β), and IL-6, as well as adiponectin and leptin, contributing to metabolic derangement and insulin resistance (13, 18, 20). Atherogenic metabolic dyslipidemia is common in chronic inflammation. Abnormalities include impaired reverse cholesterol transport ability of the HDL, increased LDL particle number, and decreased LDL size (21–23). Animal and human models have demonstrated innate immunity as well as experimental *in vivo* induction of inflammation *via* bolus of an inflammatory cytokine such as TNF-α or IL-6, results in release of adipokines and generation of peripheral insulin resistance (24–27). Moreover, anti-inflammatory therapies such as aspirin, colchicine, and more recently canakinumab have been effective in CVD treatment, supporting the critical role of inflammation in CVD (28–32).

One of the most common co-morbid conditions associated with psoriasis is psoriatic arthritis (PsA). Epidemiological data indicate that almost one-third patients with psoriasis also have prevalent PsA (33). Similar to psoriasis, PsA is associated with increased prevalence of traditional cardiovascular risk factors, greater subclinical CVD assessed as vascular inflammation (VI) by 18-FDG PET/CT and ultrasound-guided carotid plaque assessment and intima-media thickness measurement, and elevated rates of major adverse cardiovascular events (MACEs) (34–38). Furthermore, like psoriasis, traditional risk factors do not fully capture the risk of CVD in PsA (39, 40).

Recently, there is growing focus on shared immunological links between atherosclerosis and several other autoimmune diseases such as systemic lupus erythematosus, inflammatory bowel disease, human immunodeficiency virus infection, rheumatoid arthritis, and psoriasis. These all carry an accelerated CVD risk, thought to be partly attributable to inflammation-driven endothelial dysfunction, lipoprotein derangement, and metabolic dysfunction stemming from chronic inflammation (41, 42). In order to speed understanding of inflammatory cardiometabolic dysfunction, psoriasis has been utilized as a human model (3) to understand the role of innate and adaptive immunity in subclinical CVD (43, 44). The clinical implications of understanding how the inflammatory processes in psoriasis contribute to cardiovascular morbidity are vast since approximately 3% of the US population has psoriasis. Furthermore, observational reports have suggested that anti-inflammatory therapies commonly used to treat psoriasis may associate with reduced cardiovascular risk (45, 46).

POTENTIAL IMMUNOLOGIC LINKS BETWEEN PSORIASIS AND CVD

Psoriasis Is Associated With Subclinical and Clinical Atherosclerosis

In the last decade, multiple studies have demonstrated an association between psoriasis and both subclinical and clinical atherosclerosis, such as VI by ^{18}F-FDG PET/CT, coronary artery calcium and non-calcified coronary plaque burden by coronary computed tomography angiography (44, 47–51). Population-based studies provide evidence of early subclinical and clinical CVD in psoriasis (2, 4, 52, 53). Research into the concept of psoriatic march (54) has led to an understanding of common cellular and molecular level links between psoriasis and atherosclerosis (55).

Common Immune Cells Between Psoriasis and Atherosclerosis

T Cells

Studies in the last two decades have established psoriasis primarily as a T-cell-mediated disorder (56–60). While initial evidence implicated a predominant role of helper T cells type 1 (Th1) through downstream activation of macrophages, neutrophils, and CD8$^+$ cytotoxic T lymphocytes (61), recent research shows the importance of the Th17 and other IL-17 producing cell types such as CD8$^+$ T cells and γδ T cells (62). Although Th1 subtype is the most studied cell-type in psoriasis, different stages of this chronic inflammatory disease employ various cells of innate and adaptive immunity (62). All the subtypes of T cells involved in pathogenesis of psoriasis are also involved in atherosclerosis (63).

Th1 Cells—Helper T Cells Type 1

Activation of the innate immune system is the key event in beginning the inflammatory cascade in psoriasis. It primarily includes differentiation of T cells into Th1 cells catalyzed by IL-12 (62). Mechanistic studies in patients with psoriasis have suggested a preference of hematopoietic progenitors toward Th1 subtype (64). Th1 cells induce psoriatic inflammation by activating neutrophils, macrophages, and CD8$^+$ cytotoxic T lymphocytes (61). Primary mediators of Th1 activity are interferon-gamma (IFN-γ), IL-2, and TNF-α, which act on keratinocytes and induce antimicrobial peptide production that subsequently continues the inflammatory cascade. Th1 cells are also critical to the process of atherosclerosis, a process thought to be primarily driven by IFN-γ, the hallmark cytokine of the Th1 response (65). In patients with unstable angina and acute coronary syndrome (ACS), Th1 cells were found to be elevated (66, 67). Furthermore, mechanistic studies have also established the role of IL-12 in the development and progression of early atherosclerotic plaques (68–70). In addition, IL-18, a Th1-promoting cytokine, has also been shown to have a role in atherosclerosis (71, 72). Finally, targeting Th1 differentiating transcription factor is shown to associate with reduced atherosclerotic plaques (73). An IL-12 stimulated activation of Th1 response with downstream release of pro-inflammatory cytokines is a common feature between psoriasis and atherosclerosis and is thought to contribute to subsequent endothelial dysfunction and T cell recruitment to the sites of atherosclerotic plaques (74). While the role of Th1 cells is profoundly studied, the function of Th2 cells remains a topic of controversy as multiple studies exist that support pro-atherosclerotic (75), atherosclerosis protective (76), and also null effect (77) of Th2 cells.

Th17 Cells—Helper T Cells Type 17

Th17 cells in psoriasis release different cytokines such as IL-17, IL-22, and TNF-α (78) and are also involved in macrophage-dependent and -independent stimulation of dendritic cells (DCs) to propagate the inflammatory response (79). They may be involved in increased production of angiogenic inflammatory mediators such as monocyte chemoattractant protein (MCP-1), nitric oxide, and vascular endothelial growth factor (80, 81). Similar to Th2 helper cells, there is conflicting data on the role of Th17 cells in atherosclerosis (82). Patients with ACS show increased Th17 cells and IL-17 compared with those with stable angina or non-cardiac chest pain (83, 84). There is mixed evidence from mechanistic models: with some mouse models supporting the pro-atherogenic role of Th17 and IL-17 (85–87), while others have found low IL-17 mRNA in atherosclerotic plaques and overall attenuated disease development with high prevalence of Th17 cells (88–90). We later discuss the emerging role of neutrophils in the IL-17 axis, a possible mechanistic link; however, further clinical and translational research is necessary to elucidate the differential roles of Th17 and neutrophils in this pathway.

Regulatory T Cells (Treg Cells)

Regulatory T cells are a subset of T lymphocytes with a primary function to inhibit T cell activation and proliferation, through both cell-contact-dependent and cell-contact-independent anti-inflammatory cytokine (mainly TGFβ and IL-10) driven mechanisms (91). Treg inhibitory function is distinctly impaired in psoriasis (92, 93), contributing to the chronic auto- inflammation in psoriasis. ACS patients are also known to have decreased levels of circulating Treg cells with reduced efficacy and increased apoptosis susceptibility (94–97). Treg cells play an anti-inflammatory role in atherosclerosis through endothelial cell modulation, plaque stabilization by decreasing macrophages and lipid content and increasing smooth muscle cell and collagen, inhibition of pro-inflammatory cytokines, and secretion of anti-inflammatory cytokines such as TGFβ, IL-10, and IL-35 (91). Identification of common targets to reverse Treg cell dysfunction or to augment their activity in psoriasis may represent treatment mechanisms for both psoriasis and atherosclerosis simultaneously.

Finally, there are several other T cell phenotypes that have been identified in psoriasis skin lesions, such as $CD4^+$, $CD8^+$ T cells, $CD146^+$, and γδ T cells (98). However, their role in psoriasis and atherosclerosis need to be further explored. While the traditional paradigm of T cell lineages might predominate shared mechanistic links between psoriasis and atherosclerosis, there is significant heterogeneity and plasticity within the T cell subtypes. T cell predominance may change in context of subtype preponderance with the natural disease course, specifically, a switch from Th1 dominated profile in early initiation phase of psoriasis to a Th17 governed response in the chronic inflammatory phase with both involved in atherosclerosis progression (99).

Dendritic Cells

In psoriasis, DCs not only act as antigen presenters and cytokine producers but also play an important part of bridging the innate and adaptive immune systems in continuing the chronic inflammation inducing cascade (43, 79). While pDCs are important in initiation of psoriasis *via* type 1 IFN responses (62, 100), mDCs are key mediators for specific Th cell expansion *via* IL-12 and IL-23 secretion (79). While new evidence suggests a role for DCs in atherosclerotic plaque build-ups, plaque vulnerability through cholesterol metabolism and adaptive immune response modulation (101), their shared role in psoriasis and atherosclerosis needs further research.

Monocytes and Macrophages

Monocytes and macrophages are cellular hallmark of atherosclerosis (1) and are also involved in pathogenesis of psoriasis (102). While macrophages are traditionally subclassified as pro-inflammatory (M1) and anti-inflammatory (M2), they are known to be plastic and adapt to the surrounding milieu according to the underlying pathological state (103, 104). Furthermore, a preclinical *in vivo* and *in vitro* study demonstrated that chronic skin inflammation in psoriasis polarizes them toward the pro-atherosclerotic phenotype (99). These cells are involved in ACS, and their increased expression and activity is also present in vulnerable plaques (105). Novel evidence has recently suggested that a complex interplay involving neutrophil–macrophage cross-talk is crucial to the process of atherosclerosis and ACS (106–108). As these cells are involved throughout the process of atherosclerosis from plaque development to complications, such as ACS, and also play a significant role in psoriasis, further research may provide new avenues for treatment of both these conditions.

Neutrophils

Despite being the most abundant white blood cell in the circulation, neutrophils have received little attention in the pathophysiology of atherosclerosis and psoriasis. Recent mouse models and clinical trials have demonstrated the mechanistic role of neutrophils in psoriasis and atherosclerosis through the IL-17 driven keratinocyte hyper-proliferation, leading to chronic skin inflammation (109, 110). Psoriasis patients are known to have higher serum levels of IL-17 compared with healthy controls; however, the paradigm of Th17 as the predominant cellular source of IL-17 in psoriatic lesions is no longer fully valid (111). Recent studies have demonstrated that cells of the innate immune system, such as neutrophils, mast cells, γδ T cells, and innate lymphoid cells, are the main sources of IL-17 in psoriasis. Furthermore, despite controversies, IL-17 is shown to have a role in atherosclerosis in clinical and mouse model-based studies (83–85, 87).

Psoriasis increases neutrophil activation and release of neutrophil-associated proteins. Proteins associated with neutrophils such as S100A8/A9 may further provide a link between psoriasis and cardiometabolic diseases (100). S100A8/A9 (MRP8/14) is released by activated neutrophils and upregulated in psoriatic lesional skin (100, 112). We demonstrated its strong association with both skin disease severity and VI (100). Collectively, evidence suggests that neutrophils and their proteins may contribute to the early atherosclerotic milieu in psoriasis and independently predict endothelial dysfunction.

A novel subtype of neutrophils, the low-density granulocytes (LDGs), are moving to the forefront of research in psoriasis and CVD pathophysiology. LDGs are characterized by high pro-inflammatory activity, altered phagocytic function, elevated type I interferon production, and high abundance in atherosclerotic plaques and plasma of psoriasis patients (113). At the gene expression level, LDGs differ from their autologous normal-density granulocytes (NDGs) counterparts, as well as from healthy control neutrophils (114–116). LDGs also differ phenotypically from NDGs. Of these differences, the most compelling is their enhanced capacity to spontaneously form neutrophil extracellular traps (NETs). This novel defense mechanism termed NETosis goes beyond classical phagocytosis, where NETs are formed as a result of release of cytosolic granule proteins bound to nuclear material catalyzed by peptidylarginine deiminase 4 (117).

Although NETs are beneficial in antimicrobial defense, they may act as a source of autoantigens and are implicated in the development of autoimmune diseases especially psoriasis, as well as other diseases including systemic lupus erythematosus, atherosclerosis, preeclampsia, acute lung injury, deep vein thrombosis, and cancer-associated thrombosis (118–121). Cholesterol crystals are shown to trigger NETosis, further potentiating atherosclerosis by macrophage priming, Th17 activation, and immune cell recruitment in plaques (108). NETs are also shown through immunochemical stains to directly induce endothelial dysfunction and plaque rupture in human carotid plaque sections (122). NETs may be involved in the initial injury of the endothelium during atherogenesis, with recent evidence demonstrating the presence of neutrophils and NETs at sites of plaque rupture and endothelial cell erosion in human carotid plaques, features which we hypothesized would be evident in early atherosclerosis in psoriasis.

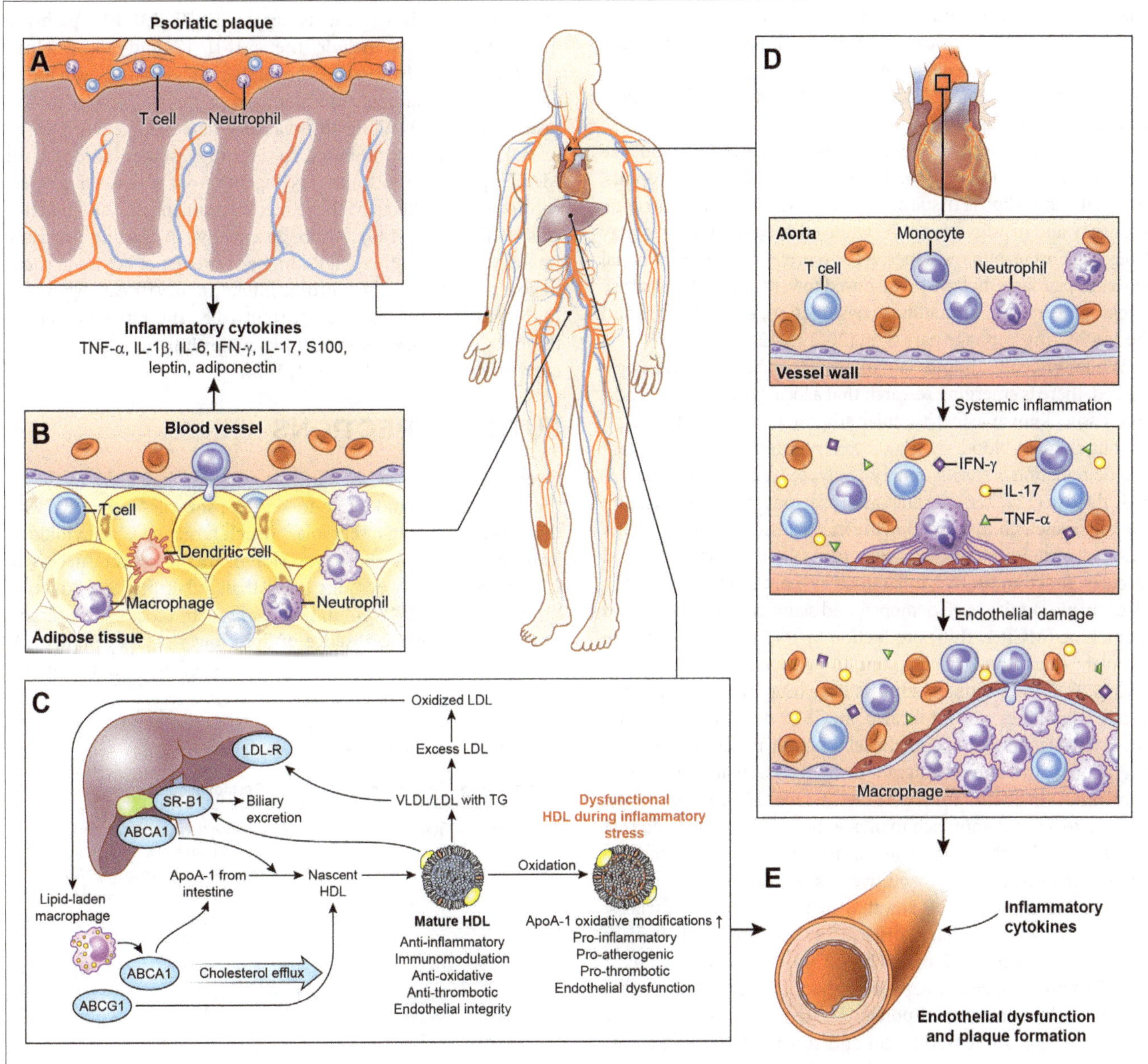

FIGURE 1 | Systemic effects of chronic low-grade inflammation in psoriasis. **(A)** Psoriasis, both cutaneous and arthritic, is a low-grade chronic, systemic inflammatory disease associated with increased circulating pro-inflammatory cytokines. **(B)** Chronic inflammation in psoriasis is associated with adipose tissue dysfunction characterized by pro-inflammatory cytokines and adipokines associated with endothelial dysfunction. **(C)** Furthermore, psoriasis exhibits a deranged lipid profile and impaired HDL function, which in combination with chronic inflammation accelerate atherosclerotic vascular disease. **(D)** The vessel wall is infiltrated through a complex interplay of pro-inflammatory cellular components, cholesterol crystals, and various lipoproteins. Over the time, with build-up of the plaque, this atherosclerotic lesion poses a significant threat to blood flow and is prone to rupture, often accelerated by inflammation leading to myocardial infarction. **(E)** Thus, psoriasis and psoriatic arthritis upregulate T-cell, neutrophil chemotaxis, and keratinocyte activation and endothelial dysfunction leading to increased atherosclerosis in blood vessels. Abbreviations: TNF-α, tumor necrosis factor-alpha; IL, interleukin; IFN-γ, interferon-gamma.

ADIPOSE DYSFUNCTION IN PSORIASIS

Systemic inflammation associated with psoriasis also contributes to inflammation of the adipose tissue (20), harboring components of the innate immune system (**Figure 1**) (63, 123). The physiological distinction between visceral and subcutaneous adiposity has been considered an important determinant in assessing CVD risk. Visceral adiposity is highly metabolically active, and its dysregulation can alter the immune cell and adipokine profile, exacerbating endothelial dysfunction. Visceral adiposity is associated with subclinical CVD measured as VI by ^{18}F-FDG PET/CT independent of cardiovascular risk factors in psoriasis (124). Furthermore, a decrease in visceral adiposity associated with an improvement of VI following 1 year of biologic anti-inflammatory therapy.

Psoriatic adipose tissue contains immune cells that influence cardiometabolic disease (20). T cells, B cells, DCs, neutrophils, mast cells, and adipose tissue macrophages (ATM) may contribute to obesity and insulin resistance, while eosinophils and Treg may protect against insulin resistance. ATM represent unique functional subset in psoriasis that are predisposed toward pro-inflammatory cytokine expression and adipose dysfunction, extending beyond the M1/M2 macrophage paradigm (20, 125, 126).

While visceral abdominal adiposity is being increasingly studied, there is emerging research that a local type of visceral adipose tissue, known as perivascular adipose tissue (PVAT), which surrounds most blood vessels (coronary arteries, the aorta, and microcirculation of the mesentery), may contribute to cardiometabolic disease (127, 128). Its anatomic proximity to the vasculature has led to research investigating the mechanisms of dysfunctional PVAT driven immune-mediated cross-talk in endothelial and vascular function under inflammatory conditions (127, 128). Mechanistic studies have demonstrated significant adipokine and chemokine (MCP-1, IL-8) production by PVAT and its ability to stimulate chemotaxis, contributing to progression of atherosclerosis (129, 130). Multiple pathways have been identified through which adipokines are implicated in CVD development—from direct vascular effects on endothelial function and smooth muscle migration to immune cell migration into the vascular wall through a potential "outside-in" inflammatory cascade (127). Recent efforts have led to a novel approach to image the PVAT and showed that it is associated with coronary inflammation in a dynamic fashion (131), with potential for prospective risk stratification.

Leptin is shown to be elevated in patients with psoriasis, to correlate with psoriasis disease severity and with indices of subclinical atherosclerosis (132, 133). We have previously exhibited an association between enhanced leptin and resistin activity with attenuated adiponectin activity in innate immune activation (24). Increased leptin and resistin promote expression of pro-inflammatory cytokines including TNF-α, IL-2, IL-6, and MCP-1, all of which are prothrombotic and drive VI through monocyte migration and macrophage activation (134). Finally, adipokines may contribute to the effect of insulin on the vasculature by contributing to changes in capillary recruitment (127).

Peri- and epicardial fat tissue are additional sources of visceral fat deposition, and a rich source of inflammatory cytokines that are associated with both subclinical and clinical coronary heart disease (128). Epicardial fat tissue has been reported to be significantly increased in psoriasis patients and may represent an independent risk factor for atherosclerosis (135).

BIOLOGIC THERAPIES

The current generation of biologic agents target cytokines critical to the pathogenesis of psoriasis, including the three known major drivers: TNF-α, IL-23, and IL-17. The majority of most effective psoriasis treatments target the IL-23/Th17 pathway. These medications include the anti-IL-17 and anti-IL23p19 agents (**Table 1**). However, as novel therapies emerge, even today, anti-TNF agents remain the standard of care in general clinical practice (43, 136). While observational data in large payer-based or veterans association-based cohorts suggest a reduced risk for MACEs primarily with anti-TNF agents, no trials assessing direct cardiovascular effects of these medications in psoriasis patients exist to date (137–140). Although effective in treating psoriasis, interestingly, these therapies have been proven of no use in rheumatoid arthritis, another chronic inflammatory disease where the IL-23/Th17 axis plays an important role. The rationale behind these contradictory findings in two major inflammatory diseases currently remains unclear (141, 142).

FUTURE DIRECTIONS

Over the last decade, remarkable progress has been made for the treatment of moderate-to-severe psoriasis, especially with the advent of biologic therapies, which target specific cytokines, immune cells, and pathways. Moreover, the recent success of CANTOS (32) has demonstrated that inflammation reduction through direct IL-1β inhibition using a monoclonal antibody, canakinumab, in the absence of lipid lowering, can reduce CV event rates. As such, the emerging field of biologic treatments

TABLE 1 | Biologic treatment options to treat psoriasis.

Biologic drug	Target cytokine	Cardiovascular effects
Etanercept Infliximab Adalimumab	Tumor necrosis factor-α	Observational data indicating better CV outcomes. RCT for subclinical cardiovascular disease (CVD) demonstrating promising results. RCT dedicated for CV events not available (139, 140, 143)
Secukinumab Ixekizumab Bimekizumab Brodalumab[a]	Interleukin-17A and interleukin-17A receptor for brodalumab	Dedicated RCT for CV events unavailable
Ustekinumab Briakinumab[a]	Interleukin-12/23p40	RCT for subclinical CVD demonstrating favorable results. Dedicated RCT unavailable (144)
Guselkumab Tildrakizumab Risankizumab	Interleukin-23p19	No data available yet for CV effects
Fezakinumab	Interleukin-22	Drug still in early development phase

[a]*Discontinued medications from the market.*

is exciting as it may provide therapeutic utility in psoriasis with added benefits of modulating CVD risk. Furthermore, completed and ongoing trials assessing the subclinical CVD in psoriasis have demonstrated promising findings (143, 144).

Finally, future research should focus on examination of complex inter-relationships between various conventional and non-conventional, inflammatory and non-inflammatory pathways to understand the heightened risk of CVD in disease conditions with underlying chronic inflammation.

CONCLUSION

Increasing evidence demonstrates an important role of immune dysfunction linking psoriasis to cardiometabolic diseases including atherosclerosis. Future efforts in patients with chronic inflammatory disease like psoriasis should focus on elucidating the complex interplay among immune cells, adipose tissue, and various biomarkers of immune dysfunction. The shared mechanistic links between psoriasis and atherosclerosis provide promising avenues in targeted treatment for both diseases, especially in light of the recent trial CANTOS (32), which demonstrated reduced incidence of recurrent cardiovascular events after treating residual inflammation in patients with known coronary artery disease.

AUTHOR CONTRIBUTIONS

AS and NM conceived and designed research. AS, AJ, HT, AD, and NM contributed to both manuscript writing and critical review.

ACKNOWLEDGMENT

We would like to acknowledge Ethan Tyler for his contribution to the figure.

REFERENCES

1. Libby P, Ridker PM, Hansson GK; Leducq Transatlantic Network on Atherothrombosis. Inflammation in atherosclerosis: from pathophysiology to practice. *J Am Coll Cardiol* (2009) 54(23):2129–38. doi:10.1016/j.jacc.2009.09.009
2. Gelfand JM, Neimann AL, Shin DB, Wang X, Margolis DJ, Troxel AB. Risk of myocardial infarction in patients with psoriasis. *JAMA* (2006) 296(14):1735–41. doi:10.1001/jama.296.14.1735
3. Harrington CL, Dey AK, Yunus R, Joshi AA, Mehta NN. Psoriasis as a human model of disease to study inflammatory atherogenesis. *Am J Physiol Heart Circ Physiol* (2017) 312(5):H867–73. doi:10.1152/ajpheart.00774.2016
4. Mehta NN, Azfar RS, Shin DB, Neimann AL, Troxel AB, Gelfand JM. Patients with severe psoriasis are at increased risk of cardiovascular mortality: cohort study using the General Practice Research Database. *Eur Heart J* (2010) 31(8):1000–6. doi:10.1093/eurheartj/ehp567
5. Brauchli YB, Jick SS, Miret M, Meier CR. Psoriasis and risk of incident myocardial infarction, stroke or transient ischaemic attack: an inception cohort study with a nested case-control analysis. *Br J Dermatol* (2009) 160(5):1048–56. doi:10.1111/j.1365-2133.2008.09020.x
6. Prodanovich S, Kirsner RS, Kravetz JD, Ma F, Martinez L, Federman DG. Association of psoriasis with coronary artery, cerebrovascular, and peripheral vascular diseases and mortality. *Arch Dermatol* (2009) 145(6):700–3. doi:10.1001/archdermatol.2009.94
7. Khot UN, Khot MB, Bajzer CT, Sapp SK, Ohman EM, Brener SJ, et al. Prevalence of conventional risk factors in patients with coronary heart disease. *JAMA* (2003) 290(7):898–904. doi:10.1001/jama.290.7.898
8. Ridker PM. Clinical application of C-reactive protein for cardiovascular disease detection and prevention. *Circulation* (2003) 107(3):363–9. doi:10.1161/01.CIR.0000053730.47739.3C
9. Mehta NN, Krishnamoorthy P, Yu Y, Khan O, Raper A, Van Voorhees A, et al. The impact of psoriasis on 10-year Framingham risk. *J Am Acad Dermatol* (2012) 67(4):796–8. doi:10.1016/j.jaad.2012.05.016
10. Mehta NN, Yu Y, Pinnelas R, Krishnamoorthy P, Shin DB, Troxel AB, et al. Attributable risk estimate of severe psoriasis on major cardiovascular events. *Am J Med* (2011) 124(8):775.e1–6. doi:10.1016/j.amjmed.2011.03.028
11. Cohen AD, Dreiher J, Shapiro Y, Vidavsky L, Vardy DA, Davidovici B, et al. Psoriasis and diabetes: a population-based cross-sectional study. *J Eur Acad Dermatol Venereol* (2008) 22(5):585–9. doi:10.1111/j.1468-3083.2008.02636.x
12. Cohen AD, Sherf M, Vidavsky L, Vardy DA, Shapiro J, Meyerovitch J. Association between psoriasis and the metabolic syndrome. A cross-sectional study. *Dermatology* (2008) 216(2):152–5. doi:10.1159/000111512
13. Davidovici BB, Sattar N, Prinz J, Puig L, Emery P, Barker JN, et al. Psoriasis and systemic inflammatory diseases: potential mechanistic links between skin disease and co-morbid conditions. *J Invest Dermatol* (2010) 130(7):1785–96. doi:10.1038/jid.2010.103
14. Langan SM, Seminara NM, Shin DB, Troxel AB, Kimmel SE, Mehta NN, et al. Prevalence of metabolic syndrome in patients with psoriasis: a population-based study in the United Kingdom. *J Invest Dermatol* (2012) 132(3 Pt 1):556–62. doi:10.1038/jid.2011.365
15. Love TJ, Qureshi AA, Karlson EW, Gelfand JM, Choi HK. Prevalence of the metabolic syndrome in psoriasis: results from the National Health and Nutrition Examination Survey, 2003–2006. *Arch Dermatol* (2011) 147(4):419–24. doi:10.1001/archdermatol.2010.370
16. Neimann AL, Shin DB, Wang X, Margolis DJ, Troxel AB, Gelfand JM. Prevalence of cardiovascular risk factors in patients with psoriasis. *J Am Acad Dermatol* (2006) 55(5):829–35. doi:10.1016/j.jaad.2006.08.040
17. Eckel RH, Krauss RM. American Heart Association call to action: obesity as a major risk factor for coronary heart disease. AHA Nutrition Committee. *Circulation* (1998) 97(21):2099–100. doi:10.1161/01.CIR.97.21.2099
18. Maresca F, Di Palma V, Bevilacqua M, Uccello G, Taglialatela V, Giaquinto A, et al. Adipokines, vascular wall, and cardiovascular disease: a focused overview of the role of adipokines in the pathophysiology of cardiovascular disease. *Angiology* (2015) 66(1):8–24. doi:10.1177/0003319713520463
19. Rao G, Powell-Wiley TM, Ancheta I, Hairston K, Kirley K, Lear SA, et al. Identification of obesity and cardiovascular risk in ethnically and racially diverse populations: a scientific statement from the American Heart Association. *Circulation* (2015) 132(5):457–72. doi:10.1161/CIR.0000000000000223
20. Rose S, Stansky E, Dagur PK, Samsel L, Weiner E, Jahanshad A, et al. Characterization of immune cells in psoriatic adipose tissue. *J Transl Med* (2014) 12:258. doi:10.1186/s12967-014-0258-2
21. McGillicuddy FC, de la Llera Moya M, Hinkle CC, Joshi MR, Chiquoine EH, Billheimer JT, et al. Inflammation impairs reverse cholesterol transport in vivo. *Circulation* (2009) 119(8):1135–45. doi:10.1161/CIRCULATIONAHA.108.810721
22. Mehta NN, Li R, Krishnamoorthy P, Yu Y, Farver W, Rodrigues A, et al. Abnormal lipoprotein particles and cholesterol efflux capacity in patients with psoriasis. *Atherosclerosis* (2012) 224(1):218–21. doi:10.1016/j.atherosclerosis.2012.06.068

23. Rosenson RS, Brewer HB Jr, Ansell BJ, Barter P, Chapman MJ, Heinecke JW, et al. Dysfunctional HDL and atherosclerotic cardiovascular disease. *Nat Rev Cardiol* (2016) 13(1):48–60. doi:10.1038/nrcardio.2015.124
24. Anderson PD, Mehta NN, Wolfe ML, Hinkle CC, Pruscino L, Comiskey LL, et al. Innate immunity modulates adipokines in humans. *J Clin Endocrinol Metab* (2007) 92(6):2272–9. doi:10.1210/jc.2006-2545
25. de la Llera Moya M, McGillicuddy FC, Hinkle CC, Byrne M, Joshi MR, Nguyen V, et al. Inflammation modulates human HDL composition and function in vivo. *Atherosclerosis* (2012) 222(2):390–4. doi:10.1016/j.atherosclerosis.2012.02.032
26. Ferguson JF, Shah RY, Shah R, Mehta NN, Rickels MR, Reilly MP. Activation of innate immunity modulates insulin sensitivity, glucose effectiveness and pancreatic beta-cell function in both African ancestry and European ancestry healthy humans. *Metabolism* (2015) 64(4):513–20. doi:10.1016/j.metabol.2014.12.007
27. Mehta NN, McGillicuddy FC, Anderson PD, Hinkle CC, Shah R, Pruscino L, et al. Experimental endotoxemia induces adipose inflammation and insulin resistance in humans. *Diabetes* (2010) 59(1):172–81. doi:10.2337/db09-0367
28. Nidorf M, Thompson PL. Effect of colchicine (0.5 mg twice daily) on high-sensitivity C-reactive protein independent of aspirin and atorvastatin in patients with stable coronary artery disease. *Am J Cardiol* (2007) 99(6):805–7. doi:10.1016/j.amjcard.2006.10.039
29. Nidorf SM, Eikelboom JW, Budgeon CA, Thompson PL. Low-dose colchicine for secondary prevention of cardiovascular disease. *J Am Coll Cardiol* (2013) 61(4):404–10. doi:10.1016/j.jacc.2012.10.027
30. Ridker PM, Cushman M, Stampfer MJ, Tracy RP, Hennekens CH. Inflammation, aspirin, and the risk of cardiovascular disease in apparently healthy men. *N Engl J Med* (1997) 336(14):973–9. doi:10.1056/NEJM199704033361401
31. Vaidya K, Arnott C, Martinez GJ, Ng B, McCormack S, Sullivan DR, et al. Colchicine therapy and plaque stabilization in patients with acute coronary syndrome: a CT Coronary Angiography Study. *JACC Cardiovasc Imag* (2018) 11(2 Pt 2):305–16. doi:10.1016/j.jcmg.2017.08.013
32. Ridker PM, Everett BM, Thuren T, MacFadyen JG, Chang WH, Ballantyne C, et al. Antiinflammatory therapy with canakinumab for atherosclerotic disease. *N Engl J Med* (2017) 377(12):1119–31. doi:10.1056/NEJMoa1707914
33. Ritchlin CT, Colbert RA, Gladman DD. Psoriatic arthritis. *N Engl J Med* (2017) 376(10):957–70. doi:10.1056/NEJMra1505557
34. Armstrong AW, Gelfand JM, Boehncke WH, Armstrong EJ. Cardiovascular comorbidities of psoriasis and psoriatic arthritis: a report from the GRAPPA 2012 annual meeting. *J Rheumatol* (2013) 40(8):1434–7. doi:10.3899/jrheum.130457
35. Eder L, Jayakar J, Shanmugarajah S, Thavaneswaran A, Pereira D, Chandran V, et al. The burden of carotid artery plaques is higher in patients with psoriatic arthritis compared with those with psoriasis alone. *Ann Rheum Dis* (2013) 72(5):715–20. doi:10.1136/annrheumdis-2012-201497
36. Kolliker Frers RA, Cosentino V, Tau J, Kerzberg EM, Urdapilleta A, Chiocconi M, et al. Immune-mediated inflammation promotes subclinical atherosclerosis in recent-onset psoriatic arthritis patients without conventional cardiovascular risk factors. *Front Immunol* (2018) 9:139. doi:10.3389/fimmu.2018.00139
37. Ogdie A, Yu Y, Haynes K, Love TJ, Maliha S, Jiang Y, et al. Risk of major cardiovascular events in patients with psoriatic arthritis, psoriasis and rheumatoid arthritis: a population-based cohort study. *Ann Rheum Dis* (2015) 74(2):326–32. doi:10.1136/annrheumdis-2014-205675
38. Rose S, Dave J, Millo C, Naik HB, Siegel EL, Mehta NN. Psoriatic arthritis and sacroiliitis are associated with increased vascular inflammation by 18-fluorodeoxyglucose positron emission tomography computed tomography: baseline report from the psoriasis atherosclerosis and cardiometabolic disease initiative. *Arthritis Res Ther* (2014) 16(4):R161. doi:10.1186/ar4676
39. Eder L, Chandran V, Gladman DD. The Framingham Risk Score underestimates the extent of subclinical atherosclerosis in patients with psoriatic disease. *Ann Rheum Dis* (2014) 73(11):1990–6. doi:10.1136/annrheumdis-2013-203433
40. Shen J, Lam SH, Shang Q, Wong CK, Li EK, Wong P, et al. Underestimation of risk of carotid subclinical atherosclerosis by cardiovascular risk scores in patients with psoriatic arthritis. *J Rheumatol* (2018) 45(2):218–26. doi:10.3899/jrheum.170025
41. Teague H, Mehta NN. The link between inflammatory disorders and coronary heart disease: a look at recent studies and novel drugs in development. *Curr Atheroscler Rep* (2016) 18(1):3. doi:10.1007/s11883-015-0557-y
42. Teague HL, Ahlman MA, Alavi A, Wagner DD, Lichtman AH, Nahrendorf M, et al. Unraveling vascular inflammation: from immunology to imaging. *J Am Coll Cardiol* (2017) 70(11):1403–12. doi:10.1016/j.jacc.2017.07.750
43. Greb JE, Goldminz AM, Elder JT, Lebwohl MG, Gladman DD, Wu JJ, et al. Psoriasis. *Nat Rev Dis Primers* (2016) 2:16082. doi:10.1038/nrdp.2016.82
44. Shaharyar S, Warraich H, McEvoy JW, Oni E, Ali SS, Karim A, et al. Subclinical cardiovascular disease in plaque psoriasis: association or causal link? *Atherosclerosis* (2014) 232(1):72–8. doi:10.1016/j.atherosclerosis.2013.10.023
45. Boehncke S, Fichtlscherer S, Salgo R, Garbaraviciene J, Beschmann H, Diehl S, et al. Systemic therapy of plaque-type psoriasis ameliorates endothelial cell function: results of a prospective longitudinal pilot trial. *Arch Dermatol Res* (2011) 303(6):381–8. doi:10.1007/s00403-010-1108-6
46. Prodanovich S, Ma F, Taylor JR, Pezon C, Fasihi T, Kirsner RS. Methotrexate reduces incidence of vascular diseases in veterans with psoriasis or rheumatoid arthritis. *J Am Acad Dermatol* (2005) 52(2):262–7. doi:10.1016/j.jaad.2004.06.017
47. Dey AK, Joshi AA, Chaturvedi A, Lerman JB, Aberra TM, Rodante JA, et al. Association between skin and aortic vascular inflammation in patients with psoriasis: a case-cohort study using positron emission tomography/computed tomography. *JAMA Cardiol* (2017) 2(9):1013–8. doi:10.1001/jamacardio.2017.1213
48. Lerman JB, Joshi AA, Chaturvedi A, Aberra TM, Dey AK, Rodante JA, et al. Coronary plaque characterization in psoriasis reveals high-risk features that improve after treatment in a prospective observational study. *Circulation* (2017) 136(3):263–76. doi:10.1161/CIRCULATIONAHA.116.026859
49. Mehta NN, Yu Y, Saboury B, Foroughi N, Krishnamoorthy P, Raper A, et al. Systemic and vascular inflammation in patients with moderate to severe psoriasis as measured by [18F]-fluorodeoxyglucose positron emission tomography-computed tomography (FDG-PET/CT): a pilot study. *Arch Dermatol* (2011) 147(9):1031–9. doi:10.1001/archdermatol.2011.119
50. Hjuler KF, Bottcher M, Vestergaard C, Botker HE, Iversen L, Kragballe K. Association between changes in coronary artery disease progression and treatment with biologic agents for severe psoriasis. *JAMA Dermatol* (2016) 152(10):1114–21. doi:10.1001/jamadermatol.2016.1984
51. Mansouri B, Kivelevitch D, Natarajan B, Joshi AA, Ryan C, Benjegerdes K, et al. Comparison of coronary artery calcium scores between patients with psoriasis and type 2 diabetes. *JAMA Dermatol* (2016) 152(11):1244–53. doi:10.1001/jamadermatol.2016.2907
52. Gelfand JM, Dommasch ED, Shin DB, Azfar RS, Kurd SK, Wang X, et al. The risk of stroke in patients with psoriasis. *J Invest Dermatol* (2009) 129(10):2411–8. doi:10.1038/jid.2009.112
53. Gelfand JM, Troxel AB, Lewis JD, Kurd SK, Shin DB, Wang X, et al. The risk of mortality in patients with psoriasis: results from a population-based study. *Arch Dermatol* (2007) 143(12):1493–9. doi:10.1001/archderm.143.12.1493
54. Boehncke WH, Boehncke S, Tobin AM, Kirby B. The 'psoriatic march': a concept of how severe psoriasis may drive cardiovascular comorbidity. *Exp Dermatol* (2011) 20(4):303–7. doi:10.1111/j.1600-0625.2011.01261.x
55. Shlyankevich J, Mehta NN, Krueger JG, Strober B, Gudjonsson JE, Qureshi AA, et al. Accumulating evidence for the association and shared pathogenic mechanisms between psoriasis and cardiovascular-related comorbidities. *Am J Med* (2014) 127(12):1148–53. doi:10.1016/j.amjmed.2014.08.008
56. Abrams JR, Lebwohl MG, Guzzo CA, Jegasothy BV, Goldfarb MT, Goffe BS, et al. CTLA4Ig-mediated blockade of T-cell costimulation in patients with psoriasis vulgaris. *J Clin Invest* (1999) 103(9):1243–52. doi:10.1172/JCI5857
57. Chamian F, Lin SL, Lee E, Kikuchi T, Gilleaudeau P, Sullivan-Whalen M, et al. Alefacept (anti-CD2) causes a selective reduction in circulating effector memory T cells (Tem) and relative preservation of central memory T cells (Tcm) in psoriasis. *J Transl Med* (2007) 5:27. doi:10.1186/1479-5876-5-27
58. Chamian F, Lowes MA, Lin SL, Lee E, Kikuchi T, Gilleaudeau P, et al. Alefacept reduces infiltrating T cells, activated dendritic cells, and inflammatory genes in psoriasis vulgaris. *Proc Natl Acad Sci U S A* (2005) 102(6):2075–80. doi:10.1073/pnas.0409569102
59. Gottlieb SL, Gilleaudeau P, Johnson R, Estes L, Woodworth TG, Gottlieb AB, et al. Response of psoriasis to a lymphocyte-selective toxin (DAB389IL-2) suggests a primary immune, but not keratinocyte, pathogenic basis. *Nat Med* (1995) 1(5):442–7. doi:10.1038/nm0595-442
60. Lowes MA, Chamian F, Abello MV, Fuentes-Duculan J, Lin SL, Nussbaum R, et al. Increase in TNF-alpha and inducible nitric oxide synthase-expressing

dendritic cells in psoriasis and reduction with efalizumab (anti-CD11a). *Proc Natl Acad Sci U S A* (2005) 102(52):19057–62. doi:10.1073/pnas.0509736102
61. Nickoloff BJ. Skin innate immune system in psoriasis: friend or foe? *J Clin Invest* (1999) 104(9):1161–4. doi:10.1172/JCI8633
62. Lowes MA, Suarez-Farinas M, Krueger JG. Immunology of psoriasis. *Annu Rev Immunol* (2014) 32:227–55. doi:10.1146/annurev-immunol-032713-120225
63. Hansson GK, Hermansson A. The immune system in atherosclerosis. *Nat Immunol* (2011) 12(3):204–12. doi:10.1038/ni.2001
64. Zhang K, Li X, Yin G, Liu Y, Tang X. Functional characterization of T cells differentiated in vitro from bone marrow-derived CD34 cells of psoriatic patients with family history. *Exp Dermatol* (2010) 19(8):e128–35. doi:10.1111/j.1600-0625.2009.01016.x
65. Hansson GK, Robertson AK, Soderberg-Naucler C. Inflammation and atherosclerosis. *Annu Rev Pathol* (2006) 1:297–329. doi:10.1146/annurev.pathol.1.110304.100100
66. Liuzzo G, Vallejo AN, Kopecky SL, Frye RL, Holmes DR, Goronzy JJ, et al. Molecular fingerprint of interferon-gamma signaling in unstable angina. *Circulation* (2001) 103(11):1509–14. doi:10.1161/01.CIR.103.11.1509
67. Methe H, Kim JO, Kofler S, Weis M, Nabauer M, Koglin J. Expansion of circulating toll-like receptor 4-positive monocytes in patients with acute coronary syndrome. *Circulation* (2005) 111(20):2654–61. doi:10.1161/CIRCULATIONAHA.104.498865
68. Davenport P, Tipping PG. The role of interleukin-4 and interleukin-12 in the progression of atherosclerosis in apolipoprotein E-deficient mice. *Am J Pathol* (2003) 163(3):1117–25. doi:10.1016/S0002-9440(10)63471-2
69. Hauer AD, Uyttenhove C, de Vos P, Stroobant V, Renauld JC, van Berkel TJ, et al. Blockade of interleukin-12 function by protein vaccination attenuates atherosclerosis. *Circulation* (2005) 112(7):1054–62. doi:10.1161/CIRCULATIONAHA.104.533463
70. Lee TS, Yen HC, Pan CC, Chau LY. The role of interleukin 12 in the development of atherosclerosis in ApoE-deficient mice. *Arterioscler Thromb Vasc Biol* (1999) 19(3):734–42. doi:10.1161/01.ATV.19.3.734
71. Elhage R, Jawien J, Rudling M, Ljunggren HG, Takeda K, Akira S, et al. Reduced atherosclerosis in interleukin-18 deficient apolipoprotein E-knockout mice. *Cardiovasc Res* (2003) 59(1):234–40. doi:10.1016/S0008-6363(03)00343-2
72. Whitman SC, Ravisankar P, Daugherty A. Interleukin-18 enhances atherosclerosis in apolipoprotein E(-/-) mice through release of interferon-gamma. *Circ Res* (2002) 90(2):E34–8. doi:10.1161/hh0202.105292
73. Buono C, Binder CJ, Stavrakis G, Witztum JL, Glimcher LH, Lichtman AH. T-bet deficiency reduces atherosclerosis and alters plaque antigen-specific immune responses. *Proc Natl Acad Sci U S A* (2005) 102(5):1596–601. doi:10.1073/pnas.0409015102
74. Libby P. Mechanisms of acute coronary syndromes and their implications for therapy. *N Engl J Med* (2013) 368(21):2004–13. doi:10.1056/NEJMra1216063
75. King VL, Szilvassy SJ, Daugherty A. Interleukin-4 deficiency decreases atherosclerotic lesion formation in a site-specific manner in female LDL receptor-/- mice. *Arterioscler Thromb Vasc Biol* (2002) 22(3):456–61. doi:10.1161/hq0302.104905
76. Huber SA, Sakkinen P, David C, Newell MK, Tracy RP. T helper-cell phenotype regulates atherosclerosis in mice under conditions of mild hypercholesterolemia. *Circulation* (2001) 103(21):2610–6. doi:10.1161/01.CIR.103.21.2610
77. King VL, Cassis LA, Daugherty A. Interleukin-4 does not influence development of hypercholesterolemia or angiotensin II-induced atherosclerotic lesions in mice. *Am J Pathol* (2007) 171(6):2040–7. doi:10.2353/ajpath.2007.060857
78. Chiricozzi A, Guttman-Yassky E, Suarez-Farinas M, Nograles KE, Tian S, Cardinale I, et al. Integrative responses to IL-17 and TNF-alpha in human keratinocytes account for key inflammatory pathogenic circuits in psoriasis. *J Invest Dermatol* (2011) 131(3):677–87. doi:10.1038/jid.2010.340
79. Nestle FO, Kaplan DH, Barker J. Psoriasis. *N Engl J Med* (2009) 361(5):496–509. doi:10.1056/NEJMra0804595
80. Numasaki M, Lotze MT, Sasaki H. Interleukin-17 augments tumor necrosis factor-alpha-induced elaboration of proangiogenic factors from fibroblasts. *Immunol Lett* (2004) 93(1):39–43. doi:10.1016/j.imlet.2004.01.014
81. Takahashi H, Numasaki M, Lotze MT, Sasaki H. Interleukin-17 enhances bFGF-, HGF- and VEGF-induced growth of vascular endothelial cells. *Immunol Lett* (2005) 98(2):189–93. doi:10.1016/j.imlet.2004.11.012
82. Liuzzo G, Trotta F, Pedicino D. Interleukin-17 in atherosclerosis and cardiovascular disease: the good, the bad, and the unknown. *Eur Heart J* (2013) 34(8):556–9. doi:10.1093/eurheartj/ehs399
83. Cheng X, Yu X, Ding YJ, Fu QQ, Xie JJ, Tang TT, et al. The Th17/Treg imbalance in patients with acute coronary syndrome. *Clin Immunol* (2008) 127(1):89–97. doi:10.1016/j.clim.2008.01.009
84. Zheng Y, Wang Z, Deng L, Zhang G, Yuan X, Huang L, et al. Modulation of STAT3 and STAT5 activity rectifies the imbalance of Th17 and Treg cells in patients with acute coronary syndrome. *Clin Immunol* (2015) 157(1):65–77. doi:10.1016/j.clim.2014.12.012
85. Erbel C, Akhavanpoor M, Okuyucu D, Wangler S, Dietz A, Zhao L, et al. IL-17A influences essential functions of the monocyte/macrophage lineage and is involved in advanced murine and human atherosclerosis. *J Immunol* (2014) 193(9):4344–55. doi:10.4049/jimmunol.1400181
86. Erbel C, Chen L, Bea F, Wangler S, Celik S, Lasitschka F, et al. Inhibition of IL-17A attenuates atherosclerotic lesion development in apoE-deficient mice. *J Immunol* (2009) 183(12):8167–75. doi:10.4049/jimmunol.0901126
87. Smith E, Prasad KM, Butcher M, Dobrian A, Kolls JK, Ley K, et al. Blockade of interleukin-17A results in reduced atherosclerosis in apolipoprotein E-deficient mice. *Circulation* (2010) 121(15):1746–55. doi:10.1161/CIRCULATIONAHA.109.924886
88. de Boer OJ, van der Meer JJ, Teeling P, van der Loos CM, Idu MM, van Maldegem F, et al. Differential expression of interleukin-17 family cytokines in intact and complicated human atherosclerotic plaques. *J Pathol* (2010) 220(4):499–508. doi:10.1002/path.2667
89. Eid RE, Rao DA, Zhou J, Lo SF, Ranjbaran H, Gallo A, et al. Interleukin-17 and interferon-gamma are produced concomitantly by human coronary artery-infiltrating T cells and act synergistically on vascular smooth muscle cells. *Circulation* (2009) 119(10):1424–32. doi:10.1161/CIRCULATIONAHA.108.827618
90. Taleb S, Tedgui A, Mallat Z. IL-17 and Th17 cells in atherosclerosis: subtle and contextual roles. *Arterioscler Thromb Vasc Biol* (2015) 35(2):258–64. doi:10.1161/ATVBAHA.114.303567
91. Meng X, Yang J, Dong M, Zhang K, Tu E, Gao Q, et al. Regulatory T cells in cardiovascular diseases. *Nat Rev Cardiol* (2015) 13:167. doi:10.1038/nrcardio.2015.169
92. Kagen MH, McCormick TS, Cooper KD. Regulatory T cells in psoriasis. *Ernst Schering Res Found Workshop* (2006) (56):193–209.
93. Sugiyama H, Gyulai R, Toichi E, Garaczi E, Shimada S, Stevens SR, et al. Dysfunctional blood and target tissue CD4+CD25high regulatory T cells in psoriasis: mechanism underlying unrestrained pathogenic effector T cell proliferation. *J Immunol* (2005) 174(1):164–73. doi:10.4049/jimmunol.174.1.164
94. Han SF, Liu P, Zhang W, Bu L, Shen M, Li H, et al. The opposite-direction modulation of CD4+CD25+ Tregs and T helper 1 cells in acute coronary syndromes. *Clin Immunol* (2007) 124(1):90–7. doi:10.1016/j.clim.2007.03.546
95. Mor A, Luboshits G, Planer D, Keren G, George J. Altered status of CD4(+) CD25(+) regulatory T cells in patients with acute coronary syndromes. *Eur Heart J* (2006) 27(21):2530–7. doi:10.1093/eurheartj/ehl222
96. Wigren M, Bjorkbacka H, Andersson L, Ljungcrantz I, Fredrikson GN, Persson M, et al. Low levels of circulating CD4+FoxP3+ T cells are associated with an increased risk for development of myocardial infarction but not for stroke. *Arterioscler Thromb Vasc Biol* (2012) 32(8):2000–4. doi:10.1161/ATVBAHA.112.251579
97. Zhang WC, Wang J, Shu YW, Tang TT, Zhu ZF, Xia N, et al. Impaired thymic export and increased apoptosis account for regulatory T cell defects in patients with non-ST segment elevation acute coronary syndrome. *J Biol Chem* (2012) 287(41):34157–66. doi:10.1074/jbc.M112.382978
98. Cai Y, Fleming C, Yan J. New insights of T cells in the pathogenesis of psoriasis. *Cell Mol Immunol* (2012) 9(4):302–9. doi:10.1038/cmi.2012.15
99. Baumer Y, Ng Q, Sanda GE, Dey AK, Teague HL, Sorokin AV, et al. Chronic skin inflammation accelerates macrophage cholesterol crystal formation and atherosclerosis. *JCI Insight* (2018) 3(1). doi:10.1172/jci.insight.97179
100. Naik HB, Natarajan B, Stansky E, Ahlman MA, Teague H, Salahuddin T, et al. Severity of psoriasis associates with aortic vascular inflammation detected by FDG PET/CT and neutrophil activation in a prospective observational study. *Arterioscler Thromb Vasc Biol* (2015) 35(12):2667–76. doi:10.1161/ATVBAHA.115.306460

101. Zernecke A. Dendritic cells in atherosclerosis: evidence in mice and humans. *Arterioscler Thromb Vasc Biol* (2015) 35(4):763–70. doi:10.1161/ATVBAHA.114.303566
102. Clark RA, Kupper TS. Misbehaving macrophages in the pathogenesis of psoriasis. *J Clin Invest* (2006) 116(8):2084–7. doi:10.1172/JCI29441
103. Moore KJ, Sheedy FJ, Fisher EA. Macrophages in atherosclerosis: a dynamic balance. *Nat Rev Immunol* (2013) 13(10):709–21. doi:10.1038/nri3520
104. Rahman K, Vengrenyuk Y, Ramsey SA, Vila NR, Girgis NM, Liu J, et al. Inflammatory Ly6Chi monocytes and their conversion to M2 macrophages drive atherosclerosis regression. *J Clin Invest* (2017) 127(8):2904–15. doi:10.1172/JCI75005
105. Ghattas A, Griffiths HR, Devitt A, Lip GY, Shantsila E. Monocytes in coronary artery disease and atherosclerosis: where are we now? *J Am Coll Cardiol* (2013) 62(17):1541–51. doi:10.1016/j.jacc.2013.07.043
106. Frodermann V, Nahrendorf M. Neutrophil-macrophage cross-talk in acute myocardial infarction. *Eur Heart J* (2017) 38(3):198–200. doi:10.1093/eurheartj/ehw085
107. Nahrendorf M, Swirski FK. Immunology. Neutrophil-macrophage communication in inflammation and atherosclerosis. *Science* (2015) 349(6245): 237–8. doi:10.1126/science.aac7801
108. Warnatsch A, Ioannou M, Wang Q, Papayannopoulos V. Inflammation. Neutrophil extracellular traps license macrophages for cytokine production in atherosclerosis. *Science* (2015) 349(6245):316–20. doi:10.1126/science.aaa8064
109. Harper EG, Guo C, Rizzo H, Lillis JV, Kurtz SE, Skorcheva I, et al. Th17 cytokines stimulate CCL20 expression in keratinocytes in vitro and in vivo: implications for psoriasis pathogenesis. *J Invest Dermatol* (2009) 129(9):2175–83. doi:10.1038/jid.2009.65
110. Johansen C, Usher PA, Kjellerup RB, Lundsgaard D, Iversen L, Kragballe K. Characterization of the interleukin-17 isoforms and receptors in lesional psoriatic skin. *Br J Dermatol* (2009) 160(2):319–24. doi:10.1111/j.1365-2133.2008.08902.x
111. Keijsers RR, Joosten I, van Erp PE, Koenen HJ, van de Kerkhof PC. Cellular sources of IL-17 in psoriasis: a paradigm shift? *Exp Dermatol* (2014) 23(11): 799–803. doi:10.1111/exd.12487
112. Kerkhoff C, Voss A, Scholzen TE, Averill MM, Zanker KS, Bornfeldt KE. Novel insights into the role of S100A8/A9 in skin biology. *Exp Dermatol* (2012) 21(11):822–6. doi:10.1111/j.1600-0625.2012.01571.x
113. Sanda GE, Belur AD, Teague HL, Mehta NN. Emerging associations between neutrophils, atherosclerosis, and psoriasis. *Curr Atheroscler Rep* (2017) 19(12):53. doi:10.1007/s11883-017-0692-8
114. Carmona-Rivera C, Kaplan MJ. Low-density granulocytes: a distinct class of neutrophils in systemic autoimmunity. *Semin Immunopathol* (2013) 35(4):455–63. doi:10.1007/s00281-013-0375-7
115. Nakou M, Knowlton N, Frank MB, Bertsias G, Osban J, Sandel CE, et al. Gene expression in systemic lupus erythematosus: bone marrow analysis differentiates active from inactive disease and reveals apoptosis and granulopoiesis signatures. *Arthritis Rheum* (2008) 58(11):3541–9. doi:10.1002/art.23961
116. Villanueva E, Yalavarthi S, Berthier CC, Hodgin JB, Khandpur R, Lin AM, et al. Netting neutrophils induce endothelial damage, infiltrate tissues, and expose immunostimulatory molecules in systemic lupus erythematosus. *J Immunol* (2011) 187(1):538–52. doi:10.4049/jimmunol.1100450
117. Brinkmann V, Reichard U, Goosmann C, Fauler B, Uhlemann Y, Weiss DS, et al. Neutrophil extracellular traps kill bacteria. *Science* (2004) 303(5663):1532–5. doi:10.1126/science.1092385
118. Delgado-Rizo V, Martinez-Guzman MA, Iniguez-Gutierrez L, Garcia-Orozco A, Alvarado-Navarro A, Fafutis-Morris M. Neutrophil extracellular traps and its implications in inflammation: an overview. *Front Immunol* (2017) 8:81. doi:10.3389/fimmu.2017.00081
119. Doring Y, Soehnlein O, Weber C. Neutrophil extracellular traps in atherosclerosis and atherothrombosis. *Circ Res* (2017) 120(4):736–43. doi:10.1161/CIRCRESAHA.116.309692
120. Qi H, Yang S, Zhang L. Neutrophil extracellular traps and endothelial dysfunction in atherosclerosis and thrombosis. *Front Immunol* (2017) 8:928. doi:10.3389/fimmu.2017.00928
121. Aldabbous L, Abdul-Salam V, McKinnon T, Duluc L, Pepke-Zaba J, Southwood M, et al. Neutrophil extracellular traps promote angiogenesis: evidence from vascular pathology in pulmonary hypertension. *Arterioscler Thromb Vasc Biol* (2016) 36(10):2078–87. doi:10.1161/ATVBAHA.116.307634
122. Quillard T, Araujo HA, Franck G, Shvartz E, Sukhova G, Libby P. TLR2 and neutrophils potentiate endothelial stress, apoptosis and detachment: implications for superficial erosion. *Eur Heart J* (2015) 36(22):1394–404. doi:10.1093/eurheartj/ehv044
123. Shah A, Mehta N, Reilly MP. Adipose inflammation, insulin resistance, and cardiovascular disease. *JPEN J Parenter Enteral Nutr* (2008) 32(6):638–44. doi:10.1177/0148607108325251
124. Rivers JP, Powell-Wiley TM, Dey AK, Rodante JA, Chung JH, Joshi AA, et al. Visceral adiposity in psoriasis is associated with vascular inflammation by 18fluorodeoxyglucose positron-emission tomography/computed tomography beyond cardiometabolic disease risk factors in an observational cohort study. *J Cardiovasc Imag* (2017) 11(2 Pt 2):349–57. doi:10.1016/j.jcmg.2017.08.014
125. Bourlier V, Zakaroff-Girard A, Miranville A, De Barros S, Maumus M, Sengenes C, et al. Remodeling phenotype of human subcutaneous adipose tissue macrophages. *Circulation* (2008) 117(6):806–15. doi:10.1161/CIRCULATIONAHA.107.724096
126. Fjeldborg K, Pedersen SB, Moller HJ, Christiansen T, Bennetzen M, Richelsen B. Human adipose tissue macrophages are enhanced but changed to an anti-inflammatory profile in obesity. *J Immunol Res* (2014) 2014:309548. doi:10.1155/2014/309548
127. Britton KA, Fox CS. Perivascular adipose tissue and vascular disease. *Clin Lipidol* (2011) 6(1):79–91. doi:10.2217/clp.10.89
128. Fitzgibbons TP, Czech MP. Epicardial and perivascular adipose tissues and their influence on cardiovascular disease: basic mechanisms and clinical associations. *J Am Heart Assoc* (2014) 3(2):e000582. doi:10.1161/JAHA.113.000582
129. Henrichot E, Juge-Aubry CE, Pernin A, Pache JC, Velebit V, Dayer JM, et al. Production of chemokines by perivascular adipose tissue: a role in the pathogenesis of atherosclerosis? *Arterioscler Thromb Vasc Biol* (2005) 25(12):2594–9. doi:10.1161/01.ATV.0000188508.40052.35
130. Karastergiou K, Evans I, Ogston N, Miheisi N, Nair D, Kaski JC, et al. Epicardial adipokines in obesity and coronary artery disease induce atherogenic changes in monocytes and endothelial cells. *Arterioscler Thromb Vasc Biol* (2010) 30(7):1340–6. doi:10.1161/ATVBAHA.110.204719
131. Antonopoulos AS, Sanna F, Sabharwal N, Thomas S, Oikonomou EK, Herdman L, et al. Detecting human coronary inflammation by imaging perivascular fat. *Sci Transl Med* (2017) 9(398):eaal2658. doi:10.1126/scitranslmed.aal2658
132. Cerman AA, Bozkurt S, Sav A, Tulunay A, Elbasi MO, Ergun T. Serum leptin levels, skin leptin and leptin receptor expression in psoriasis. *Br J Dermatol* (2008) 159(4):820–6. doi:10.1111/j.1365-2133.2008.08742.x
133. Robati RM, Partovi-Kia M, Haghighatkhah HR, Younespour S, Abdollahimajd F. Increased serum leptin and resistin levels and increased carotid intima-media wall thickness in patients with psoriasis: is psoriasis associated with atherosclerosis? *J Am Acad Dermatol* (2014) 71(4):642–8. doi:10.1016/j.jaad.2014.06.006
134. Ouchi N, Parker JL, Lugus JJ, Walsh K. Adipokines in inflammation and metabolic disease. *Nat Rev Immunol* (2011) 11(2):85–97. doi:10.1038/nri2921
135. Wang X, Guo Z, Zhu Z, Bao Y, Yang B. Epicardial fat tissue in patients with psoriasis: a systematic review and meta-analysis. *Lipids Health Dis* (2016) 15:103. doi:10.1186/s12944-016-0271-y
136. Mansouri B, Patel M, Menter A. Biological therapies for psoriasis. *Expert Opin Biol Ther* (2013) 13(12):1715–30. doi:10.1517/14712598.2013.853739
137. Rungapiromnan W, Yiu ZZN, Warren RB, Griffiths CEM, Ashcroft DM. Impact of biologic therapies on risk of major adverse cardiovascular events in patients with psoriasis: systematic review and meta-analysis of randomized controlled trials. *Br J Dermatol* (2017) 176(4):890–901. doi:10.1111/bjd.14964
138. Wu JJ, Choi YM, Bebchuk JD. Risk of myocardial infarction in psoriasis patients: a retrospective cohort study. *J Dermatolog Treat* (2015) 26(3):230–4. doi:10.3109/09546634.2014.952609
139. Wu JJ, Joshi AA, Reddy SP, Batech M, Egeberg A, Ahlehoff O, et al. Anti-inflammatory therapy with tumor necrosis factor inhibitors is associated with reduced risk of major adverse cardiovascular events in psoriasis. *J Eur Acad Dermatol Venereol* (2018). doi:10.1111/jdv.14951
140. Wu JJ, Poon KY, Channual JC, Shen AY. Association between tumor necrosis factor inhibitor therapy and myocardial infarction risk in patients

with psoriasis. *Arch Dermatol* (2012) 148(11):1244–50. doi:10.1001/archdermatol.2012.2502

141. McInnes IB, Buckley CD, Isaacs JD. Cytokines in rheumatoid arthritis – shaping the immunological landscape. *Nat Rev Rheumatol* (2016) 12(1):63–8. doi:10.1038/nrrheum.2015.171
142. Yago T, Nanke Y, Kawamoto M, Kobashigawa T, Yamanaka H, Kotake S. IL-23 and Th17 disease in inflammatory arthritis. *J Clin Med* (2017) 6(9):E81. doi:10.3390/jcm6090081
143. Gelfand JM, Joshi A, Shin D, Dey A, Torrigian D, Rader D, et al. A trial to determine the effect of psoriasis treatment (adalimumab, phototherapy, and placebo) on cardiometabolic disease: the vascular inflammation in psoriasis (VIP) trial. *J Invest Dermatol* (2017) 138(5):S67. doi:10.1016/j.jid.2018.03.400
144. Gelfand JM, Takeshita J, Dey A, Shin D, Noe MH, Fuxench ZC, et al. A phase IV, randomised, double-blind, placebocontrolled crossover study of the effects of ustekinumab on vascular inflammation in psoriasis (the VIP-U TRIAL). *J Invest Med* (2018) 66(3):697. doi:10.1136/jim-2018-000730.1

6

Long Non-Coding RNAs Play a Role in the Pathogenesis of Psoriatic Arthritis by Regulating MicroRNAs and Genes Involved in Inflammation and Metabolic Syndrome

Marzia Dolcino[1], Andrea Pelosi[2], Piera Filomena Fiore[2], Giuseppe Patuzzo[1], Elisa Tinazzi[1], Claudio Lunardi[1†] and Antonio Puccetti[3†]*

[1] Department of Medicine, University of Verona, Verona, Italy, [2] Immunology Area, Pediatric Hospital Bambino Gesù, Rome, Italy, [3] Department of Experimental Medicine – Section of Histology, University of Genova, Genova, Italy

***Correspondence:**
Claudio Lunardi
claudio.lunardi@univr.it

†These authors have contributed

Psoriatic arthritis (PsA) is an inflammatory arthritis, characterized by inflammation of entheses and synovium, leading to joint erosions and new bone formation. It affects 10–30% of patients with psoriasis, and has an estimated prevalence of approximately 1%. PsA is considered to be primarily an autoimmune disease, driven by autoreactive T cells directed against autoantigens present in the skin and in the joints. However, an autoinflammatory origin has recently been proposed. Long noncoding RNAs (lncRNAs) are RNAs more than 200 nucleotides in length that do not encode proteins. LncRNAs play important roles in several biological processes, including chromatin remodeling, transcription control, and post-transcriptional processing. Several studies have shown that lncRNAs are expressed in a stage-specific or lineage-specific manner in immune cells that have a role in the development, activation, and effector functions of immune cells. LncRNAs are thought to play a role in several diseases, including autoimmune disorders. Indeed, a few lncRNAs have been identified in systemic lupus erythematosus, rheumatoid arthritis, and psoriasis. Although several high-throughput studies have been performed to identify lncRNAs, their biological and pathological relevance are still unknown, and most transcriptome studies in autoimmune diseases have only assessed protein-coding transcripts. No data are currently available on lncRNAs in PsA. Therefore, by microarray analysis, we have investigated the expression profiles of more than 50,000 human lncRNAs in blood samples from PsA patients and healthy controls using Human Clariom D Affymetrix chips, suitable to detect rare and low-expressing transcripts otherwise unnoticed by common sequencing methodologies. Network analysis identified lncRNAs targeting highly connected genes in the PsA transcriptome. Such genes are involved in molecular pathways crucial for PsA pathogenesis, including immune response, glycolipid metabolism, bone remodeling, type 1 interferon, wingless related integration site, and tumor necrosis factor signaling. Selected lncRNAs were validated by RT-PCR in an expanded cohort of patients. Moreover, modulated genes belonging to meaningful pathways were validated by RT-PCR in PsA PBMCs and/or by ELISA in PsA sera. The findings indicate that lncRNAs are involved in PsA pathogenesis by regulating both microRNAs and genes and open new avenues for the identification of new biomarkers and therapeutical targets.

Keywords: psoriatic arthritis, gene expression, long non-coding RNAs, gene module, protein–protein interaction network

INTRODUCTION

Psoriatic arthritis (PsA) is a chronic, immune-mediated, asymmetric inflammatory arthritis characterized by inflammation at tendon or ligament insertion sites into bone (enthesitis) and by synovitis, eventually leading to joint erosions and new bone formation (1).

Up to 30% of patients with skin psoriasis may develop PsA and its prevalence is estimated in 1% in the general population. PsA shares genetic and clinical features with other forms of seronegative spondyloarthritis (2, 3). Diagnostic criteria for PsA have not been validated, but the Classification Criteria for PsA (CASPAR criteria), published in 2006, define PsA for the purpose of enrolling patients in clinical trials and provide guidance to clinicians (4, 5). Therefore, the diagnosis of PsA is mainly performed on clinical features after the exclusion of other seronegative arthritides and no diagnostic tests are available so far.

The pathogenesis of PsA is still poorly understood and both autoinflammation and autoimmunity are believed to play a pivotal role in the disease. Synovial tissue in PsA is characterized by T-cell infiltrate, by marked angiogenesis, and by synovial hyperplasia with increased secretion of cytokines and proteases, which may amplify the local inflammatory process eventually leading to joint destruction (6). Tumor necrosis factor-alpha (TNF-α) is a very important inflammatory mediator and has been implicated in the pathogenesis of articular damage in PsA (6). TNF-α inhibitors are currently used in PsA treatment; however, a high percentage of PsA patients does not respond to TNF-α antagonists (1, 7). Therefore, other cytokines have recently become targets of biological agents, such as interleukin-12 (IL-12), interleukin-23 (IL-23), and interleukin-17 (IL-17) (1, 7). Indeed IL-17 plays a fundamental role in disease development and progression (8).

We have reported the findings of the transcriptome analysis in paired synovial tissue and peripheral blood cells of patients with PsA (9). The upregulation of Th-17 cells related genes and of type I interferon (IFN) inducible genes in PsA patients strengthened the hypothesis that PsA has a strong autoimmune origin, since the coactivity of type I IFN and IL-17 pathways is typical of autoimmunity (9). Moreover, we confirmed these findings with a miRNA microarray analysis in PBMCs of PsA patients showing that pathway enrichment analysis on gene targets of deregulated microRNAs (miRNAs) revealed signaling pathways typically implicated in PsA, such as TNF, mitogen-activated protein (MAP) kinase, and wingless related integration site (WNT) cascades (10).

By this study we wanted to provide a more in-depth knowledge on the epigenetic mechanisms that regulate the PsA pathogenesis by analyzing the expression profiles of long non-coding RNAs (lncRNAs) in the same cohort of patients that we studied in our previous work (10). lncRNAs are important molecules that regulate gene expression through multiple mechanisms and are involved in immune and inflammatory pathways (11). As far as we know, no study has yet taken into consideration lncRNAs expression profiles in PsA patients and only a few data have been reported the deregulation of some lncRNAs in psoriasis (12, 13).

Moreover, in this study we offer a sophisticated and integrated analysis of lncRNAs, miRNAs, and gene expression profiles in PsA patients that allows to identify lncRNAs that regulate transcripts effectively modulated in the disease and that are involved in pathogenetically relevant molecular pathways.

MATERIALS AND METHODS

Patients

We studied a cohort of 10 patients (6 males and 4 females, mean age: 53.5 years) affected by PsA, attending the Unit of Autoimmune Diseases, at the University Hospital of Verona, Italy. All patients fulfilled the CASPAR criteria for the diagnosis of PsA: inflammatory musculoskeletal involvement combined with at least three features: (1) evidence of current psoriasis, personal history of psoriasis, and family history of psoriasis in unaffected patients; (2) affected nails (onycholysis and pitting); (3) dactylitis; (4) negative rheumatoid factor (RF); and (5) radiographic evidence of new juxta-articular bone formation (excluding osteophytes) (4). All the patients underwent clinical examination and laboratory evaluation comprehensive of inflammatory markers, such as C-reactive protein and erythrocytes sedimentation rate; RF and anti-cyclic citrullinated peptide antibody detected by ELISA test; antinuclear antibody detected by indirect immunofluorescence on HeLa-derived HEp-2 cells; and genetic screening for the association with the allele HLA-B27. All patients underwent the following instrumental investigations: ultrasonography with Power Doppler to investigate subclinical enthesopathy and synovitis in asymptomatic patients, conventional radiography, magnetic resonance imaging, and scintigraphy. The radiological features of peripheral PsA included asymmetric distribution, participation of distal interphalangeal joints, periostitis, bone density preservation, bone ankylosis, and pencil-in-cup deformity.

The patients were affected by cutaneous or nails psoriasis and were enrolled in the study at diagnosis of peripheral PsA before starting immunosuppressive treatment.

All the participants to the study signed a written informed consent and the local Ethical Committee of the University Hospital of Verona, Verona, Italy, had approved the study protocol. All the investigations have been performed according to the principles of the Helsinki declaration.

Microarray Analysis

Blood samples were collected in BD Vacutainer K2EDTA tubes using a 21-gauge needle. PBMCs were obtained upon stratification on Lympholyte® cell separation density gradient (Cedarlane, Burlington, ON, Canada). PBMCs composition was similar between patients and controls. Total RNA extraction from PBMCs was performed with miRNeasy mini kit following manufacturer's protocol (Qiagen GmbH, Hilden, Germany). 500 ng of total RNA were used for sample preparation starting from 5 ml of blood. cRNA preparation, samples hybridization and scanning were performed following the Affymetrix (Affymetrix, Santa Clara, CA, USA) provided protocols, by Cogentech Affymetrix microarray unit (Campus IFOM IEO, Milan, Italy). All samples were hybridized on Human Clariom D (Thermo Fisher Scientific) gene chip and were analyzed using the Transcriptome Analysis Console 4.0 software (Applied Biosystem, Foster City, CA, USA by Thermo Fisher Scientific, Waltham, MA, USA).

The Human Clariom D arrays allow to interrogate more than 540,000 transcripts sourced from the largest number of public databases starting from as little as 100 pg of total RNA.

The Signal Space Transformation-Robust Multi-Array Average algorithm was applied to background-adjust, normalize, and log-transform signals intensity.

Relative gene expression levels of each transcript were validated applying a One-Way analysis of variance ($p \leq 0.01$) and multiple testing correction. Coding genes and lncRNAs that displayed an expression level at least 1.5-fold different in the test sample versus control sample ($p \leq 0.01$) were carried forward in the analysis.

The targets (including microRNAs and genes) of all the lncRNAs that satisfied the above-mentioned FC and *p*-value criteria were screened using NPInter v3.0.[1] This database allows the efficient recovery of all lncRNAs interactions experimentally validated by high-throughput experimental technologies (14, 15).

The list of gene targets of miRNAs that were targeted by significantly modulated lncRNAs was obtained using the FunRich database[2] (16).

Protein–Protein Interaction (PPI) Network Construction and Network Clustering

The Search Tool for the Retrieval of Interacting Genes (STRING version 10.5[3]) was used to obtain PPIs pairs that were validated by experimental studies (17) and to construct the PPI networks. Network topological analysis was performed using the Cytoscape software[4] (18).

High-flow areas (highly connected regions) of the network were detected using the MCODE plugin of Cytoscape, based on the thresholds of *k*-core = 3 and node score cutoff = 0.2.

Gene Functional Classification and Enrichment Analysis

Genes were functionally classified into canonical biological processes (BPs) on the basis of the gene ontology (GO) annotations.[5]

Biological processes and Pathways enrichment analysis was performed employing FunRich (hypergeometric *p*-value ≤0.05).

Real-Time PCR

lncRNAs Modulated in PsA

For each sample, 500 ng of total RNA was treated with 1 unit of DNase I Amplification Grade (Invitrogen; Carlsbad, CA, USA) according to the manufacturer's protocol. First-strand cDNA was generated using the SuperScript IV First-Strand Synthesis System (Invitrogen; Carlsbad, CA, USA) with random hexamers, according to the manufacturer's protocol. Real-time PCR was performed in triplicate with PowerUp™ Sybr® Green reagent (Applied Biosystems; Foster City, CA, USA) in a QuantStudio 6 Flex system (Applied Biosystems; Foster City, CA, USA). Relative expression levels were calculated for each sample after normalization against the geometric mean of the housekeeping genes GAPDH and beta-actin (ACTB) expression. The ΔΔCt method was used for comparing relative fold expression differences. The data are expressed as fold changes with respect to healthy.

Genes Modulated in PsA

First-strand cDNA was generated using the SuperScript III First-Strand Synthesis System for RT-PCR Kit (Invitrogen), with random hexamers, according to the manufacturer's protocol. PCR was performed in a total volume of 25 μl containing 1× Taqman Universal PCR Master mix, no AmpErase UNG, and 2.5 μl of cDNA; pre-designed, gene-specific primers, and probe sets for each gene were obtained from Assay-on-Demande Gene Expression Products (Applied Biosystems).

Real-time PCR reactions were carried out in a two-tube system and in singleplex. The real-time amplifications included 10 min at 95°C (AmpliTaq Gold activation), followed by 40 cycles at 95°C for 15 s and at 60°C for 1 min. Thermocycling and signal detection were performed with 7500 Sequence Detector (Applied Biosystems). Signals were detected according to the manufacturer's instructions and the relative expression levels were calculated as it has been previously described (9).

Detection of Soluble Mediators in Sera of PsA Patients

Serum levels of glypican-4, IFN-γ, Wnt-2, mTOR, TNF-α, SPD-1, NFKB p65, NOTCH1, omentin, and adiponectin were detected using commercially available ELISA kits that were supplied by antibodies-online (glypican-4, Wnt-2, and mTOR), LifeSpan BioSciences (TNF-α, NFKB p65, and omentin), IBL International (IFN-γ), R&D (adiponectin), and Ray Biotech (sPD-1).

Plasmid Construction and Luciferase Reporter Assay

The plasmids to knockdown LINC00909 and LINC00657 were purchased from GenePharma (Shanghai, China).

Human HEK (human embryonic kidney) 293 T cells (1.5×10^4) grown in a 96-well plate were co-transfected with 150 ng of empty vector, 50 ng of firefly luciferase reporter comprising the lncRNAs mut vectors, (Promega, Madison, WI, USA) using Lipofectamie 2000 (Invitrogen, USA). Cells were harvested 48 h after transfection and analyzed using the Dual-Luciferase Reporter Assay System (Promega) according to the manufacturer's protocol.

RESULTS

High-Throughput Long Non-Coding RNA and Gene Expression Profiling in Peripheral Blood Mononuclear Cells of PsA

In order to evaluate the potential role played by lncRNAs in PsA pathogenesis, we performed a gene array study using the Clariom D human gene chip that enabled us to analyze, at the same time, both conventional gene and lncRNA expression profiles.

[1] http://www.bioinfo.org/NPInter/ (Accessed: November 16, 2017).
[2] www.funrich.org/ (Accessed: December 15, 2017).
[3] http://string-db.org/ (Accessed: February 06, 2018).
[4] www.cytoscape.org (Accessed: February 15, 2018).
[5] www.geneontology.org (Accessed: January 19, 2018).

We compared the lncRNA expression profiles of PBMC samples obtained from 10 PsA patients with 10 PBMC samples obtained from age and sex matched healthy donors and we found that 259 lncRNAs satisfied the Bonferroni-corrected p value criterion ($p \leq 0.01$) and the fold change criterion (FC $\geq |1.5|$), displaying robust and statistically significant variation between PsA and healthy controls samples (Table S1 in Supplementary Material). The study was implemented by the analysis of conventional gene expression profiles in the same PsA samples and we found that 1,922 differently expressed genes satisfied the above-mentioned criteria. The complete list of modulated genes can be found in Table S2 in Supplementary Material. In both cases, the arrays were validated by real-time PCR. LncRNAs LUCAT1 and TRIM55-1 were validated by real-time PCR in the entire series of patients analyzed. Significantly different expression levels were found for all tested lncRNAs in PsA as compared to healthy controls (see Figure S1 in Supplementary Material).

Moreover, real-time PCR analysis for seven lncRNAs was carried out in an expanded panel of PsA patients (20 patients) and healthy controls (20 subjects). A significant modulation of all these lncRNAs was found in all tested patients thus confirming gene array results (see **Figure 1**).

To gain meaningful insights on the potential role played by modulated lncRNAs in PsA pathogenesis, the complete list of modulated lncRNA was filtered, extracting only those transcripts for which a bona fide target annotations was present in NPInter. By this method 92 lncRNAs were selected (Table S3 in Supplementary Material) and, simultaneously, the list of all gene and microRNA targets of the selected lncRNAs, experimentally validated by high-throughput technologies, was extracted from the same database.

To corroborate our results we narrowed down our analysis to modulate lncRNA that targeted genes that were significantly modulated in the array and miRNAs that we found deregulated in our previous analysis of PsA PBMCs from the same cohort of patients (10) (**Table 1**). In particular, we found that 15 of these miRNAs modulated in PsA (hsa-miR-130a-3p, hsa-miR-148a-3p, hsa-miR-151a-5p, hsa-miR-17-5p, hsa-miR-186-5p, hsa-miR-199a-3p, hsa-miR-199a-5p, hsa-miR-28-5p, hsa-miR-3135b, hsa-miR-320c, hsa-miR-320d, hsa-miR-331-3p, hsa-miR-423-5p, hsa-miR-451a, and hsa-miR-92a-3p) were targeted by selected lncRNAs. We then extracted from the FunRich database the annotated gene targets of the above-mentioned miRNAs selecting only transcripts that also resulted when modulated in the Clariom D array (Table S4 in Supplementary Material). **Table 2** recapitulates the above-selected lncRNAs and targets.

In summary, we selected only those lncRNAs, that targeted miRNAs and genes with evidence of modulation in our PsA samples to trace, with a good confidence, lncRNAs–miRNAs–genes interactions that are expected to be established in the course of PsA.

To validate our results we conducted a LINC00909siRNA and a LINC00657siRNA silencing in human 293 T cells, to explore whether this knockdown altered the expression levels of selected miRNAs targeted by LINC00909 (miR-148a-3p and mir-28-5p) and by LINC00657 (miR-130a-3p and miR-17-5p). We observed that the silencing of the two lncRNAs significantly increased the level of expression of their targeted miRNAs.

The registered percentages of increase were: 70 ± 3.8 and 78 ± 1.4% for miR-148a-3p and mir-28-5p, respectively, and 75 ± 2.3 and 80 ± 1.53% for miR-130a-3p and miR-17-5p, respectively.

PPI Network of Modulated lncRNAs in PsA

The lncRNA expression profiling of PsA PBMCs was integrated with a network analysis. We, therefore, inspected, by a bioinformatic methodology, all the functional and experimentally validated interactions among the protein products of genes targeted by lncRNAs and by the 15 above-mentioned miRNAs (230 genes) that were selected as previously described. Then, taking in account of these interactions, we constructed a PPI network which showed a good PPI enrichment p-value (0.00041). In the obtained network 229 of the above-mentioned genes (nodes), were connected by 195 pairs of interactions (edges). Since 229 out of 230 of lncRNAs and miRNAs gene targets that we used as input for the network analysis, resulted connected in the PPI network, we could observe that the selected lncRNAs may act in an integrated fashion in the disease.

We then imported in Cytoscape the PPI network, adding to its scaffold the lncRNAs-genes, miRNAs-genes, and lncRNAs–miRNAs interactions that we selected as we explained above. Thus, we obtained an implemented network that is showed in **Figure 2**. A topological analysis of this network was performed to highlight lncRNAs that were highly connected to the PPI network genes (i.e., targeting a large number of PPI-network genes) also considering all the lncRNA–gene interactions mediated by the selected miRNAs (i.e., lncRNA–miRNA–gene interactions). By this approach we could select seven lncRNAs, including EPB41L4A-AS1, LA16c-360H6.3, LINC00657, LINC00909, RP11-1100L3.8, RP11-539L10.3, and RP11-403I13.5 that displayed the highest connectivity in the network. As shown in **Figures 3A–G** (where genes of the PPI network are ordered around a circle based on their degree of connectivity, i.e., number of edges) the above-mentioned lncRNAs directly or indirectly targeted genes that, in most cases, were distributed in areas of the network characterized by a high degree of connectivity. This observation indicated that, since these lncRNAs targeted highly interconnected genes, they may have a broad effect in the disease that goes beyond the modulation of single target gene(s).

Modular Analysis of Genes and lncRNAs Modulated in PsA

In a second part of our analysis we wanted to dissect the global impact of lncRNAs on the entire PsA transcriptome (i.e., on the 1,922 modulated genes in PsA). Since the targeting of genes with more interacting partners may have a broader impact on the global transciptome than the modulation of few isolated genes, we aimed to inspect if the modulated lncRNAs may display connections with highly interacting genes in PsA. To this purpose, we built the PPI network that included the protein products of all modulated genes in PsA that showed experimentally validated interactions obtaining a wide network containing 1,637 nodes and 9,415 edges and showing a very good PPI enrichment p-value ($p < 10–16$). Then we performed a modular analysis to find areas

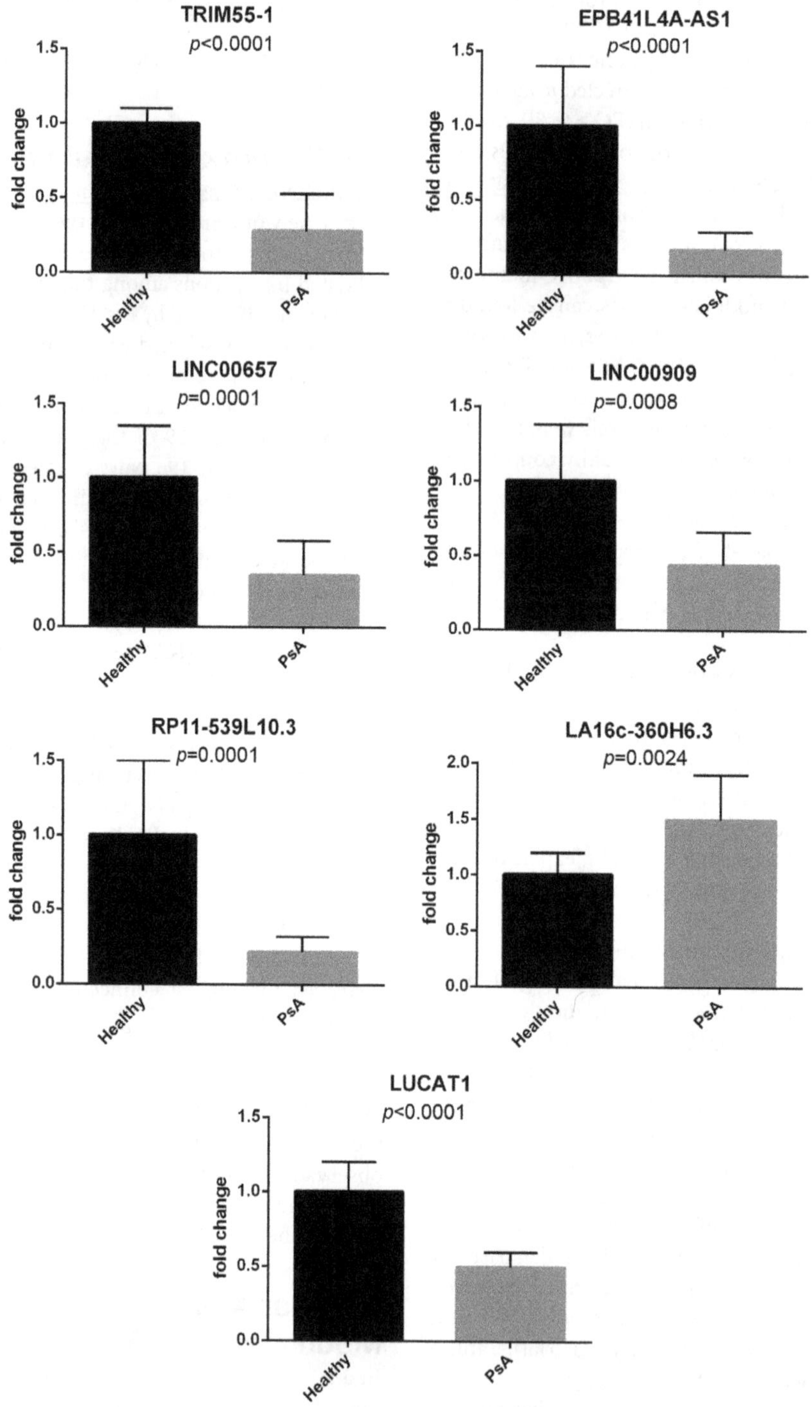

FIGURE 1 | Expression of selected long non-coding RNAs in an expanded panel of psoriatic arthritis patients (20 patients) and healthy controls (20 subjects). Bars indicate SD.

of the network that included the most highly connected genes (modules). By this analysis we could extract 16 modules (M1–M16, see Table S5 in Supplementary Material). All the 16 modules were imported in Cytoscape along with all the previously selected interactions with miRNAs and modulated lncRNAs that we also considered in the network analysis described in the previous paragraph. The graphical visualization of genes connected in modules and their interactions with lncRNAs showed that the majority of the 16 modules (10/16) were directly or indirectly targeted by modulated lncRNAs, including M1, M2, M4, M5,

TABLE 1 | Selected modulated long non-coding RNAs in psoriatic arthritis patients versus healthy controls.

ID	Fold change	*p*-value	Gene symbol	mRNA accession
TC0500008318.hg.1	−2.37	0.0026	EPB41L4A-AS1	ENST00000413221.2
TC0700007000.hg.1	−2.02	0.0015	HOTAIRM1	ENST00000616712
TC0600008510.hg.1	−2.25	0.0087	KCNQ5-IT1	ENST00000445310
TC0700013567.hg.1	2.05	0.0013	LINC00174	ENST00000416366
TC0700007277.hg.1	2.46	0.0001	LINC00265	ENST00000340510.4
TC1500007707.hg.1	−1.58	0.0089	LINC00593	ENST00000558385.1
TC2000008995.hg.1	−2.27	0.0017	LINC00657	ENST00000565493
TC1800009043.hg.1	−1.84	0.0025	LINC00909	ENST00000577806
TC0200007199.hg.1	2.27	0.0007	LINC00486	ENST00000414054
TC0100009691.hg.1	−1.97	0.0003	RP11-403I13.5	ENST00000443018.1
TC0200010127.hg.1	−3.24	<0.0001	RP11-171I2.4	ENST00000605334.1
TC0200011420.hg.1	−2.68	0.0005	AC133528.2	ENST00000433036.1
TC0400009914.hg.1	−2.37	0.0027	RP11-539L10.3	ENST00000513179.1
TC0500009465.hg.1	−1.74	0.007	RP11-779O18.3	ENST00000523005.1
TC0800007847.hg.1	−14.9	<0.0001	AC084082.3	ENST00000517961.2
TC1100011278.hg.1	1.91	0.0003	RP11-867G23.3	ENST00000501708.1
TC1200006772.hg.1	−1.86	0.0044	RP11-75L1.1	ENST00000541404.1
TC1200010732.hg.1	−3.11	0.0058	RP11-1100L3.8	ENST00000564363.1
TC1400006719.hg.1	−2.54	0.0066	RP11-468E2.5	ENST00000558478.1
TC1400009275.hg.1	−1.61	0.0027	RP11-930O11.2	ENST00000560296.1
TC1600009188.hg.1	2.21	0.0021	LA16c-360H6.3	ENST00000574245.1
TC1700007241.hg.1	2.64	0.0008	RP11-283C24.1	ENST00000578585.1
TC2100007843.hg.1	−1.78	0.0016	AF131217.1	ENST00000430247.1
TC2200008462.hg.1	−3.38	0.0058	RP3-430N8.10	ENST00000602955.1
TC1500010312.hg.1	−2.52	0.0064	RP11-815J21.2	ENST00000561409.1
TC1800007426.hg.1	−3.49	0.0032	RP11-1151B14.4	ENST00000591360.1
TC1900011833.hg.1	1.81	0.0031	CTB-25B13.12	ENST00000588225.1
TC1900007159.hg.1	−1.77	0.0084	CTB-55O6.10	ENST00000590715.1
TC1200008393.hg.1	−1.74	0.0028	RP11-981P6.1	ENST00000552778.1
TC1200008425.hg.1	−2.1	0.0024	RP11-796E2.4	ENST00000499685.2
TC1400009962.hg.1	−2.61	0.0006	RP11-471B22.2	ENST00000555853.1
TC1600006833.hg.1	2.16	0.0024	RP11-77H9.5	ENST00000564919.1
TC1400009667.hg.1	1.88	0.0092	RP4-693M11.3	ENST00000557304.1
TC1000009009.hg.1	−1.6	0.0098	RP11-498B4.5	ENST00000433600.1
TC1400010386.hg.1	1.71	0.0064	CTD-3051D23.4	ENST00000553344.2
TC1200008527.hg.1	−2.91	0.0065	RP11-256L6.3	ENST00000551849.1
TC0200007485.hg.1	1.61	0.0048	AC016722.4	ENST00000429761.1
TC1400007002.hg.1	1.95	0.0041	CTD-2002H8.2	ENST00000557322.1
TC0500008150.hg.1	−2.4	0.0066	CTD-2260A17.1	ENST00000512866.1
TC0600010636.hg.1	−1.89	0.0005	RP3-406P24.3	ENST00000415144.1

M8, M10, M11, M12, M14, and M15 (**Figure 4**). Moreover, we could observe that the vast majority of modules was targeted by the above-mentioned lncRNAs that included LINC00909 (targeting 9/10 modules) LINC00657 (targeting 8/10 modules), EPB41L4A-AS1, RP11-539L10.3 (targeting 7/10 modules), LA16c-360H6.3, RP11-403I13.5, and RP11-1100L3.8 (targeting 5/10 modules) (Table S6 in Supplementary Material).

Functional Analysis of the Targeted Modules and Their Targeting lncRNAs

To dissect the possible role played by the module-targeting-lncRNAs we performed a functional classification of genes included in the 10 targeted modules, based on the GO classification criteria. **Figure 5** recapitulates all the most relevant GO BPs in which the genes of targeted modules are classified.

M1 was the most targeted module and 35 lncRNAs showed direct or indirect connections with it (see Table S6 in Supplementary Material). The 88 genes included in this module were mostly related to translation, mRNA splicing, and protein ubiquitination GO BPs. Among genes included in protein ubiquitination, nine genes belonged to the "proteasome-mediated ubiquitin-dependent protein catabolic process" BP, including CUL1, CUL3, FBXW5, FBXW7, FBXL19, HECTD3, NEDD4L, RNF126, and UBE2A. Interestingly, it has been recently observed that ubiquitin–proteasome-mediated protein degradation plays a role in modulating the balance between bone formation and bone resorption, since it is involved in signaling pathways that are crucial for bone homeostasis like RANK/NF-κB pathway and the Wnt/β-catenin pathway (19). In addition CUL3 is also associated with the "Wnt signaling pathway" BP. 12 genes were targeted in the M1, including CUL5, TRA2B, SRRM1, ASB6, HNRNPUL1, CPSF7, HNRNPC, NUDT21, UPF1, and the above-mentioned FBXL19, NEDD4L, and FBXW7. UPF1 was the most targeted gene in M1. It is critical for the activity of Regnase-1 also called MCPIP1 (monocyte chemotactic protein-1-induced protein-1), a crucial molecule that regulates immune response avoiding over-activation of the immune system (20). Interestingly, the gene FBXL19 represents

TABLE 2 | Long non-coding RNAs (LncRNAs) and their targets modulated in psoriatic arthritis.

LncRNAs	Gene targets	miRNA targets
LINC00174	CPSF7	
LINC00265	IGF2BP2	
LINC00593	UPF1	
LINC00657	CPSF7, FXR1, HNRNPC, NUDT21 UPF1, ZC3H7B	hsa-miR-130a-3p hsa-miR-17-5p hsa-miR-186-5p hsa-miR-199a-3p hsa-miR-199a-5p hsa-miR-28-5p hsa-miR-320c hsa-miR-320d hsa-miR-331-3p hsa-miR-423-5p hsa-miR-451a
LINC00909	UPF1	hsa-miR-130a-3p hsa-miR-148a-3p hsa-miR-28-5p hsa-miR-320c hsa-miR-320d
LINC00486	FXR1, UPF1	
EPB41L4A-AS1	CPSF7, UPF1	hsa-miR-130a-3p hsa-miR-17-5p
HOTAIRM1	CPSF7, UPF1	
KCNQ5-IT1	CPSF7, UPF1	
RP11-403I13.5		hsa-miR-92a-3p
RP11-171I2.4	CPSF7	
AC133528.2	CPSF7	
RP11-539L10.3		hsa-miR-148a-3p hsa-miR-199a-3p
RP11-779O18.3	HNRNPC, UPF1, ZC3H7B	
AC084082.3	CPSF7, NUDT21, UPF1	hsa-miR-331-3p
RP11-867G23.3	UPF1, IGF2BP2	
RP11-75L1.1	UPF1	
RP11-1100L3.8	UPF1	hsa-miR-17-5p hsa-miR-423-5p
RP11-468E2.5	UPF1	
RP11-930O11.2	UPF1	
LA16c-360H6.3	IGF2BP2	hsa-miR-17-5p
RP11-283C24.1	UPF1	
AF131217.1	UPF1	
RP3-430N8.10		hsa-miR-331-3p
RP11-815J21.2		hsa-miR-186-5p
RP11-1151B14.4	UPF1	
CTB-25B13.12	UPF1	
CTB-55O6.10	CPSF7, UPF1	
RP11-981P6.1	CPSF7, UPF1, ZC3H7B	
RP11-796E2.4	UPF1	hsa-miR-3135b
RP11-471B22.2	CPSF7, IGF2BP2, UPF1, ZC3H7B	
RP11-77H9.5	CPSF7, HNRNPC, IGF2BP2, UPF1	
RP4-693M11.3	UPF1	
RP11-498B4.5	UPF1	
CTD-3051D23.4	IGF2BP2	
RP11-256L6.3	NUDT21, UPF1	
AC016722.4	CPSF7, UPF1, ZC3H7B	
CTD-2002H8.2	CPSF7, HNRNPC, NUDT21, UPF1, ZC3H7B	
CTD-2260A17.1		hsa-miR-151a-5p
RP3-406P24.3	CPSF7	

a susceptibility locus for PsA (21). Finally, other two genes of M1, TRIM32, and HERC5 play a role in the innate immune response and, in particular, HERC5 activates IRF3 (22).

M2 was targeted by 6 lncRNAs and included 40 genes that were mainly involved in cell division, inflammatory response (i.e., CCR7, CXCR1, CXCR2, PF4, and PPBP/CXCL7), tumor necrosis factor (TNF)-mediated signaling pathway (i.e., TNFRSF1B, TNFSF12, TNFRSF12A, and PSMA7), and Wnt signaling pathway (i.e., AXIN1, DVL3, GNB2, PPP2R5C, PSMA4, PSMB1, PSMC4, PSMD4, and RNF146) BPs. Interestingly, the expression of CXCL7 is increased in Rheumatoid arthritis (AR) synovia (23). Moreover AXIN2 another gene included in M2 is related to the intramembranous ossification BP. Eight genes were targeted in M2, including ADCY3, GNAI1, PSME3, PSMF1, RELA, TRAF3, and the above-mentioned TNFRSF1B and CCR7. In particular, the expression of CCR7 is stimulated by TNF-α and interleukin 1-beta in osteoclasts (24). Moreover, RELA is involved in peripheral regulatory T cell-induced tolerance (25) and TRAF3 is required for T cell and invariant natural killer T cell effector functions (26). In addition, TRAF3 is also involved in limiting osteoclastogenesis, indeed RANKL-induced degradation of TRAF3 enhances TNF-induced osteoclastogenesis (27).

M4 was targeted by seven lncRNAs and included 57 genes that were mainly involved in cell division, DNA repair, endocytosis, mitochondrial translation, mRNA export from nucleus, regulation of glycolytic process, and transcription. In addition, this module included two genes (i.e., MRE11A and XRCC6) associated with the BP "positive regulation of type I interferon production" and the gene POU2F2/OCT2 that increases the differentiation of antibodies secreting activated B cells (28). In this module the genes GBF1, MYBL2, RAD23A, and WASL were targeted.

M5 was targeted by the RP11-403I13.5 lncRNA and included 19 genes. Protein targeting to ER and translation were the most represented BPs in this module.

M8 was targeted by four lncRNAs (EPB41L4A-AS1, LINC00657, LINC00909, and RP11-539L10.3) and in this module seven genes were connected, including BRPF3, TAF12, TAF2, TAF7, TBPL1, TRIM24, and BPTF almost associated with the "translation" BP. Among these, BPTF is important for the homeostasis of T cells and is crucial for the maintenance and function of regulatory T (Treg) cells (29).

M10 was targeted by 8 lncRNAs and included 49 genes. These genes were associated with many BPs, including cell proliferation, signal transduction, transcription, Wnt signaling pathway (i.e., BCL9L, FZD6, LRP6, ATP6V0C, BCL9, and PYGO2), vasculogenesis (i.e., ENG and TGFBR2), bone resorption (i.e., TCIRG1), negative regulation of bone mineralization (i.e., SRGN), osteoblast differentiation (i.e., LGR4), and osteoblast development (i.e., LRP5). Several genes were associated with BPs related to glucose homeostasis like, for example, PPARGC1A (cellular glucose homeostasis), GSK3A (cellular response to insulin), IGF1R (insulin receptor signaling pathway), RAF1 (insulin secretion), and RAP1A (positive regulation of glucose import). In addition other genes were classified into BPs related to adaptive immune response like T cell differentiation (i.e., RIT1 and TCF7), and T cell cytokine production (KDELR1) and B cell homeostasis (SOS1). In M10 12 genes were targeted, including SHOC2, CCNL1, CDK13, MED16, MMS19, and the above-mentioned FZD6, PYGO2, KDELR1, PPARGC1A, RAP1A, SOS1, and TGFBR2.

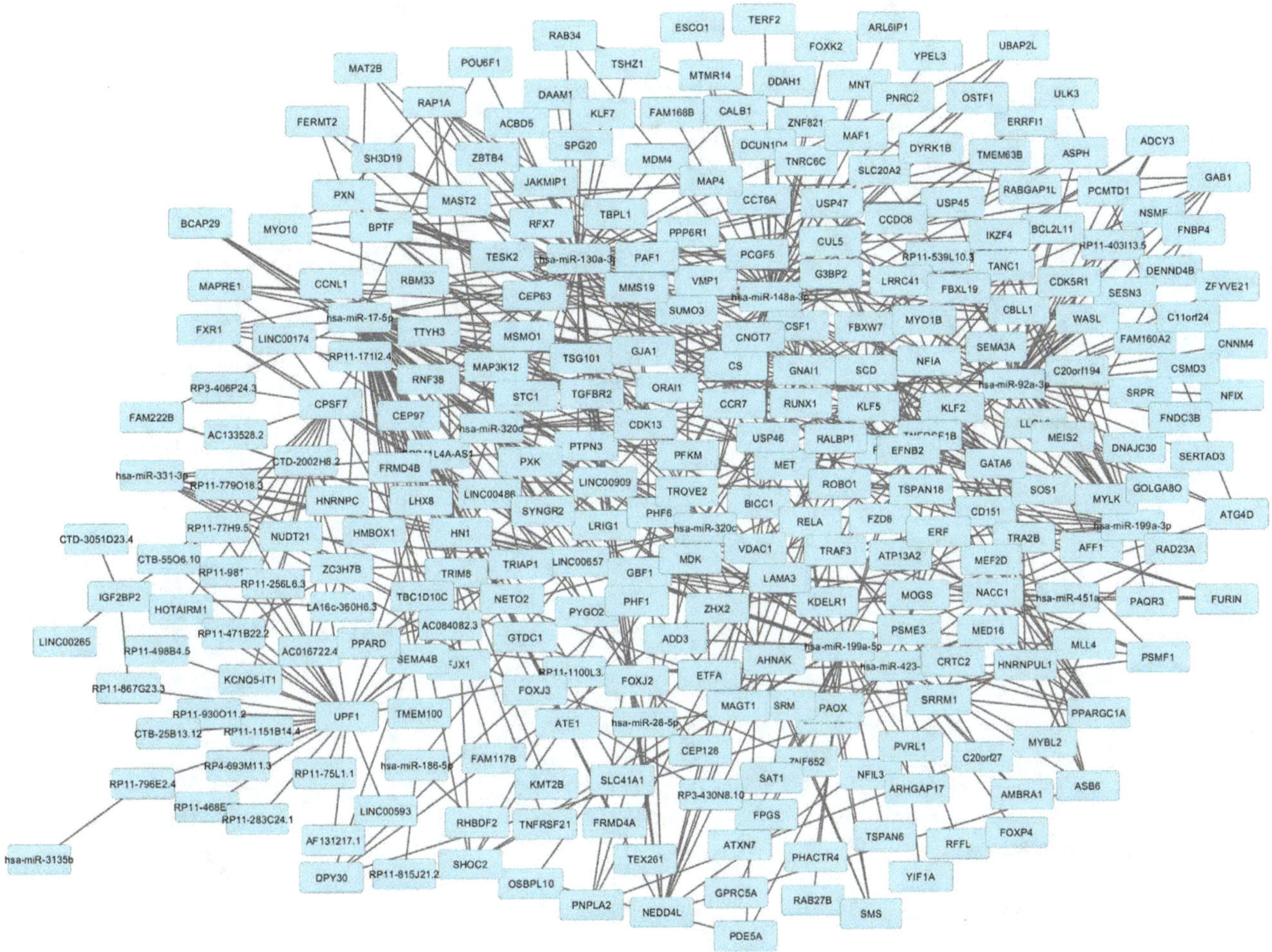

FIGURE 2 | Protein–protein interaction (PPI)-network of differently expressed genes in psoriatic arthritis (PsA) targeted by the selected long non-coding RNAs and microRNAs modulated in PsA.

M11 was targeted by 2 lncRNAs and included 28 genes. A large number of these genes were assigned to "lipid metabolic process" (i.e., PLCD3, PPAP2B, SLC27A1, and TBL1X), "phospholipid metabolic process" (i.e., AGPAT2, LPCAT3, LPCAT4, and PPAP2C), and to "phosphatidylinositol biosynthetic process" (CDIPT, MTMR14, PI4K2B, and PIK3C2B) BPs. Interestingly, two genes namely CARM1 and FASN were associated with "endochondral bone morphogenesis" and "osteoblast differentiation" BPs, respectively. In this module, TERF2, YPEL3, and the above-mentioned MTMR14 were targeted.

M12 was targeted by 6 lncRNAs and included 30 genes. We observed that several genes of this module classified in BPs related to the immune response, including SPI1/PU.1 (lymphoid progenitor cell differentiation), CD244 and KLRF1 (innate immune response), CD226 (positive regulation of natural killer cell cytokine production), CD7 (T cell activation), CD247 (T cell receptor signaling pathway), GBP1 (regulation of T cell receptor signaling pathway), CD79A (B cell activation), GBP1, GBP2, and CIITA (type I interferon signaling pathway), HCST, LILRB2, and KLRB1 (regulation of immune response), GZMA (immune response) and SPI1/PU.1 (lymphoid progenitor cell differentiation), and CIITA (positive regulation of MHC class I and of MHC class II biosynthetic process). In particular, the transcription factor SPI1/PU.1 is crucial for the development of interleukin-9-producing helper T cells (Th9) (30, 31) that have been recently involved in the PsA pathogenesis (32).

Moreover five genes, including DAG1, COL14A1, LAMA2, LAMA3, and LAMC1 were associated with the "extracellular matrix organization" BP. LAMA3 and FAM168B were targeted in this module.

M14 was targeted by three lncRNAs and included 14 genes that were mainly associated with protein targeting to mitochondrion (TOMM20 and TOMM40), protein import into mitochondrial inner membrane (TIMM22), ATP biosynthetic process (ATP5I), apoptosis (BCL2L11 and CASP4), and in Wnt signaling pathway (TLE1 and TLE3) BPs. In this module the genes BCL2L11 and VDAC1 were targeted.

Finally, M15 was targeted by 6 lncRNAs and included 44 genes. In this module, we observed the presence of genes classified in several BPS, including cell division (TUBA1C, TFDP1, CEP192,

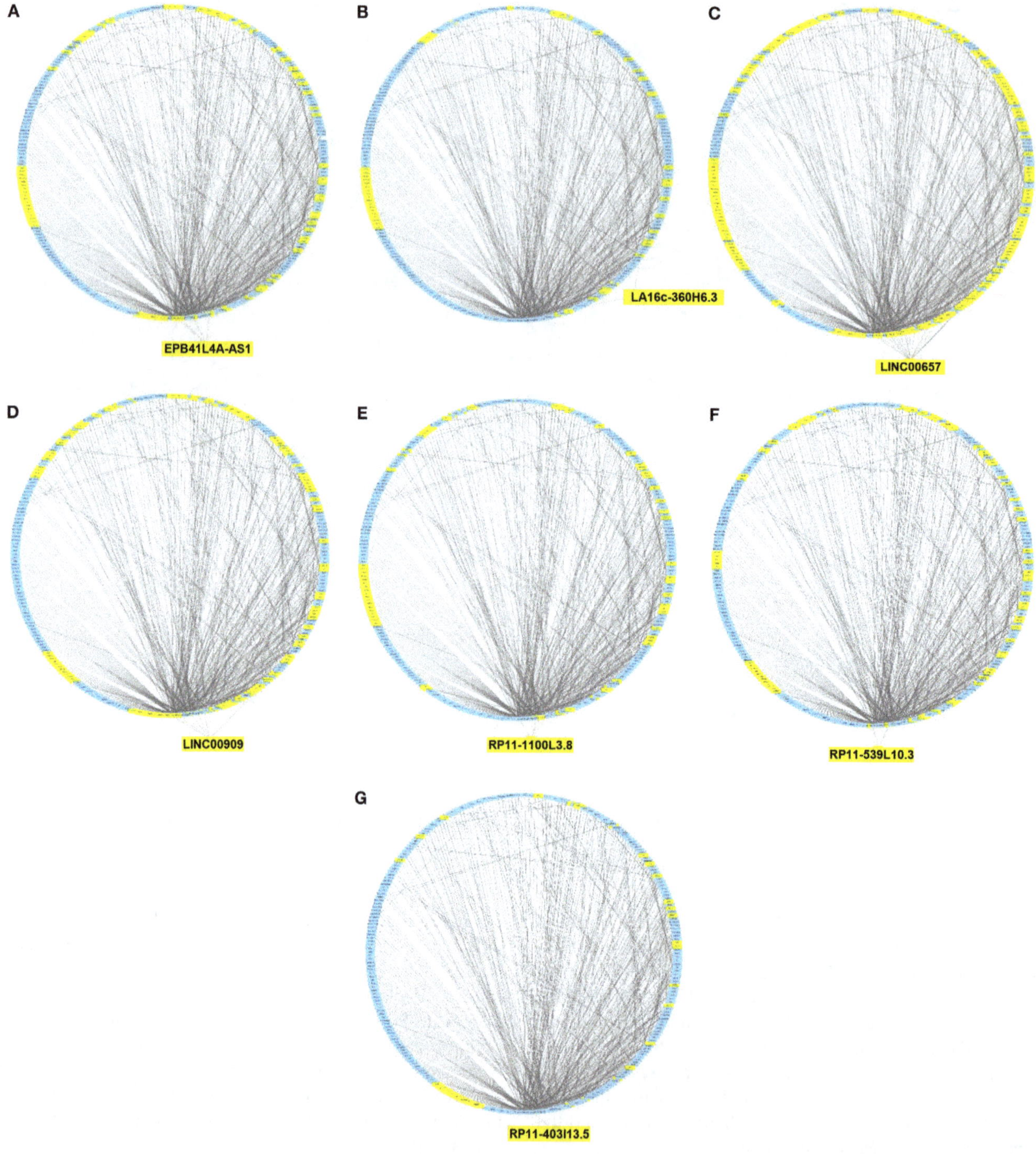

FIGURE 3 | Protein–protein interaction (PPI) network of differently expressed genes targeted by selected microRNAs and long non-coding RNAs (lncRNAs). Graphical representation of the connections among genes in the PPI network and EPB41L4A-AS1 **(A)**, LA16c-360H6.3 **(B)**, LINC00657 **(C)**, LINC00909 **(D)**, RP11-1100L3.8 **(E)**, RP11-539L10.3 **(F)**, and RP11-403I13.5 **(G)**. In the PPI network all genes are ordered around a circle based on their degree of connectivity (i.e., number of edges). Genes directly or indirectly targeted by the lncRNAs are highlighted in yellow.

CEP63, and MAPRE1) glycolytic process (PFKL, PFKM, and PKM), Wnt signaling pathway (MARK2, CTNNBIP1, EIF2C1, and TNRC6C), osteoblast differentiation (ASF1A and MAPK11), and regulation of type I interferon-mediated signaling pathway (CDC37). Genes targeted in this module were: AHNAK, CALB1, CCT6A, CEP63, CEP97, GAB1, MAPRE1, PFKM, and TNRC6C.

CALB1 plays a role in differentiation and matrix formation in osteoblasts (33), GAB1 is important for normal postnatal bone

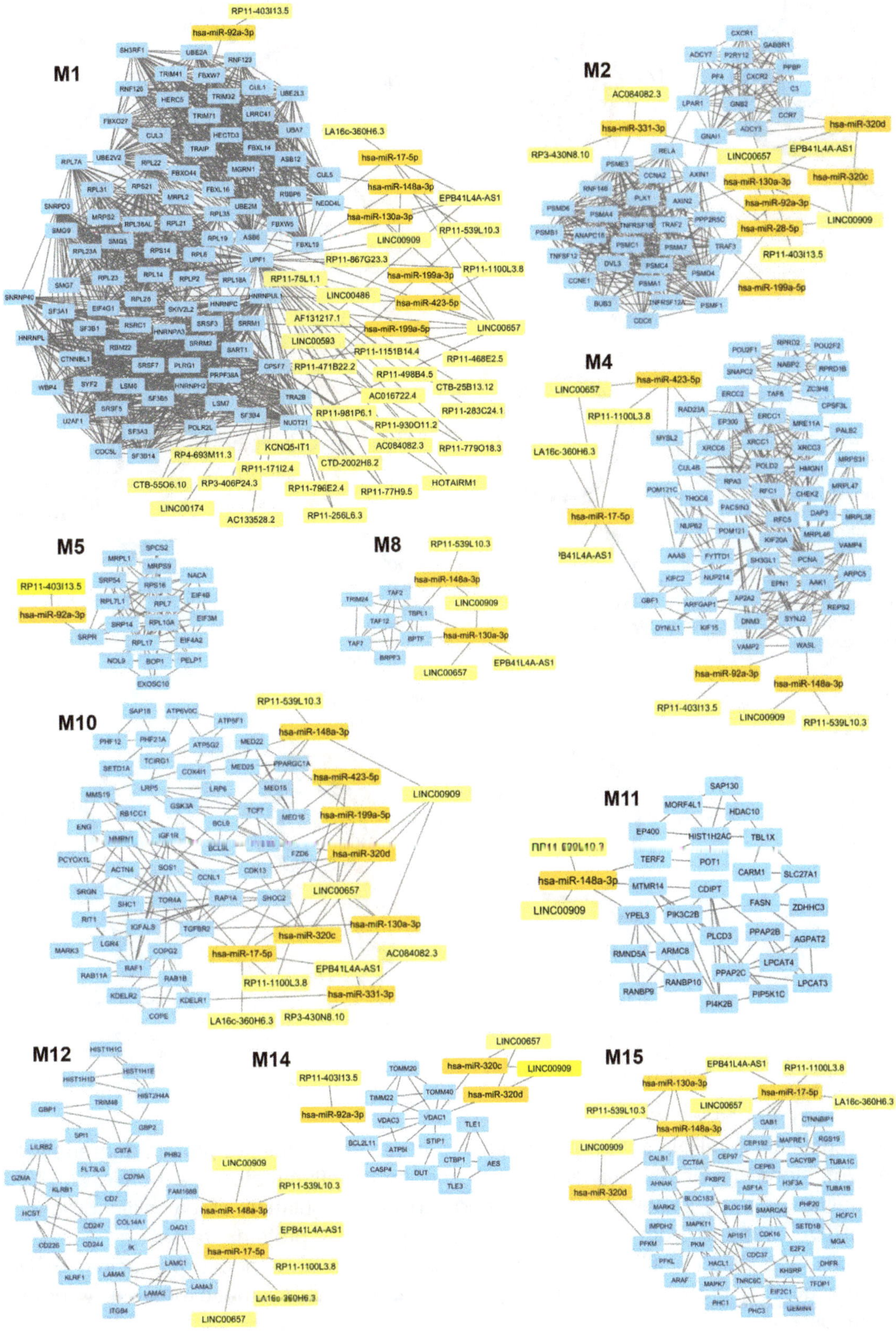

FIGURE 4 | Gene modules that are targeted by the selected long non-coding RNAs (lncRNAs) modulated in psoriatic arthritis. In each module (M) genes are represented by light blue rectangles whereas targeting microRNAs and lncRNAs are represented by orange and yellow rectangles, respectively.

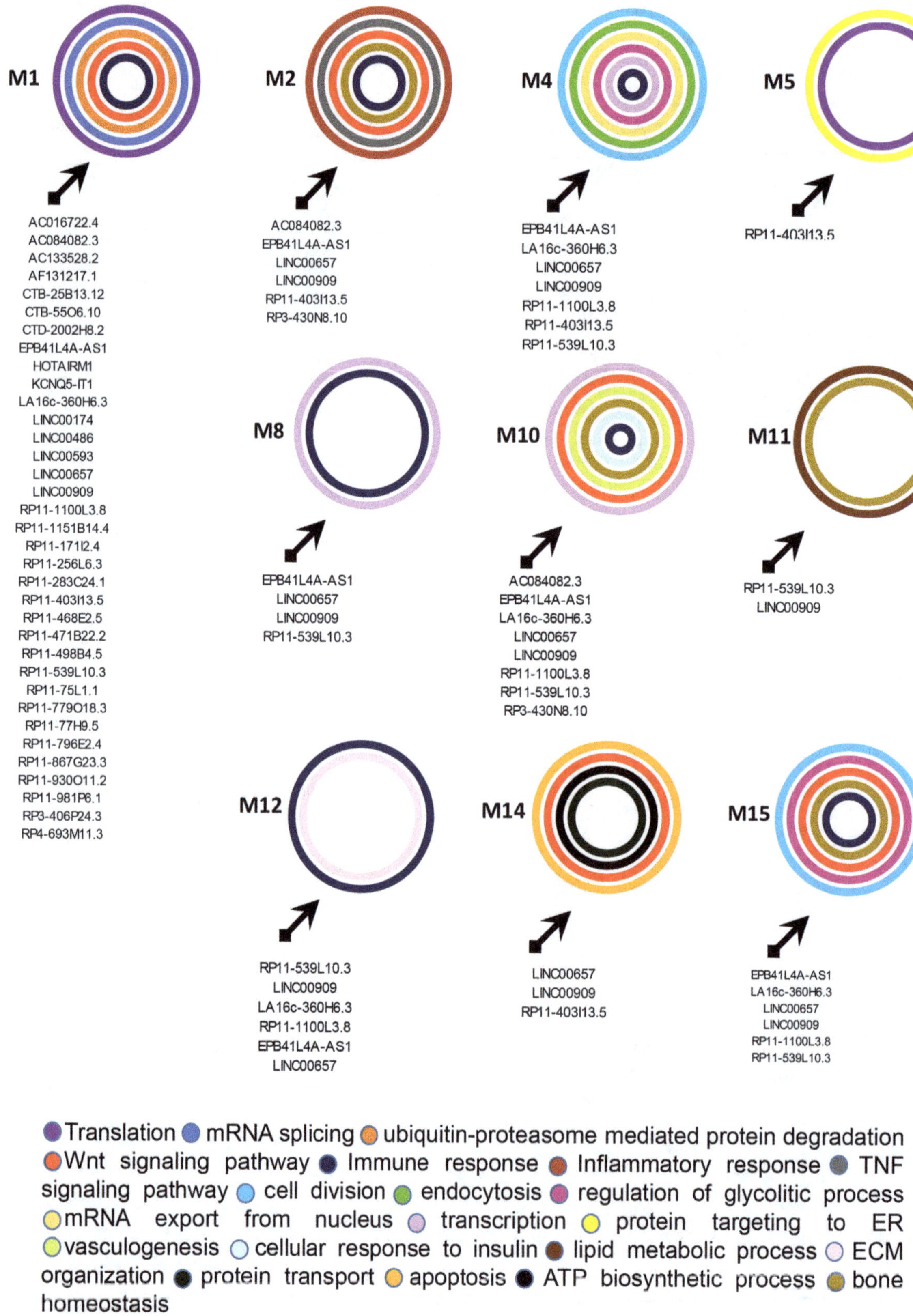

FIGURE 5 | Functional classification of genes included in the targeted modules. Graphical representation of long non-coding RNAs targeting the gene modules and of the most relevant biological processes (BPs) in which genes in each module can be classified. The BPs are represented by colored circles (each color corresponds to a different BP). The size of circles does not correspond to the number of genes that are classified in each BP.

homeostasis (34) and MAPRE1 regulates cell–cell adhesion-induced osteoblast differentiation (35).

Since disease can be viewed as the result of perturbations of complex signaling networks, a pathway enrichment analysis was performed, in each module, using FUnrich. This analysis showed that the most represented enriched pathways were related to immune response (including signaling of both adaptive and innate immune response, type I interferon and gamma interferon signaling), bone homeostasis, metabolism, and cell adhesion.

The results obtained are shown in **Figure 6**, which shows a schematic representation of the most relevant enriched signaling pathways ($p \leq 0.05$).

To provide experimental evidence that pathways identified by the throughput analysis of modulated genes and lncRNAs in PsA are active in the disease, we performed a two step validation of the presented results. Indeed, first we validated by real-time PCR the modulation of genes ascribed to several signaling pathways, including SH3GL1, EPN1, and NUP214 (mTOR signaling), TRAF2, TNFRSF1B, and RELA (TNF/NF-κB signaling), MAPK7 and MAPK11 (toll-like receptors signaling), TCF7, BCL9, and LRP6 (Wnt signaling), MED15, ENG, and ACTN4 (glypican signaling), GSK3A, IGF1R, and PARGC1A (insulin signaling), and CIITA IFI27 and MYD88 (type I interferon signaling). All the tested transcripts were overexpressed in PsA patients when compared to healthy subjects (see Figure S2 in Supplementary Material).

Second, in the sera of patients with PsA, we evaluated the presence of several molecules associated with the pathways modulated in PsA. Indeed, we decided to quantify the serum levels of glypican-4, IFN-γ, Wnt-2, mTOR, TNF-α, sPD-1, NFKB p65, NOTCH1, omentin, and adiponectin. **Figure 7** shows the concentration of these molecules in the sera of the PsA patients. The serum levels of all the tested molecules were significantly increased in PsA patients when compared to healthy donors with the exception of adiponectin and omentin that were significantly decreased in PsA sera.

DISCUSSION

Psoriatic arthritis is a chronic inflammatory arthritis that affects 10–30% of patients with skin psoriasis. IL-17, TNF-α, and type I IFNs play a fundamental role in the pathogenesis of the disease and monoclonal antibodies targeting IL-17 and TNF-α along with IL-12/IL-23 are the main biotechnological treatments that have a dramatic good response in PsA and in skin psoriasis. As we have previously reported (9), the involvement of the mentioned cytokines is typical of an autoimmune process and support the hypothesis of the autoimmune origin of the disease. In particular, IL-17 is able to synergize with TNF-α, IL-22, and other cytokines, including IL-6 and IL-8, in sustaining the inflammatory process at different sites and in favoring the development of comorbidities that are typical of psoriasis, such as PsA, metabolic syndrome, obesity, and cardiovascular disease.

Long non-coding RNAs control gene expression at multiple levels, including epigenetic regulation, chromatin remodeling, and post-transcriptional gene regulation. Accumulating evidences indicate that lncRNAs can be involved in different types of immune-mediated human diseases, including autoimmune diseases (11). The role played by lncRNAs in PSA pathogenesis has not been elucidated yet and a comprehensive analysis of lncRNA expression profiles in PsA has not been performed. We, therefore, aimed to identify lncRNA expression signatures associated with PsA, analyzing the expression of a vast array of lncRNA in PBMC cells from PsA patients by microarray analysis.

The applied criteria for the selection of modulated lncRNAs included a multiple step process that combined the lncRNAs expression analysis to the conventional gene expression and miRNAs profiling in the same cohort of patients.

By this approach we were able to select deregulated lncRNAs that were as much as possible correlated to the PsA transcriptome.

Through a complex network analysis of the whole set of molecular interactions among modulated genes and lncRNAs we further wanted to select those lncRNAs that targeted modules of most highly connected genes in the PsA interactome, since they may have a major impact on PsA gene modulation. That, for example, has led us to favor lncRNAs with high connectivity rather than poorly connected lncRNAs (even) with higher fold change. The functional analysis of the above-mentioned highly connected modules revealed that the modulated lncRNAs targeted genes involved in BPs that play a pivotal role in the PsA pathogenesis such as, for example, immune response (including B and T cell activation) inflammatory response, TNF, Wnt and type I interferon-mediated signaling, bone resorption, bone mineralization, and glyco-lipid metabolic process (see Results), thus indicating that the selected lncRNAs regulated the three major aspects of the disease, including skin involvement, osteo-articular features, and metabolic syndrome.

As it has recently acquired in molecular biology, diseases are now viewed in the context of signaling pathways perturbation. We, therefore, performed a pathway enrichment analysis of all targeted gene modules and, by this approach we reached a non-ambiguous identification of important pathways that can be modulated by the selected lncRNAs. Our analysis confirmed that these lncRNAs play a role in the regulation of signaling pathways associated with both adaptive and immune response and with autoimmune diseases (i.e., type I interferon signaling pathway). In addition, they regulate important signaling involved in bone homeostasis including glypican, syndecan, and Wnt pathways.

Moreover, these results revealed the presence in PsA of lncRNAs that modulate the signaling pathway associated with influenza, thus highlighting the possible role played by influenza viruses in triggering PsA and suggesting the possible involvement of an epigenetic control. The selected lncRNAs were involved in the modulation of lipid metabolism pathway (see Results, module M11), and it is well known that dyslipidemia is frequently associated with PsA (36) and, in particular, patients with PsA have been shown to have elevated cholesterol levels (37) and increase risk of cardiovascular disease.

Another deregulated signaling pathway is the S6K1 (S6 kinase 1) and mTOR (mammalian target of rapamycin) pathway (see Results, modules M1, M4, and M5), a nutrient sensing system that respond to nutrient overload leading to insulin resistance, obesity, and diabetes (38, 39). These observations suggest that lncRNAs may also

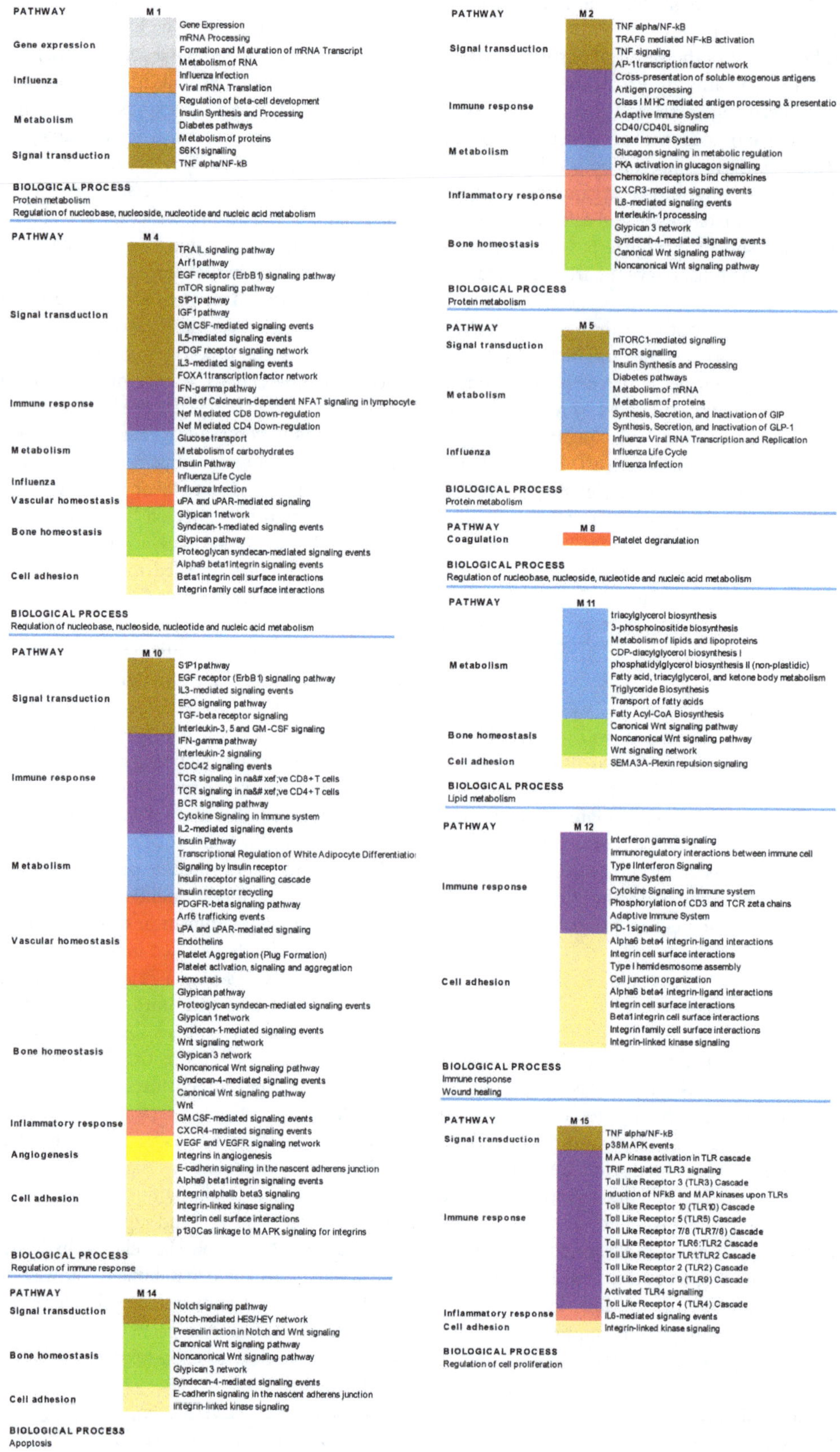

FIGURE 6 | Biological processes and pathways enrichment analysis of the targeted modules. Selection of the different enriched pathways ($p < 0.05$) in the 10 targeted modules (M). Pathways that are enriched in more than one module are labeled by the same color in the different modules.

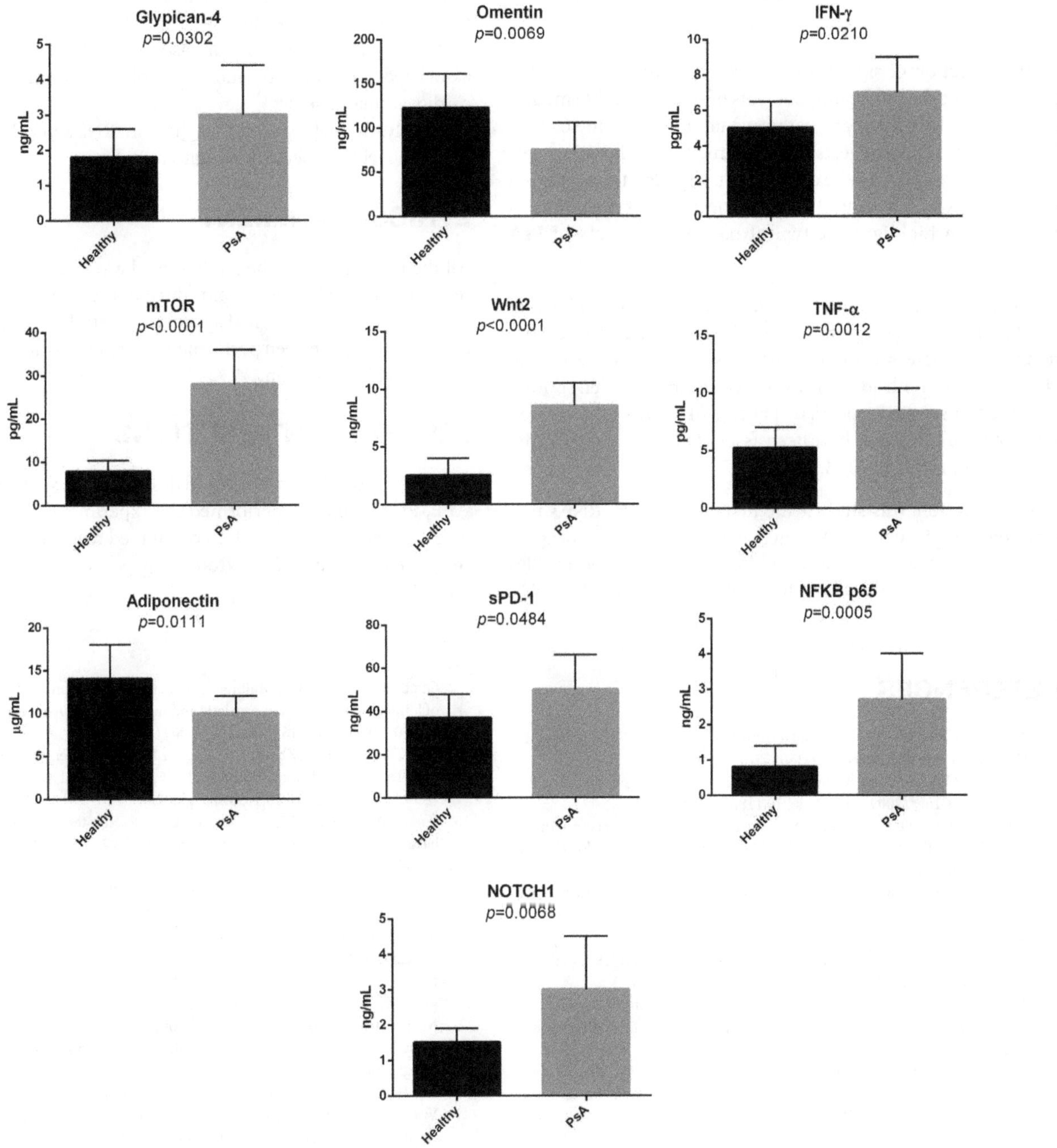

FIGURE 7 | Serum levels of selected molecules in psoriatic arthritis (PsA) patients and in normal subjects. The histograms represent the mean of the results obtained in 20 healthy donors and in 20 PsA patients.

be involved in the metabolic syndrome frequently associated with PsA. Hyperuricemia is another feature of metabolic syndrome and is also known to be more frequent in psoriatic subjects than in the normal population. In humans, purines are metabolized into uric acid, which is a strong stimulator of innate immunity. In this regard, hyperuricemia may increase uric acid crystallization in and around joints, thereby inducing PsA in psoriatic subjects, thus representing an independent risk factor for PsA. Activation of pathways modulation of genes involved in related to nucleobase, nucleoside, nucleotide, and nucleic acid metabolism (modules M1, M4, and M8) may reflect this particular aspect of PsA.

Finally, lncRNAs control several pathways involved in cell adhesion (see Results, modules M4, M10, M11, M12, M14, and M15). The modulation of these pathways may contribute to the increased mucosal permeability of the gut that has been observed in PsA, even in the absence of bowel pathology (40). Indeed, bowel disease is six times more frequent in patients with PsA. Since an altered intestinal barrier is a feature of PsA, the presence of gastrointestinal involvement in PsA should be carefully investigated during the diagnostic work up.

The detection of significantly different serum levels in PsA patients compared to healthy subjects of several soluble mediators, ascribed to the main pathways targeted by the selected lncRNAs, strongly suggests that they modulate signaling networks that are active in the disease. In particular, the increased serum levels of glypican-4 and the decrease of adiponectin and omentin highlight the typical metabolic aspects of PsA patients.

Indeed glypican-4 has been considered a novel adipokine that boosts insulin signaling and, interestingly glypican-4 levels are significantly increased in obese patients with insulin resistance (41). Moreover, both adiponectin and omentin have been showed decreased in sera from psoriatic patients (42, 43) and decreased levels of both molecules have been associated with, and involved in, metabolic syndrome (44, 45).

In conclusion, this study is the first report on lncRNAs that may exert an epigenetic control on PsA pathogenesis. The original approach that integrates genes and lncRNAs expression profiles presented in the study, allows to identify deregulated lncRNAs that modulate crucial molecular signaling associated with the typical features of the disease. These findings further support that PsA is an autoimmune disease with systemic inflammation associated with obesity and metabolic syndrome leading to cardiovascular disease.

Finally, we may suggest that these lncRNAs may be useful to design novel therapeutic strategies in PsA.

ETHICS STATEMENT

All the participants to the study signed a written informed consent and the local Ethical Committee of the University Hospital of Verona, Verona, Italy, had approved the study protocol. All the investigations have been performed according to the principles of the Helsinki declaration.

AUTHOR CONTRIBUTIONS

APU, CL, and MD conceived and designed the experiments. MD, APE, PF, GP, and ET performed the experiments. MD and APE analyzed the data. GP and ET contributed reagents and collected the patients' samples. MD wrote the paper with input from APU and CL.

REFERENCES

1. Ritchlin CT, Colbert RA, Gladman DD. Psoriatic arthritis. *N Engl J Med* (2017) 376:2095–6. doi:10.1056/NEJMra1505557
2. Fitzgerald O, Winchester R. Psoriatic arthritis: from pathogenesis to therapy. *Arthritis Res Ther* (2009) 11:214. doi:10.1186/ar2580
3. Rahman P, Elder JT. Genetic epidemiology of psoriasis and psoriatic arthritis. *Ann Rheum Dis* (2005) 64(Suppl 2):ii37–9; discussion ii40–1. doi:10.1136/ard.2004.030775
4. Mease P. Psoriatic arthritis and spondyloarthritis assessment and management update. *Curr Opin Rheumatol* (2013) 25:287–96. doi:10.1097/BOR.0b013e32835fd8d5
5. Moll JM, Wright V. Psoriatic arthritis. *Semin Arthritis Rheum* (1973) 3:55–78. doi:10.1016/0049-0172(73)90035-8
6. Robinson H, Kelly S, Pitzalis C. Basic synovial biology and immunopathology in psoriatic arthritis. *J Rheumatol Suppl* (2009) 83:14–6. doi:10.3899/jrheum.090212
7. Costa L, Perricone C, Chimenti MS, Del Puente A, Caso P, Peluso R, et al. Switching between biological treatments in psoriatic arthritis: a review of the evidence. *Drugs R D* (2017) 17:509–22. doi:10.1007/s40268-017-0215-7
8. Krueger JG, Brunner PM. Interleukin-17 alters the biology of many cell types involved in the genesis of psoriasis, systemic inflammation and associated comorbidities. *Exp Dermatol* (2018) 27:115–23. doi:10.1111/exd.13467
9. Dolcino M, Ottria A, Barbieri A, Patuzzo G, Tinazzi E, Argentino G, et al. Gene expression profiling in peripheral blood cells and synovial membranes of patients with psoriatic arthritis. *PLoS One* (2015) 10:e0128262. doi:10.1371/journal.pone.0128262
10. Pelosi A, Lunardi C, Fiore PF, Tinazzi E, Patuzzo G, Argentino G, et al. MicroRNA expression profiling in psoriatic arthritis. *Biomed Res Int* (2018) 2018:7305380. doi:10.1155/2018/7305380
11. Wu GC, Pan HF, Leng RX, Wang DG, Li XP, Li XM, et al. Emerging role of long noncoding rnas in autoimmune diseases. *Autoimmun Rev* (2015) 14:798–805. doi:10.1016/j.autrev.2015.05.004
12. Ahn R, Gupta R, Lai K, Chopra N, Arron ST, Liao W. Network analysis of psoriasis reveals biological pathways and roles for coding and long non-coding rnas. *BMC Genomics* (2016) 17:841. doi:10.1186/s12864-016-3188-y
13. Gupta R, Ahn R, Lai K, Mullins E, Debbaneh M, Dimon M, et al. Landscape of long noncoding rnas in psoriatic and healthy skin. *J Invest Dermatol* (2016) 136:603–9. doi:10.1016/j.jid.2015.12.009
14. Wu T, Wang J, Liu C, Zhang Y, Shi B, Zhu X, et al. Npinter: the noncoding rnas and protein related biomacromolecules interaction database. *Nucleic Acids Res* (2006) 34:D150–2. doi:10.1093/nar/gkj025
15. Yuan J, Wu W, Xie C, Zhao G, Zhao Y, Chen R. Npinter v2.0: an updated database of ncrna interactions. *Nucleic Acids Res* (2014) 42:D104–8. doi:10.1093/nar/gkt1057
16. Pathan M, Keerthikumar S, Ang CS, Gangoda L, Quek CY, Williamson NA, et al. Funrich: an open access standalone functional enrichment and interaction network analysis tool. *Proteomics* (2015) 15:2597–601. doi:10.1002/pmic.201400515
17. Jensen LJ, Kuhn M, Stark M, Chaffron S, Creevey C, Muller J, et al. String 8 – a global view on proteins and their functional interactions in 630 organisms. *Nucleic Acids Res* (2009) 37:D412–6. doi:10.1093/nar/gkn760
18. Cline MS, Smoot M, Cerami E, Kuchinsky A, Landys N, Workman C, et al. Integration of biological networks and gene expression data using cytoscape. *Nat Protoc* (2007) 2:2366–82. doi:10.1038/nprot.2007.324
19. Vriend J, Reiter RJ. Melatonin, bone regulation and the ubiquitin-proteasome connection: a review. *Life Sci* (2016) 145:152–60. doi:10.1016/j.lfs.2015.12.031
20. Takeuchi O. Endonuclease regnase-1/monocyte chemotactic protein-1-induced protein-1 (mcpip1) in controlling immune responses and beyond. *Wiley Interdiscip Rev RNA* (2018) 9:e1449. doi:10.1002/wrna.1449
21. Chandran V. The genetics of psoriasis and psoriatic arthritis. *Clin Rev Allergy Immunol* (2013) 44:149–56. doi:10.1007/s12016-012-8303-5
22. Sanchez-Tena S, Cubillos-Rojas M, Schneider T, Rosa JL. Functional and pathological relevance of herc family proteins: a decade later. *Cell Mol Life Sci* (2016) 73:1955–68. doi:10.1007/s00018-016-2139-8
23. Yeo L, Adlard N, Biehl M, Juarez M, Smallie T, Snow M, et al. Expression of chemokines cxcl4 and cxcl7 by synovial macrophages defines an early stage of rheumatoid arthritis. *Ann Rheum Dis* (2016) 75:763–71. doi:10.1136/annrheumdis-2014-206921
24. Lee J, Park C, Kim HJ, Lee YD, Lee ZH, Song YW, et al. Stimulation of osteoclast migration and bone resorption by c-c chemokine ligands 19 and 21. *Exp Mol Med* (2017) 49:e358. doi:10.1038/emm.2017.100
25. Messina N, Fulford T, O'Reilly L, Loh WX, Motyer JM, Ellis D, et al. The

nf-kappab transcription factor rela is required for the tolerogenic function of foxp3(+) regulatory t cells. *J Autoimmun* (2016) 70:52–62. doi:10.1016/j.jaut.2016.03.017

26. Yi Z, Wallis AM, Bishop GA. Roles of traf3 in t cells: many surprises. *Cell Cycle* (2015) 14:1156–63. doi:10.1080/15384101.2015.1021524
27. Yao Z, Lei W, Duan R, Li Y, Luo L, Boyce BF. Rankl cytokine enhances tnf-induced osteoclastogenesis independently of tnf receptor associated factor (traf) 6 by degrading traf3 in osteoclast precursors. *J Biol Chem* (2017) 292:10169–79. doi:10.1074/jbc.M116.771816
28. Emslie D, D'Costa K, Hasbold J, Metcalf D, Takatsu K, Hodgkin PO, et al. Oct2 enhances antibody-secreting cell differentiation through regulation of il-5 receptor alpha chain expression on activated b cells. *J Exp Med* (2008) 205:409–21. doi:10.1084/jem.20072049
29. Wu B, Wang Y, Wang C, Wang GG, Wu J, Wan YY. Bptf is essential for t cell homeostasis and function. *J Immunol* (2016) 197:4325–33. doi:10.4049/jimmunol.1600642
30. Guggino G, Lo Pizzo M, Di Liberto D, Rizzo A, Cipriani P, Ruscitti P, et al. Interleukin-9 over-expression and t helper 9 polarization in systemic sclerosis patients. *Clin Exp Immunol* (2017) 190:208–16. doi:10.1111/cei.13009
31. Koch S, Sopel N, Finotto S. Th9 and other il-9-producing cells in allergic asthma. *Semin Immunopathol* (2017) 39:55–68. doi:10.1007/s00281-016-0601-1
32. Karczewski J, Dobrowolska A, Rychlewska-Hanczewska A, Adamski Z. New insights into the role of t cells in pathogenesis of psoriasis and psoriatic arthritis. *Autoimmunity* (2016) 49:435–50. doi:10.3109/08916934.2016.1166214
33. Bellido T, Huening M, Raval-Pandya M, Manolagas SC, Christakos S. Calbindin-d28k is expressed in osteoblastic cells and suppresses their apoptosis by inhibiting caspase-3 activity. *J Biol Chem* (2000) 275:26328–32. doi:10.1074/jbc.M003600200
34. Weng T, Mao F, Wang Y, Sun Q, Li R, Yang G, et al. Osteoblastic molecular scaffold gab1 is required for maintaining bone homeostasis. *J Cell Sci* (2010) 123:682–9. doi:10.1242/jcs.058396
35. Pustylnik S, Fiorino C, Nabavi N, Zappitelli T, da Silva R, Aubin JE, et al. Eb1 levels are elevated in ascorbic acid (aa)-stimulated osteoblasts and mediate cell-cell adhesion-induced osteoblast differentiation. *J Biol Chem* (2013) 288:22096–. doi:10.1074/jbc.M113.481515
36. Yim KM, Armstrong AW. Updates on cardiovascular comorbidities associated with psoriatic diseases: epidemiology and mechanisms. *Rheumatol Int* (2017) 37:97–105. doi:10.1007/s00296-016-3487-2
37. Wu S, Li WQ, Han J, Sun Q, Qureshi AA. Hypercholesterolemia and risk of incident psoriasis and psoriatic arthritis in us women. *Arthritis Rheumatol* (2014) 66:304–10. doi:10.1002/art.38227
38. Gulati P, Thomas G. Nutrient sensing in the mtor/s6k1 signalling pathway. *Biochem Soc Trans* (2007) 35:236–8. doi:10.1042/BST0350236
39. Um SH, D'Alessio D, Thomas G. Nutrient overload, insulin resistance, and ribosomal protein s6 kinase 1, s6k1. *Cell Metab* (2006) 3:393–402. doi:10.1016/j.cmet.2006.05.003
40. Holden W, Orchard T, Wordsworth P. Enteropathic arthritis. *Rheum Dis Clin North Am* (2003) 29:513–530, viii. doi:10.1016/S0889-857X(03)00043-7
41. Zhu HJ, Pan H, Cui Y, Wang XQ, Wang LJ, Li NS, et al. The changes of serum glypican4 in obese patients with different glucose metabolism status. *J Clin Endocrinol Metab* (2014) 99:E2697–701. doi:10.1210/jc.2014-2018
42. Campanati A, Ganzetti G, Giuliodori K, Marra M, Bonfigli A, Testa R, et al. Serum levels of adipocytokines in psoriasis patients receiving tumor necrosis factor-α inhibitors: results of a retrospective analysis. *Int J Dermatol* (2015) 54:839–45. doi:10.1111/ijd.12706
43. Zhang C, Zhu KJ, Liu JL, Xu GX, Liu W, Jiang FX, et al. Omentin-1 plasma levels and omentin-1 expression are decreased in psoriatic lesions of psoriasis patients. *Arch Dermatol Res* (2015) 307:455–9. doi:10.1007/s00403-015-1549-z
44. Frankenberg ADV, Reis AF, Gerchman F. Relationships between adiponectin levels, the metabolic syndrome, and type 2 diabetes: a literature review. *Arch Endocrinol Metab* (2017) 61:614–22. doi:10.1590/2359-3997000000316
45. Tan BK, Adya R, Randeva HS. Omentin: a novel link between inflammation, diabesity, and cardiovascular disease. *Trends Cardiovasc Med* (2010) 20:143–8. doi:10.1016/j.tcm.2010.12.002

7

Epidermal mTORC1 Signaling Contributes to the Pathogenesis of Psoriasis and Could Serve as a Therapeutic Target

*Claudia Buerger**

Department of Dermatology, Venerology and Allergology, Clinic of the Goethe University, Frankfurt am Main, Germany

Correspondence:
Claudia Buerger
claudia.buerger@kgu.de

Although modern biologics targeting different inflammatory mediators show promising therapeutic success, comprehensive knowledge about the molecular events in psoriatic keratinocytes that contribute to the pathogenesis and could serve as therapeutic targets is still scarce. However, recent efforts to understand the deregulated signal transduction pathways have led to the development of small molecule inhibitors e.g., tofacitinib targeting the Jak/Stat cascade that opens additional therapeutic options. Recently, the PI3-K/Akt/mTOR signaling pathway has emerged as an important player in the control of epidermal homeostasis. This review summarizes the current knowledge on the role of this pathway in the pathogenesis of psoriasis, especially the epidermal manifestation of the disease and discusses current approaches to target the pathway therapeutically.

Keywords: psoriasis, mTORC1, keratinocytes, rapamycin, topical agent

INTRODUCTION

Psoriasis is a common, chronic inflammatory skin disease that affects 2–3% of the population and is associated with a reduced quality of life and a shortened life expectancy due to the association with the metabolic syndrome and cardiovascular pathologies (1). Clinically psoriasis presents with red, scaly plaques, which mostly affect predilection sites such as extensor surfaces of forearms and shins, umbilical, perianal, retro-auricular regions, and scalp (2). These plaques are characterized by epidermal hyperproliferation with impaired keratinocyte differentiation, extravasation of lymphocytes, and angio(neo)genesis. Currently it is assumed that sustained activation of plasmacytoid dendritic cells by epidermal antigens due to skin trauma or infection is the first step in the pathogenesis of psoriasis (3). This induces the maturation of myeloid dendritic cells, which in turn promote via secretion of IL-6, IL-12, and IL-23 the differentiation of T cells into Th1 and Th17 cells (4). Their effector cytokines such as IL-17, IL-22, and TNF-α induce and maintain hallmarks of psoriasis such as keratinocyte proliferation, and disturbed differentiation, leading to epidermal acanthosis, hyperkeratosis, and parakeratosis (5). Activated keratinocytes in turn produce important proinflammatory cytokines and chemokines that are able to recruit a broad spectrum of inflammatory cells from the vascular system. Thus, a "vicious circle" of excessive immune response, epidermal hyperproliferation, and neovascularization is initiated, which leads to the complex clinical appearance of psoriasis (6). The immunological events leading to the described epidermal changes are well understood and various "biologics" against different inflammatory cytokines such as TNF-α, IL-17A, or IL-12/IL-23 show promising results in the therapy of psoriasis (7). However, comprehensive knowledge about the intracellular epidermal processes induced by the immunological network, and which could serve as potential therapeutic targets, is still missing. There is some evidence that signaling pathways such as Stat1, Stat2, and Stat3 (8–10), MAPK family kinases (11–14), Wnt5a (15), or NF-kB (16–20) are dysregulated in the psoriatic epidermis and some of them have been targeted by molecular inhibitors (21, 22).

THE PI3-K/Akt/mTOR SIGNALING CASCADE

The serine/threonine kinase Akt, also known as protein kinase B (PKB), represents a crucial signaling point in eukaryotic cells and plays a central role in the regulation of cellular processes such as growth, proliferation, and metabolism (23). One of the main downstream mediators of Akt is the mTOR signaling pathway. mTOR (mechanistic target of rapamycin) occurs in two different multiprotein complexes, both of which possess the mTOR kinase as a catalytic subunit and share some regulatory proteins (mLST8, Deptor), while other proteins are complex-specific. Specific to the mTOR complex 1 (mTORC1) is the scaffold protein Raptor, which regulates the assembly and localization of the complex. This complex can be inhibited by rapamycin (24). The rapamycin-insensitive mTOR complex 2 (mTORC2), on the other hand, additionally consists of the scaffold proteins Rictor and Protor1/2 and phosphorylates Akt on Ser473 (25) and thus regulates proliferation and cell growth.

After ligand binding to cognate receptors such as tyrosine kinase receptors (RTK) or G-protein-coupled receptors (GPCR) phosphatidylinositol 3-kinase (PI3-K) becomes activated either directly or via adaptor proteins like the insulin receptor substrate 1 (IRS-1) (**Figure 1**). PI3-K mediates the synthesis of 3′-phosphoinositides (PIP_3) at the plasma membrane, which act as lipid-second messengers and recruit Akt and the phosphoinositol-dependent-kinase (PDK1) to the membrane. PDK1 can then activate Akt by phosphorylation on Thr308. For complete activation of Akt, phosphorylation of Ser473 by mTORC2 is required. Fully activated Akt is then able to phosphorylate a large number of signal molecules with different functions in the control of growth, proliferation, metabolism, or apoptosis (26). Akt and other signal molecules regulate the TSC complex, consisting of TSC1 and 2 (**Figure 1**). This complex is an important regulator of mTOR by acting as a GTPase-activating protein for Rheb (Ras homolog enriched in brain). The GTP-bound form of Rheb interacts directly with mTOR and activates the complex (27, 28). Furthermore, Akt phosphorylates the proline-rich Akt substrate of 40 kDa (PRAS40), whose inhibitory interaction with mTOR is then dissolved (29), so that the mTOR kinase is fully activated.

By phosphorylation of downstream molecules, mTORC1 regulates the biosynthesis of macromolecules necessary for cellular growth and proliferation. By phosphorylating two key proteins of translation initiation S6 kinase-1 (S6K-1) and eukaryotic initiation factor 4E (eIF-4E) binding protein-1 (4E-BP1), mTORC1 controls the rate of protein biosynthesis (30). In particular, mTORC1 regulates the translation of mRNAs with a so-called 5′TOP (5'terminal oligopyrimidine) motifs. These mRNAs mainly code for ribosomal proteins and components of the translation machinery (31), so that mTORC1 activity also contributes to the general synthesis of proteins in this way. Furthermore, mTORC1 controls the synthesis of lipids through regulation of the transcription factor SREBP (32), the production of nucleotides (33), and inhibits catabolic processes such as autophagy (34).

mTOR SIGNALING IN PSORIASIS

Recently attention has been drawn to the PI3-K/Akt/mTORC1 cascade as a regulator of epidermal homeostasis and its putative role in inflammatory skin diseases. Akt is highly activated in all epidermal layers of psoriatic lesions (35), except the basal Ki-67 positive layer that represents dividing cells (36). This may be explained either by psoriatic keratinocytes that keep their proliferative pathways turned on, even after leaving the basal layer. Alternatively, Akt could prevent cellular apoptosis, which also contributes to the fast maturation process of psoriatic keratinocytes (37). Inhibition of PI-3K/Akt could be a promising therapeutic strategy as the Vitamin D analog 1α, 25-dihydroxyvitamin D3-3-bromoacetate (BE) reversed IL-22-induced psoriasiform changes *in vitro* (38).

Our group showed for the first time that the central mediator of Akt signaling, the kinase mTOR, is hyperactivated in lesional and nonlesional skin of psoriasis patients, while downstream signaling molecules such as S6K-1, the ribosomal protein S6, and 4E-BP1 are only activated in suprabasal layers in lesional skin (39, 40). Furthermore, it was shown that additional components of mTORC1 such as Rheb and Raptor are overexpressed in psoriatic skin and others such as PRAS40 are hyperactivated (40). That hyperactivated mTORC1 signaling is indeed an important aspect in psoriasis, showed the work by Shirsath et al.: In a genetic mouse model of psoriasis, PUVA treatment not only ameliorated the histological psoriasis score, but also normalized mTORC1 signaling (41). The divergent localization of the activated signal components in the epidermis points toward a pathophysiological contribution of deregulated mTORC1 signaling in psoriasis. For example, the hyperactivation of mTORC1 in the basal layer may indicate a role during the enhanced proliferation of psoriatic keratinocytes, while the suprabasal hyperactivation points toward a role in aberrant differentiation. Using different *in vitro* approaches our group showed that healthy keratinocytes switch off Akt/mTORC1 signaling as soon as differentiation is initiated. This appears to be associated with proliferation control, as Ki-67 positive cells in the basal layer of healthy skin also showed mTOR activity. Thus, inactivation of mTOR seems to be a prerequisite for keratinocytes to initiate terminal differentiation. In contrast, in an inflammatory environment such as psoriasis, the mTORC1 cascade is aberrantly activated in all epidermal layers. We were able to show that IL-1β, IL-17A, TNF-α, and in particular a mix of these cytokines leads to activation of the mTORC1 signaling cascade. In addition, the pathway might be activated by miRNAs that are deregulated in psoriatic skin (42, 43), or by mechanosensitive molecules such as polycysteins (44).

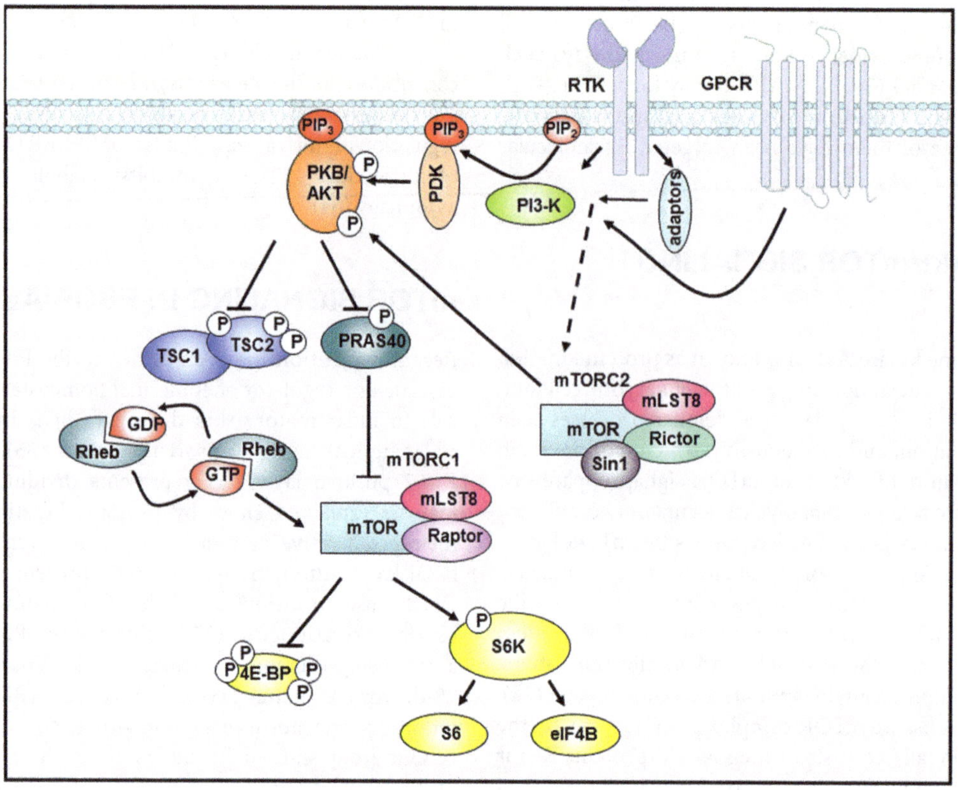

FIGURE 1 | The PI3-K/Akt/mTOR signaling cascade. Stimulation of receptor tyrosine kinases (RTK) and G-protein-coupled receptors (GPCR) leads to activation of PI3-K, which then synthesizes PIP_3 in the membrane. Subsequently, Akt is recruited to the membrane and phosphorylated by PDK-1 and mTORC2. The activated Akt kinase phosphorylates various substrates such as PRAS40, which is then inactivated and releases mTORC1. In addition, TSC2 is inhibited so that the downstream GTPase Rheb remains GTP-bound and can activate mTORC1. The fully activated mTORC1 complex then activates proteins of the translation machinery by phosphorylating S6K-1 or 4E-BP1 [adapted from Manning et al. (23)].

The latter could explain the predilection of psoriatic plaques to sites of increased mechanical stress such as elbows and knees. Our group could prove that continuous mTORC1 activity contributes to the proliferation of keratinocytes and simultaneously inhibits proper keratinocyte maturation. Thus, we suggest a model where mTORC1 signal transduction functions as a central switch between keratinocyte proliferation and differentiation (**Figure 2**). This model is supported by findings from Mitra et al. showing that IL-22 regulates keratinocyte proliferation via the Akt/mTOR cascade (45).

Apart from this model also other mechanisms, how epidermal mTORC hyperactivation can contribute to the pathogenesis of psoriasis are being discussed. Patel et al. could show that the release of pro-inflammatory mediators such as IL-6, CXCL8, or VEGF by keratinocytes is mediated via mTORC (46). Another mechanism by which hyperactive PI3-K/Akt/mTORC1 signaling might contribute to the pathogenesis of psoriasis could be through inhibiting autophagy (47). Autophagy and more specifically nucleophagy is an important mechanism during keratinocyte differentiation and maturation into corneocytes. Thus, high mTORC1 activity inhibits nuclear degradation and contributes to parakeratosis (retention of nuclei), one of the hallmarks of psoriasis (48).

Although not the main focus of this review, it has to be mentioned that mTORC1 signaling also has important functions in the innate (49) and adaptive immune system (50–52). Specifically a role for mTORC1 and 2 has been attributed to the regulation of immune cell energy metabolism and thereby to the control of their function and differentiation (53). Deregulated mTORC1 signaling was found in peripheral blood mononuclear cells (PBMCs) of psoriasis patients (54), which seems to contribute to their pathological behavior (55). Regulatory T-cells from psoriasis patients show increased mTOR phosphorylation and treatment with methotrexate reduces mTOR activation (56). In addition, a novel vitamin D analog reduced mTORC1 activity in activated memory T cells form psoriasis patients and thus contributed to the immunosuppressive effect of the drug (57).

mTOR SIGNALING AS A THERAPEUTIC TARGET IN PSORIASIS

The mTOR complex is also interesting because of its inhibitor rapamycin (sirolimus), which was isolated from Streptomyces hygroscopicus in 1975 (58). This bacterial strain was first found in the soil of Rapa Nui Island (Easter Island), after

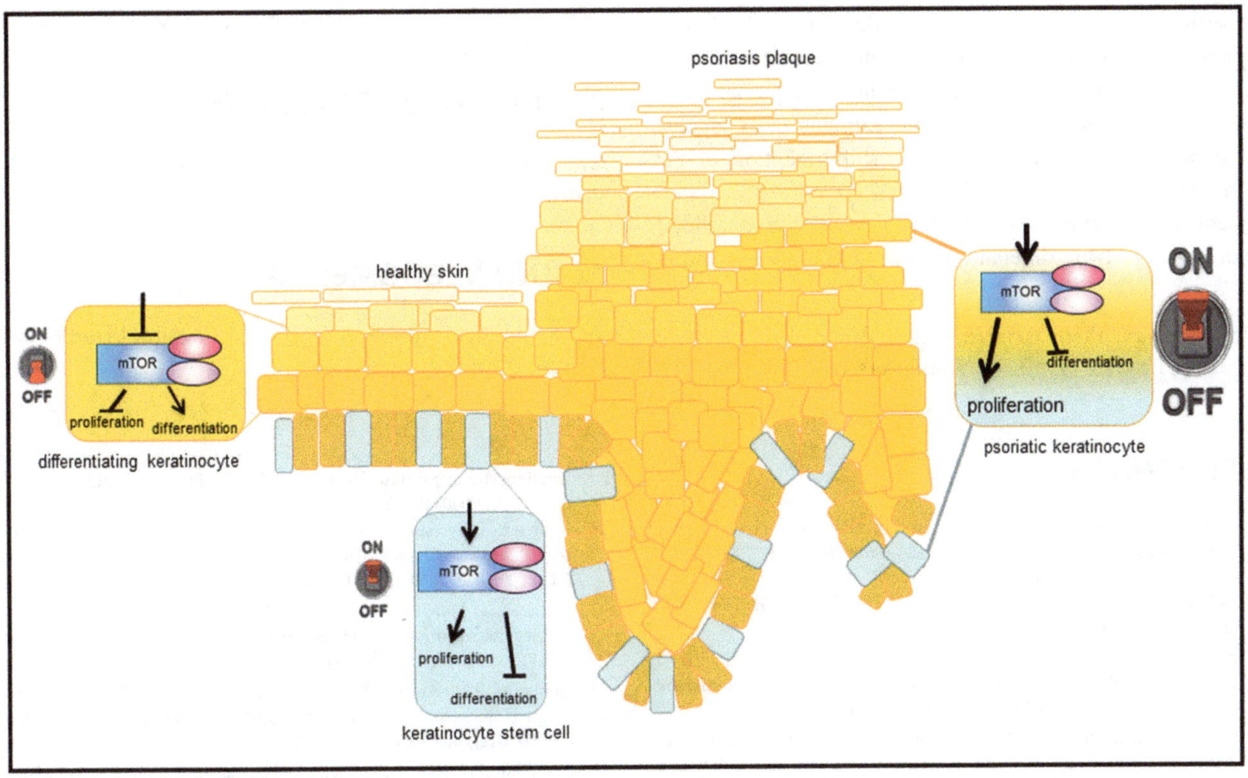

FIGURE 2 | Model, how mTORC1 signaling controls epidermal homeostasis and contributes to psoriasis. In healthy, basal keratinocytes, mTORC1 signaling pathway is active and controls proliferation while blocking differentiation. When cells leave the proliferative, basal compartment, mTORC1 is switched off and differentiation is enabled. Under inflammatory conditions, such as in psoriasis, mTORC1 is permanently activated, which leads to massive proliferation in the basal layer and disturbed keratinocyte differentiation in suprabasal layers, resulting in the phenotypic changes typical of psoriasis.

which the substance was named. Even before the kinase mTOR was identified as a target protein of rapamycin in 1994 (59), rapamycin was known for its anti-proliferative properties on lymphoid cells and associated immunosuppressive properties (60). Rapamycin is therefore still used to prevent transplant rejection (61) and restenosis after implantation of stents in coronary vessels (62). In addition, anti-tumor effects of rapamycin and its analogs (rapalogs) have been under investigation (63, 64).

It is particularly interesting that rapamycin has also been tested for its antiproliferative and immunosuppressive properties in a few small studies in psoriasis patients. Systemic administration of everolimus (a derivative of sirolimus) was successful in a single patient (65), whereas a larger study showed good results for sirolimus in combination with cylosporin therapy (66). In addition, in a renal transplant patient with refractory psoriasis, everolimus ameliorated skin lesions (67). Remarkably, only limited new substances for topical anti-psoriatic therapy have been developed in recent years and new product launches mostly consisted of derivatives or further developments of established agents (68). Thus, the establishment of new substances for topical application is desirable. In one small trial topical treatment with rapamycin led to a significant improvement of the clinical score, while the thickness of the plaques was unchanged (69). To further explore this therapeutic option, the effectiveness of topical rapamycin was investigated in the imiquimod-induced psoriasis mouse model, which showed activation mTORC1 signaling similar to human psoriasis (70, 71). Mice treated with rapamycin showed a significant improvement in clinical appearance (redness, swelling, and flaking), reduced angioneogenesis and normalization of epidermal thickness compared to the control group. While the imiquimod-treated mice showed a clear activation of mTORC1 and downstream molecules, rapamycin reduced the activity to the level of untreated mice. Rapamycin normalized the expression and distribution of differentiation markers such as keratins, involucrin, and loricrin. In addition, the influx of innate immune cells into the draining lymph nodes was partially reduced by rapamycin treatment (71). In the same mouse model rapamycin treatment also restored the expression of tropomyosins, which are downregulated in psoriatic lesion and could also contribute to the disease (72).

Rapamycin is an allosteric inhibitor, that requires binding to its intracellular receptor, FKBP12, to selectively inhibit some, but not all functions of mTORC1 (73). mTORC2 is considered rapamycin-insensitive, although it can be inhibited by chronic rapamycin treatment in some cell types (74).

To inhibit all functions of both complexes, selective ATP-competitive inhibitors of mTOR were developed (75, 76). As they are efficiently inhibiting both mTOR complexes and thus inhibit Akt signaling, they could be interesting therapeutic compounds in psoriasis. The same rationale was applied, by Chamcheu et al., that showed efficient inhibition of PI3-K, mTOR, and S6K-1 by Delphinidin, an antioxidant plant pigment (77). Topical Delphinidin was able to ameliorate symptoms in two different psoriasiform mouse models (77, 78).

In summary, there is increasing evidence that specifically topical application of mTORC inhibitors can be a successful strategy for anti-psoriatic therapies and underline the need to further explore the mTORC1 signaling pathway as a therapeutic target in psoriasis.

AUTHOR CONTRIBUTIONS

CB conceptualized and wrote the manuscript and created the figures.

ACKNOWLEDGMENTS

We would like to thank Anke König for critical reading of the manuscript.

REFERENCES

1. Boehncke WH. Systemic inflammation and cardiovascular comorbidity in psoriasis patients: causes and consequences. *Front Immunol.* (2018) 9:579. doi: 10.3389/fimmu.2018.00579
2. Boehncke WH, Schon MP. Psoriasis. *Lancet* (2015) 386:983–94. doi: 10.1016/S0140-6736(14)61909-7
3. Lande R, Gregorio J, Facchinetti V, Chatterjee B, Wang YH, Homey B, et al. Plasmacytoid dendritic cells sense self-DNA coupled with antimicrobial peptide. *Nature* (2007) 449:564–9. doi: 10.1038/nature06116
4. Zaba LC, Fuentes-Duculan J, Eungdamrong NJ, Abello MV, Novitskaya I, Pierson KC, et al. Psoriasis is characterized by accumulation of immunostimulatory and Th1/Th17 cell-polarizing myeloid dendritic cells. *J Invest Dermatol.* (2009) 129:79–88. doi: 10.1038/jid.2008.194
5. Boehncke WH, Brembilla NC. Unmet needs in the field of psoriasis: pathogenesis and treatment. *Clin Rev Allergy Immunol.* (2017) 55:295–311 doi: 10.1007/s12016-017-8634-3
6. Lowes MA, Russell CB, Martin DA, Towne JE, Krueger JG. The IL-23/T17 pathogenic axis in psoriasis is amplified by keratinocyte responses. *Trends Immunol.* (2013) 34:174–81. doi: 10.1016/j.it.2012.11.005
7. Conrad C, Gilliet M. Psoriasis: from pathogenesis to targeted therapies. *Clin Rev Allergy Immunol.* (2018) 54:102–13. doi: 10.1007/s12016-018-8668-1
8. Hald A, Andrés RM, Salskov-Iversen ML, Kjellerup RB, Iversen L, Johansen C. STAT1 expression and activation is increased in lesional psoriatic skin. *Br J Dermatol.* (2013) 168:302–10. doi: 10.1111/bjd.12049
9. Johansen C, Rittig AH, Mose M, Bertelsen T, Weimar I, Nielsen J, et al. STAT2 is involved in the pathogenesis of psoriasis by promoting CXCL11 and CCL5 production by keratinocytes. *PLoS ONE* (2017) 12:e0176994. doi: 10.1371/journal.pone.0176994
10. Calautti E, Avalle L, Poli V. Psoriasis: a STAT3-centric view. *Int J Mol Sci.* (2018) 19:E17. doi: 10.3390/ijms19010171
11. Johansen C, Funding AT, Otkjaer K, Kragballe K, Jensen UB, Madsen M, et al. Protein expression of TNF-alpha in psoriatic skin is regulated at a posttranscriptional level by MAPK-activated protein kinase 2. *J Immunol.* (2006) 176:1431–8. doi: 10.4049/jimmunol.176.3.1431
12. Mavropoulos A, Rigopoulou EI, Liaskos C, Bogdanos DP, Sakkas LI. The role of p38 MAPK in the aetiopathogenesis of psoriasis and psoriatic arthritis. *Clin Dev Immunol.* (2013) 2013:569751. doi: 10.1155/2013/569751
13. Mose M, Kang Z, Raaby L, Iversen L, Johansen C. TNFalpha- and IL-17A-mediated S100A8 expression is regulated by p38 MAP. *Exp Dermatol.* (2013) 22:476–81. doi: 10.1111/exd.12187
14. Tarutani M, Nakajima K, Takaishi M, Ohko K, Sano S. Epidermal hyperplasia induced by Raf-MAPK signaling requires Stat3 activation. *J Dermatol Sci.* (2013) 72:110–5. doi: 10.1016/j.jdermsci.2013.06.007
15. Zhang Y, Tu C, Zhang D, Zheng Y, Peng Z, Feng Y, et al. Wnt/beta-catenin and Wnt5a/Ca pathways regulate proliferation and apoptosis of keratinocytes in psoriasis lesions. *Cell Physiol Biochem.* (2015) 36:1890–902. doi: 10.1159/000430158
16. Bertelsen T, Iversen L, Johansen C. The human IL-17A/F heterodimer regulates psoriasis-associated genes through IkappaBzeta. *Exp Dermatol.* (2018) 27:1048–1052. doi: 10.1111/exd.13722
17. Bertelsen T, Ljungberg C, Boye Kjellerup R, Iversen L, Johansen C. IL-17F regulates psoriasis-associated genes through IkappaBzeta. *Exp Dermatol.* (2017) 26:234–241. doi: 10.1111/exd.13182
18. Goldminz AM, Au SC, Kim N, Gottlieb AB, Lizzul PF. NF-kappaB: an essential transcription factor in psoriasis. *J Dermatol Sci.* (2013) 69:89–94. doi: 10.1016/j.jdermsci.2012.11.002
19. Moorchung N, Kulaar JS, Chatterjee M, Vasudevan B, Tripathi T, Dutta V. Role of NF-κB in the pathogenesis of psoriasis elucidated by its staining in skin biopsy specimens. *Int J Dermatol.* (2014) 53:570–4. doi: 10.1111/ijd.12050
20. Yan S, Xu Z, Lou F, Zhang L, Ke F, Bai J, et al. NF-kappaB-induced microRNA-31 promotes epidermal hyperplasia by repressing protein phosphatase 6 in psoriasis. *Nat Commun.* (2015) 6:7652. doi: 10.1038/ncomms8652
21. Pettus LH, Wurz RP. Small molecule p38 MAP kinase inhibitors for the treatment of inflammatory diseases: novel structures and developments during 2006-2008. *Curr Top Med Chem.* (2008) 8:1452–67. doi: 10.2174/156802608786264245
22. Welsch K, Holstein J, Laurence A, Ghoreschi K. Targeting JAK/STAT signalling in inflammatory skin diseases with small molecule inhibitors. *Eur J Immunol.* (2017) 47:1096–107. doi: 10.1002/eji.201646680
23. Manning BD, Cantley LC. AKT/PKB signaling: navigating downstream. *Cell* (2007) 129:1261–74. doi: 10.1016/j.cell.2007.06.009
24. Laplante M, Sabatini DM. mTOR signaling in growth control and disease. *Cell* (2012) 149:274–93. doi: 10.1016/j.cell.2012.03.017
25. Sarbassov DD, Guertin DA, Ali SM, Sabatini DM. Phosphorylation and regulation of Akt/PKB by the rictor-mTOR complex. *Science* (2005) 307:1098–101. doi: 10.1126/science.1106148
26. Manning BD, Toker A. AKT/PKB signaling: navigating the network. *Cell* (2017) 169:381–405. doi: 10.1016/j.cell.2017.04.001
27. Manning BD, Cantley LC. Rheb fills a GAP between TSC and TOR. *Trends Biochem Sci.* (2003) 28:573–6. doi: 10.1016/j.tibs.2003.09.003
28. Long X, Lin Y, Ortiz-Vega S, Yonezawa K, Avruch J. Rheb binds and regulates the mTOR kinase. *Curr Biol.* (2005) 15:702–13. doi: 10.1016/j.cub.2005.02.053
29. Sancak Y, Thoreen CC, Peterson TR, Lindquist RA, Kang SA, Spooner E, et al. PRAS40 is an insulin-regulated inhibitor of the mTORC1 protein kinase. *Mol Cell* (2007) 25:903–15. doi: 10.1016/j.molcel.2007.03.003
30. Ben-Sahra I, Manning BD. mTORC1 signaling and the metabolic control of cell growth. *Curr Opin Cell Biol.* (2017) 45:72–82. doi: 10.1016/j.ceb.2017.02.012
31. Thoreen CC, Chantranupong L, Keys HR, Wang T, Gray NS, Sabatini DM. A unifying model for mTORC1-mediated regulation of mRNA translation. *Nature* (2012) 485:109–13. doi: 10.1038/nature11083

32. Porstmann T, Santos CR, Griffiths B, Cully M, Wu M, Leevers S, et al. SREBP activity is regulated by mTORC1 and contributes to Akt-dependent cell growth. *Cell Metab.* (2008) 8:224–36. doi: 10.1016/j.cmet.2008.07.007
33. Ben-Sahra I, Howell JJ, Asara JM, Manning BD. Stimulation of de novo pyrimidine synthesis by growth signaling through mTOR and S6K1. *Science* (2013) 339:1323–8. doi: 10.1126/science.1228792
34. Egan D, Kim J, Shaw RJ, Guan KL. The autophagy initiating kinase ULK1 is regulated via opposing phosphorylation by AMPK and mTO. *Autophagy* (2011) 7:643–4. doi: 10.4161/auto.7.6.15123
35. Madonna S, Scarponi C, Pallotta S, Cavani A, Albanesi C. Anti-apoptotic effects of suppressor of cytokine signaling 3 and 1 in psoriasis. *Cell Death Dis.* (2012) 3:e334. doi: 10.1038/cddis.2012.69
36. Buerger C, Richter B, Woth K, Salgo R, Malisiewicz B, Diehl S, et al. Interleukin-1beta interferes with epidermal homeostasis through induction of insulin resistance: implications for psoriasis pathogenesis. *J Invest Dermatol.* (2012) 132:2206–14. doi: 10.1038/jid.2012.123
37. Calautti E, Li J, Saoncella S, Brissette JL, Goetinck PF. Phosphoinositide 3-kinase signaling to Akt promotes keratinocyte differentiation versus death. *J Biol Chem.* (2005) 280:32856–65. doi: 10.1074/jbc.M506119200
38. Datta Mitra A, Raychaudhuri SP, Abria CJ, Mitra A, Wright R, Ray R, et al. 1alpha,25-Dihydroxyvitamin-D3-3-bromoacetate regulates AKT/mTOR signaling cascades: a therapeutic agent for psoriasis. *J Invest Dermatol.* (2013) 133:1556–64. doi: 10.1038/jid.2013.3
39. Buerger C, Malisiewicz B, Eiser A, Hardt K, Boehncke WH. Mammalian target of rapamycin and its downstream signalling components are activated in psoriatic skin. *Br J Dermatol.* (2013) 169:156–9. doi: 10.1111/bjd.12271
40. Buerger C, Shirsath N, Lang V, Berard A, Diehl S, Kaufmann R, et al. Inflammation dependent mTORC1 signaling interferes with the switch from keratinocyte proliferation to differentiation. *PLoS ONE* (2017) 12:e0180853. doi: 10.1371/journal.pone.0180853
41. Shirsath N, Mayer G, Singh TP, Wolf P. 8-methoxypsoralen plus UVA (PUVA) therapy normalizes signalling of phosphorylated component of mTOR pathway in psoriatic skin of K5.hTGFbeta1 transgenic mice. *Exp Dermatol.* (2015) 24:889–91. doi: 10.1111/exd.12779
42. Xu L, Leng H, Shi X, Ji J, Fu J, Leng H. MiR-155 promotes cell proliferation and inhibits apoptosis by PTEN signaling pathway in the psoriasis. *Biomed Pharmacother.* (2017) 90:524–30. doi: 10.1016/j.biopha.2017.03.105
43. A R, Yu P, Hao S, Li Y. MiR-876–5p suppresses cell proliferation by targeting Angiopoietin-1 in the psoriasis. *Biomed Pharmacother.* (2018) 103:1163–9. doi: 10.1016/j.biopha.2018.04.145
44. Gargalionis AN, Malakou LS, Adamopoulos C, Piperi C, Theohari I, Nokhbehsaim M, et al. Polycystin-1 downregulation induces ERK-dependent mTOR pathway activation in a cellular model of psoriasis. *Biochim Biophys Acta* (2018) 1864:3468–76. doi: 10.1016/j.bbadis.2018.07.036
45. Mitra A, Raychaudhuri SK, Raychaudhuri SP. IL-22 induced cell proliferation is regulated by PI3K/Akt/mTOR signaling cascade. *Cytokine* (2012) 60:38–42. doi: 10.1016/j.cyto.2012.06.316
46. Patel AB, Tsilioni I, Weng Z, Theoharides TC. TNF stimulates IL-6, CXCL8 and VEGF secretion from human keratinocytes via activation of mTOR, inhibited by tetramethoxyluteolin. *Exp Dermatol.* (2018) 27:135–43. doi: 10.1111/exd.13461
47. Varshney P, Saini N. PI3K/AKT/mTOR activation and autophagy inhibition plays a key role in increased cholesterol during IL-17A mediated inflammatory response in psoriasis. *Biochim Biophys Acta* (2018) 1864 (5 Pt A):1795–803. doi: 10.1016/j.bbadis.2018.02.003
48. Akinduro O, Sully K, Patel A, Robinson DJ, Chikh A, McPhail G, et al. Constitutive autophagy and nucleophagy during epidermal differentiation. *J Invest Dermatol.* (2016) 136:1460–70. doi: 10.1016/j.jid.2016.03.016
49. Weichhart T, Hengstschläger M, Linke M. Regulation of innate immune cell function by mTOR. *Nat Rev Immunol.* (2015) 15:599–614. doi: 10.1038/nri3901
50. Jones RG, Pearce EJ. MenTORing immunity: mTOR signaling in the development and function of tissue-resident immune cells. *Immunity* (2017) 46:730–42. doi: 10.1016/j.immuni.2017.04.028
51. Powell JD, Pollizzi KN, Heikamp EB, Horton MR. Regulation of immune responses by mTOR. *Annu Rev Immunol.* (2012) 30:39–68. doi: 10.1146/annurev-immunol-020711-075024
52. Yang H, Wang X, Zhang Y, Liu H, Liao J, Shao K, et al. Modulation of TSC-mTOR signaling on immune cells in immunity and autoimmunity. *J Cell Physiol.* (2014) 229:17–26. doi: 10.1002/jcp.24426
53. Linke M, Fritsch SD, Sukhbaatar N, Hengstschläger M, Weichhart T. mTORC1 and mTORC2 as regulators of cell metabolism in immunity. *FEBS Lett.* (2017) 591:3089–103. doi: 10.1002/1873-3468.12711
54. Ochaion A, Bar-Yehuda S, Cohen S, Barer F, Patoka R, Amital H, et al. The anti-inflammatory target A(3) adenosine receptor is over-expressed in rheumatoid arthritis, psoriasis and Crohn's disease. *Cell Immunol.* (2009) 258:115–22. doi: 10.1016/j.cellimm.2009.03.020
55. Huang T, Lin X, Meng X, Lin M. Phosphoinositide-3 kinase/protein kinase-B/mammalian target of rapamycin pathway in psoriasis pathogenesis. A potential therapeutic target? *Acta Derm Venereol.* (2014) 94:371–9. doi: 10.2340/00015555-1737
56. Yan K, Xu W, Huang Y, Zhang Z, Huang Q, Xin KZ, et al. Methotrexate restores the function of peripheral blood regulatory T cells in psoriasis vulgaris via the CD73/AMPK/mTOR pathway. *Br J Dermatol.* (2018) 179:896–905 doi: 10.1111/bjd.16560
57. Datta-Mitra A, Mitra A, Ray R, Raychaudhuri SP, Kundu-Raychaudhuri S. 1,25-Dihydroxyvitamin D3-3-bromoacetate, a novel vitamin D analog induces immunosuppression through PI3K/Akt/mTOR signaling cascade. *Int Immunopharmacol.* (2013) 17:744–51. doi: 10.1016/j.intimp.2013.08.009
58. Sehgal SN, Baker H, VÉZina C. Rapamycin (AY-22,989), a new antifungal antibiotic. IFermentation I. isolation and characterization. *J Antibiot* (1975) 28:727–32.
59. Sabatini DM, Erdjument-Bromage H, Lui M, Tempst P, Snyder SH. RAFT1: a mammalian protein that binds to FKBP12 in a rapamycin-dependent fashion and is homologous to yeast TORs. *Cell* (1994) 78:35–43. doi: 10.1016/0092-8674(94)90570-3
60. Calne RY, Collier DS, Lim S, Pollard SG, Samaan A, White DJ, et al. Rapamycin for immunosuppression in organ allografting. *Lancet* (1989) 334:227. doi: 10.1016/S0140-6736(89)90417-0
61. McMahon G, Weir MR, Li XC, Mandelbrot DA. The evolving role of mTOR inhibition in transplantation tolerance. *J Am Soc Nephrol.* (2011) 22:408–15. doi: 10.1681/ASN.2010040351
62. Habib A, Finn AV. Antiproliferative drugs for restenosis prevention. *Interv Cardiol Clin.* (2016) 5:321–9. doi: 10.1016/j.iccl.2016.02.002
63. Meng LH, Zheng XF. Toward rapamycin analog (rapalog)-based precision cancer therapy. *Acta Pharmacol Sin.* (2015) 36:1163–9. doi: 10.1038/aps.2015.68
64. Li J, Kim SG, Blenis J. Rapamycin: one drug, many effects. *Cell Metab.* (2014) 19:373–9. doi: 10.1016/j.cmet.2014.01.001
65. Frigerio E, Colombo MD, Franchi C, Altomare A, Garutti C, Altomare GF. Severe psoriasis treated with a new macrolide: everolimus. *Br J Dermatol.* (2007) 156:372–4. doi: 10.1111/j.1365-2133.2006.07602.x
66. Reitamo S, Spuls P, Sassolas B, Lahfa M, Claudy A, Griffiths CE, et al. Efficacy of sirolimus (rapamycin) administered concomitantly with a subtherapeutic dose of cyclosporin in the treatment of severe psoriasis: a randomized controlled trial. *Br J Dermatol.* (2001) 145:438–45. doi: 10.1046/j.1365-2133.2001.04376.x
67. Wei KC, Lai PC. Combination of everolimus and tacrolimus: a potentially effective regimen for recalcitrant psoriasis. *Dermatol Ther.* (2015) 28:25–7. doi: 10.1111/dth.12176
68. Wu JJ, Lynde CW, Kleyn CE, Iversen L, van der Walt JM, Carvalho A, et al. Identification of key research needs for topical therapy treatment of psoriasis - a consensus paper by the International Psoriasis Council. *J Eur Acad Dermatol Venereol.* (2016) 30:1115–9. doi: 10.1111/jdv.13614
69. Ormerod AD, Shah SA, Copeland P, Omar G, Winfield A. Treatment of psoriasis with topical sirolimus: preclinical development and a randomized, double-blind trial. *Br J Dermatol.* (2005) 152:758–64. doi: 10.1111/j.1365-2133.2005.06438.x
70. Chamcheu JC, Chaves-Rodriquez MI, Adhami VM, Siddiqui IA, Wood GS, Longley BJ, et al. Upregulation of PI3K/AKT/mTOR, FABP5 and PPARbeta/delta in human psoriasis and imiquimod-induced murine psoriasiform dermatitis model. *Acta Derm Venereol.* (2016) 96:854–6. doi: 10.2340/00015555-2359

71. Bürger C, Shirsath N, Lang V, Diehl S, Kaufmann R, Weigert A, et al. Blocking mTOR signalling with rapamycin ameliorates imiquimod-induced psoriasis in mice. *Acta Derm Venereol.* (2017) 97:1087–94. doi: 10.2340/00015555-2724
72. Gao M, Si X. Rapamycin ameliorates psoriasis by regulating the expression and methylation levels of Tropomyosin via ERK1/2 and mTOR pathways *in vitro* and *in vivo*. *Exp Dermatol.* (2018) 27:1112–9. doi: 10.1111/exd.13745
73. Thoreen CC, Kang SA, Chang JW, Liu Q, Zhang J, Gao Y, et al. An ATP-competitive mammalian target of rapamycin inhibitor reveals rapamycin-resistant functions of mTORC1. *J Biol Chem.* (2009) 284:8023–32. doi: 10.1074/jbc.M900301200
74. Sarbassov DD, Ali SM, Sengupta S, Sheen JH, Hsu PP, Bagley AF, et al. Prolonged rapamycin treatment inhibits mTORC2 assembly and Akt/PK. *Mol Cell* (2006) 22:159–68. doi: 10.1016/j.molcel.2006.03.029
75. Liu Q, Chang JW, Wang J, Kang SA, Thoreen CC, Markhard A, et al. Discovery of 1-(4-(4-propionylpiperazin-1-yl)-3-(trifluoromethyl)phenyl)-9-(quinolin-3-yl)benz o[h][1,6]naphthyridin-2(1H)-one as a highly potent, selective mammalian target of rapamycin (mTOR) inhibitor for the treatment of cancer. *J Med Chem.* (2010) 53:7146–55. doi: 10.1021/jm101144f
76. Liu Q, Wang J, Kang SA, Thoreen CC, Hur W, Ahmed T, et al. Discovery of 9-(6-aminopyridin-3-yl)-1-(3-(trifluoromethyl)phenyl)benzo[h][1,6]naphthyridin-2(1H)-one (Torin2)as a potent, selective, and orally available mammalian target of rapamycin (mTOR) inhibitor for treatment of cancer. *J Med Chem.* (2011) 54:1473–80. doi: 10.1021/jm101520v
77. Chamcheu JC, Adhami VM, Esnault S, Sechi M, Siddiqui IA, Satyshur KA, et al. Dual inhibition of PI3K/Akt and mTOR by the dietary antioxidant delphinidin ameliorates psoriatic features *in-vitro* and in an imiquimod-induced psoriasis-like disease in mice. *Antioxid Redox Signal.* (2016) 26:49–69 doi: 10.1089/ars.2016.6769
78. Pal HC, Chamcheu JC, Adhami VM, Wood GS, Elmets CA, Mukhtar H, et al. Topical application of delphinidin reduces psoriasiform lesions in the flaky skin mouse model by inducing epidermal differentiation and inhibiting inflammation. *Br J Dermatol.* (2015) 172:354–64. doi: 10.1111/bjd.13513

8

Human Leukocyte Antigen-Class I Alleles and the Autoreactive T Cell Response in Psoriasis Pathogenesis

*Jörg Christoph Prinz**

Department of Dermatology, University Clinics, Ludwig-Maximilian-University of Munich, Munich, Germany

Correspondence:
Jörg Christoph Prinz
joerg.prinz@med.uni-muenchen.de

Psoriasis is a complex immune-mediated inflammatory skin disease characterized by T-cell-driven epidermal hyperplasia. It occurs on a strong genetic predisposition. The human leukocyte antigen (HLA)-class I allele *HLA-C*06:02* on psoriasis susceptibility locus 1 (PSORS1 on 6p21.3) is the main psoriasis risk gene. Other HLA-class I alleles encoding HLA molecules presenting overlapping peptide repertoires show associations with psoriasis as well. Outside the major histocompatibility complex region, genome-wide association studies identified more than 60 psoriasis-associated common gene variants exerting only modest individual effects. They mainly refer to innate immune activation and the interleukin-23/$T_{h/c}$17 pathway. Given their strong risk association, explaining the role of the HLA-risk alleles is essential for elucidating psoriasis pathogenesis. Psoriasis lesions develop upon epidermal infiltration, activation, and expansion of CD8$^+$ T cells. The unbiased analysis of a paradigmatic Vα3S1/Vβ13S1-T-cell receptor from a pathogenic epidermal CD8$^+$ T-cell clone of an *HLA-C*06:02*$^+$ psoriasis patient had revealed that HLA-C*06:02 directs an autoimmune response against melanocytes through autoantigen presentation, and it identified a peptide form ADAMTS-like protein 5 as an HLA-C*06:02-presented melanocyte autoantigen. These data demonstrate that psoriasis is an autoimmune disease, where the predisposing HLA-class I alleles promote organ-specific inflammation through facilitating a T-cell response against a particular skin-specific cell population. This review discusses the role of HLA-class I alleles in the pathogenic psoriatic T-cell immune response. It concludes that as a principle of T-cell driven HLA-associated inflammatory diseases proinflammatory traits promote autoimmunity in the context of certain HLA molecules that present particular autoantigens.

Keywords: psoriasis, pathogenesis, autoreactive T cells, human leukocyte antigen association, HLA-C*06:02, T-cell receptor, autoimmunity, autoantigens

INTRODUCTION

Psoriasis is a complex T-cell mediated skin disease. Skin lesions are characterized by sharply demarcated heavily scaling inflammatory plaques which result from T-cell driven epidermal hyperplasia. T cells infiltrating psoriasis skin lesions display a T-helper/cytotoxic cell ($T_{h/c}$) 17 phenotype producing the $T_{h/c}$17 signature cytokines interleukin (IL)-17A, IL-22, and IFN-γ (1, 2). They promote keratinocyte proliferation, accumulation of neutrophilic granulocytes, and the production of antimicrobial peptides and other inflammatory cytokines and chemokines. Activation and differentiation

---

Abbreviations: TCR, T-cell receptor; GWAS, genome-wide association study; HLA, human leukocyte antigen; MHC, major histocompatibility complex; ADAMTSL5, ADAMTS-like protein 5.

of the lesional psoriatic $T_{h/c}17$ response is maintained by IL-23 that is produced by local dendritic cells and keratinocytes. By today, blocking IL-17A or IL-23 represents the most efficient treatment modality (3).

Psoriasis is multifactorial and involves the interaction of individual genotypes with environmental, infectious, and lifestyle factors. The human leukocyte antigen (HLA)-class I allele *HLA-C*06:02* is the main psoriasis risk gene (4–6). Functional clustering of common variants associated with psoriasis highlighted the roles of interferon signaling and the NF-κB cascade and of regulatory elements related to $CD4^+$ and $CD8^+$ T cell maturation, development, and activation including the IL-23 pathway and $T_{h/c}17$ differentiation (7). Thus, understanding psoriasis pathogenesis has to explain the role of HLA-C*06:02 within the complex genetic background predisposing to psoriasis. Therefore, this review will focus on the functional implications of the main HLA psoriasis risk gene, *HLA-C*06:02*.

HLA-CLASS I ASSOCIATION OF PSORIASIS: THE MAIN GENETIC RISK

The most significant association signal observed in psoriasis genome-wide association studies that satisfied the genome-wide significance threshold of $P < 5.0 \times 10^{-8}$ (8) was observed within the major histocompatibility complex (MHC) region (7, 9–13). The highly polymorphic nature and density of genes and the extensive linkage disequilibrium that exists within the MHC, however, had initially hampered the identification of the causal gene that confers psoriasis susceptibility in the HLA region. Sequence-based methods in large samples finally proved *HLA-C*06:02* as the main psoriasis risk gene (4, 6). *HLA-C*06:02* defines early onset, severity and familial clustering of psoriasis (14–16). Unlike HLA-class II-associated autoimmune diseases psoriasis shows no evidence of interactions between different HLA alleles. *HLA-C*06:02* contributes a non-additive risk effect and represents a true HLA-class I risk gene (17).

Interpreting HLA associations has to consider that the frequency of alleles can differ between populations. The prevalence and incidence of psoriasis shows ethnic and geographic variations. A relatively high prevalence of psoriasis in European countries and in the USA (0.5–6.5%) contrasts with a low prevalence in East Asian countries (0.2–0.3%) (18, 19). Given the strong risk effect of *HLA-C*06:02*, the ethnic allele frequency spectra of *HLA-C*06:02* may at least partially explain the heterogeneity of psoriasis in different ethnic populations. This highlights the need to use population-specific reference panels made by deep sequencing to impute MHC alleles and amino acids (8). The strong psoriasis risk of *HLA-C*06:02* allele has been validated in worldwide populations including Europeans (17, 20), East (6, 21), and South Asians (22), with odds ratios of as high as 3.0–10.0. HLA fine-mapping analysis using the HLA imputation method successfully identified multiple other less obviously associated HLA-class I and class II variants that confer psoriasis risk independently from *HLA-C*06:02* (20). Aside from *HLA-C*06:02* psoriasis associated with *HLA-C*12:03*, *HLA-C*07:01*, *HLA-C*07:02*, *HLA-C*07:04*, *HLA-B*27*, and *HLA-B*57*. Further associations were seen with *HLA-B* amino acid positions 9, 67, and 116, *HLA-A* amino acid 95, and *HLA-DQα1* amino acid position 53 which are all localized within the HLA antigen binding region (6, 20, 21, 23). Although *HLA-C*06:02* and the AA position 67 of *HLA*-B are shared between Caucasian and Chinese populations, other independent HLA-risk variants differ between the two populations. *HLA-A*02:07*, which corresponds to the cysteine residue at HLA-A position 99, shows a strong association in Chinese but is very rare or absent in Europeans, whereas *HLA-B*07* shows a strong association in Caucasians while it is very rare in Chinese. The other HLA variants are common in both Caucasian and Chinese, but show population-specific associations, *HLA-A*02:01* for Caucasian and the AA positions 114 and 144 of HLA-A for Chinese. These population-specific effects contribute significantly to the ethnic diversity of psoriasis prevalence (12).

The Japanese population has unique characteristics. Psoriasis prevalence in Japan is one of the lowest compared with worldwide populations (0.1–0.3%) (24–27), and *HLA-C*06:02* is almost absent within the Japanese population (<0.5%) (21). Due to low allele frequency in the Japanese population, the impact of *HLA-C*06:02* on psoriasis susceptibility in Japanese psoriasis patients was less apparent compared with that seen in other populations (2.3% in psoriasis cases and 0.4% in controls). Still, a Japanese-specific reference panel showed increased odds ratios for *HLA-C*06:02*, *HLA-C*12:02*, and *HLA-C*07:04* in the Japanese psoriasis population (21).

Interestingly, several of the psoriasis-associated HLA-class I alleles are also significantly increased in Crohn's disease (*HLA-C*06:02*, *HLA-C*12:02*) and ulcerative colitis (*HLA-C*12:02*, *HLA-C*07:02*) (28). *HLA-B*27* predisposes for ankylosing spondylitis, inflammatory bowel disease, and psoriasis arthritis, creating an overlapping HLA-class I risk pattern although no autoantigens have been identified in these diseases.

FUNCTIONAL ASPECTS OF HLA-CLASS I ALLELES IN PSORIASIS

Genetic variation in HLA genes within the MHC locus is associated with many immune-mediated inflammatory diseases (IMIDs): virtually any autoimmune condition is associated with particular HLA-class I or class II alleles (29–31). For most of these diseases, the HLA association explains more disease risk than any other gene locus. While IMIDs share many of the non-HLA loci, the associated HLA-class I and/or class II alleles are usually disease specific (32). This attributes the HLA alleles with a high degree of disease specificity and pleads for a direct causal role in the pathogenesis of the respective IMID. The association with *HLA-C*06:02* in psoriasis is particularly intriguing because only 3 of more than 12,000 different HLA-class I alleles show a strong disease linkage: *HLA-B*27* with ankylosing spondylitis, *HLA-B*51* with Behçet's disease, and HLA-*C*06:02* with psoriasis.

Human leukocyte antigen-class I molecules are expressed by all nucleated cells. They present peptide antigens of usually 8–10 amino acids to αβ T-cell receptors (TCRs) of $CD8^+$ T cells (33). The antigenic peptides are derived from cytoplasmic proteins, i.e., proteins produced within the cells. They are processed from the parent proteins by the proteasome for loading into the peptide-binding groove of the HLA-class I molecules. The complex of peptide and HLA-class I molecule is transported to the cell membrane for recognition by CD8$^+$ T cells (34, 35). Accordingly, an HLA-class I-restricted immune response must be directed against a particular target cell which expresses the antigenic protein within the cytoplasm.

Human leukocyte antigen alleles are extremely polymorphic. Sequence variation is concentrated in the α1 and α2 domains that contain the binding sites for peptide antigens and interact with the TCR. HLA polymorphisms result in variable peptide-binding grooves. They contain two or three specific acceptor sites or pockets which bind specific amino acid side chains of peptides and thus define the spectrum of antigenic peptides a particular HLA molecule can present (35, 36). Due to the diverse acceptor sites, different HLA molecules select different peptide repertoires for presentation (37, 38), although the binding specificities may overlap (39, 40). Because the peptide residues in between the anchors may be flexibly occupied a single HLA-class I molecule can theoretically display between $6 \times 20^{5-7}$ different decamer peptides (36, 41, 42).

The amino acid motifs of peptides presented by HLA-C*06:02 and several other HLA-class I molecules have recently been characterized in detail (43–45). Nonamer peptides presented by HLA-C*06:02 show select amino acids at the anchor residues 2 and 9, and a potentially secondary anchor at residue 7 (**Table 1**). The dominant amino acids are arginine at residue 2, leucine, valine, and less preferred isoleucine and methionine at residue 9, and arginine at residue 7. As a particular feature, HLA-C*06:02 has very negatively charged pockets defining peptides with large positively charged amino acids at residue 2 (B-pocket) and 7 (E-pocket) and thus selects a distinct repertoire of positively charged peptides. The studies of Di Marco et al. (43) and Mobbs et al. (44) further provided an estimate of the spectrum of self-peptides presented by HLA-C*06:02 and other HLA-C molecules. Depending on the experimental approach peptide elution identified between 1,000 and 3,000 different self-peptides from HLA-C*06:02 expressed in a B-cell line (43, 44). Thus, a substantial part of the cellular proteome should be immunologically visible to CD8$^+$ T cells (44).

According to the peptide-binding pattern *HLA-C*06:02* was assigned to the same HLA supertype as other psoriasis-associated HLA alleles including *HLA-C*07:01*, *HLA-C*07:02*, and *HLA-B*27* (43). All of them utilize the same anchor residues and present peptide repertoires that may partly overlap (**Table 1**) (43–45). HLA-C*06:02 further shares the strong negative charge of the E-pocket with HLA-C*12:03 (44) which has several similar functional domains and peptide-binding pockets as HLA-C*06:02 (46) and constitutes another potential HLA-risk allele for psoriasis and psoriatic arthritis (20, 23). Thus, several psoriasis-associated HLA-class I molecules have overlapping peptide-binding properties and might replace each other in conferring psoriasis risk. Due to the strength of association, *HLA-C*06:02* may be considered the representative HLA-risk allele within this spectrum and should therefore be particularly suitable for analyzing the role of HLA in psoriasis pathogenesis.

TABLE 1 | Amino acids at anchor residues 2 and 9 of peptide antigens and ADAMTS-like protein 5 (ADAMTSL5) presented by psoriasis-associated human leukocyte antigen (HLA) molecules.

HLA molecule	Residue 2	Residue 9
HLA-C*06:02	R/Y/K[a]	L/V/I/Y/F/M
HLA-C*07:01	R/T/N	L/F/Y/M
HLA-C*07:02	R/Y/K	L/Y/F/M
HLA-B*27	R	L
ADAMTSL5 peptide	R	L

[a]*One letter amino acid code; font size approximately reflects the relative frequency of the respective amino acid observed at this position in peptides eluted from the HLA molecules according to Ref. (44–45).*

THE TARGET CELL AND AUTOANTIGENS OF AN HLA-C*06:02-RESTRICTED PATHOGENIC PSORIATIC T CELL RESPONSE

Heritability is an estimation of how much variation in a disease can be explained by particular genetic variants. Genetic information then has to be combined with functional analysis to allow for a precise definition of the particular role of certain genes in disease. The actual immunological role of HLA-class I molecules suggests that HLA-C*06:02 may predispose to psoriasis by presentation of an autoantigen from a skin-specific cell population. Identification of target cell and potential autoantigens of the psoriatic immune response therefore appeared as the major challenge for clarifying psoriasis pathogenesis.

This approach requires the TCRs of the pathogenic T-cell response. The paired α- and β-chains of TCRs define both HLA restriction and fine peptide specificity of a T cell (47). Because of the high diversity of the human TCR repertoire any two T cells expressing the same αβ-TCR heterodimer likely arose from a common progenitor T cell (48). In response to antigen stimulation, T cells become activated and undergo clonal expansion at the site of antigen exposure. In the obvious absence of infections, expanded TCR clonotypes are commonly viewed to characterize those T cells relevant for the pathogenesis of IMIDs (48, 49).

Psoriasis lesions develop upon epidermal infiltration and activation of CD8$^+$ T cells (50, 51). Marked oligoclonality of the T-cell populations within psoriatic skin lesions indicated that psoriatic T-cell activation is driven by locally presented antigens (52–56). Lesional T-cell clones were strictly associated with psoriatic skin lesions and reappeared in relapsing psoriasis (52, 56). T-cell clonality was definitely proven by single cell TCR analysis and particular evident for CD8$^+$ T cells in lesional epidermis (52, 54). Accordingly, the clonal TCRs likely characterized those CD8$^+$ T cells which mediate psoriatic inflammation. To identify potential targets of the pathogenic psoriatic T-cell response we expressed the paired α- and β-chains of clonal CD8$^+$ T cells from the psoriatic T-cell infiltrate along with human CD8 α and β chains in a T-hybridoma cell line that reports on TCR signaling through the expression of super green fluorescence protein under control of NFAT (**Figure 1**) (57, 58). Consequently, these TCR hybridomas carried the specificity of the pathogenic psoriatic

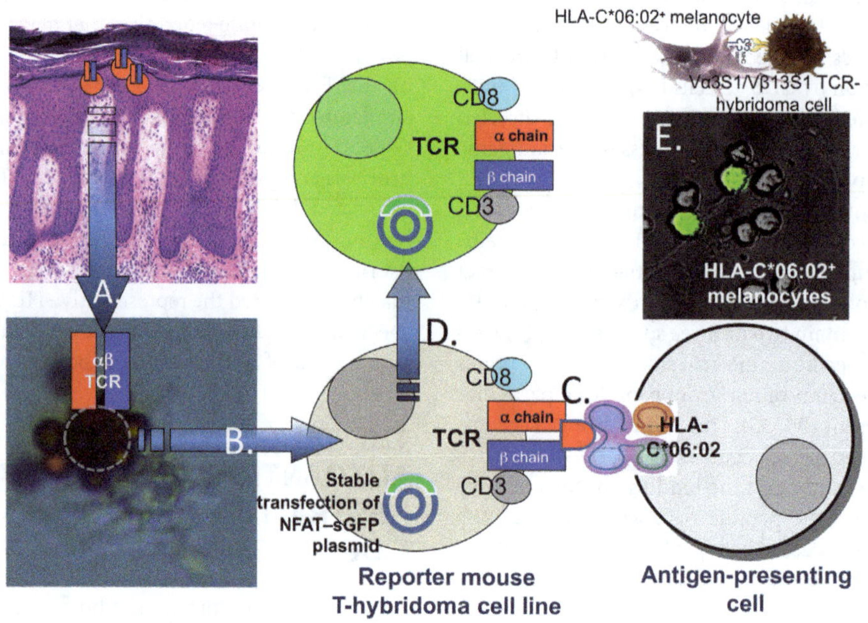

FIGURE 1 | Proof of the HLA-C*06:02-restricted autoimmune response against melanocytes in psoriasis. Following separation of epidermis and dermis of lesional biopsies from HLA-C*06:02$^+$ psoriasis patients CD8$^+$ T cells (A) were isolated from epidermal cell suspensions using magnetic beads coated with CD8 antibodies. The arrow "A" points to a CD8$^+$ T cells (encircled) isolated from lesional psoriatic epidermis which is rosetted by magnetic beads with a melanocyte attached. T-cell receptor (TCR) α and β chain mRNA of single T cells was transcribed into cDNA and sequenced by a newly developed method for single cell TCR analysis (54), cloned into expression plasmids and (B) expressed in a TCR$^{\alpha-\beta-}$ mouse reporter T-hybridoma cell line stably transfected with a plasmid for super green fluorescent protein under control of NFAT (57–59). The TCR hybridoma cells were cocultured with various primary cell types or cell lines either positive or negative for HLA-C*06:02 (C). Upon TCR ligation, the hybridoma cells produce green fluorescent protein which was visualized by UV-fluorescence microscopy or FACS analysis (D). (E) Shows the activation of the Vα3S1/Vβ13S1-TCR hybridoma by spindle-shaped HLA-C*06:02$^+$ primary melanocytes in a coculture experiment.

T cells and allowed for an unbiased, i.e., hypothesis-free analysis of the immunologic targets of the pathogenic psoriatic immune response.

Using a paradigmatic Vα3S1/Vβ13S1-TCR from an epidermal CD8$^+$ T-cell clone of an *HLA-C*06:02*-positive psoriasis patient, we could identify melanocytes as HLA-C*06:02-restricted target cells of the psoriatic immune response (**Figure 1**) (59). By means of plasmid-encoded peptide libraries, we then determined the amino acid pattern of HLA-C*06:02-presented peptide ligands of the Vα3S1/Vβ13S1-TCR. Nonamer peptides that ligated the Vα3S1/Vβ13S1-TCR displayed arginine at residues 2 and 7, and leucine at residue 9 and thus corresponded to the conserved amino acid pattern which is preferentially presented by HLA-C*06:02 and other psoriasis-associated HLA-class I molecules (**Table 1**) (43–45). Screening the human proteome and the transcriptome of melanocytes with this particular amino acid pattern identified several peptides from natural human proteins which ligated the Vα3S1/Vβ13S1-TCR. Only a peptide from ADAMTS-like protein 5 (ADAMTSL5), however, was immunogenic in the context of the full-length parent protein and unlike the other peptides could be generated through proteasomal cleavage and NH_2-terminal ERAP1 trimming. Knock-down and mutation experiments finally confirmed the role of ADAMTSL5 as melanocyte autoantigen (59). Blood lymphocytes of more than two-thirds of psoriasis patients but not healthy controls responded to ADAMTSL5 stimulation by production of the psoriasis key cytokines, IL-17 or IFN-γ (59). These data proved psoriasis as a true T-cell mediated autoimmune disease. They indicate that HLA-C*06:02 predisposes to psoriasis by mediating an autoimmune response against melanocytes through autoantigen presentation. The pathogenic psoriatic Vα3S1/Vβ13S1-TCR now represents a unique opportunity for understanding the immunopathogenesis not only of psoriasis but also of mechanisms of autoimmunity in general, since it is still unique in medical research: In no other autoimmune disease a similar approach has yet been successful to identify target cells and autoantigens.

The unbiased analysis of a pathogenic psoriatic TCR differs from other hypothesis-driven approaches for the identification of psoriatic autoantigens. Some of them were based on sequence homologies between proteins from keratinocytes and *S. pyogenes* (60, 61), a major infectious psoriasis trigger (62). The pleiotropic multifunctional 37 amino acid molecule LL37, which is generated by extracellular cleavage of the C-terminal part of the 170 amino acid Cathelicidin antimicrobial peptide (63) was proposed a potential autoantigen because LL37 peptides induced strong T-cell responses in psoriasis (64). Verification of the potential autoantigenic character for all these potential autoantigens was based on peptide stimulation assays. Several of the candidate peptides had been chosen according to HLA-C*06:02 anchor motifs. The insights into TCR polyspecificity, however, would predict that peptides designed this way will likely induce T-cell activation irrespective of pathogenic relevance (42). Furthermore, some of the proposed LL37 peptides did not contain the appropriate anchor amino acid residues for binding to HLA-C*06:02 (44). Without confirming that an HLA-class I-presented peptide can be generated from the parent protein by antigen processing and presentation pathways within the target cell, a role as autoantigen for CD8+ T cells should therefore be interpreted with care.

DISCUSSION

Defining the functional role of the main psoriasis risk gene, *HLA-C*06:02*, allowed for re-defining the architecture of the pathogenic psoriatic immune response. It proposes an HLA-centered pathogenetic model for psoriasis and other HLA-associated IMIDs where a particular HLA allele represents the causal risk gene (65). In psoriasis, HLA-C*06:02 facilitates a T-cell mediated skin-specific autoimmune response. The identification of melanocytes as organ-specific autoimmune target cells of an HLA-C*06:02-restricted immune response and of ADAMTSL5 as a melanocytic autoantigen using a pathogenic psoriatic Vα3S1/Vβ13S1-TCR provided direct experimental evidence for the autoimmune nature of psoriatic inflammation, and it explained why psoriatic inflammation primarily affects the skin (66). The predisposing HLA allele appears as an essential precondition for a tissue- and antigen-specific autoimmune response by its capacity for presentation of select autoantigens. By itself, however, autoantigen presentation is likely not sufficient for causing disease onset but requires the additive effects of common gene variants in genes which provide the costimulatory signals for activation of the actual autoimmune response. The list of common risk gene variants in psoriasis affecting proinflammatory pathways, peptide epitope trimming, IL-23 signaling and $T_{h/c}17$ differentiation is long. It includes genes related to type I interferon signaling (*ELMO1, TYK2, SOCS1, IFIH1/MDA5, RNF114, IRF4, RIG1/DDX58, IFNLR1/IL28RA*, and *IFNGR2*), activation of NF-κB pathways (*TNFAIP3, TNIP1, TYK2, REL, NFkBIA, CARD14, CARM1, UBE2L3*, and *FBXL19*), N-terminal antigen trimming (*ERAP1*), CD8+ T-cell differentiation (*ETS1, RUNX3, TNFRSF9, MBD2*, and *IRF4*), and the IL-23/IL-17A axis (*IL23R, IL12B, IL12RB, IL23A, IL23R, TYK2, STAT3, STAT5A/B, SOCS1, ETS1, TRAF3IP2, KLF4*, and *IF3*). These genetic traits may augment responsiveness of innate immune mechanisms, provide a proinflammatory environment, and generate sufficient costimulatory signals which may finally exceed the thresholds for activation, differentiation and maintenance of the pathogenic autoreactive T-cell response in psoriasis (65, 66). Overall, these insights support that proinflammatory genetic traits may promote autoimmunity in the presence of the appropriate HLA molecules which present a particular autoantigen.

AUTHOR CONTRIBUTIONS

JP has drafted and written the manuscript.

REFERENCES

1. Lowes MA, Kikuchi T, Fuentes-Duculan J, Cardinale I, Zaba LC, Haider AS, et al. Psoriasis vulgaris lesions contain discrete populations of Th1 and Th17 T cells. *J Invest Dermatol* (2008) 128:1207–11. doi:10.1038/sj.jid.5701213
2. Perera GK, Di Meglio P, Nestle FO. Psoriasis. *Annu Rev Pathol* (2012) 7: 385–422. doi:10.1146/annurev-pathol-011811-132448
3. Girolomoni G, Strohal R, Puig L, Bachelez H, Barker J, Boehncke WH, et al. The role of IL-23 and the IL-23/TH 17 immune axis in the pathogenesis and treatment of psoriasis. *J Eur Acad Dermatol Venereol* (2017) 31:1616–26. doi:10.1111/jdv.14433
4. Nair RP, Stuart PE, Nistor I, Hiremagalore R, Chia NV, Jenisch S, et al. Sequence and haplotype analysis supports HLA-C as the psoriasis susceptibility 1 gene. *Am J Hum Genet* (2006) 78:827–51. doi:10.1086/503821
5. Tiilikainen A, Lassus A, Karvonen J, Vartiainen P, Julin M. Psoriasis and HLA-Cw6. *Br J Dermatol* (1980) 102:179–84. doi:10.1111/j.1365-2133.1980.tb05690.x
6. Zhou F, Cao H, Zuo X, Zhang T, Zhang X, Liu X, et al. Deep sequencing of the MHC region in the Chinese population contributes to studies of complex disease. *Nat Genet* (2016) 48:740–6. doi:10.1038/ng.3576
7. Tsoi LC, Stuart PE, Tian C, Gudjonsson JE, Das S, Zawistowski M, et al. Large scale meta-analysis characterizes genetic architecture for common psoriasis associated variants. *Nat Commun* (2017) 8:15382. doi:10.1038/ncomms15382
8. Matzaraki V, Kumar V, Wijmenga C, Zhernakova A. The MHC locus and genetic susceptibility to autoimmune and infectious diseases. *Genome Biol* (2017) 18:76. doi:10.1186/s13059-017-1207-1
9. Sheng Y, Jin X, Xu J, Gao J, Du X, Duan D, et al. Sequencing-based approach identified three new susceptibility loci for psoriasis. *Nat Commun* (2014) 5:4331. doi:10.1038/ncomms5331
10. Tang H, Jin X, Li Y, Jiang H, Tang X, Yang X, et al. A large-scale screen for coding variants predisposing to psoriasis. *Nat Genet* (2014) 46:45–50. doi:10.1038/ng.2827
11. Tsoi LC, Spain SL, Ellinghaus E, Stuart PE, Capon F, Knight J, et al. Enhanced meta-analysis and replication studies identify five new psoriasis susceptibility loci. *Nat Commun* (2015) 6:7001. doi:10.1038/ncomms8001
12. Yin X, Low HQ, Wang L, Li Y, Ellinghaus E, Han J, et al. Genome-wide meta-analysis identifies multiple novel associations and ethnic heterogeneity of psoriasis susceptibility. *Nat Commun* (2015) 6:6916. doi:10.1038/ncomms7916
13. Zuo X, Sun L, Yin X, Gao J, Sheng Y, Xu J, et al. Whole-exome SNP array identifies 15 new susceptibility loci for psoriasis. *Nat Commun* (2015) 6:6793. doi:10.1038/ncomms7793
14. Gudjonsson JE, Karason A, Antonsdottir A, Runarsdottir EH, Hauksson VB, Upmanyu R, et al. Psoriasis patients who are homozygous for the HLA-Cw*0602 allele have a 2.5-fold increased risk of developing psoriasis compared with Cw6 heterozygotes. *Br J Dermatol* (2003) 148:233–5. doi:10.1046/j.1365-2133.2003.05115.x
15. Gudjonsson JE, Karason A, Antonsdottir AA, Runarsdottir EH, Gulcher JR, Stefansson K, et al. HLA-Cw6-positive and HLA-Cw6-negative patients with psoriasis vulgaris have distinct clinical features. *J Invest Dermatol* (2002) 118:362–5. doi:10.1046/j.0022-202x.2001.01656.x
16. Henseler T, Christophers E. Psoriasis of early and late onset: characterization of two types of psoriasis vulgaris. *J Am Acad Dermatol* (1985) 13:450–6. doi:10.1016/S0190-9622(85)70188-0
17. Lenz TL, Deutsch AJ, Han B, Hu X, Okada Y, Eyre S, et al. Widespread non-additive and interaction effects within HLA loci modulate the risk of autoimmune diseases. *Nat Genet* (2015) 47:1085–90. doi:10.1038/ng.3379
18. Chandran V, Raychaudhuri SP. Geoepidemiology and environmental factors of psoriasis and psoriatic arthritis. *J Autoimmun* (2010) 34:J314–21. doi:10.1016/j.jaut.2009.12.001

19. Parisi R, Symmons DP, Griffiths CE, Ashcroft DM; Identification and Management of Psoriasis and Associated ComorbidiTy (IMPACT) Project Team. Global epidemiology of psoriasis: a systematic review of incidence and prevalence. *J Invest Dermatol* (2013) 133:377–85. doi:10.1038/jid.2012.339
20. Okada Y, Han B, Tsoi LC, Stuart PE, Ellinghaus E, Tejasvi T, et al. Fine mapping major histocompatibility complex associations in psoriasis and its clinical subtypes. *Am J Hum Genet* (2014) 95:162–72. doi:10.1016/j.ajhg.2014.07.002
21. Mabuchi T, Ota T, Manabe Y, Ikoma N, Ozawa A, Terui T, et al. HLA-C*12:02 is a susceptibility factor in late-onset type of psoriasis in Japanese. *J Dermatol* (2014) 41:697–704. doi:10.1111/1346-8138.12569
22. Chandra A, Lahiri A, Senapati S, Basu B, Ghosh S, Mukhopadhyay I, et al. Increased risk of psoriasis due to combined effect of HLA-Cw6 and LCE3 risk alleles in Indian population. *Sci Rep* (2016) 6:24059. doi:10.1038/srep24059
23. Fitzgerald O, Haroon M, Giles JT, Winchester R. Concepts of pathogenesis in psoriatic arthritis: genotype determines clinical phenotype. *Arthritis Res Ther* (2015) 17:115. doi:10.1186/s13075-015-0640-3
24. Kubota K, Kamijima Y, Sato T, Ooba N, Koide D, Iizuka H, et al. Epidemiology of psoriasis and palmoplantar pustulosis: a nationwide study using the Japanese national claims database. *BMJ Open* (2015) 5:e006450. doi:10.1136/bmjopen-2014-006450
25. Naito R, Imafuku S. Distinguishing features of body mass index and psoriasis in men and women in Japan: a hospital-based case-control study. *J Dermatol* (2016) 43:1406–11. doi:10.1111/1346-8138.13439
26. Takahashi H, Tsuji H, Takahashi I, Hashimoto Y, Ishida-Yamamoto A, Iizuka H. Prevalence of obesity/adiposity in Japanese psoriasis patients: adiposity is correlated with the severity of psoriasis. *J Dermatol Sci* (2009) 54:61–3. doi:10.1016/j.jdermsci.2008.11.011
27. Takahashi H, Tsuji H, Takahashi I, Hashimoto Y, Ishida-Yamamoto A, Iizuka H. Prevalence of obesity/adiposity in Japanese psoriasis patients: adiposity is correlated with the severity of psoriasis. *J Dermatol Sci* (2009) 55:74–6. doi:10.1016/j.jdermsci.2009.04.003
28. Goyette P, Boucher G, Mallon D, Ellinghaus E, Jostins L, Huang H, et al. High-density mapping of the MHC identifies a shared role for HLA-DRB1*01:03 in inflammatory bowel diseases and heterozygous advantage in ulcerative colitis. *Nat Genet* (2015) 47:172–9. doi:10.1038/ng.3176
29. De Bakker PI, Raychaudhuri S. Interrogating the major histocompatibility complex with high-throughput genomics. *Hum Mol Genet* (2012) 21:R29–36. doi:10.1093/hmg/dds384
30. Fernando MM, Stevens CR, Walsh EC, De Jager PL, Goyette P, Plenge RM, et al. Defining the role of the MHC in autoimmunity: a review and pooled analysis. *PLoS Genet* (2008) 4:e1000024. doi:10.1371/journal.pgen.1000024
31. Horton R, Wilming L, Rand V, Lovering RC, Bruford EA, Khodiyar VK, et al. Gene map of the extended human MHC. *Nat Rev Genet* (2004) 5:889–99. doi:10.1038/nrg1489
32. Stokkers PC, Reitsma PH, Tytgat GN, Van Deventer SJ. HLA-DR and -DQ phenotypes in inflammatory bowel disease: a meta-analysis. *Gut* (1999) 45:395–401. doi:10.1136/gut.45.3.395
33. Townsend AR, Rothbard J, Gotch FM, Bahadur G, Wraith D, McMichael AJ. The epitopes of influenza nucleoprotein recognized by cytotoxic T lymphocytes can be defined with short synthetic peptides. *Cell* (1986) 44:959–68. doi:10.1016/0092-8674(86)90019-X
34. Blum JS, Wearsch PA, Cresswell P. Pathways of antigen processing. *Annu Rev Immunol* (2013) 31:443–73. doi:10.1146/annurev-immunol-032712-095910
35. Neefjes J, Jongsma ML, Paul P, Bakke O. Towards a systems understanding of MHC class I and MHC class II antigen presentation. *Nat Rev Immunol* (2011) 11:823–36. doi:10.1038/nri3084
36. Rock KL, Reits E, Neefjes J. Present yourself! By MHC class I and MHC class II molecules. *Trends Immunol* (2016) 37:724–37. doi:10.1016/j.it.2016.08.010
37. Falk K, Rotzschke O, Stevanovic S, Jung G, Rammensee HG. Allele-specific motifs revealed by sequencing of self-peptides eluted from MHC molecules. *Nature* (1991) 351:290–6. doi:10.1038/351290a0
38. Falk K, Rotzschke O, Stevanovic S, Jung G, Rammensee HG. Pool sequencing of natural HLA-DR, DQ, and DP ligands reveals detailed peptide motifs, constraints of processing, and general rules. *Immunogenetics* (1994) 39:230–42. doi:10.1007/BF00188785
39. Ou D, Mitchell LA, Tingle AJ. HLA-DR restrictive supertypes dominate promiscuous T cell recognition: association of multiple HLA-DR molecules with susceptibility to autoimmune diseases. *J Rheumatol* (1997) 24:253–61.
40. Sette A, Sidney J. Nine major HLA class I supertypes account for the vast preponderance of HLA-A and -B polymorphism. *Immunogenetics* (1999) 50:201–12. doi:10.1007/s002510050594
41. Mason D. A very high level of crossreactivity is an essential feature of the T-cell receptor. *Immunol Today* (1998) 19:395–404. doi:10.1016/S0167-5699(98)01299-7
42. Sewell AK. Why must T cells be cross-reactive? *Nat Rev Immunol* (2012) 12:669–77. doi:10.1038/nri3279
43. Di Marco M, Schuster H, Backert L, Ghosh M, Rammensee HG, Stevanovic S. Unveiling the peptide motifs of HLA-C and HLA-G from naturally presented peptides and generation of binding prediction matrices. *J Immunol* (2017) 199:2639–51. doi:10.4049/jimmunol.1700938
44. Mobbs JI, Illing PT, Dudek NL, Brooks AG, Baker DG, Purcell AW, et al. The molecular basis for peptide repertoire selection in the human leucocyte antigen (HLA) C*06:02 molecule. *J Biol Chem* (2017) 292:17203–15. doi:10.1074/jbc.M117.806976
45. Rasmussen M, Harndahl M, Stryhn A, Boucherma R, Nielsen LL, Lemonnier FA, et al. Uncovering the peptide-binding specificities of HLA-C: a general strategy to determine the specificity of any MHC class I molecule. *J Immunol* (2014) 193:4790–802. doi:10.4049/jimmunol.1401689
46. Helms C, Saccone NL, Cao L, Daw JA, Cao K, Hsu TM, et al. Localization of PSORS1 to a haplotype block harboring HLA-C and distinct from corneodesmosin and HCR. *Hum Genet* (2005) 118:466–76. doi:10.1007/s00439-005-0048-2
47. Davis MM, Bjorkman PJ. T-cell antigen receptor genes and T-cell recognition. *Nature* (1988) 334:395–402. doi:10.1038/334395a0
48. Newell EW, Davis MM. Beyond model antigens: high-dimensional methods for the analysis of antigen-specific T cells. *Nat Biotechnol* (2014) 32:149–57. doi:10.1038/nbt.2783
49. Woodsworth DJ, Castellarin M, Holt RA. Sequence analysis of T-cell repertoires in health and disease. *Genome Med* (2013) 5:98. doi:10.1186/gm502
50. Conrad C, Boyman O, Tonel G, Tun-Kyi A, Laggner U, De Fougerolles A, et al. Alpha1beta1 integrin is crucial for accumulation of epidermal T cells and the development of psoriasis. *Nat Med* (2007) 13:836–42. doi:10.1038/nm1605
51. Di Meglio P, Villanova F, Navarini AA, Mylonas A, Tosi I, Nestle FO, et al. Targeting CD8(+) T cells prevents psoriasis development. *J Allergy Clin Immunol* (2016) 138(274–276):e276. doi:10.1016/j.jaci.2015.10.046
52. Chang JC, Smith LR, Froning KJ, Schwabe BJ, Laxer JA, Caralli LL, et al. CD8+ T cells in psoriatic lesions preferentially use T-cell receptor V beta 3 and/or V beta 13.1 genes. *Proc Natl Acad Sci U S A* (1994) 91:9282–6. doi:10.1073/pnas.91.20.9282
53. Diluvio L, Vollmer S, Besgen P, Ellwart JW, Chimenti S, Prinz JC. Identical TCR beta-chain rearrangements in streptococcal angina and skin lesions of patients with psoriasis vulgaris. *J Immunol* (2006) 176:7104–11. doi:10.4049/jimmunol.176.11.7104
54. Kim SM, Bhonsle L, Besgen P, Nickel J, Backes A, Held K, et al. Analysis of the paired TCR alpha- and beta-chains of single human T cells. *PLoS One* (2012) 7:e37338. doi:10.1371/journal.pone.0037338
55. Menssen A, Trommler P, Vollmer S, Schendel D, Albert E, Gurtler L, et al. Evidence for an antigen-specific cellular immune response in skin lesions of patients with psoriasis vulgaris. *J Immunol* (1995) 155:4078–83.
56. Vollmer S, Menssen A, Prinz JC. Dominant lesional T cell receptor rearrangements persist in relapsing psoriasis but are absent from nonlesional skin: evidence for a stable antigen-specific pathogenic T cell response in psoriasis vulgaris. *J Invest Dermatol* (2001) 117:1296–301. doi:10.1046/j.0022-202x.2001.01494.x
57. Seitz S, Schneider CK, Malotka J, Nong X, Engel AG, Wekerle H, et al. Reconstitution of paired T cell receptor alpha- and beta-chains from microdissected single cells of human inflammatory tissues. *Proc Natl Acad Sci U S A* (2006) 103:12057–62. doi:10.1073/pnas.0604247103
58. Siewert K, Malotka J, Kawakami N, Wekerle H, Hohlfeld R, Dornmair K. Unbiased identification of target antigens of CD8+ T cells with combinatorial

libraries coding for short peptides. *Nat Med* (2012) 18:824–8. doi:10.1038/nm.2720
59. Arakawa A, Siewert K, Stohr J, Besgen P, Kim SM, Ruhl G, et al. Melanocyte antigen triggers autoimmunity in human psoriasis. *J Exp Med* (2015) 212:2203–12. doi:10.1084/jem.20151093
60. Besgen P, Trommler P, Vollmer S, Prinz JC. Ezrin, maspin, peroxiredoxin 2, and heat shock protein 27: potential targets of a streptococcal-induced autoimmune response in psoriasis. *J Immunol* (2010) 184:5392–402. doi:10.4049/jimmunol.0903520
61. Gudmundsdottir AS, Sigmundsdottir H, Sigurgeirsson B, Good MF, Valdimarsson H, Jonsdottir I. Is an epitope on keratin 17 a major target for autoreactive T lymphocytes in psoriasis? *Clin Exp Immunol* (1999) 117:580–6. doi:10.1046/j.1365-2249.1999.01013.x
62. Valdimarsson H, Thorleifsdottir RH, Sigurdardottir SL, Gudjonsson JE, Johnston A. Psoriasis – as an autoimmune disease caused by molecular mimicry. *Trends Immunol* (2009) 30:494–501. doi:10.1016/j.it.2009.07.008
63. Kahlenberg JM, Kaplan MJ. Little peptide, big effects: the role of LL-37 in inflammation and autoimmune disease. *J Immunol* (2013) 191:4895–901. doi:10.4049/jimmunol.1302005
64. Lande R, Botti E, Jandus C, Dojcinovic D, Fanelli G, Conrad C, et al. The antimicrobial peptide LL37 is a T-cell autoantigen in psoriasis. *Nat Commun* (2014) 5:5621. doi:10.1038/ncomms6621
65. Prinz JC. Autoimmune aspects of psoriasis: heritability and autoantigens. *Autoimmun Rev* (2017) 16:970–9. doi:10.1016/j.autrev.2017.07.011
66. Prinz JC. Melanocytes: target cells of an HLA-C*06:02-restricted autoimmune response in psoriasis. *J Invest Dermatol* (2017) 137:2053–8. doi:10.1016/j.jid.2017.05.023

9

Psoriasis, Cardiovascular Events and Biologics: Lights and Shadows

*Giuseppina Caiazzo[1], Gabriella Fabbrocini[1], Roberta Di Caprio[1], Annunziata Raimondo[1], Emanuele Scala[1], Nicola Balato[1] and Anna Balato[2]**

[1] Department of Clinical Medicine and Surgery, University of Naples Federico II, Napoli, Italy,

[2] Department of Advanced Biomedical Sciences, University of Naples Federico II, Napoli, Italy

Correspondence:
Anna Balato
annabalato@yahoo.it

Nowadays, it is well established a link between psoriasis and cardiovascular (CV) diseases. A series of different overlapping mechanisms including inflammation, homeostasis dysregulation, and genetic susceptibility are thought to underlie this association. Advances in understanding the molecular patterns involved in the complex scenario of psoriasis have highlighted a tight correlation with atherosclerosis. Indeed, common profiles are shared in term of inflammatory cytokines and cell types. In the last decade, the management of psoriasis patients has been revolutionized with the introduction of biological therapies, such as tumor necrosis factor-alpha (TNF-α), interleukin (IL)-12/23, and IL-17 inhibitors. In clinical setting, the effectiveness of these therapies as well as the incidence of CV events is related to the type of biologics. In particular, anti-TNF-α agents seem to reduce these events in psoriasis patients whereas anti-IL-12/23 agents related CV events reduction still remain to clarify. It has to be taken into account that IL-12/23 inhibitors have a shorter post-marketing surveillance period. An even more restricted observational time is available for anti-IL-17 agents. IL-17 is associated with psoriasis, vascular disease, and inflammation. However, IL-17 role in atherosclerosis is still debated, exerting both pro-atherogenic and anti-atherogenic effects depending on the specific context. In this review, we will discuss the differences between the onset of CV events in psoriasis patients, referred to specific biological therapy and the underlying immunological mechanism. Given the development of new therapeutic strategies, the investigation of these inhibitors impact on heart failure outcome is extremely important.

Keywords: anti-IL12/23, anti-IL17, anti-tumor necrosis factor-alpha, atherosclerosis, cardiovascular risk, psoriasis

PSORIASIS AND CARDIOVASCULAR (CV) EVENTS

The relationship between psoriasis (Pso) and an increased incidence of major adverse cardiovascular events (MACEs) has been observed for decades, since McDonald and Calabresi first demonstrated that the risk associated with arterial and vascular diseases was 2.2 times higher in more of 300 hospitalized patients with Pso compared with controls with other dermatological conditions (1). Since

---

Abbreviations: CI, confidence interval; CRP, C-reactive protein; CT, computed tomography; CV, cardiovascular; CVD, cardiovascular disease; FDG, ^{18}F-fluoro-deoxyglucose; GPRD, General Practice Research Database; HDL, high-density lipoprotein; IFN, interferon; IL, interleukin; IMT, intima-media thickness; IRs, incidence rates; LDL, low-density lipoprotein; MACEs, major adverse cardiovascular events; MCP, monocyte chemoattractant protein; MI, myocardial infarction; MTX, methotrexate; OR, odds ratio; PASI, psoriasis area severity index; PET, positron emission tomography; RBP4, retinol-binding protein 4; RCTs, random control trials; Th, T helper; TNF, tumor necrosis factor; TNFi, TNF-α inhibitors; V-CAM, vascular cell adhesion molecule; VEGF, vascular endothelial growth factor.

then, several studies have confirmed these findings, convincingly proving that patients with Pso have an effective higher risk of developing severe CV events, such as myocardial infarction (MI) and stroke (2). In 2006, using the General Practice Research Database (GPRD) source, Gelfand et al. suggested that Pso is an independent risk factor for acute MI and cardiovascular disease (CVD), particularly in young patients, and that this risk is most significant in patients with severe disease (3). In 2007, Ludwig and colleagues also identified Pso as a possible independent risk factor for CVD development founding a significantly increased prevalence and severity of the CVD indicator coronary artery calcification factor in these patients (4). In addition, increases in the prevalence of other independent "traditional" risk factors for CVD, including smoking, excess alcohol intake, as well as obesity, hypertension, dyslipidemia, and insulin resistance (the common underlying factors of metabolic syndrome), have been also reported in psoriatic patients (5–7). However, despite the evidences, some studies failed to find a significant independent association between Pso and CVD (8, 9). In 2015, using the same population-based GPRD, Parisi et al. conducted a series of multivariable analyses on patients with incident Pso concluding that neither Pso nor severe Pso are associated with a risk of MACE even after adjustment for traditional CVD risk factors (10). To date, the debate is whether or not this link represents a causal relationship or is a predisposition due to the underlying risk factors exhibited by patients with severe Pso (9, 10). The main hypothesis is that chronic inflammation which occurs in Pso is more than skin deep and results in a "psoriatic march" driving systemic mechanisms that are shared with other chronic inflammatory diseases, including atherosclerosis (**Figure 1**) (11–14). This concept was introduced for the first time in 2011 by Boehncke and colleagues to describe how systemic psoriatic inflammation may lead to insulin resistance as well as endothelial cell dysfunction, causing atherosclerosis, the major pathological change preceding MI and stroke development (15). Indeed, psoriatic patients with altered glucose metabolism and insulin resistance showed an increased arterial stiffness compared with healthy subjects, with a positive correlation between arterial stiffness and Pso disease duration (16, 17). Understanding why Pso may be a risk factor for atherosclerosis requires a basic understanding of their shared pathogenic features. In 2012, Flammer and Ruschitzka proposed the theory of "two plaques for one syndrome" since molecular mechanisms as well as pro-inflammatory cytokine profile of psoriatic lesions are remarkably similar to that of atherosclerosis ones, with a comparable inflammatory infiltrate of T cells, macrophages, and monocytes (18, 19). In addition, both diseases display a common pattern of T-cell activation, with T helper (Th)1 and Th17 cytokine upregulation, as well as increased local and systemic expression of adhesion molecules and endothelins (19). Thus, there are displacements of inflammatory cells between lesional psoriatic skin, peripheral circulation, and atheromatous plaques of coronary vasculature caused by the releasing cytokines derived from the skin and inflammatory mediators derived from Pso lesions into the circulation, together with an upregulation of cell adhesion molecules (20). Moreover, Pso-associated pro-inflammatory cytokines, such as interferon (IFN)-γ, tumor necrosis factor-alpha (TNF-α), and interleukin (IL)-17, have been found increased in atherosclerotic plaques and sera of patients with unstable CVD (21, 22). Similarly, increased expression of well known CV biomarkers, including monocyte chemoattractant protein (MCP)-1 and macrophage-derived chemokines, have been measured in the lesional skin and serum of psoriatic patients suggesting shared inflammatory pathways linking Pso and CVD (23). Recently, Kolliker Frers et al. have demonstrated that pro-atherogenic inflammation marker C-reactive protein (CRP) and soluble intercellular adhesion molecule-1 levels are increased also in psoriatic patients with no CV history or traditional CV risk factors, compared with healthy subjects, as well as in patients with recent-onset PsA, even in the absence of CV risks. These data reinforce the concept that that the degree of atherosclerosis tendency might be related to the amount of the inflammatory psoriatic burden and highlight the importance of primary prevention in Pso also in those psoriatic patients with no history of CV events (24).

THERAPEUTIC IMPLICATIONS

The growing body of evidences pointing to increases in MI and CV events in psoriatic patients has raised the question whether treating cutaneous disease might also prevent heart attacks and decrease CVD risk development. Moreover, the postulated hypothesis that inflammatory cascade activated in Pso contributes to the atherosclerotic process has laid the groundwork for supposing that the anti-inflammatory Pso therapy could theoretically improve also atherosclerosis and reduce the risk of MACE (25). Prodanovich et al. first reported that treatment with methotrexate (MTX), especially when used at low doses and in combination with folic acid supplementation, was able to reduce the rate of vascular disease in patients with Pso or rheumatoid arthritis (RA) (26). A subsequent meta-analysis of 10 studies confirmed these data concluding that the use of MTX resulted in 21% lower risk of CVD and 18% lower risk of MI (27). Moreover, data from a large health-care system in USA proved that decreased MI risk in psoriatic patients treated with MTX was greater than those receiving topical therapy (28). In 2013, using a population-based Danish cohort, an observational study found that the risk of MACE development decreased in psoriatic patients in treatment with MTX compared with other non-biological agents, including oral retinoids, cyclosporine, and phototherapy (29). Indeed, treatment with cyclosporine, leading to impaired renal function and hypertension, may negatively affect the MACE profile in these patients by increasing the risk of hypertension and dyslipidemia (30). For that reason, in psoriatic patients, cyclosporine should only be used for a limited period and should be substituted with another systemic agent once the skin condition is improved (20). Similarly, acitretin, the most commonly agent used to treat generalized pustular Pso, it has been associated with an increased risk of hypertension, hyperlipidemia, and CVD even if several investigations have shown that retinoids also improve and ameliorate the formation of atherosclerotic plaques (31, 32). Moreover, Boehncke et al. found that also treatment with fumaric acid esters resulted in an improvement of CV risk biomarkers in patients with moderate-to-severe plaque-type Pso. In particular, the authors

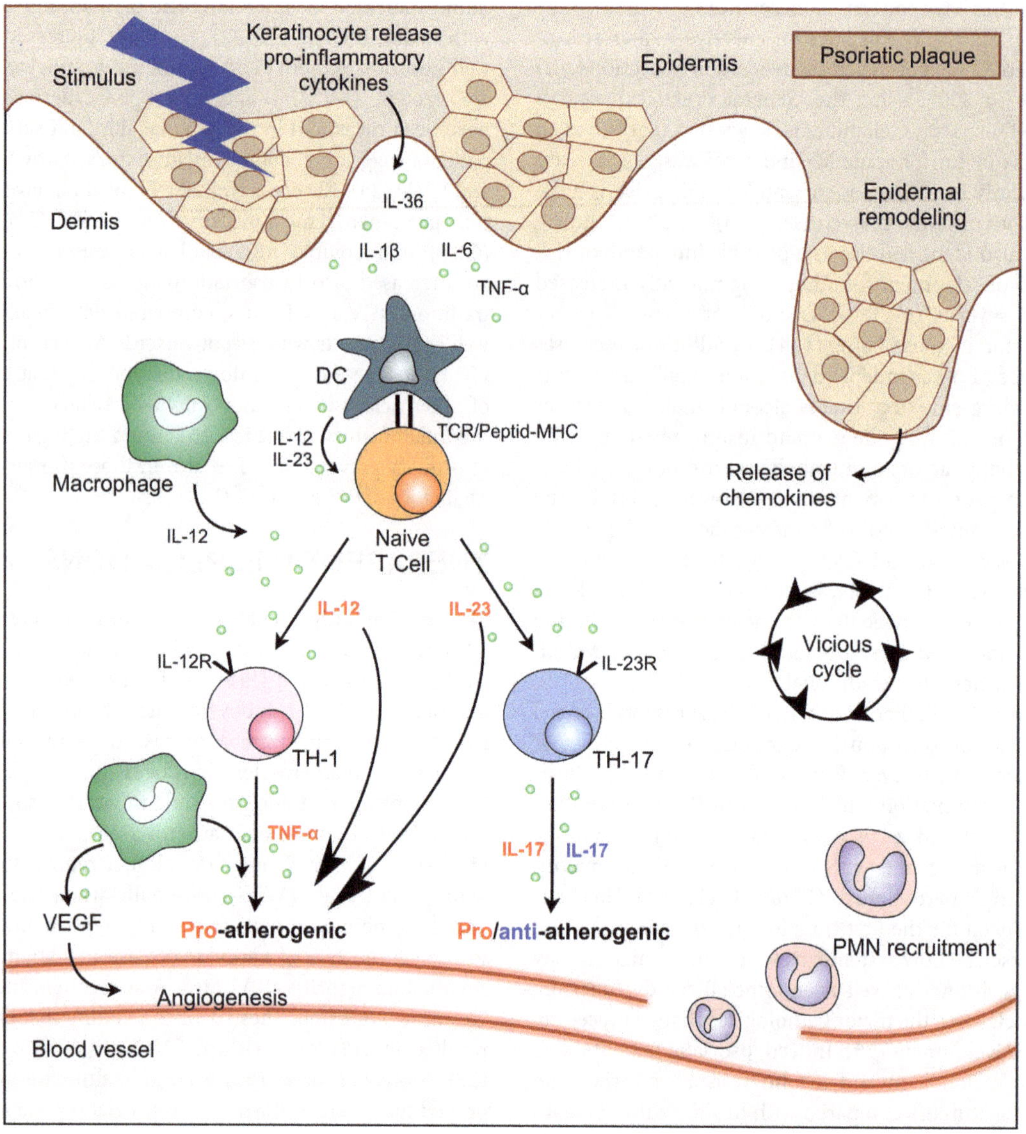

FIGURE 1 | Interactions between main cell types and cytokines present in psoriasis plaque showing their functional significance in atherosclerosis process. Abbreviations: DC, dendritic cell; IL, interleukin; MHC, major histocompatibility complex; PMN, polymorphonuclear; TCR, T cell receptor; Th, T helper; TNF, tumor necrosis factor; VEGF, vascular endothelial growth factor.

demonstrated that a continuous systemic therapy with fumaric acid esters, behind reducing Pso severity, was able to improve the endothelial vasodilator function, reduce serum levels of CRP, and increase the potentially cardioprotective adiponectin (33). However, it has been with the introduction of biological therapies that Pso treatment expectations and long-term control have greatly improved and the idea that these therapies, more than the systemic ones, might reduce the risk of CVD reinforced (34). To date, although several biological therapies have been approved and licensed for the treatment of Pso, their CV safety profile is not yet well established (35). Currently, it is unclear whether any of these therapies, which include TNF-α inhibitors (TNFi) (infliximab, etanercept, and adalimumab); inhibitors of the p40 subunit common to IL-12 and IL-23 (ustekinumab and briakinumab); IL-17A inhibitors (secukinumab and ixekizumab), and its receptor antagonist (brodalumab) could alter the risk of CVD development (35). Thus, the aim of this review has been to evaluate whether possible associations exist between currently licensed biological therapies and risk of MACEs in adult patients with Pso.

PSORIASIS AS IMMUNE-MEDIATED DISEASE

Psoriasis is an immune-mediated inflammatory skin disorder that affects 2.5% of the population worldwide. While the exact etiology of psoriasis is unknown, genetic and environmental factors are important in disease development (36, 37). Moreover, the immune system plays a crucial role in the overall disease pathogenesis, with various innate and adaptive immune cells and pro-inflammatory mediators involved at different stages of the disease (38). T cells are known to be the main actors in the pathogenesis, in particular Th1 and Th17 lymphocytes contribute through the inflammatory cytokines release that promote further recruitment of immune cells, keratinocyte proliferation, and inflammation (39). More specifically, CD4+ and CD8+ T cells with an IL-17-secretory phenotype are important contributors owing to their production of the pro-inflammatory cytokines IL-17, IL-22, and TNFα (40). For over 30 years, Pso was thought to involve a Th1 response, driven by the cytokines IFN-γ and IL-12; however, the discovery of the Th17 cell population has revolutionized the complex scenario of Pso. Indeed, the IL-23/Th17 cell signaling axis effects on keratinocytes and infiltrating immune cells in the skin has shaped the current disease model of Pso. Therefore, psoriatic disease is understood as a patterned response to chronic activation of the IL-23/Th17 axis (36). Recently, it has been identified T-regulatory cells expressing IL-17A in which, Foxp3 expression is progressively lost, whereas RORγ expression is increased (39, 40). This process is upregulated by IL-23 and concurring to the chronic inflammation seen in Pso. In particular, IL-23 regulates the maintenance of Th17 cells, whereas IL-17 and TNF mediate effector functions of innate (TNF) and adaptive (TNF, IL-17) immune cells.

EFFECTS OF BIOLOGICAL THERAPY ON CV RISK IN PSORIATIC PATIENTS

Anti-TNF-α Agents

Pso is considered a T cell-mediated immune disease with a mixed Th1/Th17 cytokines environment. The interplay of these cytokines has a central role in the disease process by causing the spread of local inflammation at systemic levels. Specifically, elevated levels of TNF-α and soluble TNF receptors have been found in lesional psoriatic skin and in the serum of patients with severe Pso, which similarly reflect those detected in congestive heart failure (CHF) patients (41–43). TNF-α activation system can lead to different outcomes: (i) the development of atherosclerosis, (ii) the deterioration of cardiac functions, and (iii) the vascular smooth muscle cell remodeling (44–46). Since 2004, US Food and Drug Administration (FDA) has approved TNFi, such as etanercept, infliximab, and adalimumab for Pso treatment. Most recently, five TNFi biosimilars have been approved by FDA for Pso: infliximab-dyyb, infliximab-abda, etanercept-szzs, adalimumab-atto, and adalimumab-adbm (47, 48). The effectiveness of these biologics in the management of psoriatic patients has been highlighted since the earliest literature (49–54). Anti-TNF-α agents can reduce the CRP, the vascular endothelial growth factor (VEGF), and the chemotactic factors (e.g., VCAM-1, E-selectin, IL-8, and MCP-1) (55, 56) as well as the Th17 cell count in the peripheral blood of psoriatic patients (49, 57). In fact, TNFi stop CD4+ T cells differentiation into Th1, Th17, and Th22 cells and the consequent release of IL-17A, IL-17F, and IL-22 (47, 58). Although the evidence indicate that TNFi are effective in reducing the systemic inflammation, it is still debated whether anti-TNF-α agents can decrease CV risk in these patients or they only represent a random association. It has been reported in literature that psoriatic patients who received TNFi showed an improvement of psoriasis area severity index (PASI) score characterized by a reduction of CV risk biomarkers (e.g., CRP, VEGF, and resistin serum levels) after 24 weeks of therapy (59). Additional studies have highlighted that the vascular function was somehow restored after 10 weeks of etanercept treatment, leading to a significant reduction in CRP levels and improvements of insulin sensitivity (60, 61). The same authors also proved that TNFi statistically led to a significant reduction ($P = 0.0001$) of retinol-binding protein 4 (RBP4) circulating levels in psoriatic patients (62). RBP4 is highly linked to subclinical atherosclerosis, due to its positive correlation to carotid intima-media thickness (IMT) indicator (61, 62). Recently, it has been assumed that psoriatic patients treated with TNFi showed IMT indicator decrease associated with appropriate therapeutic responses (63). Another experimental study has reported the aortic inflammation reduction by ^{18}F-fluoro-deoxyglucose (FDG)-positron emission tomography/computed tomography (CT) in 30 psoriatic patients who received adalimumab (64). Similarly, the TNFi effects on the development of atherosclerosis has been studied in 58 psoriatic patients during a 13-month period by CT imaging (65). In addition, the patients who did not received TNFi showed a significant progression of the coronary calcification, while the TNFi-treated group did not. Another research based on echocardiographic data confirmed the improvement of the myocardial function in 18 psoriatic subjects treated with TNFi and IL12/23 inhibitors (66). Likewise, right ventricular systolic function was improved in a 30-month study of 44 psoriatic patients treated with TNFi (67). Therefore, anti-TNF-α agents might be identified as CV protective factors together with statin drug, female gender, and age (68). However, no therapeutic effect of TNFi has been demonstrated in CHF patients classified as grade III–IV by the New York Heart Association. Initially, etanercept seemed to have beneficial effects in heart failure patients (69). Subsequently, a large study consisting of 1,500 patients with symptomatic heart failure has shown no relation to mortality or hospitalizations after treatment with etanercept (70). Other clinical trials have reported a higher percentage of mortality in CHF patients who received infliximab at 10 mg/kg (higher dose than that used in Pso and RA) than the controls (71, 72). These preliminary discovers have provided the evidence for the contraindication against the use of TNFi in CHF patients. Nowadays, anti-TNF-α drugs are not contraindicated in patients with heart diseases other than CHF (34). Random control trials (RCTs) including severe psoriatic patients who received at least one of TNFi, resulted in a number of MACEs (35, 73–76). Overall, the pooled analysis confirmed that no statistically significant difference exists between patients treated with biologics or placebo (35) (**Table 1**). Considering TNFi separately, there was also no statistically significant difference in patients receiving etanercept, infliximab, or adalimumab (35). In addition, the incidence rates (IRs) of MACEs were reduced by the use of anti-TNF-α agents respect to conventional therapies (28, 29, 77, 78). The use of TNFi for patients with Pso or psoriatic arthritis was associated with a 55% reduction in the incidence of MI compared

TABLE 1 | Main randomized controlled trials and meta-analysis studies on the rates of major adverse cardiovascular events (MACEs) in psoriatic patients treated with biological agents.

Biological agents	Reference	No. of patients or trials	MACE risk (IR or OR)	Follow-up period
TNFi	Rungapiromnan et al. (35)	18 RCTs comparing TNFi (4 adalimumab, 9 etanercept, 5 infliximab) vs placebo	OR, 0.67 (95% CI, 0.10–4.63, $P = 0.69$)	8–50 weeks
Ustekinumab (anti-IL12/23p40)	Reich et al. (82, 83)	1582 ustekinumab vs 732 placebo-treated patients	IR, 0.3%; (95% CI, 0.1–0.70) vs 0.0% (95% CI, 0.0–0.5%)	20 weeks
	Tzellos et al. (84)	9 RCTs (ustekinumab vs placebo)	OR, 3.96 (95% CI, 0.51–30.41; $P = 0.19$)	30 weeks
	Rungapiromnan et al. (35)	7 RCTs (ustekinumab vs placebo)	OR, 4.48 (95% CI, 0.24–84.77; $P = 0.32$)	30 weeks
Briakinumab (anti-IL12/23p40)	Langley et al. (85)	1258 briakinumab vs 624 placebo-treated patients	IR, 1.33% (95% CI, 0.43–3.10) vs 0.60% (95% CI, 0.35–0.94)	12 weeks
	Tzellos et al. (86)	9 RCTs (briakinumab vs placebo)	OR, 4.47 (95% CI, 0.69–28.89; $P = 0.12$)	30 weeks
Ustekinumab and Briakinumab	Tzellos et al. (86)	9 RCTs (ustekinumab and briakinumab vs placebo)	OR, 4.23, (95% CI, 1.07–16.75; $P = 0.04$)	30 weeks
Secukinumab (anti-IL17)	van de Kerkhof et al. (87) Egeberg et al. (88)	10 phase II/III clinical trials 196 patients	IR, 0.35% (95% CI, 0.10–0.90) IR, 3.1% (95% CI, 1.1–8.1)	52 weeks 104 weeks
Ixekizumab (anti-IL-17)	Strober et al. (89)	7 RCTs (UNCOVER-1, -2, and -3 plus an additional 4 phase I–III studies)	38 [0.6][a]	60 weeks
Brodalumab (anti-IL17R)	Papp et al. (90)	1 phase III clinical trial (AMAGINE-1)	5 (1.0)[b]	52 weeks

IR, incidence rate; OR, odds ratio; CI, confidence interval; RCTs, randomized controlled trials.
[a]MACE occurring in ≥1 patient, n [IR].
[b]n (exposure-adjusted event rate per 100 patient-years).

with those patients who were only treated with topical therapy (28). Similarly, psoriatic patients treated with TNFi displayed a significantly lower risk of MI when compared with MTX (79). Furthermore, treatment with TNFi is associated with an 11% reduced CV risk every 6 months of additional treatment (79). On the other hand, some authors suggested that these therapies do not seem to reduce the risk of MI, because they increase patients' weight and cholesterol levels after 3 or 6 months of therapy (66, 79, 80). These results could be related to a subsequently biological effect of TNFi due to neutralization of TNF-α cachetic properties (81). On the contrary, stable lipids levels were found in psoriatic patients treated with adalimumab, etanercept, or infliximab for 13 months (65). Psoriatic patients randomized to adalimumab or non-systemic treatment (topical therapies or phototherapy) showed no changes in total cholesterol, high-density lipoprotein, low-density lipoprotein, or triglycerides after 15 weeks of treatment (64). Despite some scientific reports overshadows TNFi role on CV risk, current studies support TNFi benefic effects on cardio metabolic parameters. To conclude, although literature remains heterogeneous, in part due to methodological differences, anti-TNF-α agents exert a protective effect on CV risk.

Anti-IL-12/23 Agents

The basis for developing anti-IL-12/23 biological drugs was encouraged by evidences that mice deficient in the subunit p40, shared by both IL-12 and IL-23, are resistant to experimentally induced autoimmune conditions, such as psoriasis (91, 92). Levels of IL-12/23p40 mRNA are more elevated in psoriatic than in healthy skin (93, 94). Cytokines induced by IL-12 (such as IFN-γ) and by IL-23 (such as IL-17A, IL-17F, and IL-22) are increased in psoriatic plaques (94). Moreover, in the last two decades, these inflammatory mediators have also been shown to contribute in CVD development. Indeed, it has been shown that serum levels of IL-12 and IL-23 are augmented in patients with CVD (95, 96). IL-12 and IL-23 are presented in atherosclerotic plaque and thereby affecting the pro-inflammatory status in these patients (96–98). Taken together, these evidences suggest that targeting IL-12/23 could represent a valid therapeutic option for psoriatic disease, with benefits on cutaneous involvement and on CV comorbidities. The efficacy of anti-IL-12/23p40 biological drugs (ustekinumab and briakinumab) for psoriasis treatment (**Table 2**) has been evaluated in two phase III RCTs and in four phase III RCTs, respectively (82, 85, 99–103). The hypothesis that these agents could possibly increase CV risk while improving cutaneous disease is unexpected. Nevertheless, safety concerns have been raised regarding the possibility of an increased risk of MACEs with the utilize of anti-IL-12/23 biological agents. We will discuss on lights and shadows of this hot question. In 2011, Reich et al. (83) evaluated this point due to the fact that in the ustekinumab clinical studies target population reported a higher rate of MACEs than placebo one. In the 1,582 ustekinumab-treated patients enrolled in the phase II and III placebo-controlled psoriasis studies, five MACE events occurred [0.3%; 95% confidence interval (CI), 0.1–0.7%] respect to no events in 732 placebo-treated patients (0.0%; 95% CI, 0.0–0.5%) (83). In particular, an important numerical imbalance in MACE rate was observed in the phase II trial with a 4:1 randomization ratio (risk difference 1.2%; 95% CI, 3.9–3.7%). However, the two phase III trials did not replicate a same high risk difference (0.2%; 95% CI, 1.2–1.2 and 0.1%; 95% CI, 0.7–0.7% for PHOENIX 1 and 2, respectively) (83) (**Table 1**). During the 12/20-week follow-up periods, MACE events did not show tendency to cluster. Indeed, the five MACEs occurred at weeks 2, 6, 10, 14, and 17 (83). The standardized IR

TABLE 2 | FDA approval biological drugs for psoriasis.

Biological drug	Biological structure	Mechanism of action	FDA approval for psoriasis (year)
Etanercept	Soluble TNFR2 coupled to Fc portion of IgG1	Anti-TNF-α	2004
Infliximab	Human/mouse chimeric IgG1 mAb	Anti-TNF-α	2006
Adalimumab	Human IgG1 mAb	Anti-TNF-α	2008
Ustekinumab	Human IgG1 mAb	Anti-p40 IL-12/23	2009
Secukinumab	Human IgG1κ mAb	Anti-IL17A	2015
Adalimumab-atto (biosimilar)	Human IgG1 mAb	Anti-TNF-α	2016
Etanercept-szzs (biosimilar)	Soluble TNFR2 coupled to Fc portion of IgG1	Anti-TNF-α	2016
Infliximab-dyyb (biosimilar)	Human/mouse chimeric IgG1 mAb	Anti-TNF-α	2016
Ixekizumab	Humanized IgG4 mAb	Anti-IL17A	2016
Adalimumab-adbm (biosimilar)	Human IgG1 mAb	Anti-TNF-α	2017
Infliximab-abda (biosimilar)	Human/mouse chimeric IgG1 mAb	Anti-TNF-α	2017
Brodalumab	Human IgG2 mAb	Anti-IL17RA	2017
Guselkumab	Human IgG1λ mAb	Anti-p19 IL-23	2017

IgG, immunoglobulin G; IL, interleukin; mAbs, monoclonal antibodies; IL-17RA, interleukin receptor A; p40, subunit 40; p19, subunit 19; TNFR2, tumor necrosis factor receptor 2; TNF-α, tumor necrosis factor; FDA, Food and Drug Administration.

in these studies ranged between 0.34 and 0.52, a rate lower than that estimated for the general population in the USA or in psoriatic patients (83). Moreover, all patients who experienced MACEs had at least three established CV risk factors. Longer term analyses demonstrated that rates of CV events remained low with up to 3 years. However, the absence of a control group precludes definitive assessment of the effect of ustekinumab on MACE risk (83). Thus, data from short-term, controlled trials give only partial information regarding the possible impact of ustekinumab on CV risk: the results suggest neither harmful nor beneficial effects. However, a smaller risk increase cannot be totally ruled out. Concerning another anti-IL-12/23p40 monoclonal antibody, briakinumab, the question is even more burning. Results from one of the four clinical trials have reported more MACE events in briakinumab-treated patients compared with placebo ones over a 12-week period (101). In details, 18 MACEs had been recorded with 4 CV deaths compared with no events in placebo group. The frequency of MACE was spread in an apparently uniform manner over time. The standardized IRs were 1.33/100 patient-years (95% CI, 0.43–3.10) respect to 0.60 (95% CI, 0.35–0.94) in the placebo-controlled phase (**Table 1**). In patients with two or more CV risk factors, the IR was more elevated (2.15 events/100 patient-years). For all these reasons, the study protocol underwent an amendment (85). Interestingly, no MACEs were reported during other two published clinical trials (briakinumab vs placebo or etanercept) as well as in another trial in which briakinumab was compared with MTX with a 52-week follow-up (82, 102, 103). However, the application for authorization to market briakinumab has been withdrawn.[1] Overall, definitive conclusions did not could be performed. For this reason, two industry-independent meta-analyses of nine randomized, double-blind, placebo-controlled, monotherapy trials have been conducted to deeper examine the possible association of MACEs with anti-IL-12/23 agents (84, 104) (**Table 1**). The meta-analysis by Ryan et al. found no increased risk of MACEs in treated patients compared with placebo ones, using the Mantel–Haenszel fixed-statistical effects model (104). On the other hand, Tzellos et al. analysis showed that the odds ratio (OR) for briakinumab- and ustekinumab-treated patients was not statistically significant (OR 4.47, 95% CI, 0.69–28.89, $P = 0.12$; OR 3.96, 95% CI, 0.51–30.41, $P = 0.19$, respectively). When combined, the OR for MACEs between patients treated with biological agents and those receiving placebo was found to be statistically significant (OR = 4.23, 95% CI, 1.07–16.75, $P = 0.04$) (84). In this case, the statistical effects model used was the Peto One-Step OR method. The divergence in these results has been attributable to the use of two different methods to estimate the risk. The Mantel–Haenszel fixed-statistical model using zero-cell corrections provides estimates for all studies, including zero event ones. This make it less suitable for meta-analysis of rare events (105–108) resulting in low statistical power. MACE event rates were estimated to be 0.28, 0.35, and 0.31% for ustekinumab, briakinumab, and both, respectively (108). It has been established that in case of an event IR of 1% or less, the best statistical approach is Peto method (105). However, the Peto OR method excluding trials with zero events from the analysis can lead to an overestimation of true relative risk. Moreover, neither the analysis by Tzellos et al. nor that by Ryan et al. have been adjusted for dropouts; this likely resulted in an overestimation of true risk (106). A large 5-year post-marketing study on the use of ustekinumab for psoriasis did not support the hypothesis of an augmented risk of MACEs (109). Moreover, an imbalance in MACE event rate has not been reported in other therapeutic indications of ustekinumab, such as psoriatic arthritis and inflammatory bowel disease (110–112). In addition, to date, the FDA has not communicated any changes regarding the prescribing for ustekinumab related to CV risk. More recently, a new meta-analysis has been performed by Rungapiromnan et al. (35) to evaluate the impact of biological therapies on risk of MACEs (**Table 1**). In this meta-analysis, they have selected RCTs in which patients received only licensed dose regimens of biological therapies. For this reason, briakinumab has been excluded from the analysis. Peto ORs with 95% CIs has been applied for statistical analysis. Regarding ustekinumab, no statistically significant difference in risk of MACEs has been reported respect to placebo (OR 4.48, 95% CI, 0.24–84.77, $P = 0.32$); similarly, comparing ustekinumab 45 mg with 90 mg the OR was not statistically significant (OR 1.00, 95% CI, 0.06–16.03, $P = 1.00$) (35). The most important limitation is that these findings were mainly based on small sample sizes and short-term follow-up (ranging from 12 to

[1] Available from: http://www.ema.europa.eu/docs/en_GB/document_library/Press_release/2011/01/WC500100769.pdf (Accessed: Febraury 8, 2018).

30 weeks). This is an important aspect to considering since it has been demonstrated that during the initial stage of therapy with ustekinumab inflammatory pro-atherogenic mediators such as IL-12/23 p40 temporarily increased and then dramatically decreased at week 32 (113, 114). Thus, other post-marketing studies and novel larger randomized controlled trials will be needed to continue the surveillance to assess the potential association connecting the use of anti-IL-12/23p40 biological drugs and increased CV risk.

Anti-IL17 Agents

In the past decade, the research has been focused on Th17 cells, which during differentiation secrete IL-17. IL-17 cytokine family consists of six members (IL-17A, B, C, D, E, and F). IL-17A (referred to here as IL-17) is among them, the major isoform (115). IL-17 is produced by Th17 cells and also by other cell subtypes, including γδ T, natural killer, etc. (116). However, interest in the Th17 population in relationship to Pso increased when numbers of circulating Th17 cells and IL-17 expression levels were found upregulated in the Pso lesional skin compared with non-lesional skin (49, 117). Recently, several anti-IL-17 agents have been developed. These primarily include anti-IL-17A monoclonal antibodies, secukinumab and ixekizumab, and brodalumab, an anti-IL-17 receptor monoclonal antibody. These biological agents that target the IL-17 signaling pathway have currently been evaluated and approved for the treatment of moderate-to-severe plaque Pso. The results reported by studies on efficacy and safety of IL-17 inhibitors are very promising. They showed the superiority of these new biological agents respect to both placebo and other biologics, such as ustekinumab and etanercept. For the first time, these trials include as end point the percentage of patient that achieving 90 or 100% of clinical improvement (PASI-90 or PASI-100, respectively) (47). In addition, although IL-17 antagonists had a higher rate of any adverse events than placebo, there was no significant difference in severe adverse events. This suggests that IL-17 antagonists are well tolerated (118). Even if the effects of IL-17 therapy on CVD in psoriatic patients is yet to be fully elucidated. Indeed, the interest on MACE is a crucial and much debated point. Likewise, Th17 pathway has a crucial role in CVD (22). Indeed, IL-17 is also involved in angiogenesis process, and on the synthesis of MMPs and CRP. Thus, in theory, Th17 cells could also play a crucial role in atherosclerotic and in CVD. Reports in atherosclerosis showed a conflicting result on IL-17 and Th17 cells in disease onset and plaque stability. IL-17 may exhibit both pro- and anti-atherogenic effects, depending on the inflammatory context (115). IL-17 pro-atherogenic effects may result from the induction of pro-inflammatory cytokines or chemokines (IL-6, GM-CSF, CCL2, and CXCL1) by endothelial cells or macrophages. The IL-17 atheroprotective effects may be dued by IFN-γ decreased and to its inhibitory effect on the expression of vascular cell adhesion molecule, this molecule is important to mediating the accumulation of monocytes and T cells within the lesions. Indeed, it was showed that IL-17, IL-21, and IL-23 were found in atherosclerotic plaques and associated with increased inflammation and plaque vulnerability (119). By contrast, Taleb et al. have reported a role for IL-17 in promoting plaque stability. Indeed, IL-17 expression in human carotid lesions was related to a fibrous phenotype with a lower macrophage and higher smooth muscle cell content (120). Despite some data suggesting increased levels of Th17 cells and IL-17 in patients with acute coronary syndromes (121, 122), the bulk of evidence indicate that circulating IL-17 levels are similar in patients with or without coronary artery disease (123). Indeed, some authors have reported that the patients with IL-17 low levels were more susceptible to the risk of death and recurrent MI (124). On the other hand, several experimental evidences and biomarker studies, which indicate a link between IL17 and instability in atherosclerotic plaques, supporting the hypothesis that in part explain the high risk of MI in Pso patients (22). Indeed, Pso patients have significantly elevated IL-17 serum levels (49) and they have a high risk to developing CV comorbidities. The conception that Th17 cytokines may provide a link between Pso and CVD comes from literature data that reporting a pathogenic role of IL-17 in Pso and examining the Th17 axis contribution into atherosclerosis (125).

As regarding secukinumab, data reported that there is a favorable safety profile in patients with moderate-to-severe plaque Pso over a total follow-up period of 52 weeks in a pooled safety analysis of 10 studies. However, at baseline, more subjects in the secukinumab groups had CV risk than comparator groups. Even if overall exposure-adjusted IRs of adjudicated MACE in secukinumab-treated subjects was comparable to etanercept-treated subjects (87). During the first 12 weeks of secukinumab studies, MACEs were reported in three patients receiving secukinumab 300 mg (0.26%), in no patients receiving etanercept, and in one patient treated with placebo. Over 52 weeks, exposure-adjusted IRs of MACEs were comparable in patients receiving secukinumab 300 mg (0.42/100 subject-years), secukinumab 150 mg (0.35/100 subject-years), and etanercept (0.34/100 subject-years), despite the presence of higher baseline CV risk factors in the two secukinumab groups (**Table 1**). All patients with a MACE had CVD risks, such as hypertension, dyslipidemia, etc. (87). In summary, from this comprehensive analysis of pooled safety data from 10 studies reported that the incidences of MACE in secukinumab-treated patients was low. A very recent real-life observational study of 195 patients (**Table 1**) treated with secukinumab for up to 2 years reported that 2% of patients suffered a CV event yielding a conspicuously elevated IR compared with findings from the secukinumab phase III clinical trial program, although the absolute numbers were very low (n = 4) (88).

The other antibody that inhibits IL-17 is ixekizumab; recently, safety data from a 12-week induction period, a 12- to 60-week maintenance period, and from all ixekizumab-treated patients were presented. The analysis of these data essentially reported similar rates of MACE between ixekizumab and etanercept and low rates of MACE with continued exposure for ixekizumab until week 60 (**Table 1**) (89). In particular, during the induction period, the between-group rates of adjudicated MACE were similar. The MACE individual components did not change substantially with longer exposure to ixekizumab. 7 of 4,035 ixekizumab-treated patients experienced vascular death. At baseline, patients subsequently developing MACE had a higher prevalence of risk factors for acute atherothrombotic events than patients without MACE. In conclusion, ixekizumab use was not associated with an increased risk of MACE. The safety profile reported in this analysis study is consistent with previous reports for ixekizumab (76, 126).

As regarding Brodalumab that selectively targets human IL-17RA and antagonizes the IL-17 pathway, it was considered safety from analysis of a prospective study, indeed incidences of serious adverse events in the induction phase were low among groups. There were no reports of MACEs during the induction phase, and only five reports (exposure-adjusted event rate of 1.0/100 patient-years) through week 52 (**Table 1**) (90). Conversely, in another phase III study, brodalumab treatment was compared with ustekinumab treatment in psoriasis, and the adverse effects were more recurrent in the brodalumab group than in the ustekinumab one. Indeed, in the AMAGINE-2 study, one death by stroke happened during the induction phase, and five deaths occurred through week 52; whereas in the AMAGINE-3 study, two deaths occurred: one from cardiac arrest and one from accidental death (127). However, the sizes of study populations, which were adequate for efficacy and common adverse event assessments, may have been inadequate to assess rare adverse events, which would require longer follow-up of large numbers of patients to better understand the safety profile of brodalumab.

Taken together, results from short-term safety and efficacy trials exploring anti-IL-17 therapy in psoriatic patients suggest no increased CVD risk compared with placebo or other classes of biologics used in Pso. Indeed, we may infer that IL-17 antagonists could possibly play an outstanding role in reducing CV morbidity. Even if there are several limitations in these clinical trials, e.g., patients highly selected, short duration of treatment with placebo or TNFi in relative few number of patients compared with the number of patients receiving IL-17 inhibitors. The advent of IL-17 biologics has improved significantly Pso disease (**Table 2**), but time will tell whether this IL-17 inhibition will also improve CVD outcomes in Pso.

CONCLUSION

Since systemic inflammation is currently considered the main cause of CVD risk in Pso, it has been thought that biological therapies might be helpful in treating not only cutaneous manifestations but have also positive or negative CV effects depending on the specific cytokine target and molecular mode of action. However, despite the recognized efficacy of biological agents in psoriasis treatment, little is known about their impact on risk of MACE in these patients. Data from meta-analyses have suggested that biological therapies including TNFi, anti-IL-12/23p40, and IL-17A agents did not have a significant impact on the risk of MACE in psoriatic patients over the short term. In particular, the use of TNFi is currently associated with a minor CVD risk in these patients, whereas the role of anti-IL-12/23p40 agents remains conflicting. Nevertheless ustekinumab, the only IL-12/23p40 inhibitor currently approved for Pso, results neutral on CV parameters. Regarding newer IL-17 inhibitors, early data have suggested no increased CVD risk respect to placebo or other classes of biologics used in psoriasis. However, because of follow-up short duration, many of these results should be interpreted with caution. Moreover, more studies, involving recruitment of a larger numbers of patients as well as a longer duration of treatment exposure, are needed to better evaluate the impact of biological therapies on the risk of MACEs in patients with Pso and to develop effective strategies for CVD prevention in these patients.

AUTHOR CONTRIBUTIONS

AB designed the manuscript structure, reviewed the scientific literature, and supervised the final version of the manuscript. GC designed the review structure and contributed to the writing of the manuscript. ES contributed to the writing of the manuscript and created graphical illustration. RC and AR reviewed the scientific literature and contributed to the writing of the manuscript. GF and NB reviewed the scientific literature and approved the final version of the manuscript.

REFERENCES

1. McDonald CJ, Calabresi P. Occlusive vascular disease in psoriatic patients. *N Engl J Med* (1973) 288:912. doi:10.1056/NEJM197304262881715
2. Samarasekera EJ, Neilson JM, Warren RB, Parnham J, Smith CH. Incidence of cardiovascular disease in individuals with psoriasis: a systematic review and meta-analysis. *J Invest Dermatol* (2013) 133:2340–6. doi:10.1038/jid.2013.149
3. Gelfand JM, Neimann AL, Shin DB, Wang X, Margolis DJ, Troxel AB. Risk of myocardial infarction in patients with psoriasis. *JAMA* (2006) 296:1735–41. doi:10.1001/jama.296.14.1735
4. Ludwig RJ, Herzog C, Rostock A, Ochsendorf FR, Zollner TM, Thaci D, et al. Psoriasis: a possible risk factor for development of coronary artery calcification. *Br J Dermatol* (2007) 156:271–6. doi:10.1111/j.1365-2133.2006.07562.x
5. Naldi L, Chatenoud L, Linder D, Belloni Fortina A, Peserico A, Virgili AR, et al. Cigarette smoking, body mass index, and stressful life events as risk factors for psoriasis: results from an Italian case-control study. *J Invest Dermatol* (2005) 125:61–7. doi:10.1111/j.0022-202X.2005.23681.x
6. Sommer DM, Jenisch S, Suchan M, Christophers E, Weichenthal M. Increased prevalence of the metabolic syndrome in patients with moderate to severe psoriasis. *Arch Dermatol Res* (2006) 298:321–8. doi:10.1007/s00403-006-0703-z
7. Padhi T, Garima. Metabolic syndrome and skin: psoriasis and beyond. *Indian J Dermatol* (2013) 58:299–305. doi:10.4103/0019-5154.113950
8. Wakkee M, Herings RM, Nijsten T. Psoriasis may not be an independent risk factor for acute ischemic heart disease hospitalizations: results of a large population-based Dutch cohort. *J Invest Dermatol* (2010) 130:962–7. doi:10.1038/jid.2009.321
9. Stern RS. Psoriasis is not a useful independent risk factor for cardiovascular disease. *J Invest Dermatol* (2010) 130:917–9. doi:10.1038/jid.2009.446
10. Parisi R, Rutter MK, Lunt M, Young HS, Symmons DPM, Griffiths CEM, et al. Psoriasis and the risk of major cardiovascular events: cohort study using the clinical practice research datalink. *J Invest Dermatol* (2015) 135:2189–97. doi:10.1038/jid.2015.87
11. Eder L, Gladman DD. Atherosclerosis in psoriatic disease: latest evidence and clinical implications. *Ther Adv Musculoskelet Dis* (2015) 7:187–95. doi:10.1177/1759720X15591801
12. Chiricozzi A, Raimondo A, Lembo S, Fausti F, Dini V, Costanzo A, et al. Crosstalk between skin inflammation and adipose tissue-derived products: pathogenic evidence linking psoriasis to increased adiposity. *Expert Rev Clin Immunol* (2016) 12:1299–308. doi:10.1080/1744666X.2016.1201423
13. Raimondo A, Lembo S, Di Caprio R, Donnarumma G, Monfrecola G, Balato N, et al. Psoriatic cutaneous inflammation promotes human monocyte differentiation into active osteoclasts, facilitating bone damage. *Eur J Immunol* (2017) 47:1062–74. doi:10.1002/eji.201646774

14. Boehncke WH. Systemic inflammation and cardiovascular comorbidity in psoriasis patients: causes and consequences. *Front Immunol* (2018) 9:579. doi:10.3389/fimmu.2018.00579
15. Boehncke WH, Boehncke S, Tobin AM, Kirby B. The 'psoriatic march': a concept of how severe psoriasis may drive cardiovascular comorbidity. *Exp Dermatol* (2011) 20:303–7. doi:10.1111/j.1600-0625.2011.01261.x
16. Gisondi P, Fantin F, Del Giglio M, Valbusa F, Marino F, Zamboni M, et al. Chronic plaque psoriasis is associated with increased arterial stiffness. *Dermatology* (2009) 218:110–3. doi:10.1159/000182256
17. Fang N, Jiang M, Fan Y. Association between psoriasis and subclinical atherosclerosis: a meta-analysis. *Medicine (Baltimore)* (2016) 95:e3576. doi:10.1097/MD.0000000000003576
18. Flammer AJ, Ruschitzka F. Psoriasis and atherosclerosis: two plaques, one syndrome? *Eur Heart J* (2012) 33:1989–91. doi:10.1093/eurheartj/ehr425
19. Davidovici BB, Sattar N, Prinz J, Puig L, Emery P, Barker JN, et al. Psoriasis and systemic inflammatory diseases: potential mechanistic links between skin disease and co-morbid conditions. *J Invest Dermatol* (2010) 130: 1785–96. doi:10.1038/jid.2010.103
20. Ryan C, Kirby B. Psoriasis is a systemic disease with multiple cardiovascular and metabolic comorbidities. *Dermatol Clin* (2015) 33:41–55. doi:10.1016/j.det.2014.09.004
21. Ghazizadeh R, Shimizu H, Tosa M, Ghazizadeh M. Pathogenic mechanisms shared between psoriasis and cardiovascular disease. *Int J Med Sci* (2010) 7:284–9. doi:10.7150/ijms.7.284
22. Chen S, Crother TR, Arditi M. Emerging role of IL-17 in atherosclerosis. *J Innate Immun* (2010) 2:325–33. doi:10.1159/000314626
23. Mehta NN, Li K, Szapary P, Krueger J, Brodmerkel C. Modulation of cardiometabolic pathways in skin and serum from patients with psoriasis. *J Transl Med* (2013) 11:194. doi:10.1186/1479-5876-11-194
24. Kolliker Frers RA, Cosentino V, Tau J, Kerzberg EM, Urdapilleta A, Chiocconi M, et al. Immune-mediated inflammation promotes subclinical atherosclerosis in recent-onset psoriatic arthritis patients without conventional cardiovascular risk factors. *Front Immunol* (2018) 9:139. doi:10.3389/fimmu.2018.00139
25. Libby P, Ridker PM, Hansson GK; Leducq Transatlantic Network on Atherothrombosis. Inflammation in atherosclerosis: from pathophysiology to practice. *J Am Coll Cardiol* (2009) 54:2129–38. doi:10.1016/j.jacc.2009.09.009
26. Prodanovich S, Ma F, Taylor JR, Pezon C, Fasihi T, Kirsner RS. Methotrexate reduces incidence of vascular diseases in veterans with psoriasis or rheumatoid arthritis. *J Am Acad Dermatol* (2005) 52:262–7. doi:10.1016/j.jaad.2004.06.017
27. Micha R, Imamura F, Wyler von Ballmoos M, Solomon DH, Hernán MA, Ridker PM, et al. Systematic review and meta-analysis of methotrexate use and risk of cardiovascular disease. *Am J Cardiol* (2011) 108:1362–70. doi:10.1016/j.amjcard.2011.06.054
28. Wu JJ, Poon KY, Channual JC, Shen AY. Association between tumor necrosis factor inhibitor therapy and myocardial infarction risk in patients with psoriasis. *Arch Dermatol* (2012) 148:1244–50. doi:10.1001/archdermatol.2012.2502
29. Ahlehoff O, Skov L, Gislason G, Lindhardsen J, Kristensen SL, Iversen L, et al. Cardiovascular disease event rates in patients with severe psoriasis treated with systemic anti-inflammatory drugs: a Danish real-world cohort study. *J Intern Med* (2013) 273:197–204. doi:10.1111/j.1365-2796.2012.02593.x
30. Hu SC, Lan CE. Psoriasis and cardiovascular comorbidities: focusing on severe vascular events, cardiovascular risk factors and implications for treatment. *Int J Mol Sci* (2017) 18:E2211. doi:10.3390/ijms18102211
31. Mottaghi A, Ebrahimof S, Angoorani P, Saboor-Yaraghi AA. Vitamin A supplementation reduces IL-17 and RORc gene expression in atherosclerotic patients. *Scand J Immunol* (2014) 80:151–7. doi:10.1111/sji.12190
32. Mahmoudi MJ, Saboor-Yaraghi AA, Zabetian-Targhi F, Siassi F, Zarnani AH, Eshraghian MR, et al. Vitamin A decreases cytotoxicity of oxidized low-density lipoprotein in patients with atherosclerosis. *Immunol Invest* (2016) 45:52–62. doi:10.3109/08820139.2015.1095208
33. Boehncke S, Fichtlscherer S, Salgo R, Garbaraviciene J, Beschmann H, Diehl S, et al. Systemic therapy of plaque-type psoriasis ameliorates endothelial cell function: results of a prospective longitudinal pilot trial. *Arch Dermatol Res* (2011) 303:381–8. doi:10.1007/s00403-010-1108-6
34. Puig L. Cardiovascular risk and psoriasis: the role of biologic therapy. *Actas Dermosifiliogr* (2012) 103:853–62. doi:10.1016/j.ad.2012.02.003
35. Rungapiromnan W, Yiu ZZN, Warren RB, Griffiths CEM, Ashcroft DM. Impact of biologic therapies on risk of major adverse cardiovascular events in patients with psoriasis: systematic review and meta-analysis of randomized controlled trials. *Br J Dermatol* (2017) 176:890–901. doi:10.1111/bjd.14964
36. Raimondo A, Balato A, Megna M, Balato N. Limitations of current monoclonal antibodies for plaque-type psoriasis and an outlook for the future. *Expert Opin Biol Ther* (2018) 18(6):605–7. doi:10.1080/14712598.2018.1479738
37. Balato A, Mattii M, Caiazzo G, Raimondo A, Patruno C, Balato N, et al. IL-36γ is involved in psoriasis and allergic contact dermatitis. *J Invest Dermatol* (2016) 136:1520–3. doi:10.1016/j.jid.2016.03.020
38. Schiattarella M, Caiazzo G, Di Caprio R, Lembo S, Raimondo A, Ayala F, et al. Paraoxonases and psoriasis: negative imbalance of anti-oxidant endogenous mechanisms. *G Ital Dermatol Venereol* (2017). doi:10.23736/S0392-0488.17.05537-7
39. Furue M, Tsuji G, Chiba T, Kadono T. Cardiovascular and metabolic diseases comorbid with psoriasis: beyond the skin. *Intern Med* (2017) 56:1613–9. doi:10.2169/internalmedicine.56.8209
40. Karczewski J, Dobrowolska A, Rychlewska-Hańczewska A, Adamski Z. New insights into the role of T cells in pathogenesis of psoriasis and psoriatic arthritis. *Autoimmunity* (2016) 49:435–50. doi:10.3109/08916934.2016.1166214
41. Baliwag J, Barnes DH, Johnston A. Cytokines in psoriasis. *Cytokine* (2015) 73:342–50. doi:10.1016/j.cyto.2014.12.014
42. Testa M, Yeh M, Lee P, Fanelli R, Loperfido F, Berman JW, et al. Circulating levels of cytokines and their endogenous modulators in patients with mild to severe congestive heart failure due to coronary artery disease or hypertension. *J Am Coll Cardiol* (1996) 28:964–71. doi:10.1016/S0735-1097(96)00268-9
43. Karbach S, Croxford AL, Oelze M, Schüler R, Minwegen D, Wegner J, et al. Interleukin 17 drives vascular inflammation, endothelial dysfunction, and arterial hypertension in psoriasis-like skin disease. *Arterioscler Thromb Vasc Biol* (2014) 34:2658–68. doi:10.1161/ATVBAHA.114.304108
44. Bozkurt B, Kribbs SB, Clubb FJ Jr, Michael LH, Didenko VV, Hornsby PJ, et al. Pathophysiologically relevant concentrations of tumor necrosis factor-α promote progressive left ventricular dysfunction and remodeling in rats. *Circulation* (1997) 97:1382–91. doi:10.1161/01.CIR.97.14.1382
45. Kubota T, McTiernan CF, Frye CS, Slawson SE, Lemster BH, Koretsky AP, et al. Dilated cardiomyopathy in transgenic mice with cardiac-specific overexpression of tumor necrosis factor-α. *Circ Res* (1997) 81:627–35. doi:10.1161/01.RES.81.4.627
46. Cesari M, Penninx BW, Newman AB, Kritchevsky SB, Nicklas BJ, Sutton-Tyrrell K, et al. Inflammatory markers and cardiovascular disease: the health, aging and body composition [health ABC] study. *Am J Cardiol* (2003) 92: 522–8. doi:10.1016/S0002-9149(03)00718-5
47. Balato A, Scala E, Balato N, Caiazzo G, Di Caprio R, Monfrecola G, et al. Biologics that inhibit the Th17 pathway and related cytokines to treat inflammatory disorders. *Expert Opin Biol Ther* (2017) 17:1363–74. doi:10.1080/14712598.2017.1363884
48. *FDA Approves Biosimilar Products*. Silver Spring, MD: US Food and Drug Administration (2018). Available from: https://www.fda.gov/Drugs/ Development Approval Process/ How Drugsare Developed and Approved/ Approval Applications/ Therapeutic Biologic Applications/ Biosimilars/ ucm580432.htm (Accessed: May 29, 2018).
49. Balato A, Schiattarella M, Di Caprio R, Lembo S, Mattii M, Balato N, et al. Effects of adalimumab therapy in adult subjects with moderate-to-severe psoriasis on Th17 pathway. *J Eur Acad Dermatol Venereol* (2014) 28:1016–24. doi:10.1111/jdv.12240
50. Caldarola G, De Simone C, Carbone A, Tulli A, Amerio P, Feliciani C. TNF and its receptors in psoriatic skin, before and after treatment with etanercept. *Int J Immunopathol Pharmacol* (2009) 22:961–6. doi:10.1177/039463200902200411
51. Cordiali-Fei P, Trento E, D'Agosto G, Bordignon V, Mussi A, Ardigò M, et al. Decreased levels of metalloproteinase-9 and angiogenic factors in skin lesions of patients with psoriatic arthritis after therapy with anti-TNF-α. *J Autoimmune Dis* (2006) 5:3–5. doi:10.1186/1740-2557-3-5

52. Strober B, Foley P, Philipp S, Zhang N, Kaur P. Evaluation of efficacy and safety of ABP 501 in a phase 3 study in subjects with moderate to severe plaque psoriasis: 52-week results. *J Am Acad Dermatol* (2016) 74(5, Suppl 1): AB249. doi:10.1016/j.jaad.2016.02.972
53. *Momenta Pharmaceuticals Announces Positive Top-Line Phase 3 Results for M923, a Proposed Humira (Adalimumab) Biosimilar [News Release].* Cambridge, MA: Momenta Pharmaceuticals, Inc (2016). Available from: http://ir.momentapharma.com/releasedetail.cfm?ReleaseID=1001255 (Accessed: January 25, 2017).
54. Kellen R, Goldenberg G. Biosimilars in psoriasis: the future or not? *Cutis* (2017) 99(2):116–20.
55. Campanati A, Orciani M, Ganzetti G, Consales V, Di Primio R, Offidani A. The effect of etanercept on vascular endothelial growth factor production by cutaneous mesenchymal stem cells from patients with psoriasis. *J Int Med Res* (2016) 44:6–9. doi:10.1177/0300060515593229
56. Henning M, Göcker Tekin H, Skov L, Egeberg A. Effects of biologic therapy on cardiovascular disease in psoriasis. *Curr Derm Rep* (2018) 7:37–42. doi:10.1007/s13671-018-0210-4
57. Gkalpakiotis S, Arenbergerova M, Gkalpakioti P, Potockova J, Arenberger P, Kraml P. Impact of adalimumab treatment on cardiovascular risk biomarkers in psoriasis: results of a pilot study. *J Dermatol* (2017) 44:363–9. doi:10.1111/1346-8138.13661
58. Goldminz AM, Suárez-Fariñas M, Wang AC, Dumont N, Krueger JG, Gottlieb AB. CCL20 and IL22 messenger RNA expression after adalimumab vs methotrexate treatment of psoriasis: a randomized clinical trial. *JAMA Dermatol* (2015) 151:837–46. doi:10.1001/jamadermatol.2015.0452
59. Boehncke S, Salgo R, Garbaraviciene J, Beschmann H, Hardt K, Diehl S, et al. Effective continuous systemic therapy of severe plaque-type psoriasis is accompanied by amelioration of biomarkers of cardiovascular risk: results of a prospective longitudinal observational study. *J Eur Acad Dermatol Venereol* (2011) 25:1187–93. doi:10.1111/j.1468-3083.2010.03947.x
60. Marra M, Campanati A, Testa R, Sirolla C, Bonfigli AR, Franceschi C, et al. Effect of etanercept on insulin sensitivity in nine patients with psoriasis. *Int J Immunopathol Pharmacol* (2007) 20:731–6. doi:10.1177/039463200702000408
61. Pina T, Armesto S, Lopez-Mejias R, Genre F, Ubilla B, Gonzalez-Lopez MA, et al. Anti-TNF-α therapy improves insulin sensitivity in non-diabetic patients with psoriasis: a 6-month prospective study. *J Eur Acad Dermatol Venereol* (2015) 29:1325–30. doi:10.1111/jdv.12814
62. Pina T, Genre F, Lopez-Mejias R, Armesto S, Ubilla B, Mijares V, et al. Anti-TNF-a therapy reduces retinol-binding protein 4 serum levels in non-diabetic patients with psoriasis: a 6-month prospective study. *J Eur Acad Dermatol Venereol* (2015) 30:92–5. doi:10.1111/jdv.13005
63. Jókai H, Szakonyi J, Kontár O, Marschalkó M, Szalai K, Kárpáti S, et al. Impact of effective tumor necrosis factor-alfa inhibitor treatment on arterial intima-media thickness in psoriasis: results of a pilot study. *J Am Acad Dermatol* (2013) 69:523–9. doi:10.1016/j.jaad.2013.06.019
64. Bissonnette R, Tardif JC, Harel F, Pressacco J, Bolduc C, Guertin MC. Effects of the tumor necrosis factor-α antagonist adalimumab on arterial inflammation assessed by positron emission tomography in patients with psoriasis: results of a randomized controlled trial. *Circ Cardiovasc Imaging* (2013) 6:83–90. doi:10.1161/CIRCIMAGING.112.975730
65. Hjuler KF, Bøttcher M, Vestergaard C, Bøtker HE, Iversen L, Kragballe K. Association between changes in coronary artery disease progression and treatment with biologic agents for severe psoriasis. *JAMA Dermatol* (2016) 152:1114–21. doi:10.1001/jamadermatol.2016.1984
66. Ahlehoff O, Hansen PR, Gislason GH, Frydland M, Bryld LE, Elming H, et al. Myocardial function and effects of biologic therapy in patients with severe psoriasis: a prospective echocardiographic study. *J Eur Acad Dermatol Venereol* (2016) 30:819–23. doi:10.1111/jdv.13152
67. Herédi E, Végh J, Pogacsas L, Gaspar K, Varga J, Kincse G. Subclinical cardiovascular disease and it's improvement after longterm TNF-alpha inhibitor therapy in severe psoriatic patients. *J Eur Acad Dermatol Venereol* (2016) 30:1531–6. doi:10.1111/jdv.13649
68. Wu JJ, Poon KY. Association of ethnicity, tumor necrosis factor inhibitor therapy, and myocardial infarction risk in patients with psoriasis. *J Am Acad Dermatol* (2013) 69(1):167–8. doi:10.1016/j.jaad.2013.02.019
69. Deswal A, Bozkurt B, Seta Y, Parilti-Eiswirth S, Hayes FA, Blosch C, et al. Safety and efficacy of a soluble P75 tumor necrosis factor receptor (Enbrel, etanercept) in patients with advanced heart failure. *Circulation* (1999) 99:3224–6. doi:10.1161/01.CIR.99.25.3224
70. Mann DL, McMurray JJ, Packer M, Swedberg K, Borer JS, Colucci WS, et al. Targeted anticytokine therapy in patients with chronic heart failure: results of the Randomized Etanercept Worldwide Evaluation (RENEWAL). *Circulation* (2004) 109:1594–602. doi:10.1161/01.CIR.0000124490.27666.B2
71. Chung ES, Packer M, Lo KH, Fasanmade AA, Willerson JT; Anti-TNF Therapy Against Congestive Heart Failure Investigators. Randomized, double-blind, placebo-controlled, pilot trial of infliximab, a chimeric monoclonal antibody to tumor necrosis factor-alpha, in patients with moderate-to-severe heart failure: results of the anti-TNF therapy against congestive heart failure (ATTACH) trial. *Circulation* (2003) 107:3133–40.
72. Pham T, Bachelez H, Berthelot JM, Blacher J, Bouhnik Y, Claudepierre P, et al. TNF alpha antagonist therapy and safety monitoring. *Joint Bone Spine* (2011) 78(Suppl 1):15–185. doi:10.1016/S1297-319X(11)70001-X
73. AbbVie. *Safety and Efficacy Study of Adalimumab in the Treatment of Plaque Psoriasis.* (2017). Available from: https://clinicaltrials.gov/show/NCT01646073 (Accessed: January 17, 2017).
74. Gottlieb AB, Matheson RT, Lowe N, Krueger GG, Kang S, Goffe BS, et al. A randomized trial of etanercept as monotherapy for psoriasis. *Arch Dermatol* (2003) 139:1627–32. doi:10.1001/archderm.139.12.1627
75. Bachelez H, van de Kerkhof PC, Strohal R, Kubanov A, Valenzuela F, Lee JH, et al. Tofacitinib versus etanercept or placebo in moderate-to-severe chronic plaque psoriasis: a phase 3 randomised non-inferiority trial. *Lancet* (2015) 386:552–61. doi:10.1016/S0140-6736(14)62113-9
76. Griffiths CE, Reich K, Lebwohl M, van de Kerkhof P, Paul C, Menter A, et al. Comparison of ixekizumab with etanercept or placebo in moderate-to-severe psoriasis (UNCOVER-2 and UNCOVER-3): results from two phase 3 randomised trials. *Lancet* (2015) 386:541–51. doi:10.1016/S0140-6736(15)60125-8
77. Solomon DH, Massarotti E, Garg R, Liu J, Canning C, Schneeweiss S. Association between disease-modifying antirheumatic drugs and diabetes risk in patients with rheumatoid arthritis and psoriasis. *JAMA* (2011) 305:2525–31. doi:10.1001/jama.2011.878
78. Abuabara K, Lee H, Kimball AB. The effect of systemic psoriasis therapies on the incidence of myocardial infarction: a cohort study. *Br J Dermatol* (2011) 165:1066–73. doi:10.1111/j.1365-2133.2011.10525.x
79. Wu JJ, Guérin A, Sundaram M, Dea K, Cloutier M, Mulani P. Cardiovascular event risk assessment in psoriasis patients treated with tumor necrosis factor-α inhibitors versus methotrexate. *J Am Acad Dermatol* (2017) 76:81–90. doi:10.1016/j.jaad.2016.07.042
80. Gisondi P, Cotena C, Tessari G, Girolomoni G. Anti-tumour necrosis factor-alpha therapy increases body weight in patients with chronic plaque psoriasis: a retrospective cohort study. *J Eur Acad Dermatol Venereol* (2008) 22:341–4. doi:10.1111/j.1468-3083.2007.02429.x
81. Cawthorn WP, Sethi JK. TNF-α and adipocyte biology. *FEBS Lett* (2007) 582:117–31. doi:10.1016/j.febslet.2007.11.051
82. Reich K, Langley RG, Papp KA, Ortonne JP, Unnebrink K, Kaul M, et al. A 52-week trial comparing briakinumab with methotrexate in patients with psoriasis. *N Engl J Med* (2011) 365:1586–96. doi:10.1056/NEJMoa1010858
83. Reich K, Langley RG, Lebwohl M, Szapary P, Guzzo C, Yeilding N, et al. Cardiovascular safety of ustekinumab in patients with moderate to severe psoriasis: results of integrated analyses of data from phase II and III clinical studies. *Br J Dermatol* (2011) 164:862–72. doi:10.1111/j.1365-2133.2011.10257.x
84. Tzellos T, Kyrgidis A, Zouboulis CC. Re-evaluation of the risk for major adverse cardiovascular events in patients treated with anti-IL-12/23 biological agents for chronic plaque psoriasis: a meta-analysis of randomized controlled trials. *J Eur Acad Dermatol Venereol* (2013) 27:622–7. doi:10.1111/j.1468-3083.2012.04500.x
85. Langley R, Valdes J, Gordon K, Papp K. P3312. Long-term safety and efficacy of ABT-874 for the treatment of moderate to severe psoriasis: interim analysis from an open-label extension study. *J Am Acad Dermatol* (2011) 64:AB148.

86. Tzellos T, Kyrgidis A, Trigoni A, Zouboulis CC. Point: major adverse cardiovascular events and anti-IL 12/23 agents. *J Am Acad Dermatol* (2014) 70(2):380–1. doi:10.1016/j.jaad.2013.07.050
87. van de Kerkhof PC, Griffiths CE, Reich K, Leonardi CL, Blauvelt A, Tsai TF, et al. Secukinumab long-term safety experience: a pooled analysis of 10 phase II and III clinical studies in patients with moderate to severe plaque psoriasis. *J Am Acad Dermatol* (2016) 75:83–98.e4. doi:10.1016/j.jaad.2016.03.024
88. Egeberg A, Ottosen MB, Gniadecki R, Broesby-Olsen S, Dam TN, Bryld LE, et al. Safety, efficacy and drug survival of biologics and biosimilars for moderate-to-severe plaque psoriasis. *Br J Dermatol* (2018) 178:509–19. doi:10.1111/bjd.16102
89. Strober B, Leonardi C, Papp KA, Mrowietz U, Ohtsuki M, Bissonnette R, et al. Short- and long-term safety outcomes with ixekizumab from 7 clinical trials in psoriasis: etanercept comparisons and integrated data. *J Am Acad Dermatol* (2017) 76:432–40. doi:10.1016/j.jaad.2016.09.026
90. Papp KA, Reich K, Paul C, Blauvelt A, Baran W, Bolduc C, et al. A prospective phase III, randomized, double-blind, placebo-controlled study of brodalumab in patients with moderate-to-severe plaque psoriasis. *Br J Dermatol* (2016) 175:273–86. doi:10.1111/bjd.14493
91. Luger D, Silver PB, Tang J, Cua D, Chen Z, Iwakura Y, et al. Either a Th17 or a Th1 effector response can drive autoimmunity: conditions of disease induction affect dominant effector category. *J Exp Med* (2008) 205:799–810. doi:10.1084/jem.20071258
92. Mitra A, Fallen RS, Lima HC. Cytokine-based therapy in psoriasis. *Clin Rev Allergy Immunol* (2013) 44:173–82. doi:10.1007/s12016-012-8306-2
93. Lee E, Trepicchio WL, Oestreicher JL, Pittman D, Wang F, Chamian F, et al. Increased expression of interleukin 23 p19 and p40 in lesional skin of patients with psoriasis vulgaris. *J Exp Med* (2004) 199:125–30. doi:10.1084/jem.20030451
94. Chan JR, Blumenschein W, Murphy E, Diveu C, Wiekowski M, Abbondanzo S, et al. IL-23 stimulates epidermal hyperplasia via TNF and IL-20R2-dependent mechanisms with implications for psoriasis pathogenesis. *J Exp Med* (2006) 203:2577–87. doi:10.1084/jem.20060244
95. Correia LCL, Andrade BB, Borges VM, Clarêncio J, Bittencourt AP, Freitas R, et al. Prognostic value of cytokines and chemokines in addition to the GRACE score in non-ST-elevation acute coronary syndromes. *Clin Chim Acta* (2010) 411:540–5. doi:10.1016/j.cca.2010.01.011
96. Abbas A, Gregersen I, Holm S, Daissormont I, Bjerkeli V, Krohg-Sørensen K, et al. Interleukin 23 levels are increased in carotid atherosclerosis. *Stroke* (2015) 46:793–9. doi:10.1161/STROKEAHA.114.006516
97. Uyemura LL, Demer SC, Castle D, Jullien JA, Berliner MK, Gately RR, et al. Cross-regulatory roles of interleukin (IL)-12 and IL-10 in atherosclerosis. *J Clin Invest* (1996) 97:2130–8. doi:10.1172/JCI118650
98. Yong K, Dogra G, Boudville N, Chan D, Adams L, Ching H, et al. Interleukin-12 is associated with arterial stiffness in healthy individuals. *Am J Hypertens* (2013) 26:159–62. doi:10.1093/ajh/hps032
99. Papp KA, Langley RG, Lebwohl M, Krueger GG, Szapary P, Yeilding N, et al. Efficacy and safety of ustekinumab, a human interleukin-12/23 monoclonal antibody, in patients with psoriasis: 52-week results from a randomised, double-blind, placebo-controlled trial (PHOENIX 2). *Lancet* (2008) 371: 1675–84. doi:10.1016/S0140-6736(08)60726-6
100. Leonardi CL, Kimball AB, Papp KA, Yeilding N, Guzzo C, Wang Y, et al. Efficacy and safety of ustekinumab, a human interleukin-12/23 monoclonal antibody, in patients with psoriasis: 76-week results from a randomised, double-blind, placebo-controlled trial (PHOENIX 1). *Lancet* (2008) 371: 1665–74. doi:10.1016/S0140-6736(08)60725-4
101. Gordon KB, Langley RG, Gottlieb AB, Papp KA, Krueger GG, Strober BE, et al. A phase III, randomized, controlled trial of the fully human IL-12/23 mAb briakinumab in moderate-to-severe psoriasis. *J Invest Dermatol* (2012) 132:304–14. doi:10.1038/jid.2011.304
102. Gottlieb AB, Leonardi C, Kerdel F, Mehlis S, Olds M, Williams DA. Efficacy and safety of briakinumab vs. etanercept and placebo in patients with moderate to severe chronic plaque psoriasis. *Br J Dermatol* (2011) 165:652–60. doi:10.1111/j.1365-2133.2011.10418.x
103. Strober BE, Crowley JJ, Yamauchi PS, Olds M, Williams DA. Efficacy and safety results from a phase III, randomized controlled trial comparing the safety and efficacy of briakinumab with etanercept and placebo in patients with moderate to severe chronic plaque psoriasis. *Br J Dermatol* (2011) 165:661–8. doi:10.1111/j.1365-2133.2011.10419.x
104. Ryan C, Leonardi CL, Krueger JG, Kimball AB, Strober BE, Gordon KB, et al. Association between biologic therapies for chronic plaque psoriasis and cardiovascular events: a meta-analysis of randomized controlled trials. *JAMA* (2011) 306:864–71. doi:10.1001/jama.2011.1211
105. Bradburn MJ, Deeks JJ, Berlin JA, Russell Localio A. Much ado about nothing: a comparison of the performance of meta-analytical methods with rare events. *Stat Med* (2007) 26:53–77. doi:10.1002/sim.2528
106. Dommasch ED, Troxel AB, Gelfand JM. Major cardiovascular events associated with anti-IL 12/23 agents: a tale of two meta-analyses. *J Am Acad Dermatol* (2013) 68:863–5. doi:10.1016/j.jaad.2013.01.011
107. Deeks JJ. Issues in the selection of a summary statistic for meta-analysis of clinical trials with binary outcomes. *Stat Med* (2002) 21:1575–600. doi:10.1002/sim.1188
108. Tzellos T, Kyrgidis A, Toulis K. Biologic therapies for chronic plaque psoriasis and cardiovascular events. *JAMA* (2011) 306:2095. doi:10.1001/jama.2011.1660
109. Kimball AB, Papp KA, Wasfi Y, Chan D, Bissonnette R, Sofen H, et al. Long-term efficacy of ustekinumab in patients with moderate-to-severe psoriasis treated for up to 5 years in the PHOENIX 1 study. *J Eur Acad Dermatol Venereol* (2012) 27:1535–45. doi:10.1111/jdv.12046
110. Gottlieb A, Menter A, Mendelsohn A, Shen Y-K, Li S, Guzzo C, et al. Ustekinumab, a human interleukin 12/23 monoclonal antibody, for psoriatic arthritis: randomised, double-blind, placebo-controlled, crossover trial. *Lancet* (2009) 373:633–40. doi:10.1016/S0140-6736(09)60140-9
111. Sandborn WJ, Feagan BG, Fedorak RN, Scherl E, Fleisher MR, Katz S, et al. A randomized trial of ustekinumab, a human interleukin-12/23 monoclonal antibody, in patients with moderate-to-severe Crohn's disease. *Gastroenterology* (2008) 135:1130–41. doi:10.1053/j.gastro.2008.07.014
112. Sandborn WJ, Gasink C, Gao L-L, Blank MA, Johanns J, Guzzo C, et al. Ustekinumab induction and maintenance therapy in refractory Crohn's disease. *N Engl J Med* (2012) 367:1519–28. doi:10.1056/NEJMoa1203572
113. Callen JP. *Are Major Adverse Cardiovascular Events Associated With Anti–IL-12/23 Therapies?* (2017). Available from: http://www.jwatch.org/jd201109160000001/2011/09/16/are-major-adverse-cardiovascular-events (Accessed: January 17, 2017).
114. Reddy M, Torres G, McCormick T, Marano C, Cooper K, Yeilding N, et al. Positive treatment effects of ustekinumab in psoriasis: analysis of lesional and systemic parameters. *J Dermatol* (2010) 37:413–25. doi:10.1111/j.1346-8138.2010.00802.x
115. Taleb S, Tedgui A, Mallat Z. IL-17 and Th17 cells in atherosclerosis: subtle and contextual roles. *Arterioscler Thromb Vasc Biol* (2015) 35:258–64. doi:10.1161/ATVBAHA.114.303567
116. Takatori H, Kanno Y, Watford WT, Tato CM, Weiss G, Ivanov II, et al. Lymphoid tissue inducer-like cells are an innate source of IL-17 and IL-22. *J Exp Med* (2009) 206:35–41. doi:10.1084/jem.20072713
117. Kagami S, Rizzo HL, Lee JJ, Koguchi Y, Blauvelt A. Circulating Th17, Th22, and Th1 cells are increased in psoriasis. *J Invest Dermatol* (2010) 130:1373–83. doi:10.1038/jid.2009.399
118. Wu D, Hou SY, Zhao S, Hou LX, Jiao T, Xu NN, et al. Efficacy and safety of interleukin-17 antagonists in patients with plaque psoriasis: a meta-analysis from phase 3 randomized controlled trials. *J Eur Acad Dermatol Venereol* (2017) 31:992–1003. doi:10.1111/jdv.14125
119. Erbel C, Dengler TJ, Wangler S, Lasitschka F, Bea F, Wambsganss N, et al. Expression of IL-17A in human atherosclerotic lesions is associated with increased inflammation and plaque vulnerability. *Basic Res Cardiol* (2011) 106:125–34. doi:10.1007/s00395-010-0135-y
120. Taleb S, Romain M, Ramkhelawon B, Uyttenhove C, Pasterkamp G, Herbin O, et al. Loss of SOCS3 expression in T cells reveals a regulatory role for interleukin-17 in atherosclerosis. *J Exp Med* (2009) 206:2067–77. doi:10.1084/jem.20090545
121. Hashmi S, Zeng QT. Role of interleukin-17 and interleukin-17-induced cytokines interleukin 6 and interleukin-8 in unstable coronary artery disease. *Coron Artery Dis* (2006) 17:699–706. doi:10.1097/01.mca.0000236288.94553.b4
122. Cheng X, Yu X, Ding YJ, Fu QQ, Xie JJ, Tang TT, et al. The Th17/Treg imbalance in patients with acute coronary syndrome. *Clin Immunol* (2008) 127:89–97. doi:10.1016/j.clim.2008.01.009

123. Eid RE, Rao DA, Zhou J, Lo SF, Ranjbaran H, Gallo A, et al. Interleukin-17 and interferon-gamma are produced concomitantly by human coronary artery-infiltrating T cells and act synergistically on vascular smooth muscle cells. *Circulation* (2009) 119:1424–32. doi:10.1161/CIRCULATIONAHA.108.827618
124. Simon T, Taleb S, Danchin N, Laurans L, Rousseau B, Cattan S, et al. Circulating levels of interleukin-17 and cardiovascular outcomes in patients with acute myocardial infarction. *Eur Heart J* (2013) 34:570–7. doi:10.1093/eurheartj/ehs263
125. Golden JB, McCormick TS, Ward NL. IL-17 in psoriasis: implications for therapy and cardiovascular co-morbidities. *Cytokine* (2013) 62:195–201. doi:10.1016/j.cyto.2013.03.013
126. Gordon KB, Blauvelt A, Papp KA, Langley RG, Luger T, Ohtsuki M, et al. Phase 3 trials of ixekizumab in moderate-to-severe plaque psoriasis. *N Engl J Med* (2016) 375:345–56. doi:10.1056/NEJMoa1512711
127. Lebwohl M, Strober B, Menter A, Gordon K, Weglowska J, Puig L, et al. Phase 3 studies comparing brodalumab with ustekinumab in psoriasis. *N Engl J Med* (2015) 373:1318–28. doi:10.1056/NEJMoa1503824

10

The Interplay Between Keratinocytes and Immune Cells in the Pathogenesis of Psoriasis

*Cristina Albanesi[1], Stefania Madonna[1], Paolo Gisondi[2] and Giampiero Girolomoni[2]**

[1] *Laboratory of Experimental Immunology, Istituto Dermopatico dell'Immacolata (IDI), IRCCS, Rome, Italy,*
[2] *Section of Dermatology, Department of Medicine, University of Verona, Verona, Italy*

Correspondence:
Giampiero Girolomoni
giampiero.girolomoni@univr.it

Psoriasis is a chronic inflammatory skin disease resulting from genetic, epigenetic, environmental, and lifestyle factors. To date, several immunopathogenic mechanisms of psoriasis have been elucidated, and, in the current model, the cross talk between autoreactive T cells and resident keratinocytes generates inflammatory and immune circuits responsible for the initiation, progression, and persistence of the disease. Several autoantigens derived from keratinocytes (i.e., LL37 cathelecidin/nucleic acid complexes, newly generated lipid antigens) have been identified, which may trigger initial activation of T cells, particularly IL-17-producing T cells, T helper (Th)1 and Th22 cells. Hence, lymphokines released in skin lesions are pivotal for keratinocyte activation and production of inflammatory molecules, which in turn lead to amplification of the local immune responses. Intrinsic genetic alterations of keratinocytes in the activation of signal transduction pathways dependent on T-cell-derived cytokines are also fundamental. The current review emphasizes the aberrant interplay of immune cells and skin-resident keratinocytes in establishing and sustaining inflammatory and immune responses in psoriasis.

Keywords: psoriasis, keratinocytes, immune cells, skin inflammation, innate immunity, adaptive immunity

INTRODUCTION

Psoriasis is a chronic inflammatory skin disorder involving both innate and adaptive immunity processes. It is caused by the infiltration of distinct effector leukocyte subpopulations in both the epidermis and dermis, which determines hyperproliferation of the epidermis with aberrant differentiation of keratinocytes (1, 2). As a consequence, the epidermis is thickened, with elongated rete ridges forming protrusions into dermis (2, 3). There has been a long debate on pathogenic functions of keratinocytes in psoriasis, and numerous studies have established that hyperproliferation and abnormal differentiation of keratinocytes is a secondary phenomenon induced by immune activation. This "immune" hypothesis, mainly based on dendritic cell (DC) and T cell pathogenic functions, has found confirmation in the efficacy of immune-targeting treatments (4–6). However, psoriasis cannot be considered uniquely as a T-cell-dependent disease, and it is now well known that keratinocytes have a crucial role in triggering the early pathogenic events, as well as in sustaining the chronic phase of the disease (1, 7). Early upstream events occurring in psoriasis include induction of innate immunity pathways and responses, and keratinocytes represent the "first-line responding" skin cells to psoriasis pathogenic environment (8). Upon activation by trigger factors, such as skin trauma and pathogens (i.e., streptococci) or drugs, respectively, keratinocytes become a source of innate immune mediators (**Figure 1A**). The latter include cationic antimicrobial peptides (AMP),

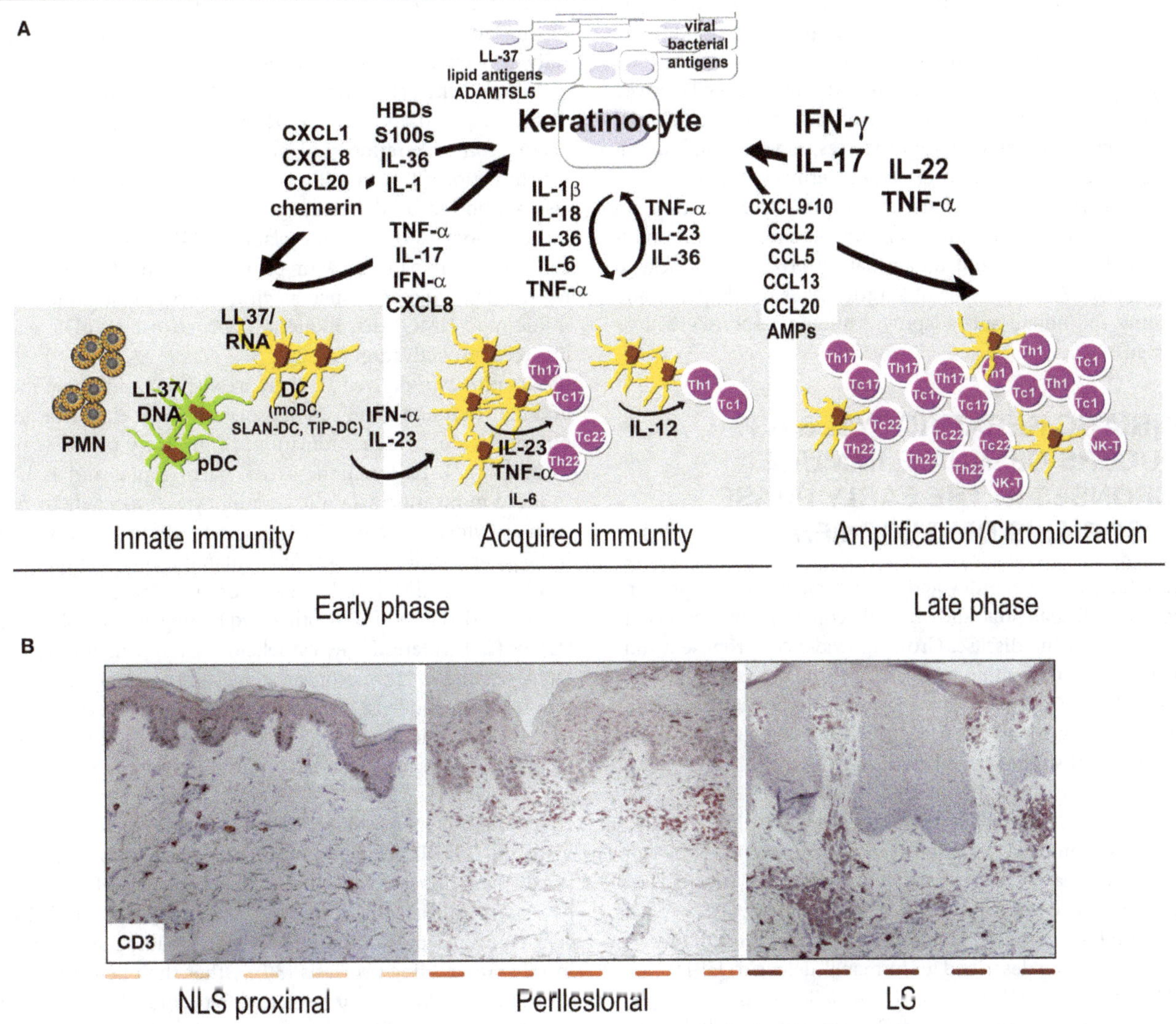

FIGURE 1 | Aberrant interplay of keratinocytes and immune cells in psoriasis. **(A)** Early upstream events in psoriasis include induction of innate immunity pathways and acquired responses, and keratinocytes represent the "key responding" skin cells by producing trigger factors, including LL37/nucleic acid complexes, lipid antigens, and ADAMTSL5, as well as pathogens of viral or bacterial origin. During this initial phase, keratinocytes also produce antimicrobial peptides (AMP), such as β-defensins (HBD) and S100 proteins, together with chemokines and cytokines of IL-1 family. Among AMP, LL37 activates plasmacytoid dendritic cells and myeloid DC (mDC), which routinely patrol uninvolved psoriatic skin, in particular, non-lesional (NLS) skin proximal to lesions, with consequent beginning of the adaptive immune phase. In early phase, SLAN-DC and TIP-DC, highly producing TNF-α, are also present. Hence, DC drive expansion of T lymphocytes, mostly Th17 and Th22 in the beginning and type-1 interferon (IFN)-γ-producing T cells, especially during the chronic phase. During acquired immunity phase, keratinocytes influence DC immune functions by producing cytokines derived from inflammasome pathway, and IL-36. T-cell infiltrate present during late/chronic phase of psoriasis establishes a cytokine milieu, mainly represented by IFN-γ, TNF-α, IL-17, IL-22, which dictates specific and pathogenic gene signatures in keratinocytes, which, thus, overexpress a number of inflammatory mediators. In parallel, under the influence of cytokines, in particular, IL-22 and IL-17, keratinocytes hyperproliferate and show altered differentiative programs. During the amplification/chronicization phase of the disease, unceasing cross-talk between keratinocytes and immune cells further amplifies inflammation and hyperplasia. **(B)** Both early and late phases of psoriasis can be found within the same psoriatic plaque, being it comprehensive of LS, perilesional and adjacent NLS areas, with markers of chronic inflammation (i.e., CD3$^+$ T accumulation in the dermis) predominantly present in LS skin [CD3 stainings have been retrieved from Ref. (48)].

cytokines of IL-1 family, and chemokines active in the recruitment of leukocyte subpopulations of innate immunity, such as plasmacytoid dendritic cells (pDC), neutrophils, mast cells, and macrophages (9, 10). Among AMP, the cathelicidin LL37 has been associated with the development of psoriasis, through its capacity to activate pDC and myeloid DC (mDC), with consequent initiation of the adaptive immune phase (10, 11). DC drive expansion of T lymphocytes, typically T helper (Th)17 and Th22 in the initial phase and interferon (IFN)-γ-producing T cells during the chronic phase of the disease (**Figure 1A**). T-cell infiltrate present in active psoriatic skin establishes a cytokine milieu that dictates specific gene signatures in keratinocytes, which, thus, overexpress several inflammatory mediators amplifying local immune reactions (12, 13). Unceasing cross-talk between keratinocytes and adaptive immunity cells further intensifies inflammation and may be essential in disease chronicity (**Figure 1A**). In addition, intrinsic or genetic alterations of keratinocytes in the activation of key signaling pathways induced by immune cell-derived cytokines may be responsible for the typical unbalance between proliferation and differentiation processes, as well as inflammatory signatures observed in psoriatic epidermis (14, 15).

In this review, we will illustrate the multiple functions of keratinocytes during the initiation, maintenance, and amplification of the immune and inflammatory programs associated with psoriasis. A critical role of keratinocytes in triggering and sustaining the innate and adaptive immune responses will be discussed.

PSORIATIC KERATINOCYTES AS INDUCERS OF INNATE IMMUNE RESPONSES IN THE EARLY PHASE OF PSORIASIS DEVELOPMENT

Much efforts have been devoted to understanding the primary pathogenic mechanisms and the cell components responsible for the onset of the disease. Growing evidences propose a fundamental role for keratinocytes. At this initial phase, pDC and neutrophils infiltrate skin plaque lesions, and psoriatic keratinocytes are deeply involved in their recruitment and activation (16). Important studies aimed at identifying the initial trigger of psoriasis demonstrated that injured keratinocytes enable pDC-, concomitantly to mDC-driven immune responses through LL37/nucleic acid complexes, highly released in psoriatic epidermis after skin trauma (11, 17). These multimeric LL37–nucleic acid complexes induce overproduction of type I IFN by pDC as well as TNF-α and IL-6 by mDC (11, 18). A similar mechanism for pDC activation has been described for human β-defensin (HBD)2 and HBD3, other two AMP released by psoriatic keratinocytes (19). Also, macrophage populations, highly present in early lesional skin, can be activated by keratinocyte-derived LL37, which promotes their differentiation toward a proinflammatory signature by recognizing the P2×7 purinergic receptor (20). Remarkably, keratinocyte-derived LL37 also regulates the expression of cytokines of IL-1 family, including IL-36γ, by keratinocytes themselves in paracrine and autocrine loops (10). Furthermore, LL37 induces CXCL8 and CXCL1 chemokines through IL-36R signaling in psoriatic keratinocytes, which would, in turn, determine the recruitment and the burst of neutrophils in lesional skin, typical of the early phase of psoriasis (10). Importantly, LL37 induces CXCL10 and CCL20 in psoriatic keratinocytes and is most likely responsible for the first flare of the acquired immunity established in later phase of psoriasis by DC and Th17 (10).

Other chemotactic factors are expressed by keratinocytes during the induction phase of psoriasis. For instance, the chemokine chemerin, which is also abundantly released by dermal fibroblasts, is responsible for migration and accumulation of BDCA-2$^+$ pDC into pre-psoriatic skin, as well as in early psoriatic lesions. Through secretion of IFN-α, pDC activate pathogenic T-cells by inducing the maturation of mDC, and by initiating the mononuclear Th1 responses, which persist in adaptive immunity (21, 22). Chemerin expression by keratinocytes and fibroblasts is lost during later stages of plaque development, and pDC disappear in fully developed psoriasis plaques (16).

Of note, the production of IFN-α by early immigrating pDC favors acquired immune responses also by suppressing IL-1 production by keratinocytes, and, therefore, by shortening skin inflammation (23). In addition, the pathogenicity of IFN-α is also supported by the findings showing its signaling signature in keratinocytes of psoriatic plaques (24), and that psoriasis is exacerbated if patients with psoriasis are treated with IFN-α for unrelated diseases, such as viral infections or tumors, or by imiquimod (IMQ) that induces IFN-α release by pDC *via* toll-like receptor activation (25, 26).

Keratinocyte-derived IL-1α represents an additional inducer of innate immune responses in psoriasis, and it can favor neutrophil and monocyte accumulation during early psoriasis papule formation. IL-1α functions as an alarm signal and is heavily induced in necrotic psoriatic keratinocytes, especially by factors such as cytosolic DNA (27). Concomitantly to IL-1α, self-DNA induces assembling of psoriatic inflammasome containing the DNA sensor AIM2, and, thus, promotes the production and release of IL-1β and IL-18, other two pathogenic member of IL-1 family (27). Interestingly, cathelicidin LL37 can interfere with DNA-sensing inflammasomes, suggesting an antagonistic function for this peptide in the autoinflammatory pathways associated to early psoriatic processes. Critical alterations in the IL-1/IL-1 receptor system have also been found in lesional psoriatic skin (28, 29), with IL-1α and IL-1β being abundant in psoriatic lesions concomitantly to the soluble isoform of the IL-1 receptor antagonist and IL-1-RII decoy receptor. These observations suggest the impairment of negative regulatory mechanisms of IL-1 system in psoriasis. Consistently, transgenic overexpression of IL-1α and IL-1 type I receptor in the skin leads to a pathogenic phenotype in mice resembling psoriasis (30). Other than activating innate immune responses, IL-1α has found to promote keratinocyte and endothelial cell proliferation and activation (31).

KERATINOCYTE INVOLVEMENT IN ADAPTIVE IMMUNE RESPONSES IN PSORIATIC SKIN

Psoriasis lesional skin shows many inflammatory CD3$^+$ T cells, which progressively accumulate in both the upper dermis and epidermis (1, 2), thus determining the typical epidermal hyperplasia and inflammation picture (**Figure 1B**). Immunophenotyping of T cells shows that they are mostly activated memory T cells expressing cutaneous lymphocyte antigen (CLA) and belongs to distinct subsets of CD4$^+$ and CD8$^+$ lymphocytes, Th1/Tc1, Th17/Tc17, and Th22/Tc22 (2). DC activation is determinant in driving T cell responses, even if keratinocytes can trigger and condition DC responses, and, thus, influence acquired immunity in psoriatic skin.

First, keratinocytes have been described as active producers of causative antigens of psoriasis, and the position of dermal mDC at the dermal–epidermal junction, as well as in the epidermis would favor the capture by mDC of keratinocyte-derived extracellular antigens for presentation to T cells, and intracellular antigens *via* cross-presentation. Recently, three autoantigens identified in keratinocytes were found to be involved in the pathogenesis of psoriasis. Among them, LL37 is recognized as autoantigen by circulating $CD4^+$ and $CD8^+$ T cells with a cytokine and skin-homing receptor profile typical of psoriatic skin T cells (IFN-γ^{high}, IL-17^{high}, CLA^+, $CCR6^+$, and $CCR10^+$), in up to 75% of psoriatic patients (32). Most recently, phospholipase A2 group IVD was identified in psoriatic keratinocytes as important player in the generation of psoriasis autoantigens (33). The latter include non-protein neolipids that are recognized by CD1a-restricted T cells, thereby inducing the production of IL-22 and IL-17A (34). These lipid antigens could be transferred from keratinocytes to neighboring antigen-presenting cells through released exosomes, similarly to what observed for $tryptase^+$ mast cells of psoriatic lesions (34). Finally, the disintegrin and metalloprotease domain containing thrombospondin type 1 motif-like 5 (ADAMTSL5), a protein modulating microfibril functions (34, 35) and identified as autoantigen presented by melanocytes in a HLA-C*06:02-restricted fashion (36), has been also recently localized in keratinocytes throughout the psoriatic epidermis (34, 37). Keratinocytes could also activate pathogenic T cells by presenting viral or bacterial products. A relevant presence of human papillomavirus-5 DNA and reactive antibodies against virus-related particles have been found in psoriasis (38). Infections by *Streptococcus* commonly associate with psoriasis, and streptococcus-derived superantigens can be presented to T lymphocytes by MHC class II-bearing keratinocytes. Psoriatic antigens are also supposed to be keratinocyte-derived molecules sharing structural homology with streptococcal proteins, which could, therefore, induce autoreactive T-cell responses against skin components (39).

Second, DC function and maturation in the psoriatic context is also depending on mediators released by keratinocytes during the innate immunity phase. Among them, IL-36 cytokines, a subgroup of IL-1 family, comprising the IL-36α, β, and γ agonists, strongly upregulated in psoriatic lesional epidermis, were found to influence DC function (40, 41). In humans, IL-36 cytokines activate mDC by increasing the proportion of cells with a strong CD83, CD86, and HLA-DR membrane expression and induce the secretion of IL-1β and IL-6, thus promoting the Th17 differentiation (42). Consistently, keratinocyte/DC cross talk mediated by IL-36 was essential in driving IMQ-induced psoriasiform dermatitis in mice. In this model, IL-36 signaling controlled the aberrant IL-23/IL-17/IL-22 axis and disease development (43). Similarly, IL-18 highly released by keratinocytes downstream to inflammasome pathway is involved in the recruitment of IL-18R-bearing DC to inflammatory sites characterized by Th1 responses, as in psoriasis. IL-18 from keratinocytes in synergy with IL-12 plays a role in the Th1 response, primarily by inducing IFN-γ in psoriatic lesions (44). In addition, recent evidence suggests that γδ T cells infiltrating can produce IL-17 *via* IL-23 in presence of IL-18 (45). Together with IL-18, mature IL-1β is also produced by keratinocytes as result of inflammasome activation, and influence DC-mediated immune responses. A number of evidence links IL-1β and Th17 pathways in psoriasis pathogenesis both in mice and in humans. Transgenic overexpression of IL-1β is responsible for massive presence of Th17 cells in the skin, as well as for the inflammatory psoriasisform phenotype of mice (46). Furthermore, the IL-23-dependent differentiation of human Th17 cells relies on the copresence of IL-1β (27).

KERATINOCYTES ARE A RESERVOIR OF INFLAMMATORY MEDIATORS, WHICH SUSTAIN PERSISTENCE OF PSORIASIS LESIONS

During the chronic phase of psoriasis, expansion and activation of T and DC subpopulations in lesional areas establishes a definite cytokine micromilieu, mostly represented by IFN-γ, IL-17, TNF-α, and IL-22. Keratinocytes bear receptors for these cytokines and potently respond by further releasing cytokines. Under the effects of these cytokines, keratinocytes also show altered proliferative and differentiation programs, as well as enhanced resistance to apoptosis (1, 47–49).

Each cytokine regulates distinct responses in keratinocytes with a certain degree of overlap in gene expression induction/inhibition. Transcriptional profiling studies conducted on lesional psoriatic skin showed that the IFN-γ-signature predominates, with the upregulated expression of approximately 400 genes dependent on signal transducer and activator of transcription 1 (STAT1), the preferential IFN-γ molecular node (50). *In vitro*, IFN-γ represents the most potent stimulus for keratinocyte inflammatory and immune activation, as it regulates the expression of approximately 1,200 genes (51). Importantly, the IFN-γ capability to induce inflammation in psoriasis was demonstrated by a study showing that IFN-γ injection in clinically uninvolved psoriatic skin determines a transcriptomic profile and inflammatory cell infiltration similar to lesional skin (51). Indeed, the same results were obtained with healthy volunteers, indicating that other cytokines specifically contribute to the psoriatic phenotype (51). IFN-γ induces in psoriatic keratinocytes key-disease mediators, such as chemokines attracting monocytes and Th1 and Th17 cells (CCL2, CCL5, CXCR3 ligands), DC (CCL13, CCL20), or $CCR10^+$ skin-homing CLA^+ T cells highly infiltrating psoriatic skin (1). HBDs and S100 proteins are also potently induced by IFN-γ in keratinocytes, alone or in synergy with TNF-α. Most of the IFN-γ-induced effects in keratinocytes are potentiated by TNF-α, which signals mainly by activating NF-κB, a transcription factor regulating gene expression frequently in collaboration with STAT1. TNF-α induces expression of ICAM-1 on keratinocytes, permitting the adhesion of circulating leukocytes. Moreover, TNF-α stimulates keratinocyte production of several chemokines active on neutrophils, T cells, and DC (CXCL1, CXCL2, CXCL8, CCL2, CCL5), as well as pro-inflammatory cytokines, such as IL-6 and IL-1, which help maintain Th17 cells (1, 2). Importantly, TNF-α induces IL-36γ in psoriasis lesions, which in turn promote expression of AMP and chemokines recruiting neutrophils and Th17 cells, as well as interfere with terminal differentiation and cornification process of psoriatic epidermis (52). The increased production of IL-36γ is also associated with the presence of Th17 lymphokines in psoriatic skin lesions, as IL-17 and IL-22 strongly induce its expression (52, 53).

Keratinocytes are also strongly influenced by IL-17 and upregulate chemokines (CXCL1, CXCL3, CXCL5, CXCL8, CCL20), AMPs (LCN2, HBD-2, S100A7), and immunomodulatory molecules, such as ICAM1, in response to this cytokine. In addition, IL-17 stimulates LL37 autoantigen production (54–56) and delay terminal differentiation of keratinocytes. IL-17 activates NF-κB, possibly through the IKBζ transcriptional regulator, as well as Act-1 intracellular pathway, which is required for IL-17 induction of keratinocyte host defense genes and inhibition of differentiative programs in keratinocytes (57). IL-17 also induces IL-19, a member of IL-20 family, which has mitogenic effects on keratinocytes themselves (58).

Th17- or Th22-derived IL-22 cytokine also acts pathogenically on psoriatic keratinocytes by promoting release of chemokines (CXCL1, CXCL2, CXCL8, CCL20), AMPs (HBD-2, HBD-3, S100 proteins), as well as inducing their proliferation and de-differentiation (59, 60). Binding of IL-22 to its receptor, the expression of which in the skin is confined to keratinocytes, mediates epidermal acanthosis through the activation of STAT3. These observations may explain the increased STAT3 expression in the epidermal compartment and the pathogenicity of STAT3 overexpression in the epidermis of transgenic mice (61). Although studies demonstrated a central role of IL-22 in psoriasis pathogenesis, this cytokine induces a limited panel of genes compared to IL-17, as detected in human lesional psoriatic skin (55), and antibodies neutralizing IL-22 failed to show a therapeutic effect in patients with psoriasis.

Collectively, IFN-γ, IL-17, TNF-α, and IL-22 can cause keratinocyte production of chemokines, cytokines, and AMPs, as well as concur to derange proliferative and differentiative programs of the epidermis. This becomes a self-amplifying loop, where these products and altered homeostasis act back on T cells, DC, and neutrophils to perpetuate the cutaneous inflammatory processes.

CONCLUSION

Currently, there are no meaningful hypotheses to explain certain typical features of psoriasis including the sharply demarcated presentation of the lesions and the more frequent localization of the lesions in certain anatomical sites (i.e., scalp, extensor body areas), although a skin/keratinocyte-specific mechanism may be involved. In contrast, the fluctuant behavior of psoriasis with phases of remission and recrudescence may be related to prevailing regulatory and effector immune mechanisms. Activated T lymphocytes are required for the development and persistence of immune responses in psoriatic skin, even though psoriasis cannot be considered uniquely as a T cell-dependent disease. In fact, the presence of type-17, type-1, and type-22 subtypes in inflamed skin could be the result of a common response to antigens, also effective in subjects not predisposed to psoriasis. Indeed, this paradox could be explained either by the presence of other not yet defined psoriasis-related cytokines in skin lesions, or by the intrinsic aberrant response of psoriatic keratinocytes to cytokines or other effector molecules. Several studies showed that genetic defects in keratinocytes are fundamental for psoriasis development. An increasing number of specific single-nucleotide polymorphisms (SNP), found in genes controlling T-cell commitment and keratinocyte inflammatory activation as well as proliferation and differentiation processes in the epidermis, has been associated with psoriasis (14). Among them, a number of SNPs were found in genes encoding molecules involved in IL-17 or TNF-α responses, even though functional studies correlating their presence to keratinocyte susceptibility to these cytokines are lacking and controversial. For instance, allelic variants were found in *NFKBIZ*, *TRAF3IP2*, and *TNFAIP3* genes (62) encoding IKBζ, Act-1 and the Act1-dependent A20 protein, respectively, all involved in IL-17 molecular signaling (57). However, no clear evidence linking these SNPs to enhanced or reduced responses of keratinocytes to IL-17 exist. In fact, Act-1 gene variants overexpressed in human keratinocytes could decrease as well as enhance Act-1-mediated IL-17 signaling, depending on the SNP type. Variants of *NFKBIZ* could also influence keratinocyte response to TNF-α since IKBζ is a transcriptional cofactor of p50 subunit of NF-κB, the main mediator of TNF-α signaling. In addition, NF-κB activity is regulated by CARD14, a protein of "signalosome" complex involved in activation of innate immunity molecules (i.e., IL-36γ, CXCL8, and CCL20), whose gene shows different allelic variants associated to psoriasis (63). Although a recent study clarified the impact of a CARD14 missense variant (Card14ΔE138), whose expression in mice determined a severe psoriatic phenotype (64), the effects of CARD14 SNPs on TNF-α- or IL-17-induced responses in keratinocytes remain to be defined.

Future studies must consider these genetic aspects, especially those concerning the relationship between genetic determinants and keratinocyte inflammatory responses to psoriasis-related cytokines. Moreover, genetic data need to be further integrated with analyses of the cytokine milieu specifically characterizing the psoriatic patient. This will permit to predict the responsiveness of psoriatic patient to a specific therapy, thus implementing a personalized medicine approach.

AUTHOR CONTRIBUTIONS

Each author has contributed in the ideation and writing of the manuscript, and each author has checked the final version of the paper.

REFERENCES

1. Albanesi C, De Pità O, Girolomoni G. Resident skin cells in psoriasis: a special look at the pathogenetic functions of keratinocytes. *Clin Dermatol* (2007) 25(6):581–8. doi:10.1016/j.clindermatol.2007.08.013
2. Chiricozzi A, Romanelli P, Volpe E, Borsellino G, Romanelli M. Scanning the immunopathogenesis of psoriasis. *Int J Mol Sci* (2018) 19(1):E179. doi:10.3390/ijms19010179
3. Sabat R, Philipp S, Höflich C, Kreutzer S, Wallace E, Asadullah K, et al. Immunopathogenesis of psoriasis. *Exp Dermatol* (2007) 16(10):779 98. doi:10.1111/j.1600-0625.2007.00629.x
4. Lowes MA, Suárez-Fariñas M, Krueger JG. Immunology of psoriasis. *Annu Rev Immunol* (2014) 32:227–55. doi:10.1146/annurev-immunol-032713-120225
5. Conrad C, Gilliet M. Psoriasis: from pathogenesis to targeted therapies. *Clin Rev Allergy Immunol* (2018) 54(1):102–13. doi:10.1007/s12016-018-8668-1

6. Hawkes JE, Chan TC, Krueger JG. Psoriasis pathogenesis and the development of novel targeted immune therapies. *J Allergy Clin Immunol* (2017) 140(3):645–53. doi:10.1016/j.jaci.2017.07.004
7. Albanesi C, Pastore S. Pathobiology of chronic inflammatory skin diseases: interplay between keratinocytes and immune cells as a target for anti-inflammatory drugs. *Curr Drug Metab* (2010) 11(3):210–27. doi:10.2174/138920010791196328
8. Büchau AS, Gallo RL. Innate immunity and antimicrobial defense systems in psoriasis. *Clin Dermatol* (2007) 25(6):616–24. doi:10.1016/j.clindermatol.2007.08.016
9. Takagi H, Arimura K, Uto T, Fukaya T, Nakamura T, Choijookhuu N, et al. Plasmacytoid dendritic cells orchestrate TLR7-mediated innate and adaptive immunity for the initiation of autoimmune inflammation. *Sci Rep* (2016) 14(6):24477–95. doi:10.1038/srep24477
10. Li N, Yamasaki K, Saito R, Fukushi-Takahashi S, Shimada-Omori R, Asano M, et al. Alarmin function of cathelicidin antimicrobial peptide LL37 through IL-36γ induction in human epidermal keratinocytes. *J Immunol* (2014) 193(10):5140–8. doi:10.4049/jimmunol.1302574
11. Ganguly D, Chamilos G, Lande R, Gregorio J, Meller S, Facchinetti V, et al. Self-RNA-antimicrobial peptide complexes activate human dendritic cells through TLR7 and TLR8. *J Exp Med* (2009) 206(9):1983–94. doi:10.1084/jem.20090480
12. Girolomoni G, Strohal R, Puig L, Bachelez H, Barker J, Boehncke WH, et al. The role of IL-23 and the IL-23/TH17 immune axis in the pathogenesis and treatment of psoriasis. *J Eur Acad Dermatol Venereol* (2017) 31(10):1616–26. doi:10.1111/jdv.14433
13. Lowes MA, Russell CB, Martin DA, Towne JE, Krueger JG. The IL-23/T17 pathogenic axis in psoriasis is amplified by keratinocyte responses. *Trends Immunol* (2013) 34(4):174–81. doi:10.1016/j.it.2012.11.005
14. Capon F. The genetic basis of psoriasis. *Int J Mol Sci* (2017) 18(12):E2526. doi:10.3390/ijms18122526
15. Harden JL, Krueger JG, Bowcock AM. The immunogenetics of Psoriasis: a comprehensive review. *J Autoimmun* (2015) 64:66–73. doi:10.1016/j.jaut.2015.07.008
16. Albanesi C, Scarponi C, Pallotta S, Daniele R, Bosisio D, Madonna S, et al. Chemerin expression marks early psoriatic skin lesions and correlates with plasmacytoid dendritic cell recruitment. *J Exp Med* (2009) 206(1):249–58. doi:10.1084/jem.20080129
17. Lande R, Gregorio J, Facchinetti V, Chatterjee B, Wang YH, Homey B, et al. Plasmacytoid dendritic cells sense self-DNA coupled with antimicrobial peptide. *Nature* (2007) 449(7162):564–9. doi:10.1038/nature06116
18. Nestle FO, Conrad C, Tun-Kyi A, Homey B, Gombert M, Boyman O, et al. Plasmacytoid predendritic cells initiate psoriasis through interferon-alpha production. *J Exp Med* (2005) 202(1):135–43. doi:10.1084/jem.20050500
19. Lande R, Chamilos G, Ganguly D, Demaria O, Frasca L, Durr S, et al. Cationic antimicrobial peptides in psoriatic skin cooperate to break innate tolerance to self-DNA. *Eur J Immunol* (2015) 45(1):203–13. doi:10.1002/eji.201344277
20. Elssner A, Duncan M, Gavrilin M, Wewers MD. A novel P2X7 receptor activator, the human cathelicidin-derived peptide LL37, induces IL-1 beta processing and release. *J Immunol* (2004) 172(8):4987–94. doi:10.4049/jimmunol.172.8.4987
21. Wittamer V, Franssen JD, Vulcano M, Mirjolet JF, Le Poul E, Migeotte I, et al. Specific recruitment of antigen-presenting cells by chemerin, a novel processed ligand from human inflammatory fluids. *J Exp Med* (2003) 198:977–85. doi:10.1084/jem.20030382
22. Liu YJ. IPC: professional type 1 interferon-producing cells and plasmacytoid dendritic cell precursors. *Annu Rev Immunol* (2005) 23:275–306. doi:10.1146/annurev.immunol.23.021704.115633
23. Christophers E, Metzler G, Rocken M. Bimodal immune activation in psoriasis. *Br J Dermatol* (2014) 170:59–65. doi:10.1111/bjd.12631
24. Yao Y, Richman L, Morehouse C, de los Reyes M, Higgs BW, Boutrin A, et al. Type I interferon: potential therapeutic target for psoriasis? *PLoS One* (2008) 3:e2737. doi:10.1371/journal.pone.0002737
25. Ketikoglou I, Karatapanis S, Elefsiniotis I, Kafiri G, Moulakakis A. Extensive psoriasis induced by pegylated interferon alpha-2b treatment for chronic hepatitis B. *Eur J Dermatol* (2005) 15:107–9.
26. Garzorz-Stark N, Lauffer F, Krause L, Thomas J, Atenhan A, Franz R, et al. Toll-like receptor 7/8 agonists stimulate plasmacytoid dendritic cells to initiate T_H17-deviated acute contact dermatitis in human subjects. *J Allergy Clin Immunol* (2018) 141(4):1320–1333.e11. doi:10.1016/j.jaci.2017.07.045
27. Dombrowski Y, Peric M, Koglin S, Kammerbauer C, Göss C, Anz D, et al. Cytosolic DNA triggers inflammasome activation in keratinocytes in psoriatic lesions. *Sci Transl Med* (2011) 3(82):82ra38. doi:10.1126/scitranslmed.3002001
28. Kupper TS, Groves RW. The interleukin-1 axis and cutaneous inflammation. *J Invest Dermatol* (1995) 105:62S–6S. doi:10.1111/1523-1747.ep12316087
29. Groves RW, Sherman L, Mizutani H, Dower SK, Kupper TS. Detection of interleukin-1 receptors in human epidermis. Induction of the type II receptor after organ culture and in psoriasis. *Am J Pathol* (1994) 145:1048–56.
30. Groves RW, Rauschmayr T, Nakamura K, Sarkar S, Williams IR, Kupper TS. Inflammatory and hyperproliferative skin disease in mice that express elevated levels of the IL-1 receptor (type I) on epidermal keratinocytes. Evidence that IL-1-inducible secondary cytokines produced by keratinocytes in vivo can cause skin disease. *J Clin Invest* (1996) 98:336–44. doi:10.1172/JCI118797
31. Bou-Dargham MJ, Khamis ZI, Cognetta AB, Sang QA. The role of Interleukin-1 in inflammatory and malignant human skin diseases and the rationale for targeting Interleukin-1 alpha. *Med Res Rev* (2017) 37(1):180–216. doi:10.1002/med.21406
32. Lande R, Botti E, Jandus C, Dojcinovic D, Fanelli G, Conrad C, et al. The antimicrobial peptide LL37 is a T-cell autoantigen in psoriasis. *Nat Commun* (2014) 3(5):5621. doi:10.1038/ncomms6621
33. Cheung KL, Jarrett R, Subramaniam S, Salimi M, Gutowska-Owsiak D, Chen YL, et al. Psoriatic T cells recognize neolipid antigens generated by mast cell phospholipase delivered by exosomes and presented by CD1a. *J Exp Med* (2016) 213(11):2399–412. doi:10.1084/jem.20160258
34. Fuentes-Duculan J, Bonifacio KM, Hawkes JE, Kunjravia N, Cueto I, Li X, et al. Autoantigens ADAMTSL5 and LL37 are significantly upregulated in active psoriasis and localized with keratinocytes, dendritic cells and other leukocytes. *Exp Dermatol* (2017) 26(11):1075–82. doi:10.1111/exd.13378
35. Bader HL, Wang LW, Ho JC, Tran T, Holden P, Fitzgerald J, et al. A disintegrin-like and metalloprotease domain containing thrombospondin type 1 motif-like 5 (ADAMTSL5) is a novel fibrillin-1-, fibrillin-2-, and heparin-binding member of the ADAMTS superfamily containing a netrin-like module. *Matrix Biol* (2012) 31(7–8):398–411. doi:10.1016/j.matbio.2012.09.003
36. Arakawa A, Siewert K, Stöhr J, Besgen P, Kim SM, Rühl G, et al. Melanocyte antigen triggers autoimmunity in human psoriasis. *J Exp Med* (2015) 212(13):2203–12. doi:10.1084/jem.20151093
37. Bonifacio KM, Kunjravia N, Krueger JG, Fuentes-Duculan J. Cutaneous expression of A disintegrin-like and metalloprotease domain containing thrombospondin type 1 motif-like 5 (ADAMTSL5) in psoriasis goes beyond melanocytes. *J Pigment Disord* (2016) 3(3):244. doi:10.4172/2376-0427.1000244
38. Favre M, Orth G, Majewski S, Baloul S, Pura A, Jablonska S. Psoriasis: a possible reservoir for human papillomavirus type 5, the virus associated with skin carcinomas of epidermodysplasia verruciformis. *J Invest Dermatol* (1998) 110(4):311–7. doi:10.1046/j.1523-1747.1998.00164.x
39. Leung DY, Travers JB, Giorno R, Norris DA, Skinner R, Aelion J, et al. Evidence for a streptococcal superantigen-driven process in acute guttate psoriasis. *J Clin Invest* (1995) 96(5):2106–12. doi:10.1172/JCI118263
40. Furue K, Yamamura K, Tsuji G, Mitoma C, Uchi H, Nakahara T, et al. Highlighting interleukin-36 signalling in plaque psoriasis and pustular psoriasis. *Acta Derm Venereol* (2018) 98(1):5–13. doi:10.2340/00015555-2808
41. Gabay C, Towne JE. Regulation and function of interleukin-36 cytokines in homeostasis and pathological conditions. *J Leukoc Biol* (2015) 97(4):645–52. doi:10.1189/jlb.3RI1014-495R
42. Foster AM, Baliwag J, Chen CS, Guzman AM, Stoll SW, Gudjonsson JE, et al. IL-36 promotes myeloid cell infiltration, activation, and inflammatory activity in skin. *J Immunol* (2014) 192(12):6053–61. doi:10.4049/jimmunol.1301481
43. Tortola L, Rosenwald E, Abel B, Blumberg H, Schäfer M, Coyle AJ, et al. Psoriasiform dermatitis is driven by IL-36-mediated DC-keratinocyte crosstalk. *J Clin Invest* (2012) 122(11):3965–76. doi:10.1172/JCI63451
44. Lee JH, Cho DH, Park HJ. IL-18 and cutaneous inflammatory diseases. *Int J Mol Sci* (2015) 16(12):29357–69. doi:10.3390/ijms161226172
45. Mielke LA, Mills KH. IL-17-producing γδ T cells and innate lymphoid cells. *Eur J Immunol* (2012) 42(9):2221–31. doi:10.1002/eji.201242569
46. Rabeony H, Pohin M, Vasseur P, Petit-Paris I, Jégou JF, Favot L, et al. IMQ-induced skin inflammation in mice is dependent on IL1R1 and MyD88 signaling but independent of the NLRP3 inflammasome. *Eur J Immunol* (2015) 45(10):2847–57. doi:10.1002/eji.201445215

47. Sestito R, Madonna S, Scarponi C, Cianfarani F, Failla CM, Cavani A, et al. STAT3-dependent effects of IL-22 in human keratinocytes are counterregulated by sirtuin 1 through a direct inhibition of STAT3 acetylation. *FASEB J* (2011) 25(3):916–27. doi:10.1096/fj.10-172288
48. Madonna S, Scarponi C, Pallotta S, Cavani A, Albanesi C. Anti-apoptotic effects of suppressor of cytokine signaling 3 and 1 in psoriasis. *Cell Death Dis* (2012) 28(3):e334. doi:10.1038/cddis.2012.69
49. Palombo R, Savini I, Avigliano L, Madonna S, Cavani A, Albanesi C, et al. Luteolin-7-glucoside inhibits IL-22/STAT3 pathway, reducing proliferation, acanthosis, and inflammation in keratinocytes and in mouse psoriatic model. *Cell Death Dis* (2016) 7(8):e2344. doi:10.1038/cddis.2016.201
50. Chiricozzi A, Romanelli M, Panduri S, Donetti E, Prignano F. Relevance of in vitro 3-D skin models in dissecting cytokine contribution to psoriasis pathogenesis. *Histol Histopathol* (2017) 32:893–8. doi:10.14670/HH-11-877
51. Johnson-Huang LM, Suárez-Fariñas M, Pierson KC, Fuentes-Duculan J, Cueto I, Lentini T, et al. A single intradermal injection of IFN-γ induces an inflammatory state in both non-lesional psoriatic and healthy skin. *J Invest Dermatol* (2012) 132:1177–87. doi:10.1038/jid.2011.458
52. Bassoy EY, Towne JE, Gabay C. Regulation and function of interleukin-36 cytokines. *Immunol Rev* (2018) 281(1):169–78. doi:10.1111/imr.12610
53. Carrier Y, Ma HL, Ramon HE, Napierata L, Small C, O'Toole M, et al. Inter-regulation of Th17 cytokines and the IL-36 cytokines in vitro and in vivo: implications in psoriasis pathogenesis. *J Invest Dermatol* (2011) 131(12):2428–37. doi:10.1038/jid.2011.234
54. Nograles KE, Zaba LC, Guttman-Yassky E, Fuentes-Duculan J, Suárez-Fariñas M, Cardinale I, et al. Th17 cytokines interleukin (IL)-17 and IL-22 modulate distinct inflammatory and keratinocyte-response pathways. *Br J Dermatol* (2008) 159:1092–102. doi:10.1111/j.1365-2133.2008.08769.x
55. Chiricozzi A, Nograles KE, Johnson-Huang LM, Fuentes-Duculan J, Cardinale I, Bonifacio KM, et al. IL-17 induces an expanded range of downstream genes in reconstituted human epidermis model. *PLoS One* (2014) 9:e90284. doi:10.1371/journal.pone.0090284
56. Harper EG, Guo C, Rizzo H, Lillis JV, Kurtz SE, Skorcheva I, et al. Th17 cytokines stimulate CCL20 expression in keratinocytes in vitro and in vivo: implications for psoriasis pathogenesis. *J Invest Dermatol* (2009) 129:2175–83. doi:10.1038/jid.2009.65
57. Muromoto R, Hirao T, Tawa K, Hirashima K, Kon S, Kitai Y, et al. IL-17A plays a central role in the expression of psoriasis signature genes through the induction of IκB-ζ in keratinocytes. *Int Immunol* (2016) 28(9):443–52. doi:10.1093/intimm/dxw011
58. Witte E, Kokolakis G, Witte K, Philipp S, Doecke WD, Babel N, et al. IL-19 is a component of the pathogenetic IL-23/IL-17 cascade in psoriasis. *J Invest Dermatol* (2014) 134:2757–67. doi:10.1038/jid.2014.308
59. Wilson NJ, Boniface K, Chan JR, McKenzie BS, Blumenschein WM, Mattson JD, et al. Development, cytokine profile and function of human interleukin 17-producing helper T cells. *Nat Immunol* (2007) 8:950–7. doi:10.1038/ni1497
60. Volpe E, Servant N, Zollinger R, Bogiatzi SI, Hupé P, Barillot E, et al. A critical function for transforming growth factor-beta, interleukin 23 and proinflammatorycytokines in driving and modulating human T(H)-17 responses. *Nat Immunol* (2008) 9:650–7. doi:10.1038/ni.1613
61. Sano S, Chan KS, Carbajal S, Clifford J, Peavey M, Kiguchi K, et al. Stat3 links activated keratinocytes and immunocytes required for development of psoriasis in a novel transgenic mouse model. *Nat Med* (2005) 11(1):43–9. doi:10.1038/nm1162
62. Tsoi LC, Spain SL, Ellinghaus E, Stuart PE, Capon F, Knight J, et al. Enhanced meta-analysis and replication studies identify five new psoriasis susceptibility loci. *Nat Commun* (2015) 6:7001. doi:10.1038/ncomms8001
63. Jordan CT, Cao L, Roberson ED, Duan S, Helms CA, Nair RP, et al. Rare and common variants in CARD14, encoding an epidermal regulator of NF-kappaB, in psoriasis. *Am J Hum Genet* (2012) 90(5):796–808. doi:10.1016/j.ajhg.2012.03.013
64. Mellett M, Meier B, Mohanan D, Schairer R, Cheng P, Satoh TK, et al. CARD14 gain-of-function mutation alone is sufficient to drive IL-23/IL-17-mediated psoriasiform skin inflammation in vivo. *J Invest Dermatol* (2018) S0022-202X (18):31874–8. doi:10.1016/j.jid.2018.03.1525

11

PSORI-CM02 Formula Increases CD4+ Foxp3+ Regulatory T Cell Frequency and Ameliorates Imiquimod-Induced Psoriasis in Mice

Haiming Chen[1,2,3,4†], Huazhen Liu[1,3,4†], Chuanjian Lu[1,3,4,5], Maojie Wang[1,3,4], Xiong Li[1,3,4], Hui Zhao[6,7], Yuhong Yan[1,3], Wanling Yu[1,3,4], Ling Han[1,3,4,5*] and Zhenhua Dai[1,3,4*]*

[1] The Second Affiliated Hospital, Guangzhou University of Chinese Medicine, Guangzhou, China, [2] Postdoctoral Programme, Guangzhou University of Chinese Medicine, Guangzhou, China, [3] Guangdong Provincial Hospital of Chinese Medicine, Guangzhou, China, [4] Guangdong Provincial Academy of Chinese Medical Sciences, Guangzhou, China, [5] Guangdong Provincial Key Laboratory of Clinical Research on Traditional Chinese Medicine Syndrome, Guangzhou, China, [6] Key Laboratory for Regenerative Medicine, Ministry of Education, Faculty of Medicine, School of Biomedical Sciences, The Chinese University of Hong Kong, Hong Kong, China, [7] Kunming Institute of Zoology Chinese Academy of Sciences-The Chinese University of Hong Kong Joint Laboratory of Bioresources and Molecular Research of Common Diseases, Hong Kong, China

***Correspondence:**
Chuanjian Lu
luchuanjian888@vip.sina.com;
Ling Han
linghan36@163.com;
Zhenhua Dai
zdai2009@hotmail.com

†These authors have contributed equally to this work.

Psoriasis is an autoimmune and inflammatory disease, which is estimated to affect 2–3% of the population in the world. PSORI-CM02 is an empirical formula of Chinese medicine optimized from Yin Xie Ling, which is widely used to treat psoriasis in China for decades. However, its antipsoriatic mechanisms are still not well understood. Here, we explored the therapeutic effects of PSORI-CM02 on psoriasis and its mechanisms of action in imiquimod-induced psoriasis-like mouse models and human HaCaT cells. In experiments *in vitro*, PSORI-CM02 significantly inhibited HaCaT cell proliferation in dose-dependent and time-dependent manners. Furthermore, it hindered the progression of HaCaT cell cycle and arrested HaCaT cells at G1 phase. On the other hand, our *in vivo* studies demonstrated that PSORI-CM02 dramatically reduced psoriasis area and severity index scores and lesion temperature in imiquimod-induced psoriatic mice. The antioxidative activities of glutathione, catalase, and superoxide dismutase were increased while oxidative activity of malonaldehyde was markedly decreased after treatments with PSORI-CM02. PSORI-CM02 also suppressed the mRNA expression of proinflammatory cytokines, including TNF-α, IL-6, and IL-17, and lowered their protein levels in the serum as well. In addition, PSORI-CM02 could reduce the expression of IKKα and NF-κB in psoriatic skin tissue. It also upregulated the proportion of CD4+ Foxp3+ regulatory T cells (Tregs) in both lymph nodes and spleens and promoted CD4+ CD25+ Treg proliferation *in vitro*. Taken together, our research demonstrated that PSORI-CM02 inhibited HaCaT cell proliferation by arresting them at G1 phase and alleviated systemic inflammation and psoriasis in mice *via* altering the oxidative/anti-oxidative status, tipping the balance between Th17 responsiveness and CD4+ Foxp3+ Treg generation, and suppressing the expression of proinflammatory cytokines as well as NF-κB signaling.

Keywords: psoriasis, inflammation, immunoregulation, regulatory T cell, PSORI-CM02

Abbreviations: CAT, catalase; DXM, dexamethasone acetate; GSH, glutathione; IMQ, imiquimod; MDA, malonaldehyde; PASI, psoriasis area and severity index; SOD, superoxide dismutase; Treg, regulatory T cell.

INTRODUCTION

Psoriasis is an autoimmune and inflammatory dermatologic disease, which affects about 2–3% of population in the world. Psoriatic pathology mainly includes thickening of epidermis, hyperproliferation of keratinocytes and parakeratosis in the epidermis with massive neutrophil infiltration in the dermis (1). Currently, the mechanisms underlying psoriasis have not been fully explored although it has been established that many factors, including genetic factors, environmental factors, immunological mechanisms, new blood vessel formation, lipid metabolism disorders, and unhealthy mentality, bear significant impacts on the occurrence of psoriasis (2). Nowadays, accumulating evidence suggests that patients with moderate or severe psoriasis may increase the risk of other diseases, including obesity, cancer, diabetes mellitus and the metabolic syndrome (3). Meanwhile, current treatments for psoriasis, such as topical therapies, phototherapies and conventional systemic therapies, are not completely satisfied by sufferers principally because of side effects and economic burden (4, 5).

During recent decades, Chinese herbal medicine, one of the traditional Chinese medicine that serves as a complementary and alternative medicine, has been used as popular strategies for treating psoriatic patients and aroused a remarkable and growing interest (6). Our previous researches have shown that Chinese herbal medicine can provide an effective therapy for psoriasis (7–10). PSORI-CM02, which was optimized based on Chinese herbal formula Yin-Xie Ling discovered by well-known professor Guo-Wei Xuan, is a novel formula of Chinese medicine that has been used to effectively treat psoriasis during recent years. PSORI-CM02 consists of five Chinese herbs (**Table 1**), including *Rhizoma curcumae*, *Radix paeoniae rubra*, *Sarcandra glabra*, *Rhizoma smilacis glabrae*, and *Fructus mume*. Currently, PSORI-CM02 formula is further undergoing a randomized, double-blinded and placebo-controlled clinical trial for treating stable psoriasis vulgaris with a syndrome pattern of blood stasis in our hospital.

The objective of our current work was to reveal the antiproliferative properties of PSORI-CM02 in human HaCaT cells *in vitro* and the therapeutic effects of PSORI-CM02 on imiquimod-induced murine psoriasis as well as its mechanisms of action. We found that PSORI-CM02 suppressed HaCaT cell proliferation by hindering their cell cycle progression at G1 phase, inhibited the expression of proinflammatory cytokines and NF-κB signaling, upregulated CD4+ Foxp3+ regulatory T cells (Tregs) *in vivo* and promoted their *in vitro* expansion as well while reducing IL-17 production and ameliorating murine psoriasis.

TABLE 1 | Constituents of PSORI-CM02.

Linnean classification	Botanical origin	Ratio
Curcumae Rhizoma	*Curcuma kwangsuensis* S.G. Lee et C.F. Liang	2
Radix Paeoniae Rubra	*Paeonia lactiflora* Pall.	3
Rhizoma Smilacis Glabrae	*Smilax glabra* Roxb.	5
Mume Fructus	*Prunus mume.* (Sieb.)Sieb.etZucc.	2
Sarcand Raeherba	*Sarcandra glabra* (Thunb.)Nakai	5

MATERIALS AND METHODS

Animals

BALB/c mice (male, weighing 20 ± 2 g) were purchased from the Center of Laboratory Animals of Southern Medical University (Guangzhou, China). Mice were housed in a standard housing room with controlled temperature (22 ± 2°C), relative humidity (45–55%), artificial light (12 h light/dark cycle), and provided free access to food and water under a specific pathogen-free environment. The animal protocols were approved by the Animal Experimental Ethics Committee of Guangdong Provincial Hospital of Chinese Medicine.

Chemicals

Minimal essential medium (MEM), fetal bovine serum (FBS), and antibiotics (penicillin–streptomycin) were purchased from Gibco (Carlsbad, CA, USA). Dexamethasone acetate (DXM) was obtained from Shanghai Xinyi Pharmaceutical Factory (Shanghai, China). Imiquimod cream was obtained from Sichuan Mingxin Pharmaceutical Co., Ltd. (Sichuan, China). Eighteen chemical standards, including citric acid, gallic acid, 5-hydroxymethylfurfural, protocatechuic acid, Quercitrin, were obtained from Shanghai Aladdin Biological Technology Co., Ltd. (Shanghai, China) or Sigma-Aldrich (St. Louis, MO, USA).

Preparation of PSORI-CM02

Five Chinese herbal components (**Table 1**) contained in PSORI-CM02 formula were purchased from Guangdong Kangmei Pharmaceutical Company Ltd. (Guangdong, China). These herbs were extracted using distilled water and the extract was concentrated and stored for the future study.

Ultrahigh-Performance Liquid Chromatography (UHPLC) Analysis

Different batches of PSORI-CM02 formula were monitored for quality control purposes by UHPLC method. Briefly, PSORI-CM02 and 18 standards (**Table 2**) were dissolved with methanol–0.1%

TABLE 2 | Eighteen chemical constituents identified in PSORI-CM02.

Peak number	Formula	Identification
1	$C_6H_8O_7$	Citric acid
2	$C_7H_6O_5$	Gallic acid
3	$C_6H_6O_3$	5-Hydroxymethylfurfural
4	$C_7H_6O_4$	Protocatechuic acid
5	$C_{16}H_{18}O_9$	Neochlorogenic acid
6	$C_{23}H_{28}O_{12}$	Oxypaeoniflorin
7	$C_{20}H_{27}NO_{11}$	Amygdalin
8	$C_{16}H_{18}O_9$	Chlorogenic acid
9	$C_9H_8O_3$	p-Coumaric acid
10	$C_{16}H_{16}O_8$	5-O-caffeoylshikimic acid
11	$C_{11}H_{10}O_5$	Isofraxidin
12	$C_{21}H_{22}O_{11}$	Neoastilbin
13	$C_{21}H_{22}O_{11}$	Astilbin
14	$C_{21}H_{22}O_{11}$	Neoisoastilbin
15	$C_{21}H_{22}O_{11}$	Isoastilbin
16	$C_{21}H_{22}O_{10}$	Engeletin
17	$C_{18}H_{16}O_8$	Rosmarinic acid
18	$C_{21}H_{20}O_{11}$	Quercitrin

formic acid. Chromatographic separation was carried out with an Accela™ UHPLC system, which was comprised of a UHPLC pump and a PDA detector with a scanning from 200 to 400 nm and recorded at 214 nm. The HPLC conditions were set as following: Column: Kintex® C18, 150 mm × 2.1 mm, 2.6 µm particle size (Phenomenax, USA); Mobile phase components: A was water with 0.1% formic acid and B was methanol; Flow rate: 250 µL/min; injection volume: 10 µL; gradient: 0–45 min, linear gradient of 10–35% A, 45–50 min, 35–46% A, 50–60 min, 46–85% A.

Cell Culture

HaCaT cell line was purchased from American Type Culture Collection (Manassas, VA, USA). HaCaT cells were cultured in MEM (Gibico, USA) medium with 10% FBS (Gibico, USA) and 100 mg/mL and 100 IU/mL penicillin/streptomycin in a humidified atmosphere (5% CO_2, 37°C).

HaCaT Cell Proliferation Assays *In Vitro*

In vitro HaCaT cell proliferation was measured using MTT assays. Briefly, HaCaT cells in logarithmic growth were collected and transferred into a 96-well microplate. After 24 h, PSORI-CM02 was added to each well to make various concentrations (125, 250, 500, and 1,000 µg/mL, respectively) with six replicate wells *per* concentration. After further incubation for 24, 48, and 72 h, 10 µL of 5 mg/mL MTT was added to each well and incubated at 37°C for an additional 4 h. The supernatant then was removed and 100 µL of DMSO was added into each well. The absorbance (A value) was measured at the wavelength of 490 nm. The cell proliferation was presented as an OD value.

Cell Cycle Analysis

HaCaT cells were placed into six-well plates at 1.0×10^6 cells/well and treated with various concentrations of PSORI-CM02 (125, 250, and 500 µg/mL) for 72 h. The cells were collected, rinsed twice with ice cold PBS and then fixed in 70% ethanol at 4°C overnight. The cells then were subject to a 30-min incubation with 250 µl of RNase A (100 µg/ml) at 37°C and propidium iodide (50 µg/ml, 500 µl) staining for 1 h. Stained cells finally were analyzed *via* a FACS-Calibur flow cytometer (BD Biosciences, San Jose, CA, USA). Three independent experiments were carried out.

Administration of Drugs

BALB/c mice were randomly grouped into six groups (n = 6 *per* group). The control groups were normal mice that were totally untreated. Vehicle and treatment groups, but not control groups, were given topical administration of imiquimod cream to induce psoriasis. Vehicle groups were administrated with distilled water while treatment groups of the mice were orally given DXM (10 mg/kg) or PSORI-CM02 (3, 6, and 12 g/kg, respectively), which was dissolved in distilled water, for a period of seven days. For *in vitro* experiments, control groups were the untreated cells in the media.

Imiquimod-Induced Psoriasis-Like Mouse Model

According to our previous studies, mice were topically administrated with a dose of 62.5 mg of 5% imiquimod cream applied to a shaved area (3 cm × 2.5 cm) on their back for seven consecutive days. The psoriasis area and severity index (PASI), which comprised parameters for skin erythema, scaling, and thickness, was employed to assess the condition of the psoriasis-like lesion on day 7. Parameters were scored independently on a scale from 0 to 4 according to the clinical signs, in which "0" represents none; "1" denotes slight; "2" means moderate; "3" depicts marked; and "4" indicates very marked clinically.

Measurement of Mouse Temperature by Infrared Thermal Image

The temperature of mice in each group was determined by the infrared thermal imager (Fluke, USA) in a quiet-state mode and photographs were analyzed by Smart View 3.2 software. Mice were then euthanized and blood samples were collected in the absence of anticoagulants and subjected to centrifugation (3,000 rpm) for 10 min to obtain serum for biochemical analyses.

Histological Analysis

The dorsal skin of the mice was harvested, fixed in 4% paraformaldehyde in PBS, and embedded in paraffin. Sections (5 µm) were then made and stained with hematoxylin and eosin (H&E) for histological analysis.

Measurements of Glutathione (GSH), Superoxide Dismutase (SOD), Catalase (CAT), and Malonaldehyde (MDA)

Skin tissues were homogenized in Tris-buffer (20 mM, pH 7.5) on ice using Ultra Turraks Homogenizer (IKA, Germany) and were subject to centrifugation (12, 000 rpm) at 4°C for 10 min. The supernatant was used to measure CAT and SOD activities and GSH and MDA levels. The protein concentration was measured using the Bradford method with BSA serving as a standard. The CAT and SOD activities and GSH and MDA levels were analyzed using commercial assay kits following the manufacturer's instructions (Jiancheng Company, Nanjing, China).

Measurements of TNF-α, IL-6, and IL-17 *via* Enzyme-linked Immunosorbent Assay (ELISA) and RT-PCR

To evaluate the serum levels of TNF-α, IL-6, and IL-17, commercially available ELISA kits (eBioscience, USA) were utilized based on the instructions. The absorbance was read at 450 nm with a microplate spectrophotometer (Multiskan GO, Thermo Fisher Scientific, USA). Total mRNA was extracted from skin tissue with Trizol reagents and mRNA was then transcribed to cDNA. The primer sequences were shown in **Table 3**. The relative mRNA expression levels of cytokines versus GAPDH were measured using an ABI 7500 Fast Real-Time PCR System (Thermo Fisher Scientific, USA).

Western Blotting Analysis

Total protein samples from skin lesion tissues were acquired with RIPA lysis buffer followed by centrifugation (12,000 rpm and 5 min) in 4°C. Protein samples were subject to fractionation by SDS-PAGE and electro-transferred to PVD membranes. The

TABLE 3 | Primer sequences of target genes.

Target gene	Primer sequence (5′ → 3′)
TNF-α (forward)	ACTGATGAGAGGGAGGCCAT
TNF-α (reverse)	CCGTGGGTTGGACAGATGAA
IL-6 (forward)	TTCTTGGGACTGATGCTGGT
IL-6 (reverse)	CCTCCGACTTGTGAAGTGGT
IL-17 (forward)	TCAAAGCTCAGCGTGTCCAA
IL-17 (reverse)	TCTTCATTGCGGTGGAGAGTC
GAPDH (forward)	CAGGTTGTCTCCTGCGACTT
GAPDH (reverse)	TATGGGGGTCTGGGATGGAA

membranes were then blocked with 5% (w/v) skim milk in TBS-T containing 0.1% Tween-20 at room temperature for 2 h and subsequently incubated with primary antibody at 4°C overnight. Then, the membranes were washed three times using TBS-T and blotted with a corresponding secondary antibody conjugated with horseradish peroxidase for 1 h. Finally, the protein bands were detected using the enhanced chemiluminescence detection reagents. The band intensity was quantified using Image J software (NIH Image, Bethesda, MD, USA).

CD4+ Foxp3+ Treg Quantification

Lymph node and spleen cells from mice were prepared after treatments with PSORI-CM02. Cells were stained for surface markers with anti-CD4-PE/CD25-FITC Abs and then an intracellular marker with anti-Foxp3-APC using intracellular fixation/permeabilization kit (eBioscience, San Diego, CA, USA). CD4+ Foxp3 Tregs were analyzed using a FACSCalibur (BD, Biosciences). Since we found that only ~94% of CD4+ CD25+ T cells were FoxP3-positive (Figure S1 in Supplementary Material) in imiquimod-induced psoriatic mice, we quantified CD4+ FoxP3+ rather than CD4+ CD25+ cell population and defined the former as Tregs.

CD4+ CD25+ Treg Proliferation *In Vitro*

Splenic cells of C57BL/6J were harvested and CD4+ CD25+ T cells were purified by high-speed cell sorting *via* a FACSAria III (BD Biosciences). The purity of the cells was typically >96%. Then, the purified Tregs were labeled with 2 μM CFSE dye (Invitrogen, Karlsruhe, Germany) at 37°C for 10 min, and cultured in 96-well plates (2×10^5 cells/well) coated with anti-CD3/anti-CD28 Abs in complete RPMI-1640 media. PSORI-CM02 (125, 250, and 500 μg/mL) was also added to the medium. After culturing for 4 days, cell proliferation was analyzed *via* FACS analyses.

Statistical Analysis

The data were statistically evaluated by a one-way analysis of variance followed by Dunnett's test and denoted as mean values ± SDs. Statistically significant differences were identified as either $P < 0.05$ or $P < 0.01$. All analyses were carried out through SPSS software (version 17.0, SPSS Inc., Chicago, IL, USA).

RESULTS

Chemical Profiles of PSORI-CM02

In order to control the quality of PSORI-CM02, we mainly detected eighteen chemical compositions of PSORI-CM02 by UHPLC analysis: citric acid, gallic acid, 5-hydroxymethylfurfural, protocatechuic acid, and so on (**Table 2**). UHPLC profiling also showed that PSORI-CM02 did not contain rapamycin and cyclosporine (Figure S2 in Supplementary Material).

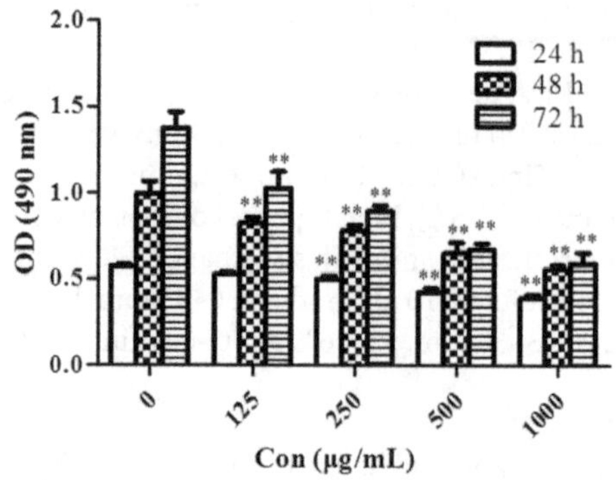

FIGURE 1 | PSORI-CM02 suppresses HaCaT cell proliferation. The proliferation of HaCaT cells *in vitro* was measured *via* MTT assays 24, 48, and 72 h after the cell culture. Data are shown as the mean values ± SDs ($n = 6$, *$P < 0.05$ and **$P < 0.01$ vs. the control group: concentration of 0 μg/ml). The results suggested that PSORI-CM02 suppressed HaCaT cell proliferation in a dose-dependent manner.

PSORI-CM02 Inhibits the Growth of HaCaT Cells

MTT assay was performed to evaluate the antiproliferative effects of PSORI-CM02 on HaCaT cells *in vitro*. As shown in **Figure 1**, PSORI-CM02 at various concentrations ranging from 125 to 1,000 μg/mL significantly suppressed HaCaT cell proliferation at all time points (24, 48, and 72 h) in a dose-dependent manner.

PSORI-CM02 Induces Cell Cycle Arrest in HaCaT Cells

Since cell cycle progression plays an essential role in cell proliferation, flow cytometry was employed to investigate cell cycle distribution in HaCaT cells after treatments of the cells with PSORI-CM02. As shown in **Figures 2A,B**, there was no significant difference in HaCaT cell cycle progression at all phases between the group treated with low concentration of PSORI-CM02 (L) and control group. Augmenting PSORI-CM02 concentration to 250 (M) or 500 (H) μg/mL increased the frequency of the cells at G1 phase while reducing their percentage at S phase. Taken together, these studies revealed that PSORI-CM02 formula induced HaCaT cell cycle arrest at G1 phase in a dose-dependent manner.

PSORI-CM02 Alleviates Clinical Symptoms and Reduces Skin Temperature of Imiquimod-Induced Psoriatic Mice

Imiquimod-induced psoriasis-like mouse models were utilized to evaluate the antipsoriatic effects of PSORI-CM02. After treatments with imiquimod cream for three days, the clinical signs of psoriasis-like lesions, including skin erythema, scaling,

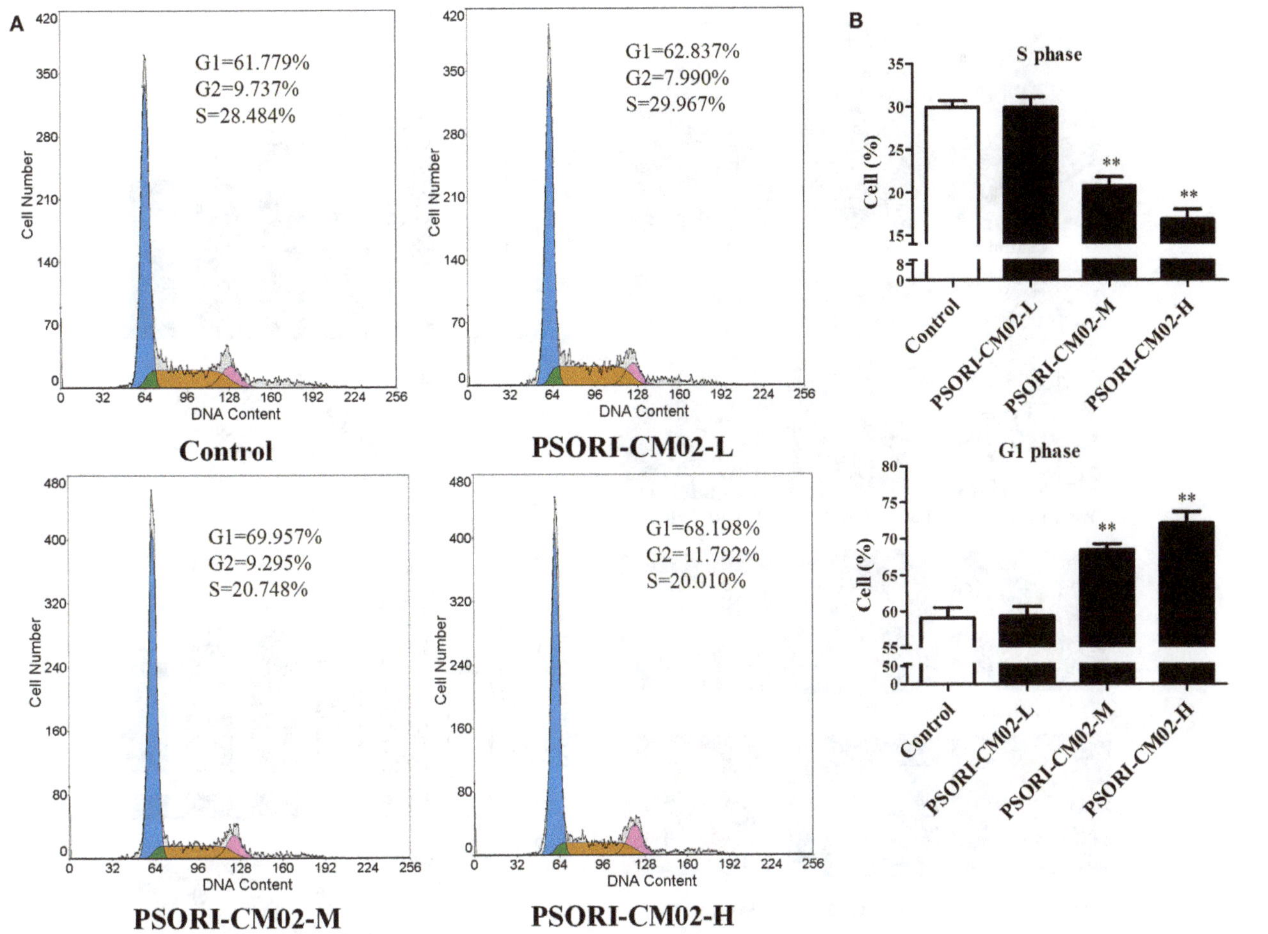

FIGURE 2 | PSORI-CM02 hinders HaCaT cell cycle progression. The cell cycles of HaCaT cells treated with PSORI-CM02 for 72 h were analyzed through flow cytometry using PI staining **(A)**. Histograms exhibited cell cycle distributions (%) in HaCaT cells **(B)**. Results represented the average proportions of S and G1 phases. Data are shown as the mean values ± SDs (n = 3, *P < 0.05 and **P < 0.01 vs. control group).

and thickness, appeared on the shaved dorsal skin, indicating that imiquimod-induced psoriasis-like mouse models were established successfully. Seven days after treatments with PSORI-CM02 or DXM, overall skin lesions were reduced and average PASI scores were decreased significantly compared with the vehicle group, as shown in **Figure 3A**. Mice treated with high doses of PSORI-CM02 appeared to be healthy except for mild psoriatic skin lesions. Histology demonstrated no liver and kidney injury in these mice (data not shown), suggesting that PSORI-CM02 is not toxic.

Since temperature assessment is one of the important indexes in inflammation, lesion temperature was measured in this study. As shown in **Figure 3B**, the psoriasis-like lesion temperature was increased significantly (P < 0.01 vs. control group) seven days following administration of imiquimod cream while PSORI-CM02 treatments lowered the temperature remarkably compared to the vehicle group.

Histological Evaluations

Histological examinations *via* H&E staining were performed on the lesion skin seven days after treatments with PSORI-CM02. As depicted in **Figure 3C**, we found significant pathological changes characterized by increased acanthosis, hyperkeratosis of the epidermis, and abundant inflammatory infiltrates in the skin of imiquimod-induced psoriatic mice. Treatments with either DXM or PSORI-CM02 ameliorated the histological skin lesions, resulting in smoother epidermis, less parakeratosis, and reduced epidermal thickening.

Effects of PSORI-CM02 on Antioxidative/Oxidative Levels of SOD, GSH, CAT, and MDA

In this study, SOD, GSH, CAT, and MDA levels in the skin were measured by the corresponding assay kits seven days after treatments. As shown in **Figures 4A–D**, imiquimod-induced psoriatic mice produced lower levels of CAT, GSH, and SOD, but a higher level of MDA than did control mice. However, upon treatments with PSORI-CM02 at medium or high doses, the antioxidative activities of GSH, CAT, and SOD were elevated significantly (P < 0.05 and P < 0.01, respectively) compared to the vehicle group. Furthermore, PSORI-CM02 at the doses of 6 and 12 g/kg were shown to obviously reduce an MDA level in the skin

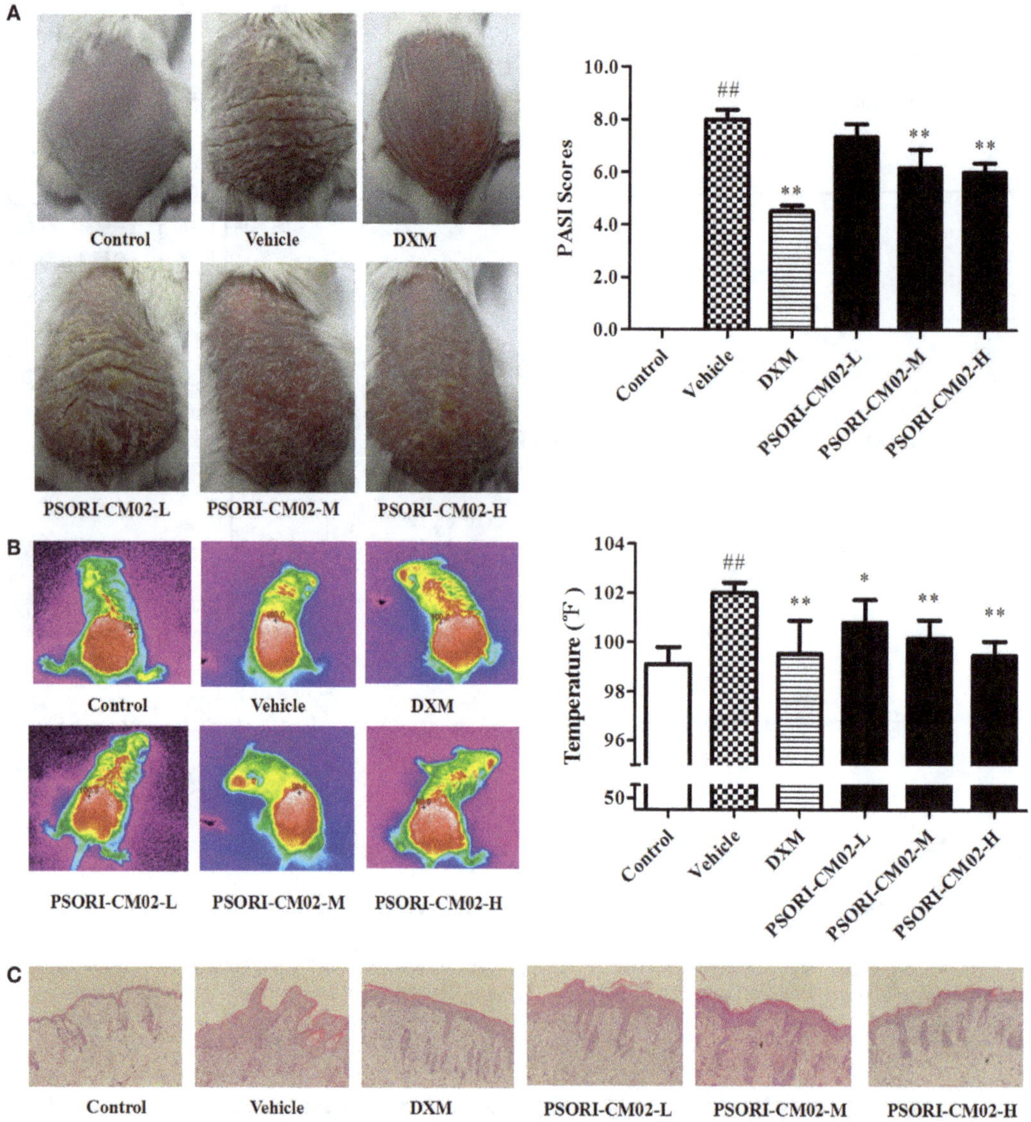

FIGURE 3 | PSORI-CM02 ameliorates murine psoriasis. Shown are macroscopic appearance and the psoriasis area and severity index (PASI) scores of the skin lesions **(A)**, the infrared thermal image of the skin tissue **(B)**, and histological evaluation of the skin tissue *via* H&E staining (magnification 100×) **(C)** in imiquimod-induced psoriasis-like mice treated without or with PSORI-CM02. Data are presented as the mean values ± SDs (n = 6, $^{\#}P < 0.05$ and $^{\#\#}P < 0.01$ vs. control group, $^{*}P < 0.05$ and $^{**}P < 0.01$ vs. vehicle group).

tissue (both $P < 0.01$). These results suggested that PSORI-CM02 effectively regulated the oxidative/antioxidative balance toward a more favorable physiological equilibrium in imiquimod-induced psoriatic mice.

PSORI-CM02 Suppresses mRNA and Protein Expressions of Proinflammatory Cytokines in Imiquimod-Treated Psoriatic Mice

Effects of PSORI-CM02 on proinflammatory cytokine expression were also observed *via* ELISA and RT-PCR seven days after PSORI-CM02 treatment. As shown in **Figures 4E–G**, the levels of TNF-α, IL-6, and IL-17 in serum in imiquimod-induced psoriatic mice (vehicle) were increased compared to the control group. Although low doses of PSORI-CM02 did not achieve statistical significance, PSORI-CM02 at medium and high doses significantly reduced the levels of proinflammatory cytokines TNF-α, IL-6, and IL-17 in the serum compared to the vehicle group.

The mRNA expressions of TNF-α, IL-6, and IL-17 in skin tissue were also determined using RT-PCR. As shown in **Figures 4H–J**, the mRNA expressions of TNF-α, IL-6, and IL-17 were augmented after treatments with imiquimod (vehicle) while administration

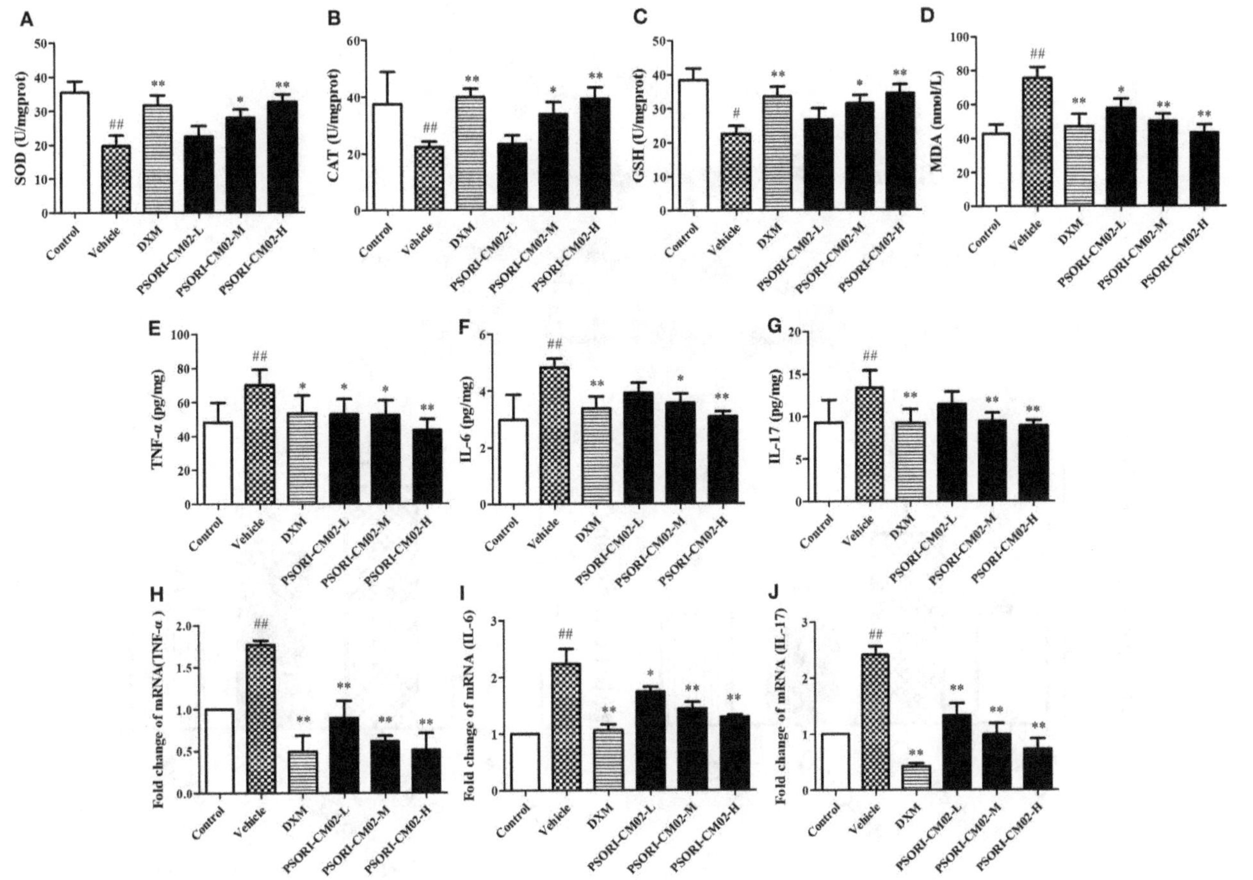

FIGURE 4 | PSORI-CM02 alters oxidative and antioxidative balance and suppresses proinflammatory cytokine expression. Effects of PSORI-CM02 on the activities of superoxide dismutase **(A)**, catalase **(B)**, glutathione **(C)**, and malonaldehyde **(D)** in homogenized skin were determined using enzymatic activity assay kits while the levels of TNF-α **(E)**, interleukin (IL)-6 **(F)**, and IL-17 **(G)** in the serum of imiquimod-induced psoriasis-like mice were evaluated by enzyme-linked immunosorbent assay kits 7 days after PSORI-CM02 treatments. The mRNA levels of TNF-α **(H)**, IL-6 **(I)**, and IL-17 **(J)** in the skin were also determined using RT-PCR. Data shown are the mean values ± SDs ($n = 6$, #$P < 0.05$ and ##$P < 0.01$ vs. control group, *$P < 0.05$ and **$P < 0.01$ vs. vehicle group).

of PSORI-CM02 at all three doses downregulated the mRNA levels of these cytokines compared with imiquimod-treated group without PSORI-CM02 (vehicle).

PSORI-CM02 Inhibits NF-κB Signaling in the Skin with Psoriasis-Like Lesions

Since PSORI-CM02 suppressed proinflammatory cytokine expression, we further explored the mechanisms underlying its antipsoriatic or anti-inflammatory effects. NF-κB signaling is a prominent therapeutic target for treating inflammatory diseases since aberrantly activated NF-κB signaling pathway contributes to inflammatory skin disorders. Thus, western blotting analysis was performed to evaluate the effects of PSORI-CM02 on NF-κB signaling pathway involving protein expression of NF-κB (P65) and IKKα. As shown in **Figure 5**, the expression of NF-κB and IKKα markedly increased after treatments with imiquimod compared to control group. In contrast, treatments with PSORI-CM02 markedly suppressed the expression of NF-κB and IKKα ($P < 0.05$ and $P < 0.01$, respectively) compared to the vehicle group.

PSORI-CM02 Upregulates CD4+ Foxp3+ Tregs in Psoriatic Mice

Regulatory T cells, a small subset of T cells, play an important role in preventing autoimmune diseases, including psoriasis. Therefore, we determined the frequency of Tregs in lymph nodes and spleens of psoriasis-like mice using FACS analyses seven days after treatments with PSORI-CM02, and the results were displayed in **Figure 6**. Treatments with either medium or high doses of PSORI-CM02 significantly augmented the frequency of CD4+ Foxp3+ Tregs in both lymph nodes and spleens compared with the vehicle group, although low doses of PSORI-CM02 only slightly increased the proportion of the Tregs.

PSORI-CM02 Promotes CD4+ CD25+ Treg Cell Proliferation *In Vitro*

Given that PSORI-CM02 could upregulate the frequency of CD4+ Foxp3+ Tregs in imuquimod-induced psoriatic mice *in vivo*, we determined its effects on Treg cell proliferation *in vitro*. FACS-sorted CD4+ CD25+ Tregs derived from naïve mice were labeled

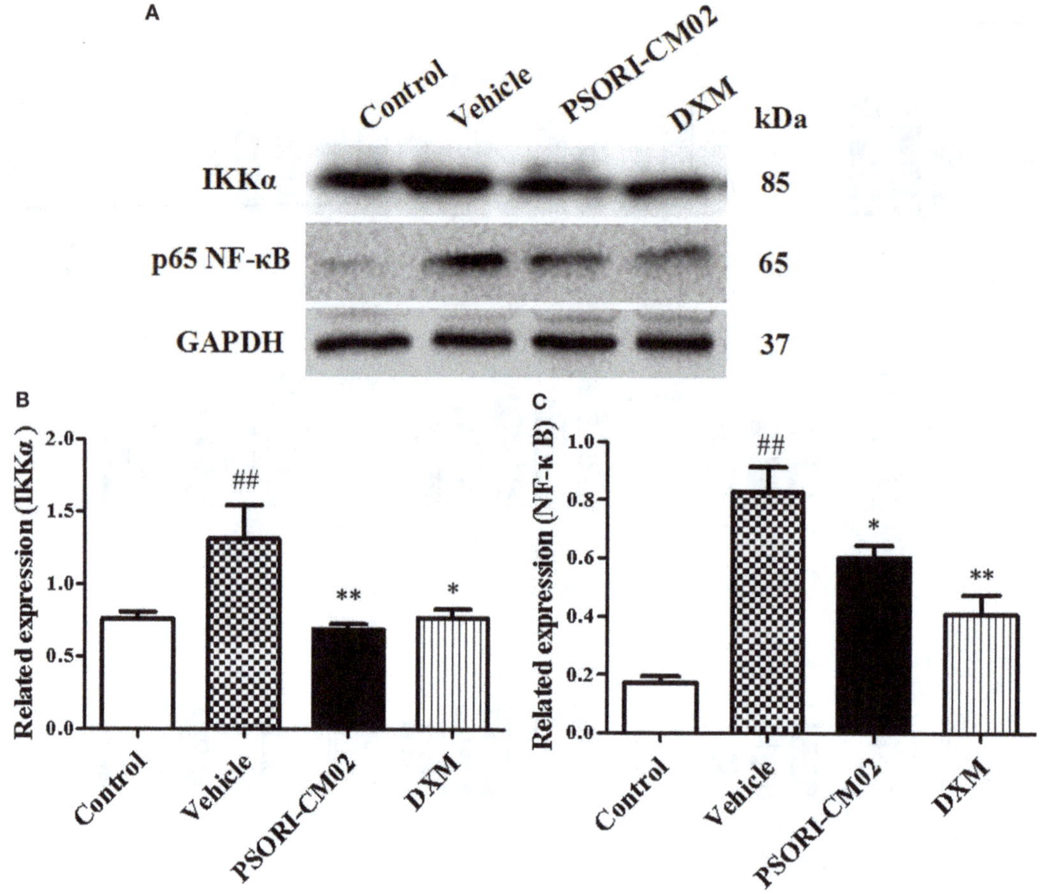

FIGURE 5 | PSORI-CM02 inhibits NF-κB expression in the skin of imiquimod (IMQ)-induced psoriasis-like mice. Impacts of PSORI-CM02 on protein expressions of IKKα and p-65 NF-κB in skin tissue of IMQ-induced psoriasis-like mice were determined using Western blotting analyses seven days after PSORI-CM02 treatments. The expression of IKKα or NF-κB was detected using Western blotting **(A)**. The densitometry analyses of the immunoblotting are shown for IKK **(B)** and NF-κB **(C)**. Data shown are the mean values ± SDs ($n = 3$, $^{\#}P < 0.05$ and $^{\#\#}P < 0.01$ vs. control group, $^{*}P < 0.05$ and $^{**}P < 0.01$ vs. vehicle group).

with CFSE and stimulated with anti-CD3 and anti-CD28 Abs in the absence or presence of PSORI-CM02 for 4 days. As shown in **Figure 7**, PSORI-CM02 significantly promoted CD4+ CD25+ Treg cell proliferation compared to the control group, suggesting that it can also expand Tregs *in vitro*.

DISCUSSION

Psoriasis is known as a chronic inflammatory dermatologic disease that affects around 2–3% of the general population (11). Although the causes for psoriasis are not fully understood, its most important pathological features include irregular epidermal hyperplasia, inflammatory infiltration and hyperplastic dermal blood vessels (12). Natural herbal medicine has been verified to be effective in preventing and treating psoriasis by attenuating aberrant proliferation and differentiation of keratinocytes (13, 14) and exerting anti-inflammatory, immunoregulatory (15, 16) and antiangiogenic effects (17). PSORI-CM02 formula is generally used for treating psoriasis in Guangdong Provincial Hospital of Chinese Medicine and has been registered (registration number: ChiCTR-IOR-15006768) for a randomized, double-blinded and placebo-controlled clinical trial. In this study, we endeavored to confirm the therapeutic effects of PSORI-CM02 formula in imiquimod-induced psoriasis-like mice and unravel its possible mechanisms of action *in vivo* as well as its antiproliferative property in HaCaT cells *in vitro*.

It is well known that cell cycle progression mediates cell growth and proliferation and that cell cycle arrest can trigger inhibition of cell proliferation and growth (18, 19). In the current study, the effects of PSORI-CM02 on cell cycle progression was analyzed using flow cytometry, and our results indicated that PSORI-CM02 suppressed HaCaT cell growth by arresting them at the G1 phase (**Figure 2B**), suggesting that PSORI-CM02 formula may attenuate imiquimod-induced murine psoriasis by inhibiting HaCaT cell growth.

It has been reported that repeatedly topical use of imiquimod in mice results in the influx of various immune cells and hyperplasia of the epidermis, generating a widely used murine model of psoriasis (20). In our study, we established the same model of imiquimod-induced psoriasis and observed that PSORI-CM02

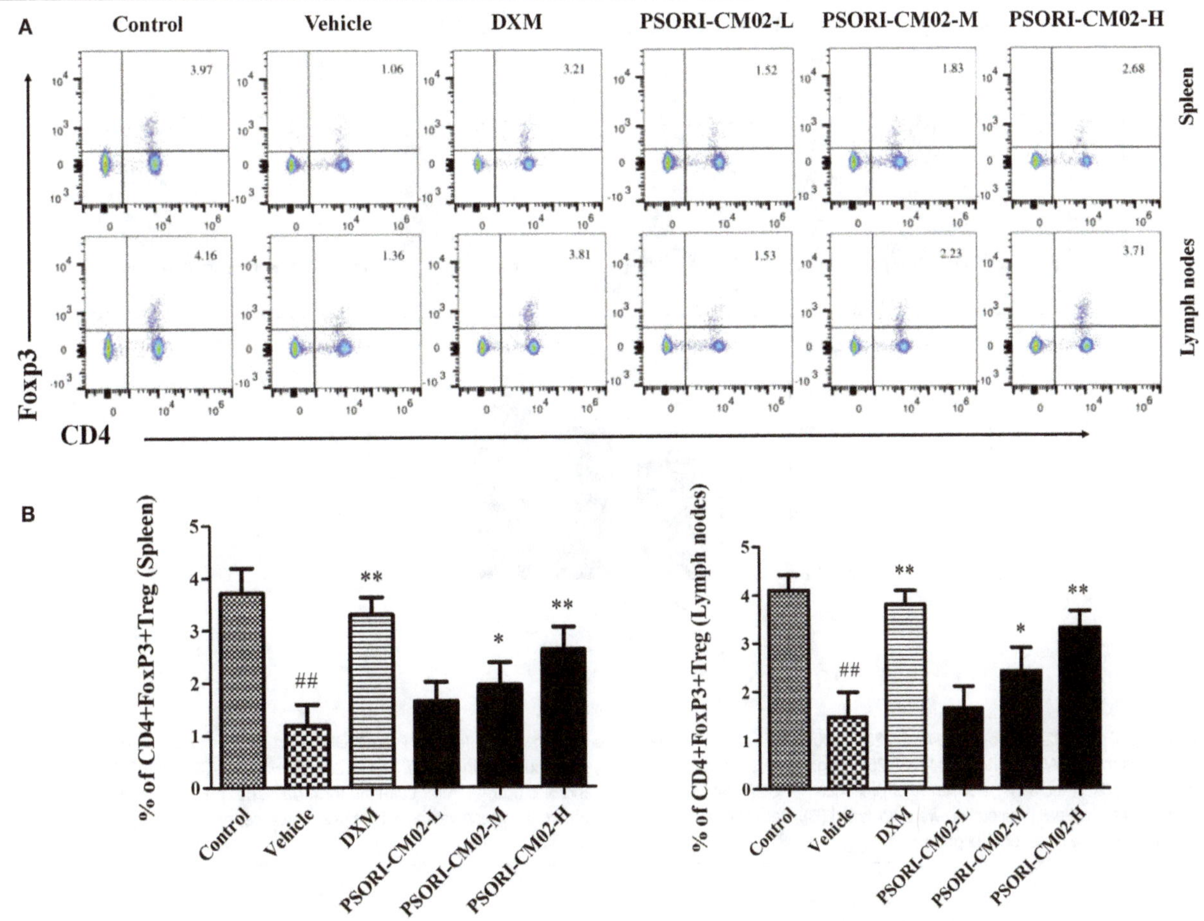

FIGURE 6 | PSORI-CM02 induces CD4+ Foxp3+ regulatory T cells (Tregs) in imiquimod (IMQ)-induced psoriasis-like mice. Effects of PSORI-CM02 on CD4+ Foxp3+ Treg frequency in spleens and lymph nodes of IMQ-induced psoriasis-like mice were observed. Spleen and lymph node cells were isolated from IMQ-induced psoriasis-like mice seven days after treatments with PSORI-CM02 or dexamethasone acetate (DXM). To quantify CD4+ Foxp3+ Tregs, cells were stained for CD4 surface and intracellular Foxp3 makers **(A)** and CD4+ Foxp3+ Treg frequency in spleen and lymph node were shown **(B)**. Data shown are the mean values ± SDs (n = 3. $^{\#}P < 0.05$ and $^{\#\#}P < 0.01$ vs. control group, $^{*}P < 0.05$ and $^{**}P < 0.01$ vs. vehicle group).

significantly lowered the PASI scores, reduced inflammatory skin temperature, and decreased the epidermal hyperplasia and epidermal thickening compared to the vehicle group, indicating that PSORI-CM02 ameliorates imiquimod-induced murine psoriasis.

We also attempted to reveal the mechanisms underlying the therapeutic effects of PSORI-CM02 on psoriasis. Production of reactive oxygen species (ROS) and weakened antioxidant system take a vital part in the pathogenesis and development of this intractable disease (21). Increased ROS production primarily affects the essential molecules in cells, such as DNA, lipid, protein, and carbohydrate. A balance between antioxidants, including SOD, CAT, and GSH, and oxidants, such as MDA, in normal skin is maintained. Malfunction of the antioxidative system and an increased production of ROS may result in skin diseases, including psoriasis (22–24). In our study, the anti-oxidative activities of SOD, CAT, and GSH were much lower in imiquimod-treated psoriatic skin than in normal skin whereas the level of oxidative MDA in the psoriatic skin was increased compared to that in the normal skin, which was consistent with the oxidative/antioxidative case of patients with psoriasis (25, 26). Treatments with PSORI-CM02 significantly increased the activities of these antioxidants, including SOD, CAT, and GSH, while decreasing the level of oxidant MDA. Therefore, PSORI-CM02 likely possesses a significant antioxidative feature, resulting in reduced free radical stress and subdued oxidative damage.

Excessive proinflammatory cytokines, such as TNF-α and IL-6, play a key role in the pathogenesis and progress of psoriasis. TNF-α released by multiple types of cells, including activated macrophages, dendritic cells, Th1/Th17 cells, cytotoxic T cells and adipocytes (27, 28), in the serum of patients with psoriasis is essential for the progression of psoriasis (29). It not only activates dendritic cells *via* NF-κB signaling, but also induces expression of adhesion molecules, angiogenic VEGF and other proinflammatory cytokines (30, 31), leading to cell proliferation and inflammation. On the other hand, IL-6 recruits neutrophils (32) and promotes the proliferation of keratinocytes in

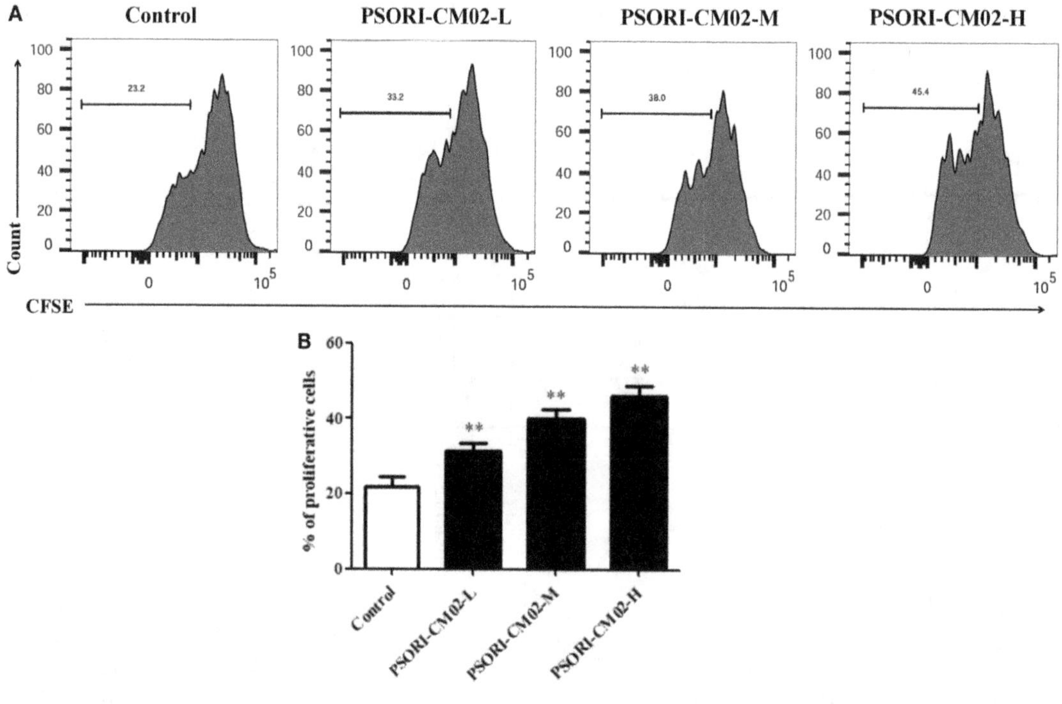

FIGURE 7 | PSORI-CM02 promotes CD4+ CD25+ regulatory T cell (Treg) cell proliferation *in vitro*. Effects of PSORI-CM02 on CD4+ CD25+ Treg cell proliferation *in vitro* were observed. FACS-sorted CD4+ CD25+ Tregs were labeled with CFSE dye and cultured in 96-well plates coated with anti-CD3/anti-CD28 Abs in complete RPMI-1640 media in the absence or presence of PSORI-CM02 (125, 250, and 500 µg/mL). After culturing for 4 days, cell proliferation was analyzed *via* FACS analyses **(A)** and cell proliferation were analyzed **(B)**. Data shown in the bar graph are the mean values ± SDs from three separate experiments (n = 3. $^{*}P < 0.05$ and $^{**}P < 0.01$ vs. control group).

imiquimod-induced psoriasis-like murine skin (33). In the serum of patients with psoriasis, the level of IL-6 is highly elevated (34). Thus, anti-IL-6 mAb has been proposed to be a novel therapeutic option for the treatment of psoriasis (35).

IL-23/IL-17 axis plays a central role in the development of various autoimmune diseases, including human psoriasis and imiquimod-induced murine psoriasis (20, 36). The number of IL-17-producing cells is elevated in mice topically administered with imiquimod (20, 37, 38). Th17 cells are proposed to be a cardinal source of IL-17 family cytokines, and IL-17 has been deemed as a critical cytokine for the establishment and maintenance of the psoriatic phenotype (39). It promotes inflammation *via* binding the receptor located on keratinocytes, dendritic cells, dermal fibroblasts, and endothelial cells (40). Our results also indicate that PSORI-CM02 ameliorates murine psoriasis by reducing IL-17 production.

NF-κB is a key inflammatory signaling pathway and a critical contributor mediating the pathogenesis and progression of psoriasis (41, 42). NF-κB signaling alters functional states of keratinocytes and immune cells *via* exerting its effects on cellular proliferation, differentiation and apoptosis as well as cytokine and chemokine production (39). When keratinocytes are stimulated with TNF-α, their NF-κB signaling pathway is activated, resulting in the overexpression and release of various proinflammatory cytokines, chemokines and enzymes (43). In our present work, we found that PSORI-CM02 significantly suppressed the expression of NF-κB and IKKα in the skin of imiquimod-simulated psoriatic mice. Thus, PSORI-CM02 exerted its therapeutic effects on murine psoriasis by inhibiting NF-κB signaling pathway.

It has been reported that the imbalance between Tregs and Th17 cells is critical for the pathogenesis and development of psoriasis (44). Tregs are essential for the immune homeostasis and tolerance because of their capability of inhibiting the function of other immune cells and inflammatory responses (45). Therefore, we quantified CD4+ Foxp3+ Tregs in spleens and lymph nodes of psoriasis-like mice *in vivo* and determined the effects of PSORI-CM02 on CD4+ CD25+ Treg proliferation *in vitro*. Our results demonstrated that PSORI-CM02 upregulated the frequency of CD4+ Foxp3+ Tregs *in vivo* and promoted *in vitro* proliferation of CD4+ CD25+ Tregs as well, indicating that these Tregs play a role in attenuation of murine psoriasis by PSORI-CM02. On the other hand, previous studies by Di et al. demonstrated that astilbin ameliorated the inflammation in imiquimod-induced psoriasis-like mice *via* suppressing Th17 cell differentiation and IL-17 secretion (16). In our study, we found that astilbin was one of the main ingredients in PSORI-CM02 formula, and that PSORI-CM02 could inhibit the expression and production of IL-17, which was partially consistent with their studies on astilbin. However, we found that PSORI-CM02 also increased Tregs *in vitro* and *in vivo* and suppressed the expression of NF-κB and IKKα. PSORI-CM02 formula was composed of numerous chemical compositions with 18 major compositions identified already. The therapeutic effect of PSORI-CM02 could be stronger than that of astilbin alone.

In conclusion, we demonstrated that PSORI-CM02 inhibited the keratinocyte proliferation through arresting HaCaT cells at G1 phase. In addition, we found that PSORI-CM02 effectively protected imiquimod-induced psoriasis-like mice from skin lesions by decreasing TNF-α, IL-6, and IL-17 levels, regulating the oxidant/antioxidant status, altering the balance between Th17 response and CD4+ Foxp3+ Treg generation, and inhibiting NF-κB signaling pathway.

ETHICS STATEMENT

This study was carried out in accordance with the recommendations of Chinese national guidelines and institutional review board of Guangdong Provincial Academy of Chinese Medical Sciences. The protocol was approved by the Institutional Animal Care and Use Committee of Guangdong Provincial Academy of Chinese Medical Sciences.

AUTHOR CONTRIBUTIONS

Conceived and designed the experiments: CL, ZD, and LH. Performed the experiments: HC, HL, MW, WY, and XL. Analyzed and interpreted the data: HC, YY, and HZ. Revised the data analysis and interpretation: HL and ZD. Wrote the article: HC, HL, and ZD. All authors have read and approved the manuscript.

REFERENCES

1. Chorachoo J, Saeloh D, Srichana T, Amnuaikit T, Musthafa KS, Sretrirutchai S, et al. Rhodomyrtone as a potential anti-proliferative and apoptosis inducing agent in HaCaT keratinocyte cells. *Eur J Pharmacol* (2016) 772:144–51. doi:10.1016/j.ejphar.2015.12.005
2. Tian S, Krueger JG, Li K, Jabbari A, Brodmerkel C, Lowes MA, et al. Meta-analysis derived (MAD) transcriptome of psoriasis defines the "core" pathogenesis of disease. *PLoS One* (2012) 7(9):e44274. doi:10.1371/journal.pone.0044274
3. Ryan C, Kirby B. Psoriasis is a systemic disease with multiple cardiovascular and metabolic comorbidities. *Dermatol Clin* (2015) 33(1):41–55. doi:10.1016/j.det.2014.09.004
4. Traub M, Marshall K. Psoriasis – pathophysiology, conventional, and alternative approaches to treatment. *Altern Med Rev* (2007) 12(4):319–30.
5. Feldman SR, Burudpakdee C, Gala S, Nanavaty M, Mallya UG. The economic burden of psoriasis: a systematic literature review. *Expert Rev Pharmacoecon Outcomes Res* (2014) 14(5):685–705. doi:10.1586/14737167.2014.933671
6. Vuorelaa P, Leinonenb M, Saikkuc P, Tammelaa P, Rauhad JP, Wennberge T, et al. Natural products in the process of finding new drug candidates. *Curr Med Chem* (2004) 11(11):1375–89. doi:10.2174/0929867043365116
7. Yu JJ, Zhang CS, Zhang AL, May B, Xue CC, Lu C. Add-on effect of Chinese herbal medicine bath to phototherapy for psoriasis vulgaris: a systematic review. *Evid Based Complement Alternat Med* (2013) 2013:673078. doi:10.1155/2013/673078
8. Zhang CS, Yu JJ, Parker S, Zhang AL, May B, Lu C, et al. Oral Chinese herbal medicine combined with pharmacotherapy for psoriasis vulgaris: a systematic review. *Int J Dermatol* (2014) 53(11):1305–18. doi:10.1111/ijd.12607
9. Yu JJ, Zhang CS, Coyle ME, Du Y, Zhang AL, Guo X, et al. Compound glycyrrhizin plus conventional therapy for psoriasis vulgaris: a systematic review and meta-analysis of randomized controlled trials. *Curr Med Res Opin* (2017) 33(2):279–87. doi:10.1080/03007995.2016.1254605
10. Zhang CS, May B, Yan Y, Yu JJ, Yao D, Chang S, et al. Terms referring to psoriasis vulgaris in the classical Chinese medicine literature: a systematic analysis. *Complement Ther Med* (2016) 25:55–60. doi:10.1016/j.ctim.2015.12.014
11. Nestle FO, Kaplan DH, Barker J. Psoriasis. *N Engl J Med* (2009) 361(5):496–509. doi:10.1056/NEJMra0804595
12. Xiao C, Zhu Z, Sun S, Gao J, Fu M, Liu Y, et al. Activation of Langerhans cells promotes the inflammation in imiquimod-induced psoriasis-like dermatitis. *J Dermatol Sci* (2017) 85(3):170–7. doi:10.1016/j.jdermsci.2016.12.003
13. Chen S, Han K, Li H, Cen J, Yang Y, Wu H, et al. Isogarcinol extracted from *Garcinia mangostana* L. ameliorates imiquimod-induced psoriasis-like skin lesions in mice. *J Agric Food Chem* (2017) 65(4):846–57. doi:10.1021/acs.jafc.6b05207
14. Tse WP, Che CT, Liu K, Lin ZX. Evaluation of the anti-proliferative properties of selected psoriasis-treating Chinese medicines on cultured HaCaT cells. *J Ethnopharmacol* (2006) 108(1):133–41. doi:10.1016/j.jep.2006.04.023
15. Zhang S, Liu X, Mei L, Wang H, Fang F. Epigallocatechin-3-gallate (EGCG) inhibits imiquimod-induced psoriasis-like inflammation of BALB/c mice. *BMC Complement Altern Med* (2016) 16(1):334. doi:10.1186/s12906-016-1325-4
16. Di TT, Ruan ZT, Zhao JX, Wang Y, Liu X, Wang Y, et al. Astilbin inhibits Th17 cell differentiation and ameliorates imiquimod-induced psoriasis-like skin lesions in BALB/c mice via Jak3/Stat3 signaling pathway. *Int Immunopharmacol* (2016) 32:32–8. doi:10.1016/j.intimp.2015.12.035
17. Wen J, Pei H, Wang X, Xie C, Li S, Huang L, et al. Gambogic acid exhibits anti-psoriatic efficacy through inhibition of angiogenesis and inflammation. *J Dermatol Sci* (2014) 74(3):242–50. doi:10.1016/j.jdermsci.2014.03.001
18. Pu L, Amoscato AA, Bier ME, Lazo JS. Dual G1 and G2 phase inhibition by a novel, selective Cdc25 inhibitor 6-chloro-7-[corrected](2-morpholin-4-ylethylamino)- quinoline-5,8-dione. *J Biol Chem* (2002) 277(49):46877–85. doi:10.1074/jbc.M207902200
19. Chao JI, Kuo PC, Hsu TS. Down-regulation of survivin in nitric oxide-induced cell growth inhibition and apoptosis of the human lung carcinoma cells. *J Biol Chem* (2004) 279(19):20267–76. doi:10.1074/jbc.M312381200
20. van der Fits L, Mourits S, Voerman JS, Kant M, Boon L, Laman JD, et al. Imiquimod-induced psoriasis-like skin inflammation in mice is mediated via the IL-23/IL-17 axis. *J Immunol* (2009) 182(9):5836–45. doi:10.4049/jimmunol.0802999
21. Popov I, Lewin G. A deficient function of the antioxidative system of the organism as an aetiopathogenetic factor in psoriasis. *Med Hypotheses* (1991) 35(3):229–36. doi:10.1016/0306-9877(91)90238-T
22. Zhou Q, Mrowietz U, Rostami-Yazdi M. Oxidative stress in the pathogenesis of psoriasis. *Free Radic Biol Med* (2009) 47(7):891–905. doi:10.1016/j.freeradbiomed.2009.06.033
23. Pastore S, Korkina L. Redox imbalance in T cell-mediated skin diseases. *Mediators Inflamm* (2010) 2010:861949. doi:10.1155/2010/861949
24. Geronikaki AA, Gavalas AM. Antioxidants and inflammatory disease: synthetic and natural antioxidants with anti-inflammatory activity. *Comb Chem High Throughput Screen* (2006) 9(6):425–42. doi:10.2174/138620706777698481
25. Baz K, Cimen MY, Kokturk A, Yazici AC, Eskandari G, Ikizoglu G, et al. Oxidant/ antioxidant status in patients with psoriasis. *Yonsei Med J* (2003) 44(6):987–90. doi:10.3349/ymj.2003.44.6.987
26. Pujari VM, Suryakar AN, Ireddy S. Oxidants and antioxidant status in psoriasis patients. *Biomed Res* (2010) 21(2):221–24.
27. Gottlieb AB, Chamian F, Masud S, Cardinale I, Abello MV, Lowes MA, et al. TNF inhibition rapidly down-regulates multiple proinflammatory pathways in psoriasis plaques. *J Immunol* (2005) 175(4):2721–9. doi:10.4049/jimmunol.175.4.2721

28. Aggarwal BB, Gupta SC, Sung B. Curcumin: an orally bioavailable blocker of TNF and other pro-inflammatory biomarkers. *Br J Pharmacol* (2013) 169(8):1672–92. doi:10.1111/bph.12131
29. Fantuzzi F, Del Giglio M, Gisondi P, Girolomoni G. Targeting tumor necrosis factor alpha in psoriasis and psoriatic arthritis. *Expert Opin Ther Targets* (2008) 12(9):1085–96. doi:10.1517/14728222.12.9.1085
30. Kupetsky EA, Mathers AR, Ferris LK. Anti-cytokine therapy in the treatment of psoriasis. *Cytokine* (2013) 61(3):704–12. doi:10.1016/j.cyto.2012.12.027
31. Bradley JR. TNF-mediated inflammatory disease. *J Pathol* (2008) 214(2): 149–60. doi:10.1002/path.2287
32. Fielding CA, McLoughlin RM, McLeod L, Colmont CS, Najdovska M, Grail D, et al. IL-6 regulates neutrophil trafficking during acute inflammation via STAT3. *J Immunol* (2008) 181(3):2189–95. doi:10.4049/jimmunol.181.3.2189
33. Grossman RM, Krueger J, Yourish D, Granelli-Piperno A, Murphy DP, May LT, et al. Interleukin 6 is expressed in high levels in psoriatic skin and stimulates proliferation of cultured human keratinocytes. *Proc Natl Acad Sci U S A* (1989) 86(16):6367–71. doi:10.1073/pnas.86.16.6367
34. Toruniowa B, Krasowska D, Koziol M, Ksiazek A, Pietrzak A. Serum levels of IL-6 in mycosis fungoides, psoriasis, and lichen planus. *Ann N Y Acad Sci* (1995) 762:432–4. doi:10.1111/j.1749-6632.1995.tb32358.x
35. Saggini A, Chimenti S, Chiricozzi A. IL-6 as a druggable target in psoriasis: focus on pustular variants. *J Immunol Res* (2014) 2014:964069. doi:10.1155/2014/964069
36. Di Cesare A, Di Meglio P, Nestle FO. The IL-23/Th17 axis in the immunopathogenesis of psoriasis. *J Invest Dermatol* (2009) 129(6):1339–50. doi:10.1038/jid.2009.59
37. Cai Y, Shen X, Ding C, Qi C, Li K, Li X, et al. Pivotal role of dermal IL-17-producing gammadelta T cells in skin inflammation. *Immunity* (2011) 35(4):596–610. doi:10.1016/j.immuni.2011.08.001
38. El Malki K, Karbach SH, Huppert J, Zayoud M, Reissig S, Schuler R, et al. An alternative pathway of imiquimod-induced psoriasis-like skin inflammation in the absence of interleukin-17 receptor a signaling. *J Invest Dermatol* (2013) 133(2):441–51. doi:10.1038/jid.2012.318
39. Lowes MA, Suarez-Farinas M, Krueger JG. Immunology of psoriasis. *Annu Rev Immunol* (2014) 32:227–55. doi:10.1146/annurev-immunol-032713-120225
40. Lynde CW, Poulin Y, Vender R, Bourcier M, Khalil S. Interleukin 17A: toward a new understanding of psoriasis pathogenesis. *J Am Acad Dermatol* (2014) 71(1):141–50. doi:10.1016/j.jaad.2013.12.036
41. Nair RP, Duffin KC, Helms C, Ding J, Stuart PE, Goldgar D, et al. Genome-wide scan reveals association of psoriasis with IL-23 and NF-kappaB pathways. *Nat Genet* (2009) 41(2):199–204. doi:10.1038/ng.311
42. Goldminz AM, Au SC, Kim N, Gottlieb AB, Lizzul PF. NF-kappaB: an essential transcription factor in psoriasis. *J Dermatol Sci* (2013) 69(2):89–94. doi:10.1016/j.jdermsci.2012.11.002
43. Tsuruta D. NF-kappaB links keratinocytes and lymphocytes in the pathogenesis of psoriasis. *Recent Pat Inflamm Allergy Drug Discov* (2009) 3(1):40–8. doi:10.2174/187221309787158399
44. Mattozzi C, Salvi M, D'Epiro S, Giancristoforo S, Macaluso L, Luci C, et al. Importance of regulatory T cells in the pathogenesis of psoriasis: review of the literature. *Dermatology* (2013) 227(2):134–45. doi:10.1159/000353398
45. Bovenschen HJ, van de Kerkhof PC, van Erp PE, Woestenenk R, Joosten I, Koenen HJ. Foxp3+ regulatory T cells of psoriasis patients easily differentiate into IL-17A-producing cells and are found in lesional skin. *J Invest Dermatol* (2011) 131(9):1853–60. doi:10.1038/jid.2011.139

12

The Interleukin-23/Interleukin-17 Axis Links Adaptive and Innate Immunity in Psoriasis

Michael P. Schön[1,2] and Luise Erpenbeck[1]**

[1] Department of Dermatology, Venereology and Allergology, University Medical Center Göttingen, Göttingen, Germany,

[2] Lower Saxony Institute of Occupational Dermatology, University Medical Center Göttingen, University of Osnabrück, Osnabrück, Germany

***Correspondence:**
Michael P. Schön
michael.schoen@med.uni-goettingen.de;
Luise Erpenbeck
luise.erpenbeck@med.uni-goettingen.de

Research into the pathophysiology of psoriasis has shed light onto many fascinating immunological interactions and underlying genetic constellations. Most prominent among these is the crosstalk between components of the innate and the adaptive immune system and the crucial role of interleukins (IL)-23 and -17 within this network. While it is clear that IL-23 drives and maintains the differentiation of Th17 lymphocytes, many aspects of the regulation of IL-23 and IL-17 are not quite as straightforward and have been unraveled only recently. For example, we know now that Th17 cells are not the only source of IL-17 but that cells of the innate immune system also produce considerable amounts of this central effector cytokine. In addition, there is IL-23-independent production of IL-17. Besides other innate immune cells, neutrophilic granulocytes prominently contribute to IL-17-related immune regulations in psoriasis, and it appears that they employ several mechanisms including the formation of neutrophil extracellular traps. Here, we strive to put the central role of the IL-23/IL-17 axis into perspective within the crosstalk between components of the innate and the adaptive immune system. Our aim is to better understand the complex immune regulation in psoriasis, a disorder that has become a model disease for chronic inflammation.

Keywords: psoriasis, interleukin-17, interleukin-23, innate immunity, adaptive immunity

INTRODUCTION

Psoriasis has evolved into an instructive model disease for many immune-mediated disorders. Numerous different types of immune cells are involved in the disease process (**Figures 1A–E**). Our increasing understanding of pathophysiological principles has facilitated the development of effective therapies. Perhaps equally important, such therapies have taught us a lot about disease mechanisms (1, 2). In consequence, both research into the pathophysiology and targeted treatments of psoriasis have been and still are progressing hand-in-hand. Psoriasis-directed precision medicine illuminates vividly how pieces of the immunological mosaic fall into place to ultimately improve our patients' lives. In this light, we here discuss immunological mechanisms governing the pathogenesis of psoriasis with a certain emphasis on links between the adaptive and the innate immune system. We believe that such interactive and dynamic links are of paramount importance for complex immune regulations in general and are key to successful therapeutic interventions.

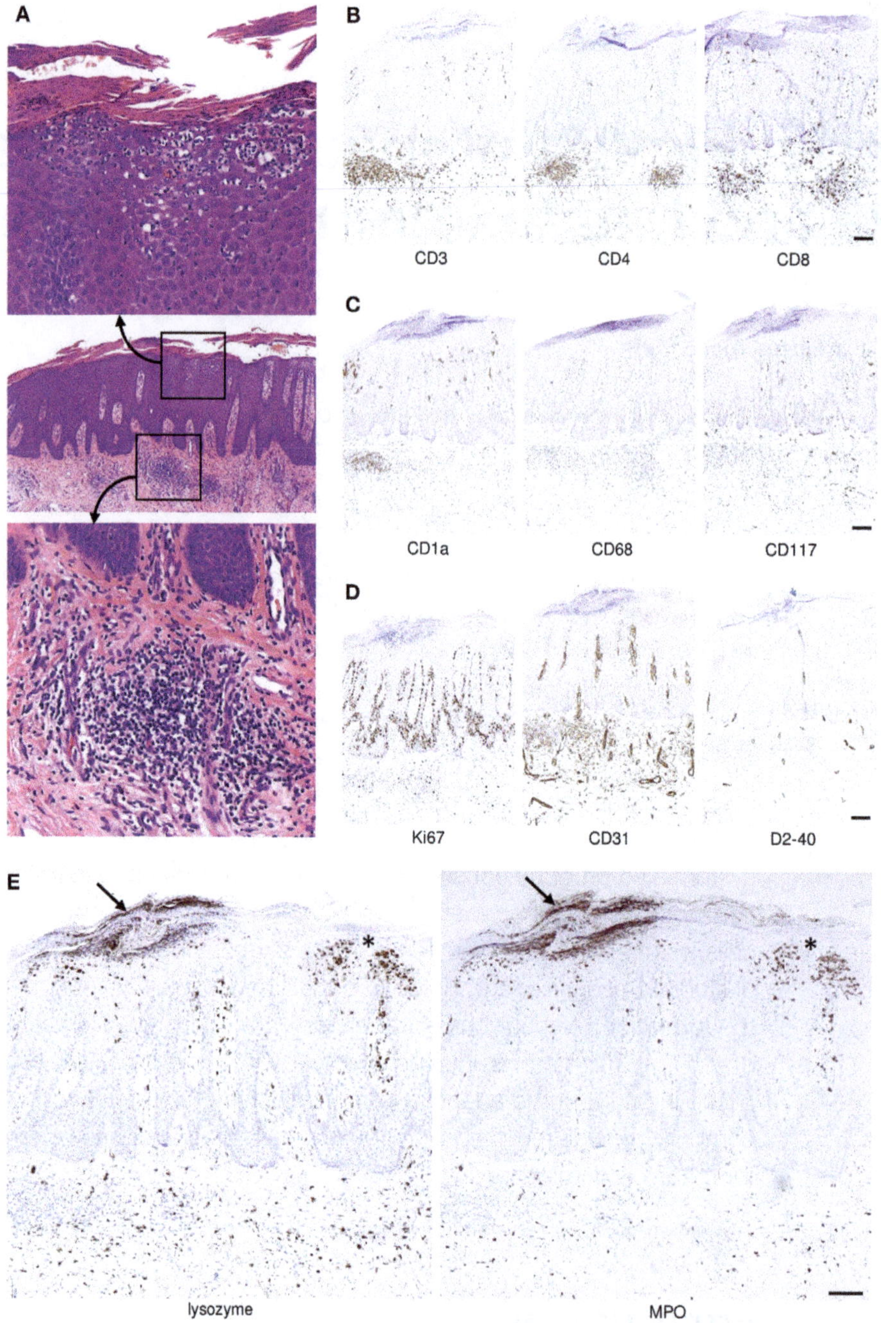

FIGURE 1 | Spatial distribution and compartmentalization of cells of the immune system in psoriatic skin. **(A)** A full-fledged psoriasis lesion was biopsied and stained with hematoxylin and eosin. Within the profoundly altered epithelial and mesenchymal compartments there are abundant cells of the adaptive and innate immune system (middle panel). The indicated magnified insets depict focal accumulations of neutrophilic granulocytes underneath and within the epidermal *stratum corneum* (upper image) and focal dermal aggregations of lymphocytes (admixed with other immunocytes; bottom image). **(B)** T cells indicated by expression of CD3 (left photomicrograph) reside within both the dermal compartment and, albeit to a lesser extent, the epidermis. CD4+ T cells are more abundant compared to CD8+ T cells, but epidermal T cells are almost exclusively CD8+. **(C)** Langerhans cells expressing CD1a are not only found in the epidermis but also within the dermal inflammatory infiltrate of psoriatic skin. The majority of macrophages expressing CD68 reside within the dermis, and a smaller proportion migrates up into higher layers of the epidermis. Mast cells expressing CD117 are present in the perivascular area and directly underneath the hyperplastic epidermis. **(D)** Highly increased proliferation of keratinocytes with some suprabasal proliferative activity is indicated by staining with Ki67, and dermal blood vessels are vastly increased in number and size as visualized by staining for CD31. By contrast, lymphatics identified by the D2–40 antibody are not significantly increased. **(E)** Neutrophilic granulocytes expressing lysozyme (left image; lysozyme is also expressed by some macrophages) and myeloperoxidase (MPO, right) migrate upward through the epidermis forming the telltale spongiform pustules of Kogoj within the *stratum spinosum* (asterisk near the right-hand margins of the images) and microabscesses of Munro directly underneath and within the *stratum corneum* (arrow near the left-hand-margin of the images). All images represent sequential sections of the same biopsy specimen. Scale bars = 100 μm.

ON THE BRINK OF UNDERSTANDING: THE LINK BETWEEN GENETICS AND IMMUNITY IN THE PATHOGENESIS OF PSORIASIS

Psoriasis is a systemic chronic inflammatory disease with primary manifestations on the skin and joints, and associations with a number of systemic comorbid diseases. The disorder has an immunogenetic basis and can be provoked by extrinsic or intrinsic stimuli. The familial occurrence of psoriasis evinces the relevance of genes for its pathogenesis (3). Several dozens of gene loci have been associated with psoriasis (so-called psoriasis susceptibility loci) (4, 5). Genome-wide association studies (GWAS), which also take into account single-nucleotide polymorphisms, associate the risk of psoriasis with genes that encode factors of antigen presentation and the innate and adaptive immune system. Psoriasis is associated with several human leukocyte antigens [HLA, also termed major histocompatibility complex (MHC)] class I genotypes. This applies to both skin psoriasis (HLA-C*06 and HLA-B*57) and psoriatic arthritis (PsA; HLA-B*27 and HLA-B*39). Patients with given HLA genotypes can be assigned to certain clinical characteristics of psoriasis as well as functional immunological parameters. Likewise, the detection of certain autoantigens depends on HLA genotypes such as HLA-C*06:02 (6). Potential autoantigens in psoriasis include peptide fragments of keratin 17 with sequence homologies to streptococcal M-proteins (7, 8), the antimicrobial peptide LL37 (9), and the melanocytic autoantigen ADAMTSL5 (10). While LL37 can activate both CD4+ T helper cells (Ths) and CD8+ cytotoxic T cells, ADAMTSL5 only activates CD8+ T cells. Interestingly, both peptides are recognized by the immune system after binding to HLA-C*06:02. This underlines the importance of certain HLA genotypes for the development of psoriasis.

A group of psoriasis-associated polymorphisms were found in genes encoding transcription factors such as REL, TYK2, STAT3, or RUNX3 (3). The transcription factor REL belongs to the NF-κB-family and is involved not only in the regulation of different inflammatory factors, but also in the regulation of keratinocyte proliferation (3, 11, 12). The Janus kinase (JAK) TYK2 is involved in the signal transduction of interferons and cytokines such as interleukin (IL)-12 and IL-23. The association with the transcription factor STAT3 is of particular interest, since STAT3 is essential for the differentiation of Th17 cells on the one hand and regulates the expression of IL-23R on the other (13). Furthermore, STAT3 activation in keratinocytes has a proliferation-promoting effect. The transcription factor RUNX3 is involved in the pathogenicity of autoreactive Th17 cells (14). Another important genetic association to psoriasis is the gene TRAF3IP2, which encodes the protein Act1, which is part of the signal cascade of IL-17.

Genome-wide association studies analyses also revealed psoriasis-associated genes encoding cytokines and cytokine receptors (3). These include the IL12B, IL23A, IL23R, and IL4/IL13 gene loci. The heterodimeric cytokine IL-23, one of the most important mediators in the immunopathogenesis of psoriasis, is composed of the gene products of IL12B (p40) and IL23A (p19).

Pustular psoriasis may represent a distinct entity, at least in a considerable proportion of cases. Recent studies have revealed associations of generalized pustular psoriasis with mutations in the genes of CARD14 and IL36RN (15–17) and, as a consequence, several studies to block either IL-36 or the IL-36 receptor (IL-36R) are underway (18). Furthermore, mutations in the AP1S3 gene, encoding the AP-1 complex subunit σ1C, which lead to a disruption of the endosomal translocation of toll-like receptor 3 (TLR3), are associated with pustular psoriasis (19).

Palmoplantar pustulosis is associated with missense mutations in CARD14, but not IL36RN (20). CARD14 is expressed by keratinocytes and endothelial cells, and mutations in this gene lead to increased activation of NF-κB. IL-36RN is a natural antagonist of the IL-1 family cytokine IL-36 (21). The consequence of mutations within the IL36RN gene is an increased production of NF-κB-regulated messengers (3, 22). IL-36 is also relevant for clonal responses of Th17 cells in patients with generalized pustular psoriasis (23). However, many patients with generalized pustular psoriasis and the vast majority of localized pustular psoriasis do not share mutations in the IL-36RN gene (24).

ADAPTIVE IMMUNITY AND THE IL-23/IL-17 AXIS IN THE PATHOGENESIS OF PSORIASIS

The pathogenesis of psoriasis is thought to be based on tight interactions between components of the innate and adaptive immune system (1, 3, 22, 25, 26). Several classical studies underscores the importance of T cells for the pathogenesis of psoriasis: the disease can be improved by cyclosporin A (27) or other drugs that inhibit the function (e.g., CD2 blockade) or recruitment (e.g., LFA-1 blockade) of T cells (28, 29). A similar effect can be achieved by IL-4, which shifts the cytokine environment toward a Th two-weighted immune response (30), with a likely attenuation of the Th17 function due to decreased IL-23 production in antigen-presenting cells (31). IL-10 can also reduce psoriatic symptoms by influencing T cell functions (32). Psoriasis can be triggered by bone marrow transplantation (33) and, like other autoinflammatory diseases, it shows the above-mentioned association with certain HLA expression patterns (34–36). Finally, psoriatic skin inflammation in animal models without pre-existing epithelial changes can be induced by certain CD4+ T cells alone (37, 38), and T cells induce psoriatic lesions in transplanted human skin (39–41). These older studies have culminated in the more recent and above-mentioned discovery of potential autoantigens in psoriasis (8–10).

In recent years, few areas in immunological science have attracted as much attention as the research on Th17 cells, a group of CD4+ T lymphocytes that differ from the "classical" Th1 and Th2 cells (42) and which were named after their production of IL-17 (**Figure 2**). Th17 cells are prominently involved in the pathogenesis of psoriasis (43–45), palmoplantar pustulosis (46), as well as other chronic inflammatory diseases (47, 48). Even healthy human skin contains some IL-17-producing T lymphocytes (49), which suggests their involvement in immune surveillance. Changes in the number and activation state of Th17 cells lead to

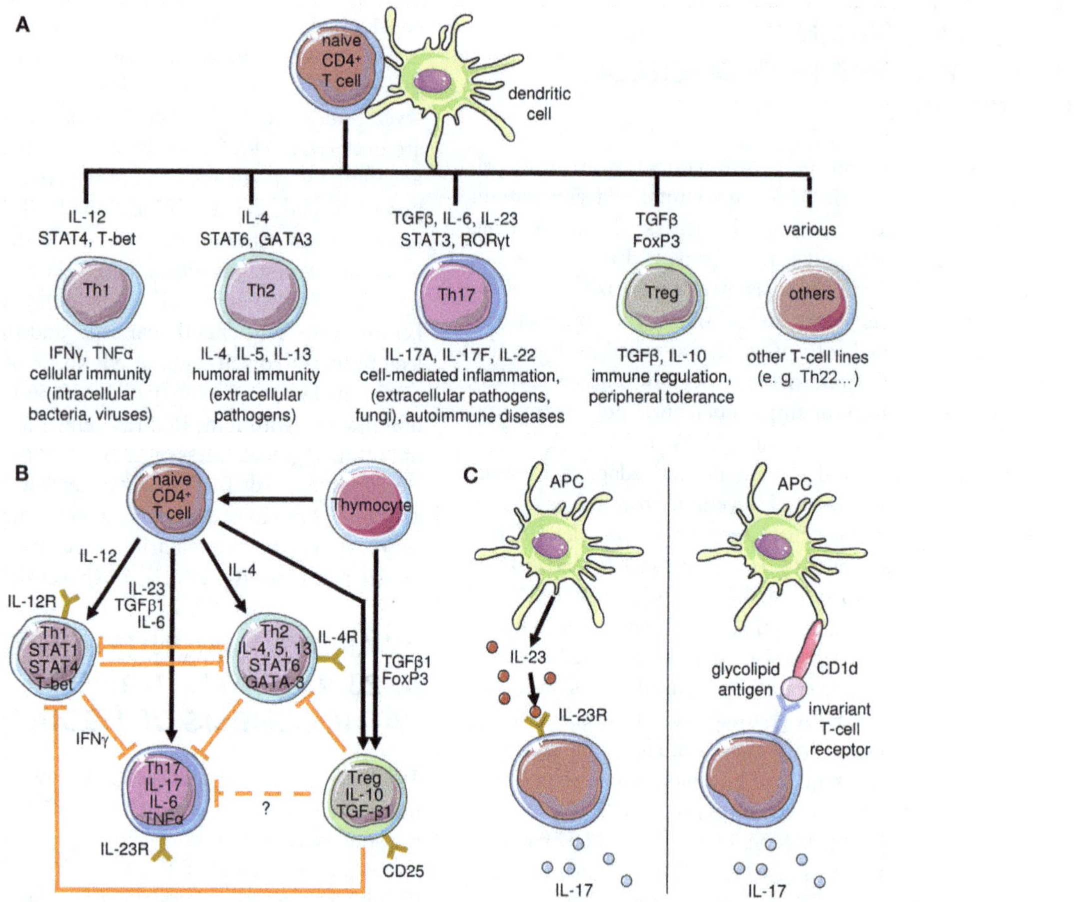

FIGURE 2 | Differentiation of T cell subsets and lineage-defining role of interleukin (IL)-23 for Th17 cells. **(A)** The differentiation of T cell subsets from naive T cells requires stimulation by dendritic cells and specific mediators. Key cytokines and transcription factors driving differentiation of the indicated populations are depicted above the respective T cell type, while their primary function is indicated below. **(B)** The differentiation of Th17 cells is embedded in a complex regulatory network. Antigen presentation by dendritic cells and cytokine stimulation lead to differentiation of effector cells including (but not limited to) Th1, Th2, or Th17, the latter induced by IL-23 in conjunction with other mediators. Regulatory T cells (Treg) inhibit differentiation and effector functions of Th1 and Th2 cells. Their effect on Th17 cells is not exactly known. **(C)** Besides the classical IL-23-dependent stimulation of IL-17 secretion (left panel), IL-23-independent induction of IL-17A may occur in response to presentation of glycolipid antigens by CD1d (right panel).

a dysbalance between these and regulatory T cells, resulting in inflammation (43, 50, 51). Circulating effector memory T cells can be stimulated by streptococcal extracts to produce Th17 cytokines and stimulate keratinocyte proliferation (50). In turn, activated keratinocytes stimulate the IL-17 production of T cells, which culminates in a positive feedback loop (52) (**Figure 3**). In psoriatic skin, IL-17 is not only produced by CD4+ Th17 cells but also by CD8+ T cells (53) and, as alluded to below, by cells of the innate immune system. IL-17A is the most important of the six known IL-17 isoforms for the pathophysiology of psoriasis (45).

Although the initiation of development from naive precursor cells has not yet been fully clarified, a robust body of evidence supports the notion that IL-23 produced by myeloid cells is essential for terminal differentiation and the preservation of Th17 cells (54–56) (**Figure 2**). This activity is conveyed *via* the IL-23 receptor expressed on naive T cells, together with other cytokines and their receptors such as TNFα, IL-1, and IL-6. This differentiation in combination and balance with Th1 cells is of central importance for the pathogenesis of psoriasis (57) and other chronic inflammatory diseases (58). The Th17-mediated inflammation can be modulated by exogenous factors such as vitamin D3 or UV radiation (59, 60), or by other cytokines such as IL-9 (61).

In addition to IL-23-dependent production of IL-17A, a series of studies has demonstrated an alternative route which is independent of IL-23 and has been described, for example, for γδ-T cells (a subset of the so-called "unconventional" T-cells) or invariant natural killer cells (62–65) (**Figure 2C**). However, implications of this alternative pathway on the course of inflammatory diseases or potential side effects following blockade of either IL-23 or IL-17 are not entirely clear yet.

In general, unconventional T-cells appear to merit further studies in the context (66). They include CD1-restricted T cells, MR1-restricted mucosal-associated invariant T cells (MAIT cells), MHC class Ib-reactive T cells, and the above-mentioned γδ

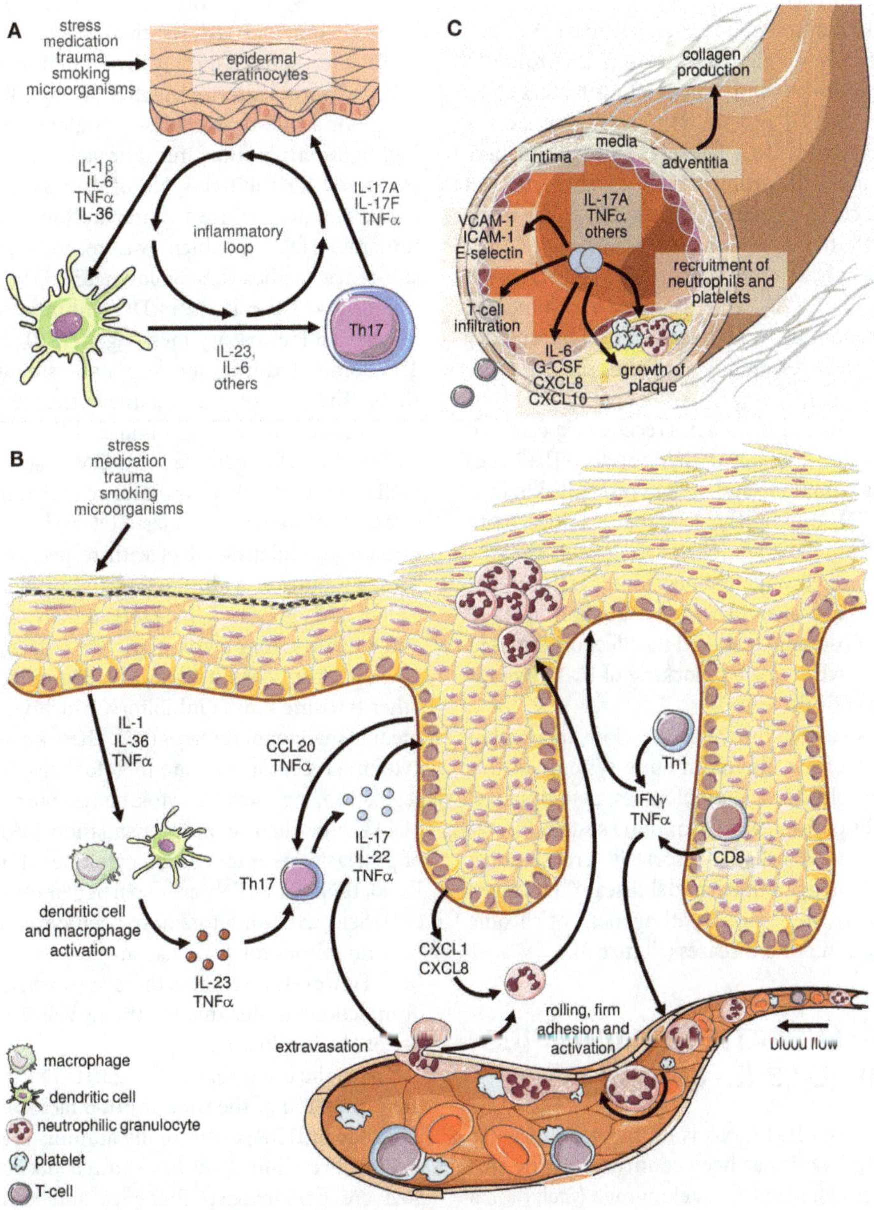

FIGURE 3 | Inflammatory loops in psoriasis involving innate and adaptive immune cells. **(A)** Inflammatory cytokines including interleukin (IL)-23 and IL-6 produced by cells of the innate immune system such as dendritic cells and macrophages facilitate the differentiation of Th17 cells. The latter secrete IL-17 and other mediators which stimulate epidermal cells to produce cytokines and chemokines that attract and activate cells of the innate immune system. The result is an inflammatory loop or "vicious circle" in which IL-23 and IL-17 play central roles. **(B)** On a larger scale, a complex network of inflammatory mediators connects virtually all resident and immigrating cells within the skin. In fact, this machinery can be considered the core of psoriasis pathophysiology. The examples depicted here (in reality, there are considerably more players orchestrating the pathophysiology of psoriasis) highlight the intertwined crosstalk of cells of the innate and the adaptive immune system with activated resident cells such as vascular endothelial cells and epidermal keratinocytes. Such interactions can explain most, if not all, hallmark features of psoriasis such as, on the one hand, recruitment, activation, spatial compartmentalization, and disease-promoting differentiation of cells of the immune system, as well as, on the other hand, pathological changes of resident tissues such as the epidermis and the cutaneous vasculature. The alterations extend to additional skin components not depicted here such as cutaneous nerves and the connective tissue. **(C)** Inflammatory mediators such as IL-17 and TNFα are present at elevated levels in the serum of psoriasis patients. Their systemic activity also facilitates vascular changes, thus contributing to the accrual and course of comorbid diseases, in particular cardiovascular disorders (depicted here is atherosclerosis).

T cells. A role of these cells in chronic inflammatory disorders is currently emerging, although actual data in psoriasis are still scant (66). For example, MAIT cells seem to be altered or activated in patients with inflammatory bowel disease, psoriasis, or autoimmune diseases (67–69). However, further studies are needed to assess the role of the other populations in psoriasis.

Innate lymphoid cells (ILCs) also appear to be promising new candidates to reveal novel aspects in the pathogenesis of psoriasis. ILCs are a heterogeneous group of innate immune cells, characterized by their lack of somatic rearrangement of antigen-specific receptors. They are divided into subsets according to their function, cytokine profile, and transcription factors (NK, ILC1, ieILC1, ILC2, ILC3, LTi, and ILCP) (70). Recent studies show considerable diversity of ILCs between and within these major subsets. Interestingly, the group 3 ILCs are characterized by the ability to produce Th17-like cytokines and express the transcription factor RORγt, traits which are reminiscent of Th17 T-cells. Even more strikingly, as a subset of group 3 ILCs is able to generate both IL-17 and IL-22 (70), it is reasonable to assume that these cells play a role in psoriasis and other chronic inflammatory diseases. Nevertheless, more research is needed to solidify these initial findings.

The still young field of IL-17 research has recently experienced a paradigm shift due to the observation that not only Th17 cells but also cells of the innate immune system and resident skin cells can secrete IL-17 (71–73). Among the cells that produce IL-17 are mast cells and neutrophilic granulocytes. It appears that the presentation of IL-17 through so-called neutrophil extracellular traps (NETs) may also play a role (74). The production of IL-17 by different cell types in psoriatic skin and its effect on different target cells could explain why targeted blocking of IL-17 by new drugs works so quickly and effectively.

The IL-23/IL-17 axis clearly illustrates the close interaction of different components of the innate immune system (in this case IL-23-producing myeloid cells, granulocytes, macrophages, and mast cells) with cells of the adaptive immune system (Th17- and IL17-producing CD8+ T cells) in psoriasis. Translational research into the immunology of this "model disease" has given us fascinating insights into the complex pathogenesis of chronic inflammation including comorbid diseases (**Figure 3**).

NOT LOST IN TRANSLATION: THERAPIES TARGETING THE IL-23/IL-17 AXIS

The discovery that the IL-23/IL-17 axis is of major importance for the pathogenesis of psoriasis has been confirmed by the efficacy of new therapeutics (1): in 2009, Ustekinumab (Stelara®), a monoclonal antibody that inhibits the p40 subunit found in both IL-12 and IL-23, was approved for the treatment of psoriasis (75). The development of this compound began when it was assumed that IL-12 was significantly involved in the development of psoriasis (76). It was somewhat fortunate that Ustekinumab also inhibited IL-23, which is now considered to be more pathogenetically relevant than IL-12 (77). Guselkumab (Tremfya®), which specifically neutralizes human IL-23 by blocking the p19 subunit, has been approved recently and shows very good efficacy against psoriasis (78). In fact, circumventing a potential unwanted effect of concomitant blocking of IL-12 (**Figure 2B**) by specific blockade of IL-23 may account, at least in part, for the seemingly higher efficacy of guselkumab as compared to ustekinumab. Several further anti-p19 antibodies, in addition to a large number of other anti-psoriatic agents, are currently in phase 3 clinical trials. The direct blockade of IL-17A by Secukinumab (Cosentyx®) and Ixekizumab (Taltz®) also leads to a convincing improvement in psoriasis (79, 80). Similarly, the blockade of the IL-17 receptor by brodalumab (Siliq®, Kyntheum®) was very effective (81, 82).

In addition to specifically targeting the IL-23/IL-17 axis, this pathway is also modulated by more broadly acting classical compounds. Two examples of orally available pharmaceuticals highlight this notion: fumaric acid esters and apremilast are registered for the treatment of psoriasis. The main component of the fumaric acid ester preparation Fumaderm® is dimethyl fumarate (DMF), which was recently approved as a single-substance medication (Skilarence®). DMF reduces the production of IL-23 and IL-12 in DC and promotes the production of the anti-inflammatory messenger IL-10 (83). It shifts the Th17/Th1 dominated immune response—similar to IL-4—toward an IL-4+ Th2 phenotype. In patients treated with DMF-containing preparations, fewer IL-17+ and IFNγ+ T cells are found, and IL-4+ Th2 cells increase (83). DMF can also reduce the endothelial recruitment of immune cells (84, 85). The phosphodiesterase 4 inhibitor apremilast (Otezla®) has a somewhat similar immunomodulating effect with respect to the IL-23/IL-17 axis. This inhibitor also diminishes the production of IL-23, IL-12, TNFα, and IFNγ and, like DMF, it increases the formation of the anti-inflammatory cytokine IL-10 (86).

New classes of immune modulators are JAK inhibitors and other tyrosine kinase inhibitors, which we know from the treatment of malignant diseases (87). These kinases are associated with cytokine receptors and are therefore also important for immune regulation, e.g., several cytokine receptors require the activation of JAKs for their signal transmission (88). In the pathogenesis of psoriasis, receptors of the cytokines IL-6, IL-12, IL-21, IL-22, IL-23, IFNα, and IFNγ are of particular importance in this respect (87). Selective inhibitors have been developed, and a number of JAK inhibitors for psoriasis are in phase 2 and 3 clinical trials (89). However, it remains to be seen whether the potential risks of infections under this treatment will limit the broad systemic use of JAK Inhibitors.

Given the importance of IL-23/IL-17 signaling in psoriasis and the expression of the transcription factor RORγt in Th17 cells, a blockade of RORγt with orally administered drugs is also aimed at (90). Pre-clinical studies showed positive results. A tangible goal are personalized therapies and prediction of individual therapeutic success of selected drugs, also known as "Precision Medicine" (91, 92).

BRIDGING THE GAP: COMMUNICATION BETWEEN INNATE AND ADAPTIVE IMMUNE SYSTEM IN PSORIASIS

While the puzzle of the multifactorial immunogenetic pathology of psoriasis is emerging ever more clearly (93), the mechanisms of its first manifestation are quite far from being understood. Infections with streptococcal bacteria and medications such as lithium or β-blockers have been described as triggers. Mechanical stress eliciting an isomorphic irritant effect (Köbner's phenomenon) may explain the symmetrical localization of psoriasis, for example, on the elbows and knees. Minimal trauma may lead to responses with rapid immigration and activation of immune cells such as neutrophilic granulocytes and T cells (71), some of which seem to react in the above-mentioned autoimmune fashion (9, 10). Amplifying feedback loops between T cells as representatives of the adaptive immune system and neutrophilic granulocytes and keratinocytes of the innate immune system finally lead to an amplification and chronification of the immune response (**Figure 3**). In addition, ILC with traits of both innate and adaptive immunocytes and the capacity to produce IL-17 and IL-22 have entered the stage very recently (94, 95).

Characteristic for keratinocytes in psoriatic plaques are their increased proliferation rate, altered differentiation and production of antimicrobial peptides and proteins (AMP). AMPs are the first line of innate immune defense. Due to their specific properties (positive charge, hydrophobicity, and amphiphilic properties) they can form pores and thus exert their antimicrobial functions. Owing to their strong pro-inflammatory properties, these peptides have also been called alarmins. Many studies have been carried out on cathelicidin (LL37), which is expressed at elevated levels in psoriatic skin (96) and has a direct stimulatory effect on keratinocytes (97). In addition, the positively charged LL37 is able to form immunostimulatory complexes with negatively charged DNA and RNA. These complexes are taken up by myeloid dendritic cells (mDC) and plasmacytoid DC (pDC), where RNA motifs stimulate TLR7 and 8 and DNA leads to the stimulation of TLR9 (98–100). TLR7/8-stimulated myeloid DC secrete the messenger substances TNFα, IL-23, and IL-12, while pDC produce large amounts of interferon α <χιτ>(93).

In addition to LL37, S100 proteins are important for the pathogenesis of psoriasis. An important stimulus for the production of S100A7 (psoriasin) and S100A15 (koebnerisin) by keratinocytes is IL-17A (101). Both AMPs have pro-inflammatory properties (102). The calgranulins, S100A8 and S100A9, are produced by myeloid cells and keratinocytes. They stimulate the proliferation and cytokine production of keratinocytes (103) and are able to facilitate a T cell-dependent autoimmune response in murine models (104). Defensins are also alarmins produced by keratinocytes in psoriasis plaques and, similar to LL37, human β-defensin 2 and 4 are known to bind DNA and stimulate pDC in a TLR9-dependent manner (105). DC performs important regulatory functions in psoriasis. Activated by alarmins of keratinocytes and neutrophils, they stimulate pathogenetically important T cells (93). Primary activation and programming of relevant Th17/Th1 and Th22 cells takes place in the lymph node. Activated DC facilitates the differentiation of naive T cells through IL-1β, IL-6, and IL-23 into Th17 cells (9). IL-12 assumes these functions for Th1 cells (which dampen Th17 activity), and TNFα and IL-6 lead to the programming of Th22 cells (**Figures 2** and **3**).

In skin lesions of psoriasis patients, CD11c+ inflammatory DC can be detected more frequently, expressing TNFα, IL-23, and iNOS (so-called TNFα- and iNOS-expressing TIP-DC) (100). Attempts to define these cells more precisely have suggested that they are not classical myeloid CD1c+ DC1 or CD141+ DC2 (100). A portion of the TIP-DC corresponds to the so-called slanDC (106). In addition, CD163+ macrophages with phenotypic properties of TIP-DC could also be detected (107). These slanDC were first detected in the blood using the specific marker slan and the expression of CD16 (108–110). They are now believed to be of monocytic origin and produce large amounts of pro-inflammatory cytokines such as IL-12, IL-23, IL-1β, and TNFα. Numerous pDCs perform stimulatory functions in psoriatic skin and are characterized by high production of interferon α (111).

NEUTROPHILS, NETs, AND MECHANISMS OF DISEASE

In addition to DC, macrophages, and T cells, neutrophilic granulocytes are a hallmark feature of psoriatic skin lesions (**Figures 1E** and **4A**). They are key effector cells of the innate immune system and they target invading microbes by phagocytosis, the generation of reactive oxygen species (ROS), as well as the release of AMPs and inflammatory mediators. While these "classical" strategies are well known for many years, the recent discovery of NETs has catapulted neutrophils back into the focus of immunological science including psoriasis research (112).

The mechanisms leading to the formation of NETs are only partially understood. It is clear that upon contact with various stimuli including bacteria, fungi, activated platelets, antigen-antibody complexes or CXCL8 (IL-8), calcium ionophores, phorbol 12-myristate 13-acetate, or lipopolysaccharide neutrophils enter a cell-death pathway that is different from apoptosis and necrosis (113–115). To this end, the neutrophils go through a series of dramatic alterations of their morphology and behavior. In the course of several hours, they stop migrating and rearrange their cytoskeleton. The nuclear and granular membranes dissolve and a mixing of granular content with chromatin occurs before NETs are finally released. On the molecular level, this pathway generally requires the production of ROS and is therefore dependent on the NADPH oxidase complex (114, 116), although ROS-independent mechanisms have also been proposed (117). In addition, there is evidence for an involvement of protein kinase C and the Raf–MEK–ERK pathway (118). NETosis relies strongly on myeloperoxidase (MPO) and neutrophil elastase (NE). NE is released from azurophilic granules into the cytosol in an MPO-dependent manner (119) and subsequently translocates to the nucleus, where it cleaves histones to decondense chromatin (120). MPO also travels to the nucleus where it synergizes with NE in promoting chromatin decondensation independent of its enzymatic activity (120). Finally, a crucial player is peptidylarginine deiminase 4, an enzyme that, after translocation to the nucleus (121), leads to (global) histone hypercitrullination and enables histone decondensation (122), a prerequisite for expelling the chromatin content of the cell in the form of NETs (**Figure 4B**).

While originally described as a method to entrap and kill bacteria, we now know that NETs play a broader role in the immune system. Free DNA of host origin, as released during NET formation, indicates a disruption of cellular integrity and therefore constitutes a potent "danger" signal. Interestingly, DNA complexed with LL-37, is much more stable and activates DCs more effectively than "naked" DNA, triggering them to produce pro-inflammatory interferons (98). In addition, LL-37 (as well as other AMPs such as human beta defensin-3 and human neutrophil peptide-1) protects neutrophil-derived DNA against nuclease degradation (123). At the same time LL37 appears to

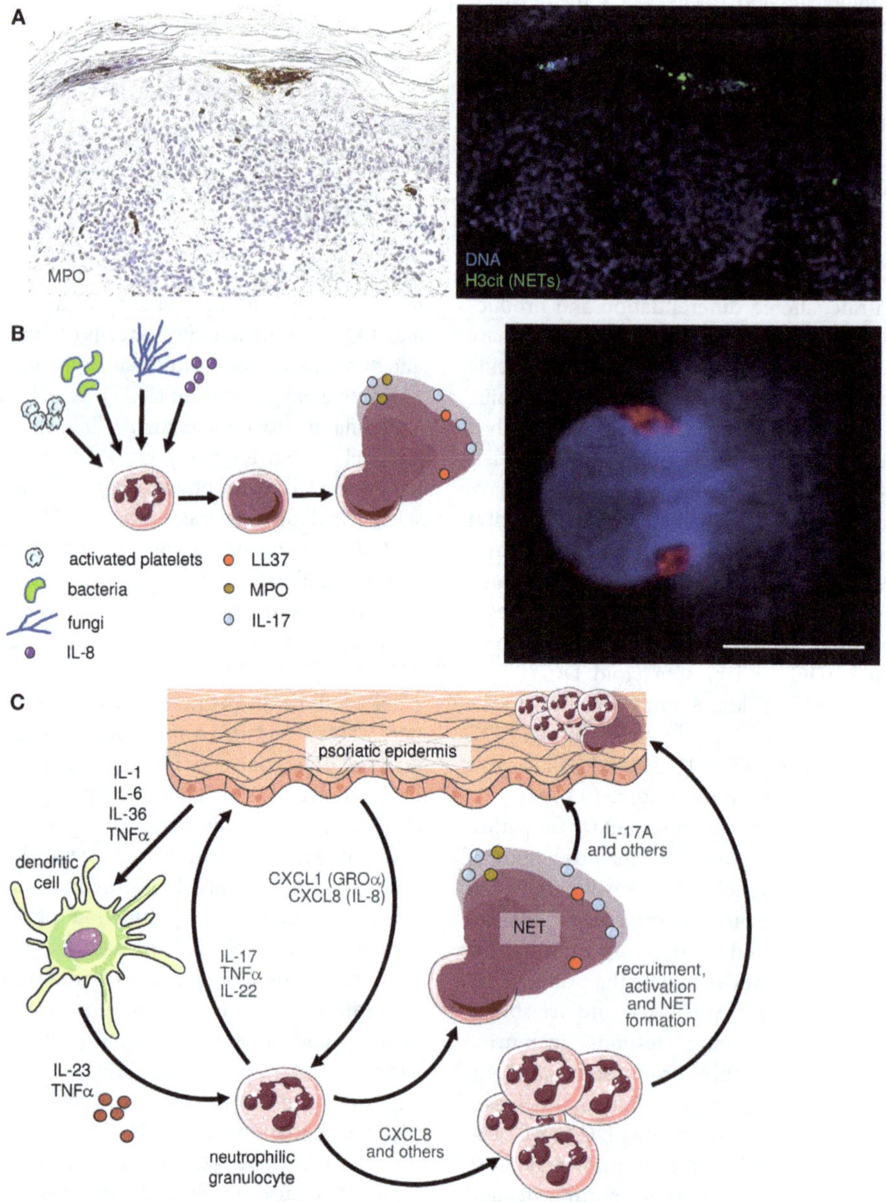

FIGURE 4 | Neutrophilic granulocytes become recruited, activated, and form neutrophil extracellular traps (NETs) in psoriatic skin. **(A)** Two consecutive sections of an early psoriatic lesion were stained by immunohistochemistry for myeloperoxidase (MPO; left photomicrograph) and by immunofluorescence for citrullinated histone-3 (H3cit; right). Within the typical subcorneal neutrophil accumulations (Munro's microabscesses) there are numerous H3cit-positive cells indicating NETosis. **(B)** Schematic of NET formation: a variety of stimuli can activate neutrophils. Consequently, their chromatin decondenses until it fills the entire cell. Finally, the cell membrane ruptures to release the NET, consisting of DNA, histones and a plethora of antimicrobial peptides, chemokines, etc. The right-hand image depicts a characteristic confocal image of a neutrophil directly after NET release (DNA staining by Hoechst in blue, membrane staining by the PHK26 dye in red). Scale bar = 10 µm. **(C)** The complex interactions between neutrophils, which are among the most prominent representatives of the innate immune system in psoriatic skin, include recruitment and activation by CXCL8 [interleukin (IL)-8], CXCL-1 (GROα), and other mediators as well as activation by cytokines such as IL-23 and TNFα. In turn, neutrophils undergo NETosis and they are thought to produce and release pro-inflammatory factors including IL-17, IL-22, CXCL8, and TNFα.

lose its antimicrobial activity when bound to DNA, implying that antimicrobial peptides may have different, mutually exclusive roles in the immune system. The high presence of AMPs within NETs indicates that most likely NETs and AMPs act in unison to either directly kill invading pathogens or to modulate the immune system.

The clinical relevance of these mechanisms becomes apparent when studying their impact in diseases like systemic lupus erythematosus (124) or autoimmune diabetes (125). In addition, NETs can directly prime T cells by reducing their activation threshold. Thus, NET-mediated priming increases T cell responses to antigens and even to suboptimal stimuli, thus providing an additional link between the innate and the adaptive immune system (126).

In autoimmune diseases featuring anti-neutrophilic cytoplasmic antibodies (ANCAs) like lupus erythematosus or ANCA-associated small-vessel vasculitis, tolerance against nuclear components of neutrophils is disrupted. In order for these ANCAs to form, neutrophil proteins such as MPO or proteinase-3 must be processed by professional antigen-presenting cells and presented to T- and B-cells. It has been shown that the structure of NETs favors the upload of neutrophilic antigens into mDCs, leading to their activation and presentation of these antigens to the effector cells of the adaptive immune system (127). The formation of antigen-antibody complexes that ensues from this process may then lead to a vicious circle as antigen-antibody complexes in turn effectively trigger NETosis. Deregulated NETosis may therefore be important for the pathophysiology of inflammatory diseases.

So what does all this mean in the context of psoriasis? While here the pathogenic importance of NETs is less well-established than in other autoimmune diseases, NETs are prominently present in both psoriatic plaques (**Figures 4A,C**) and psoriatic pustules (112). Research into the contribution of NETs and neutrophils in general to the pathogenesis of psoriasis is hampered by the fact that the currently most popular mouse model, namely that of imiquimod-induced dermatitis, does not reflect the importance of neutrophils in human psoriasis (128). In this model, γδ-T cells are the primary source of IL-17, limiting its suitability to study neutrophils or NETs in murine skin (129). So far only neutrophil depletion in flaky skin mice has provided evidence for the involvement of neutrophils in a psoriasis-like phenotype in an animal model (129). The use of other animal models, for example, IL-23-induced psoriasis-like skin inflammation will hopefully help to overcome this limitation (130).

NEUTROPHILS, IL-17, AND OTHER CYTOKINES

While it was long assumed that Th17 cells were the most important sources of IL-17 in psoriasis, there is accumulating evidence that cells of the innate immune system like neutrophils, mast cells, γδ T cells, and ILCs are major sources of IL-17 (74, 131). Similar to Th17 cells, neutrophils possess the machinery to produce IL-17. In humans, two models of psoriasis-like inflammation (leukotriene B4 application or repeated tape stripping) have shown the coexpression of the IL-17-associated transcription factor RORγt and IL-17 (71, 131). In neutrophils, incubation with keratinocytes (72) or IL-23 induced IL-17 and IL-22 in an mTOR-dependent manner (126). However, to what extent neutrophil-produced IL-17 stimulates inflammatory reactions and the mechanism of IL-17-release, in particular within the context of NET formation, still remains enigmatic (74). It appears likely that IL-17 is released alongside NETs and may even be displayed on them, as IL-17 co-localizes with indirect immunohistochemical markers of NETs in psoriatic tissue and Munro's microabscesses (74).

Interleukin-17 stimulates many pro-inflammatory and immunomodulatory functions including production of IL-6 and IL-8 (CXCL8) but also TNFα, IL-1, CXCL10, and CCL20 (112, 132). In turn, IL-8 promotes the recruitment and activation of neutrophils and has long been known to trigger NETosis (133, 134). In addition, interaction of CCL20 with its corresponding receptor CCR6 is enhanced in chronic inflammatory diseases such as inflammatory bowel disease and may augment the recruitment of Il-17-producing cells such as Th17 T-cells (135, 136).

Neutrophils themselves produce a number of cytokines such as TNFα, IL-12 or, again, IL-8 (CXCL8), in addition to the aforementioned IL-17, which may add to the overall pro-inflammatory environment, recruitment of additional leukocytes, and NET production (137), creating a vicious circle that can be efficiently intercepted by modern therapies directed against the key cytokines IL-23 and IL-17 as well as TNFα in psoriasis (**Figure 4C**). In fact, IL-17 and TNFα have been shown to synergistically regulate cytokine levels, for example, upregulating beta-defensins and, yet again, IL-8, and to exert synergistic effects both on keratinocytes (138) and on melanocytes (139). One may hypothesize that the reason IL-17 blockade and TNFα-inhibition have similarly strong effects in patients is the abolition of this synergism.

WHAT CAN WE EXPECT?

Psoriasis remains a fascinating entity, and while we have been able to solve some of the mysteries surrounding this disease, many aspects still remain enigmatic. Among the most mesmerizing novel concepts in the disease mechanisms are the emerging roles of "young" immune cells such as ILCs and nonconventional T-cells, whose role in immunology we are only just beginning to understand. Just as importantly, we have learned that cells such as neutrophils and mast cells may have a central role in psoriasis that reaches beyond the originally described functions of innate immune cells and may in fact bridge the innate and the adaptive immune system. Last but not least, "classical" psoriasis-associated cells such as certain Ths keep presenting us with surprising findings when it comes to the complex, often synergistic effects of chemokines.

These exciting developments show potential for novel therapeutic approaches. While we have already come very far in applying our knowledge and generating new therapies that make a vast difference in patients' quality of life, the inhibition of all or some of the above-mentioned mediators theoretically present therapeutic opportunities. For example, inhibition of IL-9 could be explored in the context of psoriasis (61). In general, medicine is moving toward more personalized therapeutic approaches. For psoriasis, this could mean targeting the cytokines most relevant for the given subtype of psoriasis. For example, while chronic plaque-type psoriasis is dominated by the IL-17/INFγ axis, pustular forms of psoriasis feature an IL-17/IL-36/IL-1 signature (140). The development of highly effective (targeted) therapies with mild to moderate side effects also allows the exploration of "early intervention" to prevent the psoriatic march which may lead to cardiovascular diseases resulting from systemic inflammation. Similar to approaches used in rheumatoid arthritis, it can be speculated that blocking inflammatory mediators early on in the disease process could intercept the evolution of psoriasis toward a more detrimental systemic disease. Such approaches may also include targeting of important resident cell types such as vascular endothelial cells (141).

The above-mentioned "novel players" in psoriasis, including ILCs, unconventional T-cells but also "old" new candidates like neutrophils (including NETs released by them) and mast cells also present interesting new targets in psoriasis. It is conceivable that targeting these cells or other factors in psoriasis may require an approach adapted to the disease stage or activity, as for example, NETs might only be present in acute inflammatory exacerbations while other cells and cytokines may dominate more chronic phases of the disease.

Whatever the future holds in stock for us and patients suffering from psoriasis, looking back on the last couple of years of psoriasis research certainly justifies optimism.

AUTHOR CONTRIBUTIONS

MS and LE jointly wrote the manuscript. They contributed equally.

REFERENCES

1. Boehncke WH, Schön MP. Psoriasis. *Lancet* (2015) 386(9997):983–94. doi:10.1016/S0140-6736(14)61909-7
2. Hawkes JE, Chan TC, Krueger JG. Psoriasis pathogenesis and the development of novel targeted immune therapies. *J Allergy Clin Immunol* (2017) 140(3):645–53. doi:10.1016/j.jaci.2017.07.004
3. Harden JL, Krueger JG, Bowcock AM. The immunogenetics of psoriasis: a comprehensive review. *J Autoimmun* (2015) 64:66–73. doi:10.1016/j.jaut.2015.07.008
4. Tsoi LC, Spain SL, Knight J, Ellinghaus E, Stuart PE, Capon F, et al. Identification of 15 new psoriasis susceptibility loci highlights the role of innate immunity. *Nat Genet* (2012) 44(12):1341–8. doi:10.1038/ng.2467
5. Das S, Stuart PE, Ding J, Tejasvi T, Li Y, Tsoi LC, et al. Fine mapping of eight psoriasis susceptibility loci. *Eur J Hum Genet* (2015) 23(6):844–53. doi:10.1038/ejhg.2014.172
6. Chen L, Tsai TF. HLA-Cw6 and psoriasis. *Br J Dermatol* (2018) 178(4): 854–62. doi:10.1111/bjd.16083
7. Thorleifsdottir RH, Sigurdardottir SL, Sigurgeirsson B, Olafsson JH, Sigurdsson MI, Petersen H, et al. Improvement of psoriasis after tonsillectomy is associated with a decrease in the frequency of circulating T cells that recognize streptococcal determinants and homologous skin determinants. *J Immunol* (2012) 188(10):5160–5. doi:10.4049/jimmunol.1102834
8. Sigmundsdottir H, Sigurgeirsson B, Troye-Blomberg M, Good MF, Valdimarsson H, Jonsdottir I. Circulating T cells of patients with active psoriasis respond to streptococcal M-peptides sharing sequences with human epidermal keratins. *Scand J Immunol* (1997) 45(6):688–97. doi:10.1046/j.1365-3083.1997.d01-438.x
9. Lande R, Botti E, Jandus C, Dojcinovic D, Fanelli G, Conrad C, et al. The antimicrobial peptide LL37 is a T-cell autoantigen in psoriasis. *Nat Commun* (2014) 5:5621. doi:10.1038/ncomms6621
10. Arakawa A, Siewert K, Stöhr J, Besgen P, Kim SM, Rühl G, et al. Melanocyte antigen triggers autoimmunity in human psoriasis. *J Exp Med* (2015) 212(13):2203–12. doi:10.1084/jem.20151093
11. Lorenz VN, Schön MP, Seitz CS. c-Rel in epidermal homeostasis: a spotlight on c-rel in cell cycle regulation. *J Invest Dermatol* (2016) 136(6):1090–6. doi:10.1016/j.jid.2016.02.003
12. Lorenz VN, Schön MP, Seitz CS. c-Rel downregulation affects cell cycle progression of human keratinocytes. *J Invest Dermatol* (2014) 134(2):415–22. doi:10.1038/jid.2013.315
13. Ghoreschi K, Laurence A, Yang XP, Tato CM, McGeachy MJ, Konkel JE, et al. Generation of pathogenic T(H)17 cells in the absence of TGF-beta signalling. *Nature* (2010) 467(7318):967–71. doi:10.1038/nature09447
14. Fu D, Song X, Hu H, Sun M, Li Z, Tian Z. Downregulation of RUNX3 moderates the frequency of Th17 and Th22 cells in patients with psoriasis. *Mol Med Rep* (2016) 13(6):4606–12. doi:10.3892/mmr.2016.5108
15. Jordan CT, Cao L, Roberson ED, Duan S, Helms CA, Nair RP, et al. Rare and common variants in CARD14, encoding an epidermal regulator of NF-kappaB, in psoriasis. *Am J Hum Genet* (2012) 90(5):796–808. doi:10.1016/j.ajhg.2012.03.013
16. Sugiura K, Muto M, Akiyama M. CARD14 c.526G>C (p.Asp176His) is a significant risk factor for generalized pustular psoriasis with psoriasis vulgaris in the Japanese cohort. *J Invest Dermatol* (2014) 134(6):1755–7. doi:10.1038/jid.2014.46
17. Zhang Z, Ma Y, Zhang Z, Lin J, Chen G, Han L, et al. Identification of two loci associated with generalized pustular psoriasis. *J Invest Dermatol* (2015) 135(8):2132–4. doi:10.1038/jid.2015.111
18. Tsai Y-C, Tsai T-F. Anti-interleukin and interleukin therapies for psoriasis: current evidence and clinical usefulness. *Ther Adv Musculoskelet Dis* (2017) 9(11):277–94. doi:10.1177/1759720X17735756
19. Setta-Kaffetzi N, Simpson MA, Navarini AA, Patel VM, Lu HC, Allen MH, et al. AP1S3 mutations are associated with pustular psoriasis and impaired toll-like receptor 3 trafficking. *Am J Hum Genet* (2014) 94(5):790–7. doi:10.1016/j.ajhg.2014.04.005
20. Mössner R, Frambach Y, Wilsmann-Theis D, Löhr S, Jacobi A, Weyergraf A, et al. Palmoplantar pustular psoriasis is associated with missense variants in CARD14, but not with loss-of-function mutations in IL36RN in European patients. *J Invest Dermatol* (2015) 135(10):2538–41. doi:10.1038/jid.2015.186
21. Bachelez H. Pustular psoriasis and related pustular skin diseases. *Br J Dermatol* (2018) 178(3):614–8. doi:10.1111/bjd.16232
22. Schakel K, Schön MP, Ghoreschi K. [Pathogenesis of psoriasis]. *Hautarzt* (2016) 67(6):422–31. doi:10.1007/s00105-016-3800-8
23. Arakawa A, Vollmer S, Besgen P, Galinski A, Summer B, Kawakami Y, et al. Unopposed IL-36 activity promotes clonal CD4(+) T-cell responses with IL-17A production in generalized pustular psoriasis. *J Invest Dermatol* (2018) 138(6):1338–47. doi:10.1016/j.jid.2017.12.024
24. Mossner R, Wilsmann-Theis D, Oji V, Gkogkolou P, Löhr S, Schulz P, et al. The genetic basis for most patients with pustular skin disease remains elusive. *Br J Dermatol* (2018) 178(3):740–8. doi:10.1111/bjd.15867
25. Nestle FO, Kaplan DH, Barker J. Psoriasis. *N Engl J Med* (2009) 361(5): 496–509. doi:10.1056/NEJMra0804595
26. Schön MP, Boehncke WH. Psoriasis. *N Engl J Med* (2005) 352(8):1899–912. doi:10.1056/NEJMra041320
27. Mueller W, Herrmann B. Cyclosporin A for psoriasis. *N Engl J Med* (1979) 301(10):555. doi:10.1056/NEJM197909063011015
28. Ellis CN, Krueger GG; Alefacept Clinical Study Group. Treatment of chronic plaque psoriasis by selective targeting of memory effector T lymphocytes. *N Engl J Med* (2001) 345(4):248–55. doi:10.1056/NEJM200107263450403
29. Schon MP. Efalizumab in the treatment of psoriasis: mode of action, clinical indications, efficacy, and safety. *Clin Dermatol* (2008) 26(5):509–14. doi:10.1016/j.clindermatol.2007.10.027
30. Ghoreschi K, Thomas P, Breit S, Dugas M, Mailhammer R, van Eden W, et al. Interleukin-4 therapy of psoriasis induces Th2 responses and improves human autoimmune disease. *Nat Med* (2003) 9(1):40–6. doi:10.1038/nm804
31. Guenova E, Skabytska Y, Hoetzenecker W, Weindl G, Sauer K, Tham M, et al. IL-4 abrogates T(H)17 cell-mediated inflammation by selective silencing of IL-23 in antigen-presenting cells. *Proc Natl Acad Sci U S A* (2015) 112(7):2163–8. doi:10.1073/pnas.1416922112
32. Asadullah K, Sterry W, Stephanek K, Jasulaitis D, Leupold M, Audring H, et al. IL-10 is a key cytokine in psoriasis. Proof of principle by IL-10 therapy: a new therapeutic approach. *J Clin Invest* (1998) 101(4):783–94. doi:10.1172/JCI1476
33. Gardembas-Pain M, Ifrah N, Foussard C, Boasson M, Saint Andre JP, Verret JL. Psoriasis after allogeneic bone marrow transplantation. *Arch Dermatol* (1990) 126(11):1523. doi:10.1001/archderm.1990.01670350139033
34. Trembath RC, Clough RL, Rosbotham JL, Jones AB, Camp RD, Frodsham A, et al. Identification of a major susceptibility locus on chromosome 6p and

evidence for further disease loci revealed by a two stage genome-wide search in psoriasis. *Hum Mol Genet* (1997) 6(5):813–20. doi:10.1093/hmg/6.5.813

35. Boehncke WH, Sterry W. Psoriasis – a systemic inflammatory disorder: clinic, pathogenesis and therapeutic perspectives. *J Dtsch Dermatol Ges* (2009) 7(11):946–52. doi:10.1111/j.1610-0387.2009.07083_supp.x
36. Burden AD, Javed S, Bailey M, Hodgins M, Connor M, Tillman D. Genetics of psoriasis: paternal inheritance and a locus on chromosome 6p. *J Invest Dermatol* (1998) 110(6):958–60. doi:10.1046/j.1523-1747.1998.00213.x
37. Breban M, Fernández-Sueiro JL, Richardson JA, Hadavand RR, Maika SD, Hammer RE, et al. T cells, but not thymic exposure to HLA-B27, are required for the inflammatory disease of HLA-B27 transgenic rats. *J Immunol* (1996) 156(2):794–803.
38. Schön MP, Detmar M, Parker CM. Murine psoriasis-like disorder induced by naive CD4+ T cells. *Nat Med* (1997) 3(2):183–8. doi:10.1038/nm0297-183
39. Wrone-Smith T, Nickoloff BJ. Dermal injection of immunocytes induces psoriasis. *J Clin Invest* (1996) 98(8):1878–87. doi:10.1172/JCI118989
40. Boyman O, Hefti HP, Conrad C, Nickoloff BJ, Suter M, Nestle FO. Spontaneous development of psoriasis in a new animal model shows an essential role for resident T cells and tumor necrosis factor-alpha. *J Exp Med* (2004) 199(5):731–6. doi:10.1084/jem.20031482
41. Boehncke WH, Dressel D, Zollner TM, Kaufmann R, et al. Pulling the trigger on psoriasis. *Nature* (1996) 379(6568):777. doi:10.1038/379777a0
42. Steinman L. A brief history of T(H)17, the first major revision in the T(H)1/T(H)2 hypothesis of T cell-mediated tissue damage. *Nat Med* (2007) 13(2):139–45. doi:10.1038/nm1551
43. Di Cesare A, Di Meglio P, Nestle FO. The IL-23/Th17 axis in the immunopathogenesis of psoriasis. *J Invest Dermatol* (2009) 129(6):1339–50. doi:10.1038/jid.2009.59
44. Lowes MA, Kikuchi T, Fuentes-Duculan J, Cardinale I, Zaba LC, Haider AS, et al. Psoriasis vulgaris lesions contain discrete populations of Th1 and Th17 T cells. *J Invest Dermatol* (2008) 128(5):1207–11. doi:10.1038/sj.jid.5701213
45. Lynde CW, Poulin Y, Vender R, Bourcier M, Khalil S. Interleukin 17A: toward a new understanding of psoriasis pathogenesis. *J Am Acad Dermatol* (2014) 71(1):141–50. doi:10.1016/j.jaad.2013.12.036
46. Murakami M, Hagforsen E, Morhenn V, Ishida-Yamamoto A, Iizuka H. Patients with palmoplantar pustulosis have increased IL-17 and IL-22 levels both in the lesion and serum. *Exp Dermatol* (2011) 20(10):845–7. doi:10.1111/j.1600-0625.2011.01325.x
47. Kebir H, Kreymborg K, Ifergan I, Dodelet-Devillers A, Cayrol R, Bernard M, et al. Human TH17 lymphocytes promote blood-brain barrier disruption and central nervous system inflammation. *Nat Med* (2007) 13(10):1173–5. doi:10.1038/nm1651
48. Neurath MF. IL-23: a master regulator in Crohn disease. *Nat Med* (2007) 13(1):26–8. doi:10.1038/nm0107-26
49. Poot J, Thewissen M, Booi D, Nieuwhof C. Characterization of skin-resident T cells using a crawl-out method and flow cytometry. *Exp Dermatol* (2013) 22(8):554–5. doi:10.1111/exd.12191
50. Noack M, Miossec P. Th17 and regulatory T cell balance in autoimmune and inflammatory diseases. *Autoimmun Rev* (2014) 13(6):668–77. doi:10.1016/j.autrev.2013.12.004
51. Chen X, Oppenheim JJ. Th17 cells and Tregs: unlikely allies. *J Leukoc Biol* (2014) 95(5):723–31. doi:10.1189/jlb.1213633
52. Muhr P, Renne J, Schaefer V, Werfel T, Wittmann M. Primary human keratinocytes efficiently induce IL-1-dependent IL-17 in CCR6+ T cells. *Exp Dermatol* (2010) 19(12):1105–7. doi:10.1111/j.1600-0625.2010.01134.x
53. Kryczek I, Bruce AT, Gudjonsson JE, Johnston A, Aphale A, Vatan L, et al. Induction of IL-17+ T cell trafficking and development by IFN-gamma: mechanism and pathological relevance in psoriasis. *J Immunol* (2008) 181(7):4733–41. doi:10.4049/jimmunol.181.7.4733
54. McGeachy MJ, Chen Y, Tato CM, Laurence A, Joyce-Shaikh B, Blumenschein WM, et al. The interleukin 23 receptor is essential for the terminal differentiation of interleukin 17-producing effector T helper cells in vivo. *Nat Immunol* (2009) 10(3):314–24. doi:10.1038/ni.1698
55. Bettelli E, Korn T, Kuchroo VK. Th17: the third member of the effector T cell trilogy. *Curr Opin Immunol* (2007) 19(6):652–7. doi:10.1016/j.coi.2007.07.020
56. Stritesky GL, Yeh N, Kaplan MH. IL-23 promotes maintenance but not commitment to the Th17 lineage. *J Immunol* (2008) 181(9):5948–55. doi:10.4049/jimmunol.181.9.5948
57. Ghoreschi K, Weigert C, Röcken M. Immunopathogenesis and role of T cells in psoriasis. *Clin Dermatol* (2007) 25(6):574–80. doi:10.1016/j.clindermatol.2007.08.012
58. Boniface K, Blom B, Liu YJ, de Waal Malefyt R. From interleukin-23 to T-helper 17 cells: human T-helper cell differentiation revisited. *Immunol Rev* (2008) 226:132–46. doi:10.1111/j.1600-065X.2008.00714.x
59. Singh TP, Schön MP, Wallbrecht K, Michaelis K, Rinner B, Mayer G, et al. 8-methoxypsoralen plus ultraviolet A therapy acts via inhibition of the IL-23/Th17 axis and induction of Foxp3+ regulatory T cells involving CTLA4 signaling in a psoriasis-like skin disorder. *J Immunol* (2010) 184(12):7257–67. doi:10.4049/jimmunol.0903719
60. Drozdenko G, Heine G, Worm M. Oral vitamin D increases the frequencies of CD38+ human B cells and ameliorates IL-17-producing T cells. *Exp Dermatol* (2014) 23(2):107–12. doi:10.1111/exd.12300
61. Singh TP, Schön MP, Wallbrecht K, Gruber-Wackernagel A, Wang XJ, Wolf P. Involvement of IL-9 in Th17-associated inflammation and angiogenesis of psoriasis. *PLos One* (2013) 8(1):e51752. doi:10.1371/journal.pone.0051752
62. Yoshiga Y, Goto D, Segawa S, Ohnishi Y, Matsumoto I, Ito S, et al. Invariant NKT cells produce IL-17 through IL-23-dependent and -independent pathways with potential modulation of Th17 response in collagen-induced arthritis. *Int J Mol Med* (2008) 22(3):369–74. doi:10.3892/ijmm_00000032
63. Cua DJ, Tato CM. Innate IL-17-producing cells: the sentinels of the immune system. *Nat Rev Immunol* (2010) 10(7):479–89. doi:10.1038/nri2800
64. Lee JS, Tato CM, Joyce-Shaikh B, Gulen MF, Cayatte C, Chen Y, et al. Interleukin-23-independent IL-17 production regulates intestinal epithelial permeability. *Immunity* (2015) 43(4):727–38. doi:10.1016/j.immuni.2015.09.003
65. Wei YL, Han A, Glanville J, Fang F, Zuniga LA, Lee JS, et al. A highly focused antigen receptor repertoire characterizes γδ T cells that are poised to make IL-17 rapidly in naive animals. *Front Immunol* (2015) 6:118. doi:10.3389/fimmu.2015.00118
66. Godfrey DI, Uldrich AP, McCluskey J, Rossjohn J, Moody DB. The burgeoning family of unconventional T cells. *Nat Immunol* (2015) 16(11):1114–23. doi:10.1038/ni.3298
67. Teunissen MBM, Yeremenko NG, Baeten DLP, Chielie S, Spuls PI, de Rie MA, et al. The IL-17A-producing CD8+ T-cell population in psoriatic lesional skin comprises mucosa-associated invariant T cells and conventional T cells. *J Invest Dermatol* (2014) 134(12):2898–907. doi:10.1038/jid.2014.261
68. Serriari NE, Eoche M, Lamotte L, Lion J, Fumery M, Marcelo P, et al. Innate mucosal-associated invariant T (MAIT) cells are activated in inflammatory bowel diseases. *Clin Exp Immunol* (2014) 176(2):266–74. doi:10.1111/cei.12277
69. Cho YN, Kee SJ, Kim TJ, Jin HM, Kim MJ, Jung HJ, et al. Mucosal-associated invariant T cell deficiency in systemic lupus erythematosus. *J Immunol* (2014) 193(8):3891–901. doi:10.4049/jimmunol.1302701
70. Simoni Y, Newell EW. Dissecting human ILC heterogeneity: more than just three subsets. *Immunology* (2018) 153(3):297–303. doi:10.1111/imm.12862
71. Keijsers RR, Hendriks AGM, van Erp PEJ, van Cranenbroek B, van de Kerkhof PCM, Koenen HJPM, et al. In vivo induction of cutaneous inflammation results in the accumulation of extracellular trap-forming neutrophils expressing RORgammat and IL-17. *J Invest Dermatol* (2014) 134(5):1276–84. doi:10.1038/jid.2013.526
72. Dyring-Andersen B, Honoré TV, Madelung A, Bzorek M, Simonsen S, Clemmensen SN, et al. Interleukin (IL)-17A and IL-22-producing neutrophils in psoriatic skin. *Br J Dermatol* (2017) 177(6):e321–2. doi:10.1111/bjd.15533
73. Schon MP. The plot thickens while the scope broadens: a holistic view on IL-17 in psoriasis and other inflammatory disorders. *Exp Dermatol* (2014) 23(11):804–6. doi:10.1111/exd.12541
74. Lin AM, Rubin CJ, Khandpur R, Wang JY, Riblett M, Yalavarthi S, et al. Mast cells and neutrophils release IL-17 through extracellular trap formation in psoriasis. *J Immunol* (2011) 187(1):490–500. doi:10.4049/jimmunol.1100123
75. Griffiths CE, Strober BE, van de Kerkhof P, Ho V, Fidelus-Gort R, Yeilding N, et al. Comparison of ustekinumab and etanercept for moderate-to-severe psoriasis. *N Engl J Med* (2010) 362(2):118–28. doi:10.1056/NEJMoa0810652
76. Nestle FO, Conrad C. The IL-12 family member p40 chain as a master switch and novel therapeutic target in psoriasis. *J Invest Dermatol* (2004) 123(6):xiv–xv. doi:10.1111/j.0022-202X.2004.23488.x

77. Teng MW, Bowman EP, McElwee JJ, Smyth MJ, Casanova JL, Cooper AM, et al. IL-12 and IL-23 cytokines: from discovery to targeted therapies for immune-mediated inflammatory diseases. *Nat Med* (2015) 21(7):719–29. doi:10.1038/nm.3895
78. Gordon KB, Duffin KC, Bissonnette R, Prinz JC, Wasfi Y, Li S, et al. A phase 2 trial of guselkumab versus adalimumab for plaque psoriasis. *N Engl J Med* (2015) 373(2):136–44. doi:10.1056/NEJMoa1501646
79. Langley RG, Elewski BE, Lebwohl M, Reich K, Griffiths CE, Papp K, et al. Secukinumab in plaque psoriasis – results of two phase 3 trials. *N Engl J Med* (2014) 371(4):326–38. doi:10.1056/NEJMoa1314258
80. Leonardi C, Matheson R, Zachariae C, Cameron G, Li L, Edson-Heredia E, et al. Anti-interleukin-17 monoclonal antibody ixekizumab in chronic plaque psoriasis. *N Engl J Med* (2012) 366(13):1190–9. doi:10.1056/NEJMoa1109997
81. Lebwohl M, Strober B, Menter A, Gordon K, Weglowska J, Puig L, et al. Phase 3 studies comparing brodalumab with ustekinumab in psoriasis. *N Engl J Med* (2015) 373(14):1318–28. doi:10.1056/NEJMoa1503824
82. Papp KA, Leonardi C, Menter A, Ortonne JP, Krueger JG, Kricorian G, et al. Brodalumab, an anti-interleukin-17-receptor antibody for psoriasis. *N Engl J Med* (2012) 366(13):1181–9. doi:10.1056/NEJMoa1109017
83. Ghoreschi K, Brück J, Kellerer C, Deng C, Peng H, Rothfuss O, et al. Fumarates improve psoriasis and multiple sclerosis by inducing type II dendritic cells. *J Exp Med* (2011) 208(11):2291–303. doi:10.1084/jem.20100977
84. Wallbrecht K, Drick N, Hund AC, Schön MP. Downregulation of endothelial adhesion molecules by dimethylfumarate, but not monomethylfumarate, and impairment of dynamic lymphocyte-endothelial cell interactions. *Exp Dermatol* (2011) 20(12):980–5. doi:10.1111/j.1600-0625.2011.01376.x
85. Hund AC, Lockmann A, Schön MP. Mutually enhancing anti-inflammatory activities of dimethyl fumarate and NF-kappaB inhibitors – implications for dose-sparing combination therapies. *Exp Dermatol* (2016) 25(2):124–30. doi:10.1111/exd.12892
86. Schafer P. Apremilast mechanism of action and application to psoriasis and psoriatic arthritis. *Biochem Pharmacol* (2012) 83(12):1583–90. doi:10.1016/j.bcp.2012.01.001
87. Ghoreschi K, Laurence A, O'Shea JJ. Janus kinases in immune cell signaling. *Immunol Rev* (2009) 228(1):273–87. doi:10.1111/j.1600-065X.2008.00754.x
88. Schwartz DM, Kanno Y, Villarino A, Ward M, Gadina M, O'Shea JJ, et al. JAK inhibition as a therapeutic strategy for immune and inflammatory diseases. *Nat Rev Drug Discov* (2017) 16(12):843–62. doi:10.1038/nrd.2017.201
89. Ghoreschi K, Gadina M. Jakpot! New small molecules in autoimmune and inflammatory diseases. *Exp Dermatol* (2014) 23(1):7–11. doi:10.1111/exd.12265
90. Patel DD, Kuchroo VK. Th17 cell pathway in human immunity: lessons from genetics and therapeutic interventions. *Immunity* (2015) 43(6):1040–51. doi:10.1016/j.immuni.2015.12.003
91. Alwan W, Nestle FO. Pathogenesis and treatment of psoriasis: exploiting pathophysiological pathways for precision medicine. *Clin Exp Rheumatol* (2015) 33(5 Suppl 93):s2–6.
92. Collins FS, Varmus H. A new initiative on precision medicine. *N Engl J Med* (2015) 372(9):793–5. doi:10.1056/NEJMp1500523
93. Lowes MA, Suárez-Fariñas M, Krueger JG. Immunology of psoriasis. *Annu Rev Immunol* (2014) 32:227–55. doi:10.1146/annurev-immunol-032713-120225
94. Villanova F, Flutter B, Tosi I, Grys K, Sreeneebus H, Perera GK, et al. Characterization of innate lymphoid cells in human skin and blood demonstrates increase of NKp44+ ILC3 in psoriasis. *J Invest Dermatol* (2014) 134(4):984–91. doi:10.1038/jid.2013.477
95. Ward NL, Umetsu DT. A new player on the psoriasis block: IL-17A- and IL-22-producing innate lymphoid cells. *J Invest Dermatol* (2014) 134(9):2305–7. doi:10.1038/jid.2014.216
96. Frohm M, Agerberth B, Ahangari G, Ståhle-Bäckdahl M, Lidén S, Wigzell H, et al. The expression of the gene coding for the antibacterial peptide LL-37 is induced in human keratinocytes during inflammatory disorders. *J Biol Chem* (1997) 272(24):15258–63. doi:10.1074/jbc.272.24.15258
97. Morizane S, Yamasaki K, Mühleisen B, Kotol PF, Murakami M, Aoyama Y, et al. Cathelicidin antimicrobial peptide LL-37 in psoriasis enables keratinocyte reactivity against TLR9 ligands. *J Invest Dermatol* (2012) 132(1):135–43. doi:10.1038/jid.2011.259
98. Lande R, Gregorio J, Facchinetti V, Chatterjee B, Wang YH, Homey B, et al. Plasmacytoid dendritic cells sense self-DNA coupled with antimicrobial peptide. *Nature* (2007) 449(7162):564–9. doi:10.1038/nature06116
99. Ganguly D, Chamilos G, Lande R, Gregorio J, Meller S, Facchinetti V, et al. Self-RNA-antimicrobial peptide complexes activate human dendritic cells through TLR7 and TLR8. *J Exp Med* (2009) 206(9):1983–94. doi:10.1084/jem.20090480
100. Zaba LC, Suárez-Fariñas M, Fuentes-Duculan J, Nograles KE, Guttman-Yassky E, Cardinale I, et al. Effective treatment of psoriasis with etanercept is linked to suppression of IL-17 signaling, not immediate response TNF genes. *J Allergy Clin Immunol* (2009) 124(5):1022–10.e1–395. doi:10.1016/j.jaci.2009.08.046
101. Hegyi Z, Zwicker S, Bureik D, Peric M, Koglin S, Batycka-Baran A, et al. Vitamin D analog calcipotriol suppresses the Th17 cytokine-induced proinflammatory S100 "alarmins" psoriasin (S100A7) and koebnerisin (S100A15) in psoriasis. *J Invest Dermatol* (2012) 132(5):1416–24. doi:10.1038/jid.2011.486
102. Batycka-Baran A, Maj J, Wolf R, Szepietowski JC. The new insight into the role of antimicrobial proteins-alarmins in the immunopathogenesis of psoriasis. *J Immunol Res* (2014) 2014:628289. doi:10.1155/2014/628289
103. Lee Y, Jang S, Min JK, Lee K, Sohn KC, Lim JS, et al. S100A8 and S100A9 are messengers in the crosstalk between epidermis and dermis modulating a psoriatic milieu in human skin. *Biochem Biophys Res Commun* (2012) 423(4):647–53. doi:10.1016/j.bbrc.2012.05.162
104. Loser K, Vogl T, Voskort M, Lueken A, Kupas V, Nacken W, et al. The toll-like receptor 4 ligands Mrp8 and Mrp14 are crucial in the development of autoreactive CD8+ T cells. *Nat Med* (2010) 16(6):713–7. doi:10.1038/nm.2150
105. Tewary P, de la Rosa G, Sharma N, Rodriguez LG, Tarasov SG, Howard OM, et al. beta-Defensin 2 and 3 promote the uptake of self or CpG DNA, enhance IFN-alpha production by human plasmacytoid dendritic cells, and promote inflammation. *J Immunol* (2013) 191(2):865–74. doi:10.4049/jimmunol.1201648
106. Hänsel A, Günther C, Ingwersen J, Starke J, Schmitz M, Bachmann M, et al. Human slan (6-sulfo LacNAc) dendritic cells are inflammatory dermal dendritic cells in psoriasis and drive strong TH17/TH1 T-cell responses. *J Allergy Clin Immunol* (2011) 127(3):787–94.e1–9. doi:10.1016/j.jaci.2010.12.009
107. Fuentes-Duculan J, Suárez-Fariñas M, Zaba LC, Nograles KE, Pierson KC, Mitsui H, et al. A subpopulation of CD163-positive macrophages is classically activated in psoriasis. *J Invest Dermatol* (2010) 130(10):2412–22. doi:10.1038/jid.2010.165
108. Schäkel K, Kannagi R, Kniep B, Goto Y, Mitsuoka C, Zwirner J, et al. 6-Sulfo LacNAc, a novel carbohydrate modification of PSGL-1, defines an inflammatory type of human dendritic cells. *Immunity* (2002) 17(3):289–301. doi:10.1016/S1074-7613(02)00393-X
109. Schäkel K, Mayer E, Federle C, Schmitz M, Riethmüller G, Rieber EP. A novel dendritic cell population in human blood: one-step immunomagnetic isolation by a specific mAb (M-DC8) and in vitro priming of cytotoxic T lymphocytes. *Eur J Immunol* (1998) 28(12):4084–93. doi:10.1002/(SICI)1521-4141(199812)28:12<4084::AID-IMMU4084>3.0.CO;2-4
110. Schäkel K, von Kietzell M, Hänsel A, Ebling A, Schulze L, Haase M, et al. Human 6-sulfo LacNAc-expressing dendritic cells are principal producers of early interleukin-12 and are controlled by erythrocytes. *Immunity* (2006) 24(5):767–77. doi:10.1016/j.immuni.2006.03.020
111. Di Meglio P, Perera GK, Nestle FO. The multitasking organ: recent insights into skin immune function. *Immunity* (2011) 35(6):857–69. doi:10.1016/j.immuni.2011.12.003
112. Schön MP, Broekaert SM, Erpenbeck L. Sexy again: the renaissance of neutrophils in psoriasis. *Exp Dermatol* (2017). 26(4):305–11. doi:10.1111/exd.13067
113. Chen K, Nishi H, Travers R, Tsuboi N, Martinod K, Wagner DD, et al. Endocytosis of soluble immune complexes leads to their clearance by FcgammaRIIIB but induces neutrophil extracellular traps via FcgammaRIIA in vivo. *Blood* (2012) 120(22):4421–31. doi:10.1182/blood-2011-12-401133
114. Fuchs TA, Abed U, Goosmann C, Hurwitz R, Schulze I, Wahn V, et al. Novel cell death program leads to neutrophil extracellular traps. *J Cell Biol* (2007) 176(2):231–41. doi:10.1083/jcb.200606027
115. Metzler KD, Fuchs TA, Nauseef WM, Reumaux D, Roesler J, Schulze I, et al. Myeloperoxidase is required for neutrophil extracellular trap formation: implications for innate immunity. *Blood* (2011) 117(3):953–9. doi:10.1182/blood-2010-06-290171

116. Bianchi M, Hakkim A, Brinkmann V, Siler U, Seger RA, Zychlinsky A, et al. Restoration of NET formation by gene therapy in CGD controls aspergillosis. *Blood* (2009) 114(13):2619–22. doi:10.1182/blood-2009-05-221606
117. Parker H, Dragunow M, Hampton MB, Kettle AJ, Winterbourn CC. Requirements for NADPH oxidase and myeloperoxidase in neutrophil extracellular trap formation differ depending on the stimulus. *J Leukoc Biol* (2012) 92(4): 841–9. doi:10.1189/jlb.1211601
118. Hakkim A, Fuchs TA, Martinez NE, Hess S, Prinz H, Zychlinsky A, et al. Activation of the Raf-MEK-ERK pathway is required for neutrophil extracellular trap formation. *Nat Chem Biol* (2011) 7(2):75–7. doi:10.1038/nchembio.496
119. Metzler KD, Goosmann C, Lubojemska A, Zychlinsky A, Papayannopoulos V. A myeloperoxidase-containing complex regulates neutrophil elastase release and actin dynamics during NETosis. *Cell Rep* (2014) 8(3):883–96. doi:10.1016/j.celrep.2014.06.044
120. Papayannopoulos V, Metzler KD, Hakkim A, Zychlinsky A. Neutrophil elastase and myeloperoxidase regulate the formation of neutrophil extracellular traps. *J Cell Biol* (2010) 191(3):677–91. doi:10.1083/jcb.201006052
121. Lewis HD, Liddle J, Coote JE, Atkinson SJ, Barker MD, Bax BD, et al. Inhibition of PAD4 activity is sufficient to disrupt mouse and human NET formation. *Nat Chem Biol* (2015) 11(3):189–91. doi:10.1038/nchembio.1735
122. Wang Y, Li M, Stadler S, Correll S, Li P, Wang D, et al. Histone hypercitrullination mediates chromatin decondensation and neutrophil extracellular trap formation. *J Cell Biol* (2009) 184(2):205–13. doi:10.1083/jcb.200806072
123. Neumann A, Völlger L, Berends ET, Molhoek EM, Stapels DA, Midon M, et al. Novel role of the antimicrobial peptide LL-37 in the protection of neutrophil extracellular traps against degradation by bacterial nucleases. *J Innate Immun* (2014) 6(6):860–8. doi:10.1159/000363699
124. Lande R, Ganguly D, Facchinetti V, Frasca L, Conrad C, Gregorio J, et al. Neutrophils activate plasmacytoid dendritic cells by releasing self-DNA-peptide complexes in systemic lupus erythematosus. *Sci Transl Med* (2011) 3(73):73ra19. doi:10.1126/scitranslmed.3001180
125. Diana J, Simoni Y, Furio L, Beaudoin L, Agerberth B, Barrat F, et al. Crosstalk between neutrophils, B-1a cells and plasmacytoid dendritic cells initiates autoimmune diabetes. *Nat Med* (2013) 19(1):65–73. doi:10.1038/nm.3042
126. Tillack K, Breiden P, Martin R, Sospedra M. T lymphocyte priming by neutrophil extracellular traps links innate and adaptive immune responses. *J Immunol* (2012) 188(7):3150–9. doi:10.4049/jimmunol.1103414
127. Sangaletti S, Tripodo C, Chiodoni C, Guarnotta C, Cappetti B, Casalini P, et al. Neutrophil extracellular traps mediate transfer of cytoplasmic neutrophil antigens to myeloid dendritic cells toward ANCA induction and associated autoimmunity. *Blood* (2012) 120(15):3007–18. doi:10.1182/blood-2012-03-416156
128. Pantelyushin S, Haak S, Ingold B, Kulig P, Heppner FL, Navarini AA, et al. Rorgammat+ innate lymphocytes and gammadelta T cells initiate psoriasiform plaque formation in mice. *J Clin Invest* (2012) 122(6):2252–6. doi:10.1172/JCI61862
129. Schön M, Denzer D, Kubitza RC, Ruzicka T, Schön MP. Critical role of neutrophils for the generation of psoriasiform skin lesions in flaky skin mice. *J Invest Dermatol* (2000) 114(5):976–83. doi:10.1046/j.1523-1747.2000.00953.x
130. Riol-Blanco L, Ordovas-Montanes J, Perro M, Naval E, Thiriot A, Alvarez D, et al. Nociceptive sensory neurons drive interleukin-23-mediated psoriasiform skin inflammation. *Nature* (2014) 510(7503):157–61. doi:10.1038/nature13199
131. Keijsers RR, Joosten I, van Erp PE, Koenen HJ, van de Kerkhof PC. Cellular sources of IL-17 in psoriasis: a paradigm shift? *Exp Dermatol* (2014) 23(11): 799–803. doi:10.1111/exd.12487
132. Teunissen MB, Koomen CW, de Waal Malefyt R, Wierenga EA, Bos JD. Interleukin-17 and interferon-gamma synergize in the enhancement of proinflammatory cytokine production by human keratinocytes. *J Invest Dermatol* (1998) 111(4):645–9. doi:10.1046/j.1523-1747.1998.00347.x
133. Gupta AK, Joshi MB, Philippova M, Erne P, Hasler P, Hahn S, et al. Activated endothelial cells induce neutrophil extracellular traps and are susceptible to NETosis-mediated cell death. *FEBS Lett* (2010) 584(14):3193–7. doi:10.1016/j.febslet.2010.06.006
134. Gupta AK, Hasler P, Holzgreve W, Gebhardt S, Hahn S. Induction of neutrophil extracellular DNA lattices by placental microparticles and IL-8 and their presence in preeclampsia. *Hum Immunol* (2005) 66(11):1146–54. doi:10.1016/j.humimm.2005.11.003
135. Kaneko S, Kondo Y, Yokosawa M, Furuyama K, Segawa S, Tsuboi H, et al. The RORgammat-CCR6-CCL20 axis augments Th17 cells invasion into the synovia of rheumatoid arthritis patients. *Mod Rheumatol* (2018):1–12. doi:10.1080/14397595.2017.1422304
136. Skovdahl HK, Granlund AV, Østvik AE, Bruland T, Bakke I, Torp SH, et al. Expression of CCL20 and its corresponding receptor CCR6 is enhanced in active inflammatory bowel disease, and TLR3 mediates CCL20 expression in colonic epithelial cells. *PLoS One* (2015) 10(11):e0141710. doi:10.1371/journal.pone.0141710
137. Savchenko AS, Borissoff JI, Martinod K, De Meyer SF, Gallant M, Erpenbeck L, et al. VWF-mediated leukocyte recruitment with chromatin decondensation by PAD4 increases myocardial ischemia/reperfusion injury in mice. *Blood* (2014) 123(1):141–8. doi:10.1182/blood-2013-07-514992
138. Chiricozzi A, Guttman-Yassky E, Suárez-Fariñas M, Nograles KE, Tian S, Cardinale I, et al. Integrative responses to IL-17 and TNF-alpha in human keratinocytes account for key inflammatory pathogenic circuits in psoriasis. *J Invest Dermatol* (2011) 131(3):677–87. doi:10.1038/jid.2010.340
139. Wang CQF, Akalu YT, Suarez-Farinas M, Gonzalez J, Mitsui H, Lowes MA, et al. IL-17 and TNF synergistically modulate cytokine expression while suppressing melanogenesis: potential relevance to psoriasis. *J Invest Dermatol* (2013) 133(12):2741–52. doi:10.1038/jid.2013.237
140. Johnston A, Xing X, Wolterink L, Barnes DH, Yin Z, Reingold L, et al. IL-1 and IL-36 are dominant cytokines in generalized pustular psoriasis. *J Allergy Clin Immunol* (2017) 140(1):109–20. doi:10.1016/j.jaci.2016.08.056
141. Zibert JR, Wallbrecht K, Schön M, Mir LM, Jacobsen GK, Trochon-Joseph V, et al. Halting angiogenesis by non-viral somatic gene therapy alleviates psoriasis and murine psoriasiform skin lesions. *J Clin Invest* (2011) 121(1):410–21. doi:10.1172/JCI41295

13

Thrombosis in Psoriasis: Cutaneous Cytokine Production as a Potential Driving Force of Haemostatic Dysregulation and Subsequent Cardiovascular Risk

Maria J. E. Visser[1], *Gareth Tarr*[1,2] *and Etheresia Pretorius*[1*]

[1] *Department of Physiological Sciences, Faculty of Science, Stellenbosch University, Stellenbosch, South Africa,*
[2] *Division of Rheumatology, Institute of Orthopaedics and Rheumatology, Winelands Mediclinic Orthopaedic Hospital, Stellenbosch, South Africa*

Correspondence:
Etheresia Pretorius
resiap@sun.ac.za
orcid.org/0000-0002-9108-2384

Psoriasis (PsO) is a common T cell-mediated inflammatory disorder of the skin with an estimated prevalence of 2%. The condition manifests most commonly as erythematous plaques covered with scales. The aetiology of PsO is multifactorial and disease initiation involves interactions between environmental factors, susceptibility genes, and innate and adaptive immune responses. The underlying pathology is mainly driven by interleukin-17. In addition, various inflammatory mediators from specific T helper (T_H) cell subsets, namely T_H1, T_H17, and T_H22, are overexpressed in cutaneous lesions and may also be detected in the peripheral blood of psoriatic patients. Moreover, these individuals are also at greater risk, compared to the general population, of developing multiple comorbid conditions. Cardiovascular disease (CVD) has been recognised as a prominent comorbidity of PsO. A potential mechanism contributing to this association may be the presence of a hypercoagulable state in these individuals. Inflammation and coagulation are closely related. The presence of chronic, low-grade systemic inflammation may promote thrombosis – one of the major determinants of CVD. A pro-inflammatory milieu may induce the expression of tissue factor, augment platelet activity, and perturb the vascular endothelium. Altogether, these changes will result in a prothrombotic state. In this review, we describe the aetiology of PsO, as well as the pathophysiology of the condition. We also consider its relationship to CVD. Given the systemic inflammatory nature of PsO, we evaluate the potential contribution of prominent inflammatory mediators (implicated in PsO pathogenesis) to establishing a prothrombotic state in psoriatic patients.

Keywords: cardiovascular disease, endothelium, hypercoagulability, platelets, psoriasis, systemic inflammation

INTRODUCTION

Psoriasis (PsO) is a chronic immune-mediated inflammatory disease of the skin, often associated with multiple comorbidities, affecting approximately 2% of the global population (1). Of those affected, 30% may develop an inflammatory arthritis (psoriatic arthritis). The reported prevalence of PsO in childhood may be up to 1.37% (2–4), while the estimated prevalence in adults ranges from 0.51% to 11.43% (3, 5, 6). Research suggests that disease development involves a complex interplay between genetic predisposition, environmental stimuli, and disordered innate and adaptive immune responses. Lesions may assume a variety of clinical forms (7), with plaque PsO being the most common disease variant. Typically, the condition manifests as well-circumscribed, erythematous papules and/or plaques covered with scales. In addition to its physical symptoms, PsO also imposes a significant psychosocial burden that may lead to anxiety, depression, and in severe cases, suicidality (8). The physical and psychological impact of PsO may significantly influence a patients' quality of life (9), as well as contribute to an increased risk of mortality in severe forms of the disease (10).

PsO is considered to be a T cell-mediated disease and the corresponding cytokine profile of psoriatic lesions indicates important roles for interferon (IFN)-α, interleukin (IL)-22, the IL-23/IL-17 axis, and tumour necrosis factor (TNF) in psoriatic pathology (11–13). In addition to localised cutaneous inflammation, these molecules have also been detected in the systemic circulation of psoriatic patients – increasing the risk of comorbidities (14–16). Considering these observations, a paradigm shift has occurred from viewing PsO as merely 'skin-deep' to viewing it as a systemic inflammatory condition that can affect various extracutaneous tissues (17). Cardiovascular disease (CVD) is a notable comorbidity in patients suffering from PsO. An increased risk of major cardiovascular events, as well as an increased CVD mortality in severe forms of the disease, has been reported in these individuals (18–22). The relationship between PsO and CVD is widely acknowledged, however, the mechanisms responsible remain uncertain.

Hypercoagulability is a potential mechanistic link accounting for the association between CVD and PsO. It is becoming increasingly clear that inflammation and coagulation are interrelated processes (23, 24). A hypercoagulable state may develop as a result of an imbalance in haemostatic and inflammatory activity mediated by pro-inflammatory cytokines. These molecules may promote the initiation of coagulation, inhibit endogenous anticoagulant systems, and impair fibrinolytic activity (24, 25). The vascular endothelium also plays a central role in clot formation, as it is located at the nexus of inflammation and coagulation. Under normal physiological conditions, the resting endothelium displays anticoagulant and anti-inflammatory effects (26, 27). This homeostasis is disrupted in inflammatory conditions as a result of pro-inflammatory cytokines perturbing the vessel wall, resulting in a transition to an activated state that favours coagulation (28).

This review will briefly discuss genetic and environmental risk factors associated with the development of PsO, as well as the pathogenesis of the condition. In addition, the literature describing the systemic inflammatory nature of PsO and its subsequent relationship to CVD will also be considered. Finally, the potential contribution of prominent inflammatory mediators in PsO, to promote a prothrombotic state, is also appraised.

THE AETIOLOGY OF PSORIASIS

Genetic Risk Factors

The important role of a genetic component in the molecular pathogenesis of PsO has been supported by various family-based studies (29), including twin studies. An increased disease concordance rate has been reported in monozygotic twins, compared to dizygotic twins (30–32). Despite this disease concordance, the incidence never reaches 100% – suggesting a role for environmental factors in addition to genetic susceptibility in PsO development. The current view is that the mode of inheritance for PsO is multifactorial. Classic genome-wide linkage analysis has identified at least nine different chromosomal regions, termed psoriasis susceptibility (*PSORS1–PSORS9*) loci, which have shown statistically significant associations with PsO (33). Multiple studies have validated *PSORS1* as the most important genomic region in PsO predisposition and that it may account for up to 35% of disease heritability (34). *PSORS1* is located on human chromosome 6p21.3 within the region of the major histocompatibility complex (MHC). *Human leukocyte antigen (HLA)-Cw*0602* has been accepted as the most likely *PSORS1* disease allele (35). The *HLA-C* gene encodes a class 1 MHC protein and participates in the priming of cluster of differentiation (CD) 8^+ T cell immune responses. More than 80 PsO susceptibility loci have been identified in genome-wide association studies (GWASs), conducted mainly on European and Asian populations (36). In 2007, in the first GWAS for PsO, two genes (*IL12B* and *IL23R*) were identified that were associated with PsO risk (37). Specific pathways implicated in PsO pathogenesis that have been identified through GWASs include interferon signalling, the IL-23 pathway, the nuclear factor kappa-light-chain-enhancer of activated B cells (NF-κB) cascade and the regulation of T cell responses (38–42).

Environmental Risk Factors

Environmental triggers play a critical role in the onset and development of PsO in genetically predisposed individuals through the interaction with genes and the induction of epigenetic modifications (43). Various environmental exposures have been associated with the initiation and/or exacerbation of psoriatic lesions. Stressful life events are well known to contribute to the initiation and aggravation of PsO. A potential explanation for stress-induced PsO onset or flares may be dysregulation of hypothalamic–pituitary–adrenal axis activity (44, 45). Obesity is another significant risk factor for PsO and body mass index has been demonstrated to correlate with disease severity (46). Potential mediators of this association may include adipokines, such as leptin and resistin, which possess pro-inflammatory actions (47). Furthermore, epidemiological studies have suggested an association between smoking and the development of PsO, based on the increased incidence of PsO reported among current and former smokers compared to non-smokers (48–50). Smoking may induce PsO by augmenting the existing systemic oxidative stress, interacting with immune cells, and altering gene expression (51, 52). Bacterial infections, specifically by *Staphylococcus aureus* and *Streptococcus pyogenes*, are recognised triggers of PsO. β-haemolytic streptococci have been isolated more frequently from throat swabs from PsO patients, compared to controls (53), and enterotoxins from *Staphylococcus aureus* have been linked to more severe PsO (54). Dysbiosis of both the gut and skin microbiome has become a recurrent theme in psoriatic individuals (55). Gut dysbiosis, characterised by a decrease in microbes with anti-inflammatory and immunomodulatory properties (56, 57), seems to be prevalent in these individuals (58, 59). An altered skin microbiome has also been associated with the condition (60, 61).

PATHOGENESIS OF PSORIASIS

Environmental factors (e.g., stress, obesity, smoking, infection, and dysbiosis) or physical trauma (the Koebner phenomenon) may perturb keratinocytes, resulting in the release of self-deoxyribonucleic acid (DNA) or self-ribonucleic acid (RNA) (62, 63). In turn, these self-nucleic acids may form a complex with the endogenous antimicrobial peptide (AMP), cathelicidin/LL37 (63). DNA-LL37 complexes activate plasmacytoid dendritic cells (pDCs), *via* Toll-like receptor (TLR) 9 signalling, which secrete high levels of IFN-α (64). In a similar fashion, RNA-LL37 complexes activate pDCs in a TLR7-dependent manner (62). Consequently, conventional dendritic cells (cDCs), which function as professional antigen-presenting cells (APCs), are activated by IFN-α. RNA-LL37 complexes also possess the capacity to activate cDCs directly, leading to the production of IL-6 and TNF by these cells. Once activated, cDCs migrate to secondary lymphoid organs and secrete IL-12 and IL-23 (65), which induce the differentiation of naïve $CD4^+$ T cells into T_H1 (66) and T_H17 (67) cells, respectively. This process provides a potential mechanism for the initiation of the inflammatory sequelae in PsO and highlights the central role of DCs to establish a link between the innate and adaptive branches of the immune system.

T_H1 cells express cytokines such as IFN-γ, IL-2, and TNF (66, 68). IFN-γ induces the expression of several chemokines and cytokines in the skin and also promotes the accumulation and infiltration of inflammatory cells (69, 70). TNF has been identified as a key regulatory molecule in the cytokine network of PsO. In addition to T_H1 cells, a distinct subset of DCs, namely TNF- and inducible nitric oxide synthase-producing DCs, also release large amounts of TNF (71). It has been suggested that TNF production mediates the proliferation of resident T cells in the development of psoriatic lesions (72). In addition, TNF regulates the expression of cell adhesion molecules, which mediate the extravasation of leukocytes, on endothelial cells and keratinocytes in psoriatic skin (73). TNF also stimulate keratinocytes to induce the expression of pro-inflammatory cytokines such as IL-6, IL-8, and TNF itself, through the activation of NF-κB (74). Furthermore, TNF may synergise with IL-17 to enhance the expression of key inflammatory genes in keratinocytes (75).

T_H17 cytokines such as IL-17A, IL-17F, and IL-22 (76, 77) are key pathogenic effectors in PsO. Therefore, PsO has been regarded as a T_H17-mediated disease. However, this paradigm is shifting towards understanding PsO as an IL-17-driven disease (78). Various other cellular sources of IL-17 exist, including $CD8^+$ T cells (comprising mucosa-associated invariant T cells and conventional T cells) (79), dermal γδ T cells (80), group 3 innate lymphoid cells (81), mast cells, and neutrophils (82). IL-17A has been shown to govern the expression of signature PsO genes in keratinocytes (83). IL-17 acts on keratinocytes to induce the expression of AMPs, such as β-defensin 2, and neutrophil chemoattractants, namely C-X-C motif chemokine ligand (CXCL)1, CXCL3, CXCL5, CXCL6, and CXCL8 (70). Specifically, IL-17F promotes neutrophil accumulation in the dermis by stimulating the release of IL-8 by keratinocytes (84). T_H17 cytokines (IL-17A, IL-22, and TNF) also cause keratinocytes to produce C-C motif chemokine ligand (CCL) 20 and its receptor, C-C motif chemokine receptor (CCR) 6, thereby facilitating the recruitment and infiltration of T_H17 cells (85). IL-17A-induced keratinocyte production of IL-19 has been shown to upregulate the production of antimicrobial proteins, namely S100 calcium-binding protein (S100)A7, S100A8, and S100A9. IL-19 and IL-17A may also interact synergistically to enhance the keratinocyte response. These observations seem to suggest IL-19 as a potentially novel component of the IL-23/IL-17 axis (86), which plays a crucial role in the development of psoriatic inflammation (87). Apart from its role in T_H17 differentiation and expansion, IL-23 has been demonstrated to induce dermal inflammation and epidermal hyperplasia – mediated through the combined effects of IL-17A (88) and IL-22 (77).

IL-22 is co-expressed with IL-17A and IL-17F by activated T_H17 cells (76, 77) as well as T_H22 cells (89). IL-22 does not affect immune cells (90) and primarily targets epithelial cells, mediating innate immune responses and contributing to wound healing (91). This cytokine has a dual nature, exhibiting both anti- and pro-inflammatory properties (92). IL-22 induces the overexpression of AMPs, such as β-defensin 2, and the S100 protein family (76, 93, 94). In addition, IL-22 has been reported to downregulate the expression of genes involved in the regulation of keratinocyte differentiation, resulting in acanthosis (94–96). As a pro-inflammatory cytokine, IL-22 stimulates keratinocyte production of chemokines (CCL2, CCL20, CXCL5, and CXCL8) (93, 94). These chemotactic agents will promote the infiltration of monocytes/macrophages (97), neutrophils (98), and T cells (99) at sites of cutaneous inflammation. A graphical representation of key cytokine circuits in the immunopathogenesis of PsO is provided in **Figure 1**.

Other cytokines that have been implicated in psoriatic inflammation include IL-9, IL-19, IL-20, IL-24, IL-33, and IL-36.

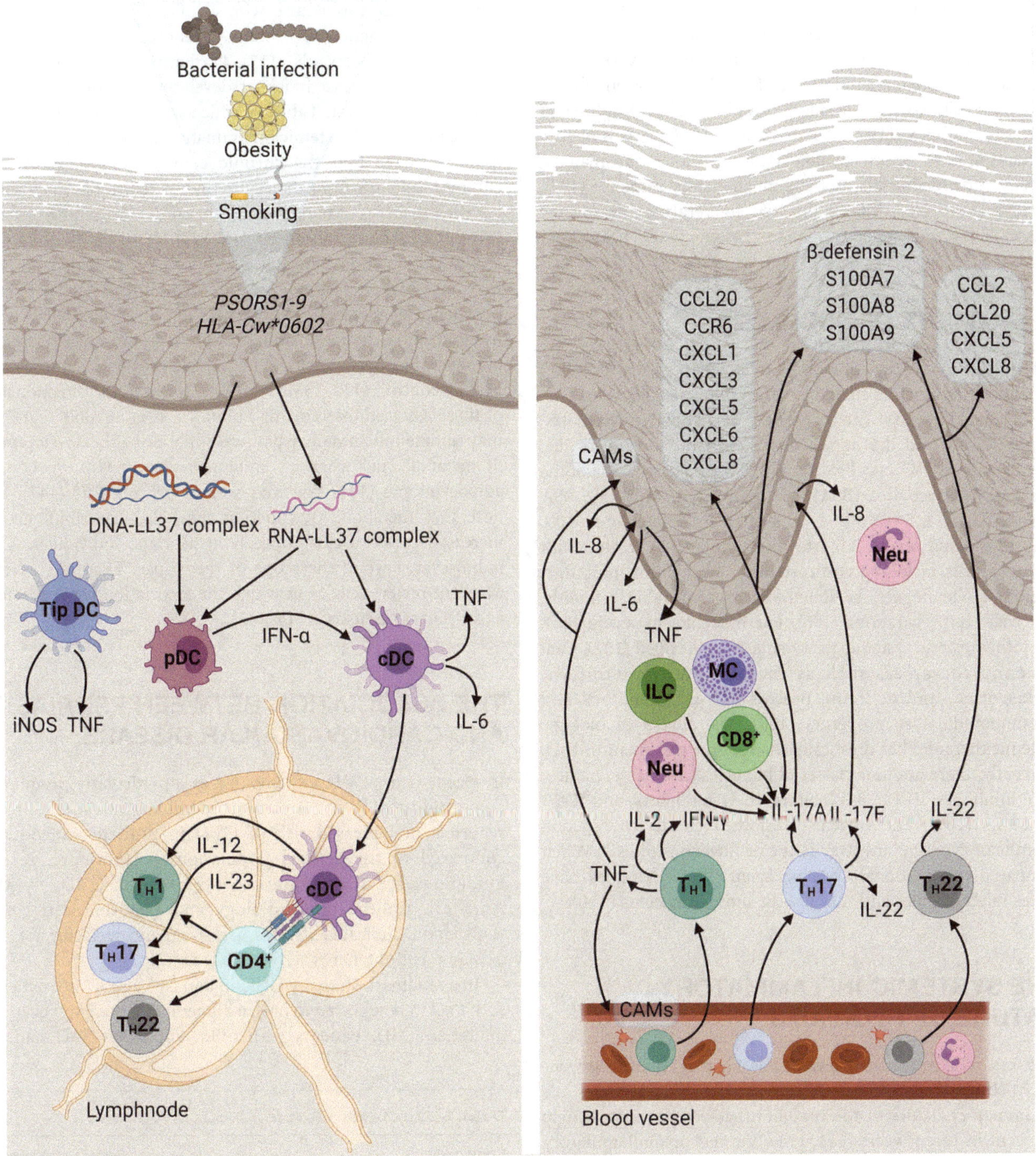

FIGURE 1 | The immunopathogenesis of PsO. A combination of genetic and environmental factors activates pDCs. In turn, cDCs activate naïve CD 4+ T cells through the presentation of an unknown antigen. Subsequently, activated CD4+ T cells differentiate into T_H1, T_H17, and T_H22 cells, which migrate to the dermis and give rise to a psoriatic plaque. Diagram created with BioRender.com. CAM, cell adhesion molecule; CCL, C-C motif chemokine ligand; CCR, C-C motif chemokine receptor; CD, cluster of differentiation; cDC, conventional dendritic cell; CXCL, C-X-C motif chemokine ligand; DNA, deoxyribonucleic acid; *HLA*, human leukocyte antigen; IFN, interferon; IL, interleukin; ILC, innate lymphoid cell; iNOS, inducible nitric oxide synthase; MC, mast cell; Neu, neutrophil; pDC, plasmacytoid dendritic cell; *PSORS*: psoriasis susceptibility; RNA, ribonucleic acid; S100, S100 calcium-binding protein; T_H, T helper; Tip DC, tumour necrosis factor- and inducible nitric oxide synthase-producing dendritic cell; TNF, tumour necrosis factor.

IL-9 has been suggested to contribute to PsO pathogenesis *via* its pro-angiogenic activity and induction of IL-17 production (100). In addition, members of the IL-20 subfamily of cytokines (IL-19, IL-20, and IL-24) have been shown to affect keratinocyte proliferation and differentiation and to induce the expression of various PsO-related molecules (101). Indeed, suppression of these cytokines resulted in alleviation of epidermal hyperplasia in psoriatic patients (102). Furthermore, IL-33 was recently demonstrated to act on keratinocytes in an autocrine manner, thereby perpetuating the psoriatic inflammatory response (103). Finally, IL-36 has been implicated in keratinocyte-specific pathways that mediate dermal inflammation in PsO (104, 105).

TREATMENT OF PSORIASIS

When determining the appropriate treatment regimen for a PsO patient, various factors should be taken into consideration, such as disease severity the presence of psoriatic arthritis, comorbidities, and the impact on the patient's quality of life. The severity of PsO may be determined by the percentage of the total body surface area (BSA) that is involved, with <3% BSA considered mild, 3–10% BSA considered moderate, and >10% BSA considered severe. Mild to moderate PsO is treated with topical agents including corticosteroids, calcineurin inhibitors, vitamin D_3 analogues, keratolytic agents, anthralin, retinoids, and coal tar preparations (106). For moderate to severe PsO, phototherapy and systemic treatments are prescribed (107). Oral systemic therapies, such as methotrexate, apremilast, cyclosporine, and acitretin, possess anti-inflammatory and immunomodulatory properties (108). The advent of biologic systemic therapies has drastically changed the treatment of PsO. Currently, there are four classes of biologicals available, namely TNF inhibitors, IL-12/23 inhibitors, IL-17 inhibitors, and IL-23 inhibitors (109). These agents exert their effects by targeting prominent cytokines involved in the pathogenesis of PsO. When compared to traditional systemic agents these therapies have better safety profiles and may also be more efficacious (110).

THE SYSTEMIC INFLAMMATORY NATURE OF PSORIASIS

PsO was initially primarily regarded as a hyperkeratotic disorder solely confined to affected skin areas. However, the systemic inflammatory nature of the condition has become increasingly apparent in recent years (111, 112). Various pro-inflammatory products are overexpressed in psoriatic skin lesions. These mediators also seem to be released into the systemic circulation of psoriatic patients and may reflect disease severity (113). Peripheral inflammation is evident by the abnormal expression of a host of inflammatory molecules in the blood of these individuals (113–116). Moreover, inflammation may also be detected at extracutaneous sites. In a pilot study by Mehta et al. (117), ^{18}F-fluorodeoxyglucose emission tomography-computed tomography was utilised to localise and quantify inflammatory activity in individuals with moderate to severe PsO. The authors detected systemic inflammation in the skin, joints, liver, and vasculature, with significantly greater aortic and hepatic inflammation in psoriatic patients compared to age- and gender-matched controls (117). Furthermore, individuals with PsO have an increased risk of developing multiple comorbid diseases (presented in **Table 1**), which serves as further evidence for the presence of systemic inflammation in the condition. It has been proposed that the chronic course of PsO, as well as common inflammatory molecules and/or pathways, may act as the driving forces of the development and/or worsening of these extracutaneous manifestations (15, 111).

Besides systemic comorbid conditions, individuals with PsO may also develop metabolic abnormalities. An increased prevalence of metabolic syndrome (MetS) – a constellation of dyslipidaemia, hypertension, insulin resistance, and visceral obesity – has been reported in psoriatic patients compared to healthy controls (132, 133, 138–140). However, the directionality of these associations remains unknown. It is possible that PsO may initiate inflammatory pathways that drive the development of metabolic disturbances. Inflamed adipose tissue produces adipocytokines (141) that may worsen existing PsO (142). We note that metabolic dysfunction may also contribute to an increased cardiovascular burden in psoriatic individuals. This is however, beyond the scope of this paper. There are several excellent review articles in which the association between MetS and PsO are discussed (143–145).

THE ASSOCIATION BETWEEN PSORIASIS AND CARDIOVASCULAR DISEASE

In recent years, CVD has emerged as a particularly prominent comorbidity of PsO. Several epidemiological studies have reported an increased risk of CVD in psoriatic individuals, compared to the general population. Furthermore, recent guidelines for the primary prevention of CVD, by the American College of Cardiology and the American Heart Association, indicated PsO as a risk-enhancing factor for the development of atherosclerotic CVD (146).

In a landmark study by Gelfand and colleagues (20), patients with PsO were reported to have a higher incidence of myocardial infarction (MI). Patients with mild and severe PsO had an

TABLE 1 | Comorbidities associated with PsO.

Comorbidity	Selected references
Chronic kidney disease	(118–120)
CVD	(18–20)
Depression	(8, 121, 122)
Diabetes	(123–125)
Inflammatory bowel disease	(126–128)
Malignancy	(129–131)
Metabolic syndrome	(132–134)
Non-alcoholic fatty liver disease	(135–137)

CVD, cardiovascular disease.

incidence of 4.04 (95% confidence interval [CI]: 3.88–4.21) and 5.13 (95% CI: 4.22–6.17) per 1000 person-years, compared to an incidence of 3.58 in healthy control subjects (95% CI: 3.52–3.65) (20). In addition, traditional CVD risk factors such as hyperlipidaemia, hypertension, and smoking were more prevalent among psoriatic individuals. PsO remained an independent risk factor for CVD, after adjusting for established CVD risk factors. Similar associations were noted in studies assessing the risk of stroke (19) and venous thromboembolism (VTE) (18) in psoriatic individuals. Gelfand et al. (19) reported an increased risk of stroke in mild (hazard ratio [HR] 1.06; 95% CI: 1.0–1.1) and severe (HR 1.43; 95% CI: 1.1–1.9) PsO, after adjusting for major risk factors (19). Furthermore, Ahlehoff and colleagues (18) reported higher incidence rates of VTE in psoriatic individuals (1.92 and 3.20 per 1000 person-years for mild and severe PsO) compared to healthy controls (1.29 per 1000 person-years) (18). In a meta-analysis by Gaeta and colleagues (147), it was shown that PsO confers an excess risk of 24% for the development of CVD (147). It has also been reported that severe disease activity contributes substantially to increased mortality due to CVD (148–150). Mehta et al. (21) identified severe PsO as an independent risk factor for CVD deaths (HR 1.57; 95% CI: 1.26–1.96), after adjusting for traditional CVD risk factors (21). Lastly, in a study by Abuabara and colleagues (149), it was determined that CVD was responsible for the highest absolute (61.9 deaths per 1000 person-years) and excess (3.1 deaths per 1000 person-years) risk in PsO patients (149).

The link between PsO and CVD may potentially be explained by the chronic course of the disease and the associated systemic inflammation. A considerable body of literature supports the notion that chronic low-grade systemic inflammation is a central theme in the pathogenesis and propagation of CVD (151–154). Moreover, elevated levels of C-reactive protein (CRP) – a sensitive marker of systemic inflammation – has been suggested as a predictor of future CVD events (155). Two landmark trials, namely the Justification for the Use of Statins in Prevention: an Intervention Trial Evaluating Rosuvastatin (JUPITER) study (156), and the Canakinumab Anti-inflammatory Thrombosis Outcome Study (CANTOS) (157), also provided evidence for a prominent role of systemic inflammation in the etiopathogenesis of CVD. In the following section, we will elaborate on the interplay between inflammation and coagulation as well as how an imbalance in these activities may promote the development of CVD – specifically *via* thrombosis.

PSORIATIC INFLAMMATION AND COAGULOPATHY

Inflammation and coagulation are interdependent processes, demonstrated by the dynamic crosstalk between these systems. Under normal physiological conditions, these systems function as protective mechanisms and are tightly regulated. However, dysregulation may result in chronic, systemic inflammation and/or thrombotic complications. In response to invading pathogens or tissue damage, inflammation ensues to eliminate the original insult and to promote wound healing and tissue repair. However, if the inflammatory process is not duly resolved; acute inflammation may transition to chronic, systemic inflammation. In turn, the sustained activation of the coagulation cascade, driven primarily by pro-inflammatory cytokines, may follow.

A particularly prominent molecule in the context of inflammation-induced coagulation is tissue factor (TF) (25). The tenase complex, comprising TF and factor VIIa, activates the extrinsic coagulation pathway, culminating in the generation of thrombin. In the final steps of coagulation, thrombin catalyses the conversion of soluble fibrinogen to insoluble fibrin. Pro-inflammatory cytokines may upregulate the expression of TF on endothelial cells and monocytes (158). In addition, inflammation favours the suppression of natural anticoagulant mechanisms, namely the antithrombin pathway, the protein C pathway, and tissue factor pathway inhibitor (TFPI) (24, 25). Finally, fibrinolytic activity may also decrease due to a continuous increase in plasminogen activator inhibitor (PAI)-1 levels stimulated by pro-inflammatory molecules (25). Thus, chronic systemic inflammation may alter the haemostatic balance to favour a prothrombotic state.

In turn, coagulation may also modulate and perpetuate the inflammatory response. Coagulation proteases may bind to protease-activated receptors on the activated endothelium, inducing the synthesis and expression of cell adhesion molecules (159, 160). These molecules play a pivotal role in the extravasation of leukocytes to sites of inflammation. Furthermore, activated coagulation factors may also elicit an inflammatory response by interacting with immune cells to induce the production of cytokines (161, 162). Thrombocytes or platelets are also increasingly recognised for their ability to mediate and regulate inflammation. Activated platelets release their granular content, which comprises a plethora of procoagulant and pro-inflammatory molecules. Platelets are also implicated in the recruitment of leukocytes and the regulation of vascular permeability (163).

From these observations, it is evident that inflammation and coagulation should not be viewed as separate entities and that an imbalance in these activities may culminate in the development of prothrombotic conditions. Thrombosis is the most common pathology underlying the three major cardiovascular conditions, namely ischaemic heart disease, ischaemic stroke, and VTE (164–166). Arterial thrombosis, which ensues after the rupture of an atherosclerotic plaque or damage to the vessel wall, may give rise to MI or stroke. Platelets play a central role in the formation of an arterial thrombus (167). In contrast, the pathomechanism of venous thrombosis, associated with deep vein thrombosis (DVT) and pulmonary embolism, is less clear. Virchow's triad describes three factors, namely hypercoagulability, endothelial dysfunction, and altered blood flow, which may predispose an individual to the development of venous thrombosis (168).

As discussed in the previous sections, PsO is characterised by chronic, systemic inflammation and accompanied by an increased risk for CVD. A potential mechanism may be the development of a prothrombotic state, *via* the action of multiple pro-inflammatory cytokines, due to psoriatic pathology. The most prominent cytokines that could play a role in the development of a prothrombotic state - IL-6, IL-17, and TNF - will be discussed below. We focus specifically on the effects of these cytokines on platelets and the endothelium. In **Figures 2** and **3** schematic representations are provided of the signalling pathways that could be initiated in platelets and endothelial cells, respectively, upon stimulation with these cytokines.

Interleukin-6

IL-6 is a pleiotropic cytokine involved in several physiological processes including the acute-phase response and antibody production (169). The effects of IL-6 are mediated *via* two receptors, namely the IL-6 receptor (IL-6R) and the signal-transducing subunit, glycoprotein (gp) 130 (169). In PsO, IL-6, combined with IL-23, contributes to the differentiation of T_H17 cells (12). The overexpression of this cytokine has been detected in psoriatic skin lesions (170) as well as in the circulation of these individuals (113, 171, 172). In addition, IL-6 signalling has been suggested to diminish regulatory T cell activity in PsO, thereby allowing the expansion of effector T cells (170). In the context of CVD, IL-6 has emerged as a pivotal mediator of thrombotic disease. Raised IL-6 levels have been found to be related to recurrent venous thrombosis (173), with detectable levels of IL-6 associated with a two-fold increase in the risk of venous thrombosis (174). The potential involvement of IL-6 in the development of adverse cardiovascular events is further supported by findings of a sub-study of the CANTOS trial. In this study, baseline IL-6 levels were associated with an increased risk of cardiovascular events. More importantly, it was demonstrated for the first time that lowering IL-6 levels – *via* the inhibition of IL-1β by canakinumab – resulted in a 15% reduction of atherothrombotic events (MI and stroke) (175).

During inflammation, IL-6 acts on hepatocytes to induce the synthesis of acute-phase proteins such as CRP, fibrinogen, and serum amyloid A (SAA) (176). Both CRP and SAA have demonstrated the ability to promote coagulation *via* the induction of TF synthesis in endothelial cells and suppression of the TFPI pathway (177, 178). With regard to fibrinogen, it has been suggested that a causal relationship exists between hyperfibrinogenaemia and thrombosis (179).

Although platelets do not express IL-6R, they have been shown to express gp130 (180, 181). Upon thrombin-induced platelet activation, the soluble form of IL-6R is secreted which can form a complex with IL-6 (180, 181). This complex may activate gp130, in a process termed trans-signalling, resulting in the activation of signal transducer and activator of transcription (STAT) 3 (181). However, IL-6 trans-signalling does not seem to affect platelet activation and/or aggregation. Nevertheless, IL-6 may promote platelet adhesion and aggregation indirectly. IL-6 inhibits the activity of a disintegrin-like and metalloprotease with thrombospondin type 1 motif, 13 (ADAMTS13) (182). ADAMTS13 is responsible for the cleavage of ultra-large von Willebrand factor multimers released by the endothelium. In the ultra-large form, these multimers are hyperreactive and may interact with platelets to induce adhesion and aggregation.

Interleukin-17

IL-17 plays a pivotal role in the innate immune response, particularly in host defence against microbial invasion (183). The IL-17 family consists of six members, namely IL-17A to IL-17F, and signalling is mediated through the IL-17 receptor (IL-17R) family that comprises five members, IL-17RA to IL-17RE (184). This pro-inflammatory cytokine has been implicated in the pathogenesis of diverse autoimmune and inflammatory diseases, including PsO (185). Indeed, IL-17 is regarded as the principal driver of psoriatic inflammation. The overexpression of this cytokine has been detected in lesional psoriatic skin, when compared to nonlesional skin (186, 187). In addition, serum levels of IL-17A are elevated in psoriatic patients (188) and may also reflect disease severity (186). With respect to cardiovascular pathology, conflicting results have been reported on the role of IL-17. Some studies have found a protective effect of IL-17 (189), while others have reported a pro-atherogenic role for IL-17 (190). Nevertheless, prothrombotic effects of IL-17 have been demonstrated. In a murine model of DVT, IL-17A was found to promote thrombus formation by enhancing platelet aggregation and neutrophil infiltration of thrombi (191). Moreover, it has been shown that targeted blocking of IL-12/23 and IL-17 resulted in improved skin phenotype and lengthened clotting times to occlusive thrombus formation in a murine model of psoriatic disease (192).

Platelets have been demonstrated to express a functional IL-17 receptor, namely IL-17RA (193). Exposing activated platelets (induced by adenosine diphosphate) to IL-17 augments platelet aggregation (193–195). This action is suggested to be mediated by the opening of the mitochondrial permeability transition pore (196) and the phosphorylation of extracellular signal-regulated kinase-2 (194, 196). Furthermore, stimulation with IL-17 causes an increased expression and accelerated externalisation of P-selectin and exposure of the $\alpha_{IIb}\beta_3$ integrin (193, 194, 196). Both of the aforementioned molecules facilitate platelet aggregation and are used as markers of platelet activation.

IL-17 may also alter the endothelium towards an activated state. IL-17RA is constitutively expressed in endothelial cells (197). It has been reported that IL-17 and TNF act synergistically to activate the endothelium, resulting in the synthesis of inflammatory mediators, and the expression of cell adhesion molecules (E-selectin and intercellular adhesion molecule-1) and TF by these cells (195). Anticoagulant activity by the endothelium also becomes diminished, as thrombomodulin expression is downregulated (195). It should be noted that IL-17 alone is not a strong inducer of inflammatory activity, however, IL-17 in concert with TNF potently induce pro-inflammatory gene expression. This effect is thought to be mediated by the ability of IL-17 to stabilise messenger RNA (198, 199). Finally, the vascular expression of CD39, an inhibitor of platelet aggregation, is also downregulated by IL-17A (195, 200).

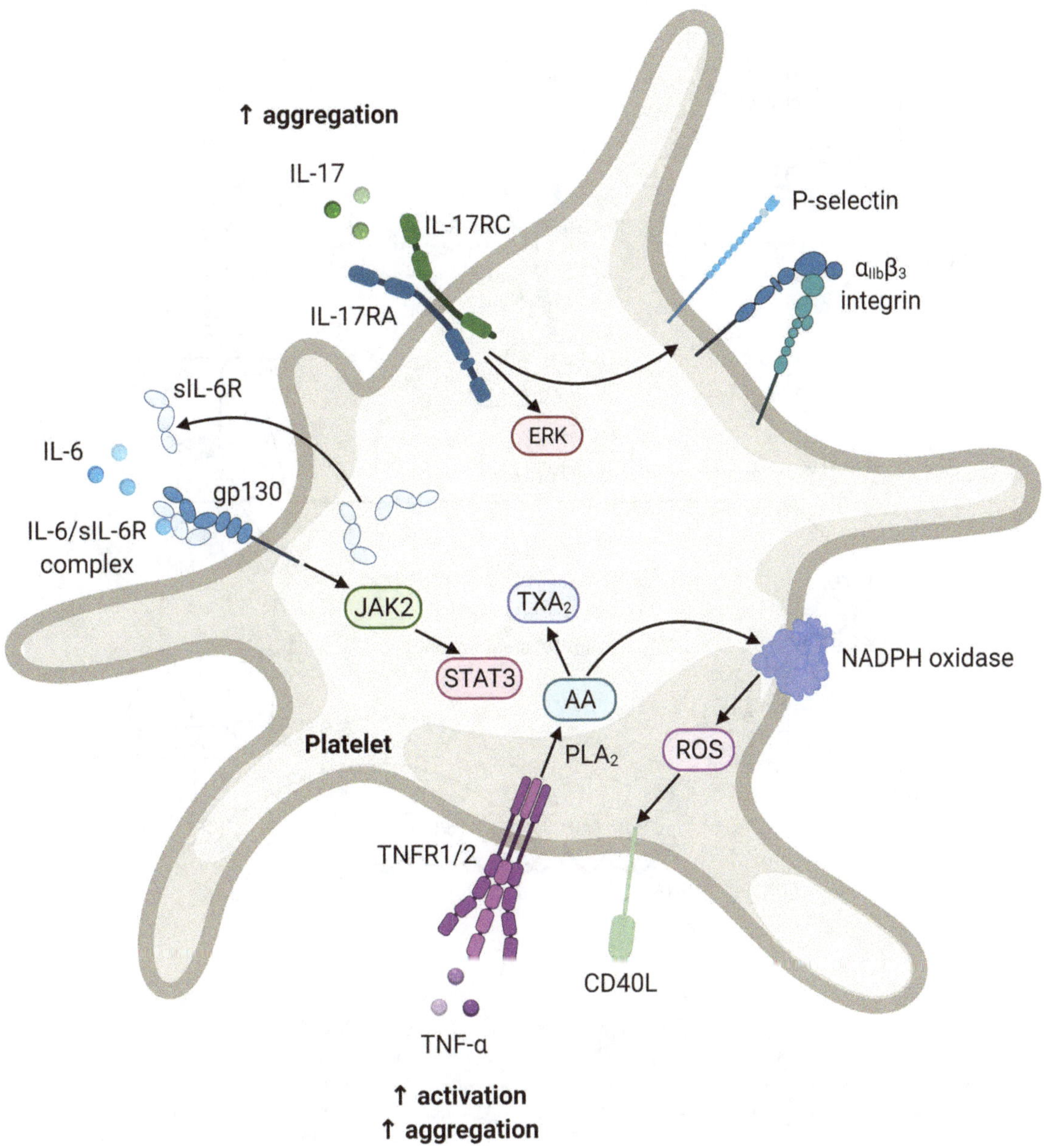

FIGURE 2 | Potential signalling pathways in platelets upon stimulation with IL-6, IL-17, and TNF. These mediators may contribute to platelet activation as well as enhancing the platelet response to agonist-induced platelet activation. Diagram created with BioRender.com. AA, arachidonic acid; CD40L, CD40 ligand; ERK, extracellular signal-regulated kinase; gp, glycoprotein; IL, interleukin; IL-17RA, interleukin-17 receptor A; IL-17RC, interleukin-17 receptor C; JAK, Janus kinase; NADPH, nicotinamide adenine dinucleotide phosphate; PLA_2, phospholipase A_2; ROS, reactive oxygen species; sIL-6R, soluble interleukin-6 receptor; STAT, signal transducer and activator of transcription; TXA_2, thromboxane A_2; TNF, tumour necrosis factor; TNFR, tumour necrosis factor receptor.

Tumour Necrosis Factor

TNF is a potent inflammatory cytokine, orchestrating various processes such as inflammation, cell differentiation, and apoptosis (201). The effects of TNF are mediated by two receptors, namely TNF receptor (TNFR) 1 and TNFR2 (202). In PsO, this cytokine amplifies the inflammatory response *via* the generation of reactive oxygen species and inducing the expression of cytokines and cell adhesion molecules (73, 203). Increased TNF activity has been detected in involved skin from psoriatic individuals (204) and TNF levels were also elevated in the serum of these individuals (113, 205). In relation to cardiovascular diseases, increased concentrations of TNF have been associated with recurrent coronary events (206), and venous thrombosis (174). In addition, TNF levels have been

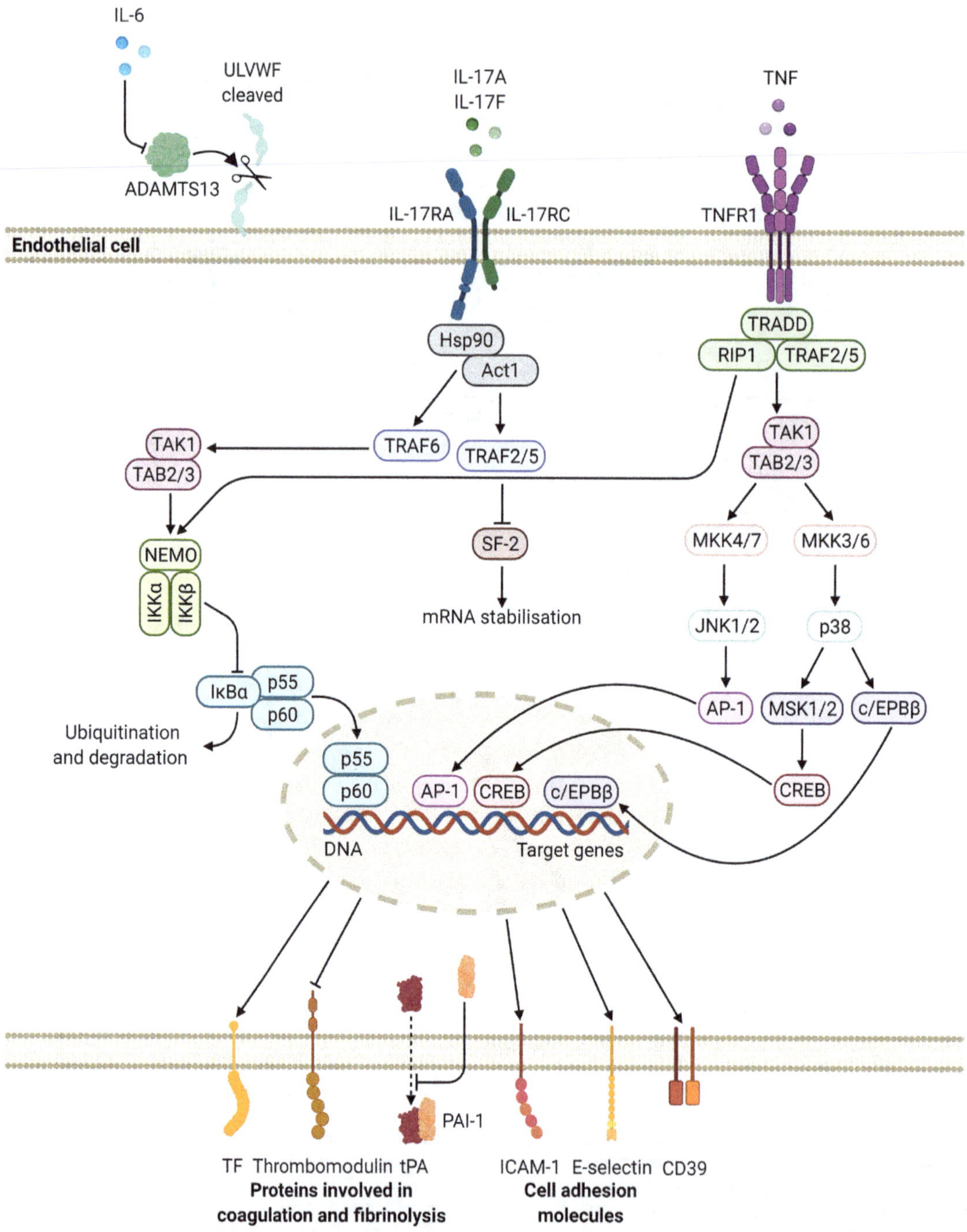

FIGURE 3 | Potential intracellular signalling pathways initiated in endothelial cells, upon stimulation with IL-6, IL-17, and TNF. These mediators may upregulate the synthesis and release of molecules that promote platelet adhesion and coagulation, while suppressing the expression of proteins involved in fibrinolysis. Altogether these changes may lead to a prothrombotic state. Diagram created with BioRender.com. ADAMTS13, a disintegrin-like and metalloprotease with thrombospondin type 1 motif, 13; AP, activator protein; c/EPB, CCAAT/enhancer-binding protein; CD, cluster of differentiation; CREB, cAMP response element binding protein; DNA, deoxyribonucleic acid; Hsp, heat shock protein; ICAM-1, intercellular adhesion molecule-1; IKBα, NF-kappa-B inhibitor alpha; IKK, inhibitor of nuclear factor kappa-B kinase; IL, interleukin; IL-17RA, interleukin-17 receptor A; IL-17RC, interleukin-17 receptor C; JNK, c-Jun N-terminal kinase; MKK, mitogen-activated protein kinase kinase; MSK, mitogen- and stress-activated protein kinase; NEMO, NF-kappa-B essential modulator; PAI-1, plasminogen activator inhibitor-1; SF, splicing factor; TF, tissue factor; TNF, tumour necrosis factor; TNFR, tumour necrosis factor receptor; tPA, tissue-type plasminogen activator; TRADD, tumour necrosis factor receptor 1-associated death domain protein; TRAF, tumour necrosis factor receptor-associated factor; RIP, receptor-interacting protein kinase; ULVWF, ultra-large von Willebrand factor.

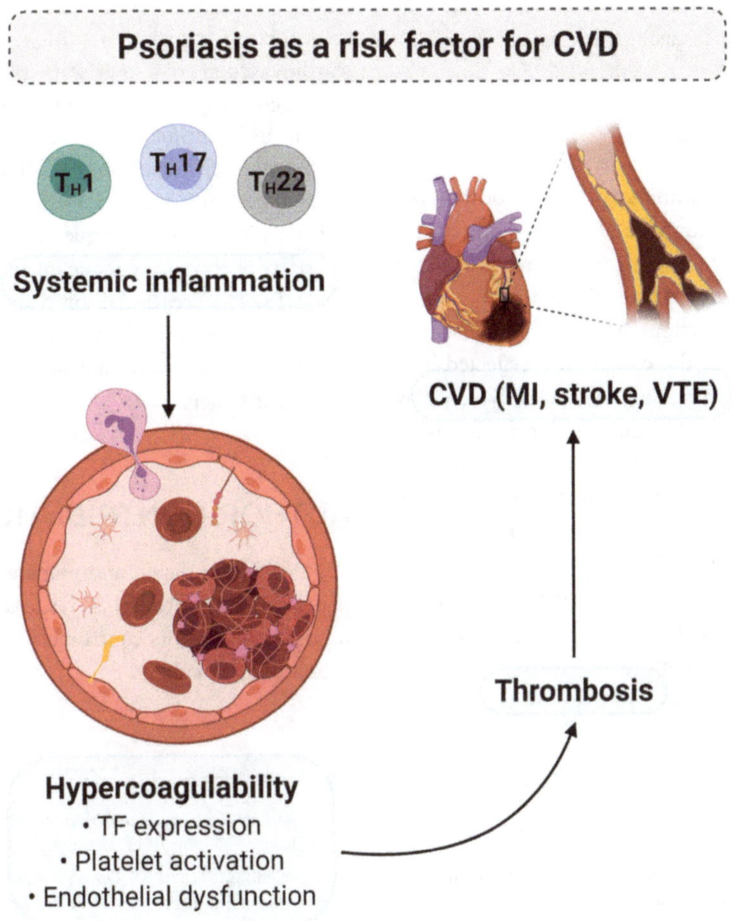

FIGURE 4 | PsO as a risk factor for CVD. Chronic low-grade systemic inflammation, due to psoriatic pathology, may contribute to the development of a hypercoagulable state. Pro-inflammatory mediators induce the expression of TF, enhance platelet activation and/or the platelet response, and endothelial dysfunction. In turn, hypercoagulability predisposes thrombosis, which is the major underlying pathology of CVD. Diagram created with BioRender.com. CVD, cardiovascular disease; MI, myocardial infarction; TF, tissue factor; T_H, T helper; VTE, venous thromboembolism.

suggested to be an independent predictor of cardiovascular events such as MI, stroke, and CVD mortality (207). Regarding the prothrombotic properties of TNF, discrepant results have been reported. In a murine model of atherothrombosis, potent antithrombotic effects of TNF were reported (208). In contrast, another study found that treatment with this cytokine resulted in accelerated thrombus formation (209).

It has been suggested that TNF may promote the (hyper) activation of platelets by interacting with TNFR1 and TNFR2, which is expressed on the platelet membrane (210). TNF may also facilitate platelet activation by stimulating the arachidonic acid pathway (210). Furthermore, CD40 ligand (CD40L) expression by activated platelets may be induced by TNF *via* an arachidonic acid-dependent oxidative stress mechanism (211, 212). In turn, CD40L enhances platelet activation and aggregation, as well as thrombus formation (213). TNF also induces the release of large von Willebrand factor multimers from endothelial cells, which propagates platelet thrombus formation (182). Nevertheless, the ability of TNF to stimulate platelet activation directly remains contested, with some studies reporting no effect (209).

TNF may alter the properties of the endothelium by inducing the synthesis of procoagulant molecules and suppressing natural anticoagulant mechanisms. Engagement of TNF with TNFR1 results in the expression of TF on the surface of endothelial cells and the subsequent deposition of fibrin (209, 214–216). In addition, the production of platelet-activating factor (PAF), by the endothelium, is also induced by TNF (217, 218). PAF induces platelet aggregation (219) and functions as a potent inflammatory mediator (220). The activity of the anticoagulant molecule, activated protein C, is dependent on the presence of functional endothelial thrombomodulin, which has been shown to be downregulated by TNF (216). Mechanistically, this inhibitory effect is mediated by downregulating the transcription of the thrombomodulin gene (209, 221). Finally, TNF inhibits fibrinolysis by induction of the PAI-1 gene (209) through the activity of NF-κB (222) and by decreasing the release of tPA (223).

CONCLUDING REMARKS

PsO is an immune-mediated inflammatory disorder of the skin, characterised by the overexpression of T_H1-, T_H17-, and T_H22-derived inflammatory cytokines. These mediators are upregulated in the lesional skin of psoriatic individuals and may also be released into the circulatory system of these patients. The systemic inflammatory nature of the condition is reflected by a multitude of dysregulated inflammatory molecules, which may give rise to various comorbidities. PsO has been identified as an independent risk factor for the development of CVD (**Figure 4**). The chronic subclinical systemic inflammation associated with the condition may predispose psoriatic individuals to thrombosis – a major determinant of CVD. Inflammatory cytokines may contribute to the development of a prothrombotic state, *via* the induction of TF, platelet activation and/or enhancing the platelet response, and endothelial dysfunction.

The exact mechanisms underlying the association between PsO and CVD remains elusive. However, it is imperative that both physicians and patients must be aware of the potential cardiovascular risk that PsO may pose. Therefore, effective management of the condition should not only aim to ameliorate cutaneous inflammation but also systemic inflammation, in order to prevent secondary comorbidities such as CVD. Finally, as pointed out in a recent review by Aksentijevich and colleagues (224), PsO presents a unique opportunity as a human model for the study of chronic systemic inflammation in the development of CVD (224). Treatment of psoriatic patients with targeted biological therapies may shed light on the contribution of specific cytokines to cardiovascular morbidity, and provide novel treatment targets.

AUTHOR CONTRIBUTIONS

MV: writing of paper, and preparation of figures. GT: editing of paper. EP: study leader, corresponding author, editing of paper, funding. All authors contributed to the article and approved the submitted version.

REFERENCES

1. Nestle FO, Kaplan DH, Barker J. Psoriasis. *New Engl J Med* (2009) 361 (5):496–509. doi: 10.1056/NEJMra0804595
2. Chen GY, Cheng YW, Wang CY, Hsu TJ, Hsu MM, Yang PT, et al. Prevalence of Skin Diseases Among Schoolchildren in Magong, Penghu, Taiwan: A Community-Based Clinical Survey. *J Formosan Med Assoc = Taiwan yi zhi* (2008) 107(1):21–9. doi: 10.1016/s0929-6646(08)60004-2
3. Michalek IM, Loring B, John SM. A Systematic Review of Worldwide Epidemiology of Psoriasis. *J Eur Acad Dermatol Venereol: JEADV* (2017) 31(2):205–12. doi: 10.1111/jdv.13854
4. Yang YC, Cheng YW, Lai CS, Chen W. Prevalence of Childhood Acne, Ephelides, Warts, Atopic Dermatitis, Psoriasis, Alopecia Areata and Keloid in Kaohsiung County, Taiwan: A Community-Based Clinical Survey. *J Eur Acad Dermatol Venereol: JEADV* (2007) 21(5):643–9. doi: 10.1111/j.1468-3083.2006.02036.x
5. Danielsen K, Olsen AO, Wilsgaard T, Furberg AS. Is the Prevalence of Psoriasis Increasing? A 30-Year Follow-Up of a Population-Based Cohort. *Br J Dermatol* (2013) 168(6):1303–10. doi: 10.1111/bjd.12230
6. Takeshita J, Gelfand JM, Li P, Pinto L, Yu X, Rao P, et al. Psoriasis in the US Medicare Population: Prevalence, Treatment, and Factors Associated With Biologic Use. *J Invest Dermatol* (2015) 135(12):2955–63. doi: 10.1038/jid.2015.296
7. Naldi L, Gambini D. The Clinical Spectrum of Psoriasis. *Clinics Dermatol* (2007) 25(6):510–8. doi: 10.1016/j.clindermatol.2007.08.003
8. Kurd SK, Troxel AB, Crits-Christoph P, Gelfand JM. The Risk of Depression, Anxiety, and Suicidality in Patients With Psoriasis: A Population-Based Cohort Study. *Arch Dermatol* (2010) 146(8):891–5. doi: 10.1001/archdermatol.2010.186
9. Armstrong AW, Schupp C, Wu J, Bebo B. Quality of Life and Work Productivity Impairment Among Psoriasis Patients: Findings From the National Psoriasis Foundation Survey Data 2003-2011. *PloS One* (2012) 7 (12):e52935. doi: 10.1371/journal.pone.0052935
10. Gelfand JM, Troxel AB, Lewis JD, Kurd SK, Shin DB, Wang X, et al. The Risk of Mortality in Patients With Psoriasis: Results From a Population-Based Study. *JAMA Dermatol* (2007) 143(12):1493–9. doi: 10.1001/archderm.143.12.1493
11. Hao J-Q. Targeting Interleukin-22 in Psoriasis. *Inflammation* (2014) 37 (1):94–9. doi: 10.1007/s10753-013-9715-y
12. Di Cesare A, Di Meglio P, Nestle FO. The IL-23/Th17 Axis in the Immunopathogenesis of Psoriasis. *J Invest Dermatol* (2009) 129(6):1339–50. doi: 10.1038/jid.2009.59
13. Grine L, Dejager L, Libert C, Vandenbroucke RE. An Inflammatory Triangle in Psoriasis: TNF, Type I IFNs and IL-17. *Cytokine Growth Factor Rev* (2015) 26(1):25–33. doi: 10.1016/j.cytogfr.2014.10.009
14. Oliveira M, Rocha B, Duarte GV. Psoriasis: Classical and Emerging Comorbidities. *Bras Dermatol* (2015) 90(1):9–20. doi: 10.1590/abd1806-4841.20153038
15. Reich K. The Concept of Psoriasis as a Systemic Inflammation: Implications for Disease Management. *J Eur Acad Dermatol Venereol: JEADV* (2012) 26 Suppl 2:3–11. doi: 10.1111/j.1468-3083.2011.04410.x
16. Takeshita J, Grewal S, Langan SM, Mehta NN, Ogdie A, Van Voorhees AS, et al. Psoriasis and Comorbid Diseases: Epidemiology. *J Am Acad Dermatol* (2017) 76(3):377–90. doi: 10.1016/j.jaad.2016.07.064
17. Davidovici BB, Sattar N, Prinz J, Puig L, Emery P, Barker JN, et al. Psoriasis and Systemic Inflammatory Diseases: Potential Mechanistic Links Between Skin Disease and Co-Morbid Conditions. *J Invest Dermatol* (2010) 130 (7):1785–96. doi: 10.1038/jid.2010.103
18. Ahlehoff O, Gislason GH, Lindhardsen J, Charlot MG, Jorgensen CH, Olesen JB, et al. Psoriasis Carries an Increased Risk of Venous Thromboembolism: A Danish Nationwide Cohort Study. *PloS One* (2011) 6(3):e18125. doi: 10.1371/journal.pone.0018125

19. Gelfand JM, Dommasch ED, Shin DB, Azfar RS, Kurd SK, Wang X, et al. The Risk of Stroke in Patients With Psoriasis. *J Invest Dermatol* (2009) 129 (10):2411–8. doi: 10.1038/jid.2009.112
20. Gelfand JM, Neimann AL, Shin DB, Wang X, Margolis DJ, Troxel AB. Risk of Myocardial Infarction in Patients With Psoriasis. *JAMA* (2006) 296 (14):1735–41. doi: 10.1001/jama.296.14.1735
21. Mehta NN, Azfar RS, Shin DB, Neimann AL, Troxel AB, Gelfand JM. Patients With Severe Psoriasis Are at Increased Risk of Cardiovascular Mortality: Cohort Study Using the General Practice Research Database. *Eur Heart J* (2010) 31(8):1000–6. doi: 10.1093/eurheartj/ehp567
22. Manolis AA, Manolis TA, Melita H, Manolis AS. Psoriasis and Cardiovascular Disease: The Elusive Link. *Int Rev Immunol* (2019) 38 (1):33–54. doi: 10.1080/08830185.2018.1539084
23. Foley JH, Conway EM. Cross Talk Pathways Between Coagulation and Inflammation. *Circ Res* (2016) 118(9):1392–408. doi: 10.1161/CIRCRESAHA.116.306853
24. Esmon CT. The Interactions Between Inflammation and Coagulation. *Br J Haematol* (2005) 131(4):417–30. doi: 10.1111/j.1365-2141.2005.05753.x
25. Levi M, van der Poll T. Two-Way Interactions Between Inflammation and Coagulation. *Trends Cardiovasc Med* (2005) 15(7):254–9. doi: 10.1016/j.tcm.2005.07.004
26. Abeyama K, Stern DM, Ito Y, Kawahara K, Yoshimoto Y, Tanaka M, et al. The N-Terminal Domain of Thrombomodulin Sequesters High-Mobility Group-B1 Protein, a Novel Antiinflammatory Mechanism. *J Clin Invest* (2005) 115(5):1267–74. doi: 10.1172/jci22782
27. Iwaki T, Cruz DT, Martin JA, Castellino FJ. A Cardioprotective Role for the Endothelial Protein C Receptor in Lipopolysaccharide-Induced Endotoxemia in the Mouse. *Blood* (2005) 105(6):2364–71. doi: 10.1182/blood-2004-06-2456
28. Bevilacqua MP, Pober JS, Majeau GR, Fiers W, Cotran RS, Gimbrone MAJr. Recombinant Tumor Necrosis Factor Induces Procoagulant Activity in Cultured Human Vascular Endothelium: Characterization and Comparison With the Actions of Interleukin 1. *Proc Natl Acad Sci USA* (1986) 83(12):4533–7. doi: 10.1073/pnas.83.12.4533
29. Abele DC, Dobson RL, Graham JB. Heredity and Psoriasis: Study of a Large Family. *JAMA Dermatol* (1963) 88(1):38–47. doi: 10.1001/archderm.1963.01590190044005
30. Duffy DL, Spelman LS, Martin NG. Psoriasis in Australian Twins. *J Am Acad Dermatol* (1993) 29(3):428–34. doi: 10.1016/0190-9622(93)70206-9
31. Grjibovski AM, Olsen AO, Magnus P, Harris JR. Psoriasis in Norwegian Twins: Contribution of Genetic and Environmental Effects. *J Eur Acad Dermatol Venereol* (2007) 21(10):1337–43. doi: 10.1111/j.1468-3083.2007.02268.x
32. Farber EM, Nall ML, Watson W. Natural History of Psoriasis in 61 Twin Pairs. *Arch Dermatol* (1974) 109(2):207–11. doi: 10.1001/archderm.109.2.207
33. Duffin KC, Chandran V, Gladman DD, Krueger GG, Elder JT, Rahman P. Genetics of Psoriasis and Psoriatic Arthritis: Update and Future Direction. *J Rheumatol* (2008) 35(7):1449–53.
34. Trembath RC, Clough RL, Rosbotham JL, Jones AB, Camp RD, Frodsham A, et al. Identification of a Major Susceptibility Locus on Chromosome 6p and Evidence for Further Disease Loci Revealed by a Two Stage Genome-Wide Search in Psoriasis. *Hum Mol Genet* (1997) 6(5):813–20. doi: 10.1093/hmg/6.5.813
35. Nair RP, Stuart PE, Nistor I, Hiremagalore R, Chia NVC, Jenisch S, et al. Sequence and Haplotype Analysis Supports HLA-C as the Psoriasis Susceptibility 1 Gene. *Am J Hum Genet* (2006) 78(5):827–51. doi: 10.1086/503821
36. Hwang ST, Nijsten T, Elder JT. Recent Highlights in Psoriasis Research. *J Invest Dermatol* (2017) 137(3):550–6. doi: 10.1016/j.jid.2016.11.007
37. Cargill M, Schrodi SJ, Chang M, Garcia VE, Brandon R, Callis KP, et al. A Large-Scale Genetic Association Study Confirms IL12B and Leads to the Identification of IL23R as Psoriasis-Risk Genes. *Am J Hum Genet* (2007) 80 (2):273–90. doi: 10.1086/511051
38. Nair RP, Duffin KC, Helms C, Ding J, Stuart PE, Goldgar D, et al. Genome-Wide Scan Reveals Association of Psoriasis With IL-23 and NF-kappaB Pathways. *Nat Genet* (2009) 41(2):199–204. doi: 10.1038/ng.311
39. Tsoi LC, Stuart PE, Tian C, Gudjonsson JE, Das S, Zawistowski M, et al. Large Scale Meta-Analysis Characterizes Genetic Architecture for Common Psoriasis Associated Variants. *Nat Commun* (2017) 8(1):15382. doi: 10.1038/ncomms15382
40. Strange A, Capon F, Spencer CC, Knight J, Weale ME, Allen MH, et al. A Genome-Wide Association Study Identifies New Psoriasis Susceptibility Loci and an Interaction Between HLA-C and ERAP1. *Nat Genet* (2010) 42 (11):985–90. doi: 10.1038/ng.694
41. Tsoi LC, Spain SL, Knight J, Ellinghaus E, Stuart PE, Capon F, et al. Identification of 15 New Psoriasis Susceptibility Loci Highlights the Role of Innate Immunity. *Nat Genet* (2012) 44(12):1341–8. doi: 10.1038/ng.2467
42. Sun LD, Cheng H, Wang ZX, Zhang AP, Wang PG, Xu JH, et al. Association Analyses Identify Six New Psoriasis Susceptibility Loci in the Chinese Population. *Nat Genet* (2010) 42(11):1005–9. doi: 10.1038/ng.690
43. Zeng J, Luo S, Huang Y, Lu Q. Critical Role of Environmental Factors in the Pathogenesis of Psoriasis. *J Dermatol* (2017) 44(8):863–72. doi: 10.1111/1346-8138.13806
44. Evers AWM, Verhoeven EWM, Kraaimaat FW, Jong EMGJD, Brouwer SJMD, Schalkwijk J, et al. How Stress Gets Under the Skin: Cortisol and Stress Reactivity in Psoriasis. *Br J Dermatol* (2010) 163(5):986–91. doi: 10.1111/j.1365-2133.2010.09984.x
45. Richards HL, Ray DW, Kirby B, Mason D, Plant D, Main CJ, et al. Response of the Hypothalamic–Pituitary–Adrenal Axis to Psychological Stress in Patients With Psoriasis. *Br J Dermatol* (2005) 153(6):1114–20. doi: 10.1111/j.1365-2133.2005.06817.x
46. Duarte GV, Oliveira M, Cardoso TM, Follador I, Silva TS, Cavalheiro CMA, et al. Association Between Obesity Measured by Different Parameters and Severity of Psoriasis. *Int J Dermatol* (2013) 52(2):177–81. doi: 10.1111/j.1365-4632.2011.05270.x
47. Johnston A, Arnadottir S, Gudjonsson JE, Aphale A, Sigmarsdottir AA, Gunnarsson SI, et al. Obesity in Psoriasis: Leptin and Resistin as Mediators of Cutaneous Inflammation. *Br J Dermatol* (2008) 159(2):342–50. doi: 10.1111/j.1365-2133.2008.08655.x
48. Armstrong AW, Harskamp CT, Dhillon JS, Armstrong EJ. Psoriasis and Smoking: A Systematic Review and Meta-Analysis. *Br J Dermatol* (2014) 170 (2):304–14. doi: 10.1111/bjd.12670
49. Li W, Han J, Choi HK, Qureshi AA. Smoking and Risk of Incident Psoriasis Among Women and Men in the United States: A Combined Analysis. *Am J Epidemiol* (2012) 175(5):402–13. doi: 10.1093/aje/kwr325
50. Naldi L, Chatenoud L, Linder D, Belloni Fortina A, Peserico A, Virgili AR, et al. Cigarette Smoking, Body Mass Index, and Stressful Life Events as Risk Factors for Psoriasis: Results From an Italian Case–Control Study. *J Invest Dermatol* (2005) 125(1):61–7. doi: 10.1111/j.0022-202X.2005.23681.x
51. Attwa E, Swelam E. Relationship Between Smoking-Induced Oxidative Stress and the Clinical Severity of Psoriasis. *J Eur Acad Dermatol Venereol* (2011) 25(7):782–7. doi: 10.1111/j.1468-3083.2010.03860.x
52. Armstrong AW, Armstrong EJ, Fuller EN, Sockolov ME, Voyles SV. Smoking and Pathogenesis of Psoriasis: A Review of Oxidative, Inflammatory and Genetic Mechanisms. *Br J Dermatol* (2011) 165 (6):1162–8. doi: 10.1111/j.1365-2133.2011.10526.x
53. Guðjónsson JE, Thorarinsson AM, Sigurgeirsson B, Kristinsson KG, Valdimarsson H. Streptococcal Throat Infections and Exacerbation of Chronic Plaque Psoriasis: A Prospective Study. *Br J Dermatol* (2003) 149 (3):530–4. doi: 10.1046/j.1365-2133.2003.05552.x
54. Tomi NS, Kränke B, Aberer E. Staphylococcal Toxins in Patients With Psoriasis, Atopic Dermatitis, and Erythroderma, and in Healthy Control Subjects. *J Am Acad Dermatol* (2005) 53(1):67–72. doi: 10.1016/j.jaad.2005.02.034
55. Visser MJE, Kell DB, Pretorius E. Bacterial Dysbiosis and Translocation in Psoriasis Vulgaris. *Front Cell Infect Microbiol* (2019) 9:7. doi: 10.3389/fcimb.2019.00007
56. Mosca A, Leclerc M, Hugot JP. Gut Microbiota Diversity and Human Diseases: Should We Reintroduce Key Predators in Our Ecosystem? *Front Microbiol* (2016) 7:455. doi: 10.3389/fmicb.2016.00455
57. Hiippala K, Jouhten H, Ronkainen A, Hartikainen A, Kainulainen V, Jalanka J, et al. The Potential of Gut Commensals in Reinforcing Intestinal Barrier Function and Alleviating Inflammation. *Nutrients* (2018) 10(8):1–23. doi: 10.3390/nu10080988

58. Codoñer FM, Ramírez-Bosca A, Climent E, Carrión-Gutierrez M, Guerrero M, Pérez-Orquín JM, et al. Gut Microbial Composition in Patients With Psoriasis. *Sci Rep* (2018) 8(1):3812. doi: 10.1038/s41598-018-22125-y
59. Eppinga H, Sperna Weiland CJ, Thio HB, van der Woude CJ, Nijsten TEC, Peppelenbosch MP, et al. Similar Depletion of Protective Faecalibacterium Prausnitzii in Psoriasis and Inflammatory Bowel Disease, But Not in Hidradenitis Suppurativa. *J Crohn's Colitis* (2016) 10(9):1067–75. doi: 10.1093/ecco-jcc/jjw070
60. Alekseyenko AV, Perez-Perez GI, De Souza A, Strober B, Gao Z, Bihan M, et al. Community Differentiation of the Cutaneous Microbiota in Psoriasis. *Microbiome* (2013) 1(1):31. doi: 10.1186/2049-2618-1-31
61. Gao Z, Tseng CH, Strober BE, Pei Z, Blaser MJ. Substantial Alterations of the Cutaneous Bacterial Biota in Psoriatic Lesions. *PloS One* (2008) 3(7):e2719. doi: 10.1371/journal.pone.0002719
62. Ganguly D, Chamilos G, Lande R, Gregorio J, Meller S, Facchinetti V, et al. Self-RNA-Antimicrobial Peptide Complexes Activate Human Dendritic Cells Through TLR7 and TLR8. *J Exp Med* (2009) 206(9):1983–94. doi: 10.1084/jem.20090480
63. Lande R, Gregorio J, Facchinetti V, Chatterjee B, Wang Y-H, Homey B, et al. Plasmacytoid Dendritic Cells Sense Self-DNA Coupled With Antimicrobial Peptide. *Nature* (2007) 449(7162):564–9. doi: 10.1038/nature06116
64. Nestle FO, Conrad C, Tun-Kyi A, Homey B, Gombert M, Boyman O, et al. Plasmacytoid Predendritic Cells Initiate Psoriasis Through Interferon-Alpha Production. *J Exp Med* (2005) 202(1):135–43. doi: 10.1084/jem.20050500
65. Oppmann B, Lesley R, Blom B, Timans JC, Xu Y, Hunte B, et al. Novel P19 Protein Engages IL-12p40 to Form a Cytokine, IL-23, With Biological Activities Similar as Well as Distinct From IL-12. *Immunity* (2000) 13 (5):715–25. doi: 10.1016/s1074-7613(00)00070-4
66. Nestle FO, Turka LA, Nickoloff BJ. Characterization of Dermal Dendritic Cells in Psoriasis. Autostimulation of T Lymphocytes and Induction of Th1 Type Cytokines. *J Clin Invest* (1994) 94(1):202–9. doi: 10.1172/jci117308
67. Zaba LC, Fuentes-Duculan J, Eungdamrong NJ, Abello MV, Novitskaya I, Pierson KC, et al. Psoriasis Is Characterized by Accumulation of Immunostimulatory and Th1/Th17 Cell-Polarizing Myeloid Dendritic Cells. *J Invest Dermatol* (2009) 129(1):79–88. doi: 10.1038/jid.2008.194
68. Austin LM, Ozawa M, Kikuchi T, Walters IB, Krueger JG. The Majority of Epidermal T Cells in Psoriasis Vulgaris Lesions can Produce Type 1 Cytokines, Interferon-Gamma, Interleukin-2, and Tumor Necrosis Factor-Alpha, Defining TC1 (Cytotoxic T Lymphocyte) and TH1 Effector Populations: A Type 1 Differentiation Bias Is Also Measured in Circulating Blood T Cells in Psoriatic Patients. *J Invest Dermatol* (1999) 113(5):752–9. doi: 10.1046/j.1523-1747.1999.00749.x
69. Johnson-Huang LM, Suárez-Fariñas M, Pierson KC, Fuentes-Duculan J, Cueto I, Lentini T, et al. A Single Intradermal Injection of IFN-γ Induces an Inflammatory State in Both non-Lesional Psoriatic and Healthy Skin. *J Invest Dermatol* (2012) 132(4):1177–87. doi: 10.1038/jid.2011.458
70. Nograles KE, Zaba LC, Guttman-Yassky E, Fuentes-Duculan J, Suarez-Farinas M, Cardinale I, et al. Th17 Cytokines Interleukin (IL)-17 and IL-22 Modulate Distinct Inflammatory and Keratinocyte-Response Pathways. *Br J Dermatol* (2008) 159(5):1092–102. doi: 10.1111/j.1365-2133.2008.08769.x
71. Lowes MA, Chamian F, Abello MV, Fuentes-Duculan J, Lin SL, Nussbaum R, et al. Increase in TNF-Alpha and Inducible Nitric Oxide Synthase-Expressing Dendritic Cells in Psoriasis and Reduction With Efalizumab (Anti-CD11a). *Proc Natl Acad Sci USA* (2005) 102(52):19057–62. doi: 10.1073/pnas.0509736102
72. Boyman O, Hefti HP, Conrad C, Nickoloff BJ, Suter M, Nestle FO. Spontaneous Development of Psoriasis in a New Animal Model Shows an Essential Role for Resident T Cells and Tumor Necrosis Factor-Alpha. *J Exp Med* (2004) 199(5):731–6. doi: 10.1084/jem.20031482
73. Terajima S, Higaki M, Igarashi Y, Nogita T, Kawashima M. An Important Role of Tumor Necrosis Factor-Alpha in the Induction of Adhesion Molecules in Psoriasis. *Arch Dermatol Res* (1998) 290(5):246–52. doi: 10.1007/s004030050299
74. Young CN, Koepke JI, Terlecky LJ, Borkin MS, Boyd SL, Terlecky SR. Reactive Oxygen Species in Tumor Necrosis Factor-Alpha-Activated Primary Human Keratinocytes: Implications for Psoriasis and Inflammatory Skin Disease. *J Invest Dermatol* (2008) 128(11):2606–14. doi: 10.1038/jid.2008.122
75. Chiricozzi A, Guttman-Yassky E, Suárez-Fariñas M, Nograles KE, Tian S, Cardinale I, et al. Integrative Responses to IL-17 and TNF-α in Human Keratinocytes Account for Key Inflammatory Pathogenic Circuits in Psoriasis. *J Invest Dermatol* (2011) 131(3):677–87. doi: 10.1038/jid.2010.340
76. Liang SC, Tan XY, Luxenberg DP, Karim R, Dunussi-Joannopoulos K, Collins M, et al. Interleukin (IL)-22 and IL-17 Are Coexpressed by Th17 Cells and Cooperatively Enhance Expression of Antimicrobial Peptides. *J Exp Med* (2006) 203(10):2271–9. doi: 10.1084/jem.20061308
77. Zheng Y, Danilenko DM, Valdez P, Kasman I, Eastham-Anderson J, Wu J, et al. Interleukin-22, a T(H)17 Cytokine, Mediates IL-23-Induced Dermal Inflammation and Acanthosis. *Nature* (2007) 445(7128):648–51. doi: 10.1038/nature05505
78. Brembilla NC, Senra L, Boehncke WH. The IL-17 Family of Cytokines in Psoriasis: IL-17A and Beyond. *Front Immunol* (2018) 9:1682. doi: 10.3389/fimmu.2018.01682
79. Teunissen MBM, Yeremenko NG, Baeten DLP, Chielie S, Spuls PI, de Rie MA, et al. The IL-17A-Producing CD8+ T-Cell Population in Psoriatic Lesional Skin Comprises Mucosa-Associated Invariant T Cells and Conventional T Cells. *J Invest Dermatol* (2014) 134(12):2898–907. doi: 10.1038/jid.2014.261
80. Cai Y, Shen X, Ding C, Qi C, Li K, Li X, et al. Pivotal Role of Dermal IL-17-Producing γδ T Cells in Skin Inflammation. *Immunity* (2011) 35(4):596–610. doi: 10.1016/j.immuni.2011.08.001
81. Villanova F, Flutter B, Tosi I, Grys K, Sreeneebus H, Perera GK, et al. Characterization of Innate Lymphoid Cells in Human Skin and Blood Demonstrates Increase of NKp44+ ILC3 in Psoriasis. *J Invest Dermatol* (2014) 134(4):984–91. doi: 10.1038/jid.2013.477
82. Lin AM, Rubin CJ, Khandpur R, Wang JY, Riblett M, Yalavarthi S, et al. Mast Cells and Neutrophils Release IL-17 Through Extracellular Trap Formation in Psoriasis. *J Immunol* (2011) 187(1):490–500. doi: 10.4049/jimmunol.1100123
83. Muromoto R, Hirao T, Tawa K, Hirashima K, Kon S, Kitai Y, et al. IL-17A Plays a Central Role in the Expression of Psoriasis Signature Genes Through the Induction of IkappaB-Zeta in Keratinocytes. *Int Immunol* (2016) 28 (9):443–52. doi: 10.1093/intimm/dxw011
84. Watanabe H, Kawaguchi M, Fujishima S, Ogura M, Matsukura S, Takeuchi H, et al. Functional Characterization of IL-17F as a Selective Neutrophil Attractant in Psoriasis. *J Invest Dermatol* (2009) 129(3):650–6. doi: 10.1038/jid.2008.294
85. Harper EG, Guo C, Rizzo H, Lillis JV, Kurtz SE, Skorcheva I, et al. Th17 Cytokines Stimulate CCL20 Expression in Keratinocytes *In Vitro* and *In Vivo*: Implications for Psoriasis Pathogenesis. *J Invest Dermatol* (2009) 129 (9):2175–83. doi: 10.1038/jid.2009.65
86. Witte E, Kokolakis G, Witte K, Philipp S, Doecke WD, Babel N, et al. IL-19 Is a Component of the Pathogenetic IL-23/IL-17 Cascade in Psoriasis. *J Invest Dermatol* (2014) 134(11):2757–67. doi: 10.1038/jid.2014.308
87. van der Fits L, Mourits S, Voerman JSA, Kant M, Boon L, Laman JD, et al. Imiquimod-Induced Psoriasis-Like Skin Inflammation in Mice Is Mediated *via* the IL-23/IL-17 Axis. *J Immunol* (2009) 182(9):5836. doi: 10.4049/jimmunol.0802999
88. Rizzo HL, Kagami S, Phillips KG, Kurtz SE, Jacques SL, Blauvelt A. IL-23-Mediated Psoriasis-Like Epidermal Hyperplasia Is Dependent on IL-17a. *J Immunol* (2011) 186(3):1495–502. doi: 10.4049/jimmunol.1001001
89. Eyerich S, Eyerich K, Pennino D, Carbone T, Nasorri F, Pallotta S, et al. Th22 Cells Represent a Distinct Human T Cell Subset Involved in Epidermal Immunity and Remodeling. *J Clin Invest* (2009) 119(12):3573–85. doi: 10.1172/jci40202
90. Wolk K, Kunz S, Witte E, Friedrich M, Asadullah K, Sabat R. IL-22 Increases the Innate Immunity of Tissues. *Immunity* (2004) 21(2):241–54. doi: 10.1016/j.immuni.2004.07.007
91. Zenewicz LA, Flavell RA. Recent Advances in IL-22 Biology. *Int Immunol* (2011) 23(3):159–63. doi: 10.1093/intimm/dxr001
92. Alabbas SY, Begun J, Florin TH, Oancea I. The Role of IL-22 in the Resolution of Sterile and Nonsterile Inflammation. *Clin Transl Immunol* (2018) 7(4):e1017–e. doi: 10.1002/cti2.1017
93. Tohyama M, Shirakata Y, Hanakawa Y, Dai X, Shiraishi K, Murakami M, et al. Bcl-3 Induced by IL-22 *via* STAT3 Activation Acts as a Potentiator of

Psoriasis-Related Gene Expression in Epidermal Keratinocytes. *Eur J Immunol* (2018) 48(1):168–79. doi: 10.1002/eji.201747017

94. Boniface K, Bernard FX, Garcia M, Gurney AL, Lecron JC, Morel F. IL-22 Inhibits Epidermal Differentiation and Induces Proinflammatory Gene Expression and Migration of Human Keratinocytes. *J Immunol* (2005) 174 (6):3695–702. doi: 10.4049/jimmunol.174.6.3695
95. Wolk K, Haugen H, Xu W, Witte E, Waggie K, Anderson M, et al. IL-22 and IL-20 Are Key Mediators of the Epidermal Alterations in Psoriasis While IL-17 and IFN-Gamma Are Not. *J Mol Med (Berlin Germany)* (2009) 87:523–36. doi: 10.1007/s00109-009-0457-0
96. Wolk K, Witte E, Wallace E, Docke WD, Kunz S, Asadullah K, et al. IL-22 Regulates the Expression of Genes Responsible for Antimicrobial Defense, Cellular Differentiation, and Mobility in Keratinocytes: A Potential Role in Psoriasis. *Eur J Immunol* (2006) 36(5):1309–23. doi: 10.1002/eji.200535503
97. Vestergaard C, Just H, Baumgartner Nielsen J, Thestrup-Pedersen K, Deleuran M. Expression of CCR2 on Monocytes and Macrophages in Chronically Inflamed Skin in Atopic Dermatitis and Psoriasis. *Acta Derm Venereol* (2004) 84(5):353–8. doi: 10.1080/00015550410034444
98. Gillitzer R, Ritter U, Spandau U, Goebeler M, Bröcker E-B. Differential Expression of GRO-α and IL-8 mRNA Psoriasis: A Model for Neutrophil Migration and Accumulation *In Vivo*. *J Invest Dermatol* (1996) 107(5):778–82. doi: 10.1111/1523-1747.ep12371803
99. Homey B, Dieu-Nosjean MC, Wiesenborn A, Massacrier C, Pin JJ, Oldham E, et al. Up-Regulation of Macrophage Inflammatory Protein-3 Alpha/CCL20 and CC Chemokine Receptor 6 in Psoriasis. *J Immunol* (2000) 164 (12):6621–32. doi: 10.4049/jimmunol.164.12.6621
100. Singh TP, Schön MP, Wallbrecht K, Gruber-Wackernagel A, Wang X-J, Wolf P. Involvement of IL-9 in Th17-Associated Inflammation and Angiogenesis of Psoriasis. *PloS One* (2013) 8(1):e51752. doi: 10.1371/journal.pone.0051752
101. Sa SM, Valdez PA, Wu J, Jung K, Zhong F, Hall L, et al. The Effects of IL-20 Subfamily Cytokines on Reconstituted Human Epidermis Suggest Potential Roles in Cutaneous Innate Defense and Pathogenic Adaptive Immunity in Psoriasis. *J Immunol* (2007) 178(4):2229–40. doi: 10.4049/jimmunol.178.4.2229
102. Wang F, Smith N, Maier L, Xia W, Hammerberg C, Chubb H, et al. Etanercept Suppresses Regenerative Hyperplasia in Psoriasis by Acutely Downregulating Epidermal Expression of Interleukin (IL)-19, IL-20 and IL-24. *Br J Dermatol* (2012) 167(1):92–102. doi: 10.1111/j.1365-2133.2012.10961.x
103. Zeng F, Chen H, Chen L, Mao J, Cai S, Xiao Y, et al. An Autocrine Circuit of IL-33 in Keratinocytes Is Involved in the Progression of Psoriasis. *J Invest Dermatol* (2021) 141(3):596–606. doi: 10.1016/j.jid.2020.07.027
104. Hernández-Santana YE, Leon G, St Leger D, Fallon PG, Walsh PT. Keratinocyte Interleukin-36 Receptor Expression Orchestrates Psoriasiform Inflammation in Mice. *Life Sci Alliance* (2020) 3(4): e201900586. doi: 10.26508/lsa.201900586
105. Goldstein JD, Bassoy EY, Caruso A, Palomo J, Rodriguez E, Lemeille S, et al. IL-36 Signaling in Keratinocytes Controls Early IL-23 Production in Psoriasis-Like Dermatitis. *Life Sci Alliance* (2020) 3(6):e202000688. doi: 10.26508/lsa.202000688
106. Elmets CA, Korman NJ, Prater EF, Wong EB, Rupani RN, Kivelevitch D, et al. Joint AAD-NPF Guidelines of Care for the Management and Treatment of Psoriasis With Topical Therapy and Alternative Medicine Modalities for Psoriasis Severity Measures. *J Am Acad Dermatol* (2021) 84(2):432–70. doi: 10.1016/j.jaad.2020.07.087
107. Armstrong AW, Read C. Pathophysiology, Clinical Presentation, and Treatment of Psoriasis: A Review. *Jama* (2020) 323(19):1945–60. doi: 10.1001/jama.2020.4006
108. Menter A, Gelfand JM, Connor C, Armstrong AW, Cordoro KM, Davis DMR, et al. Joint American Academy of Dermatology-National Psoriasis Foundation Guidelines of Care for the Management of Psoriasis With Systemic Nonbiologic Therapies. *J Am Acad Dermatol* (2020) 82(6):1445–86. doi: 10.1016/j.jaad.2020.02.044
109. Griffiths CEM, Armstrong AW, Gudjonsson JE, Barker JNWN. Psoriasis. *Lancet* (2021) 397(10281):1301–15. doi: 10.1016/S0140-6736(20)32549-6
110. Kaushik SB, Lebwohl MG. Review of Safety and Efficacy of Approved Systemic Psoriasis Therapies. *Int J Dermatol* (2019) 58(6):649–58. doi: 10.1111/ijd.14246
111. Grozdev I, Korman N, Tsankov N. Psoriasis as a Systemic Disease. *Clinics Dermatol* (2014) 32(3):343–50. doi: 10.1016/j.clindermatol.2013.11.001
112. Korman NJ. Management of Psoriasis as a Systemic Disease: What Is the Evidence? *Br J Dermatol* (2020) 182(4):840–8. doi: 10.1111/bjd.18245
113. Arican O, Aral M, Sasmaz S, Ciragil P. Serum Levels of TNF-Alpha, IFN-Gamma, IL-6, IL-8, IL-12, IL-17, and IL-18 in Patients With Active Psoriasis and Correlation With Disease Severity. *Mediators Inflammation* (2005) 2005 (5):273–9. doi: 10.1155/mi.2005.273
114. Bai F, Zheng W, Dong Y, Wang J, Garstka MA, Li R, et al. Serum Levels of Adipokines and Cytokines in Psoriasis Patients: A Systematic Review and Meta-Analysis. *Oncotarget* (2018) 9(1):1266–78. doi: 10.18632/oncotarget.22260
115. Cataldi C, Mari NL, Lozovoy MAB, Martins LMM, Reiche EMV, Maes M, et al. Proinflammatory and Anti-Inflammatory Cytokine Profiles in Psoriasis: Use as Laboratory Biomarkers and Disease Predictors. *Inflammation Res: Off J Eur Histamine Res Soc [et al]* (2019) 68(7):557–67. doi: 10.1007/s00011-019-01238-8
116. Rashmi R, Rao KS, Basavaraj KH. A Comprehensive Review of Biomarkers in Psoriasis. *Clin Exp Dermatol* (2009) 34(6):658–63. doi: 10.1111/j.1365-2230.2009.03410.x
117. Mehta NN, Yu Y, Saboury B, Foroughi N, Krishnamoorthy P, Raper A, et al. Systemic and Vascular Inflammation in Patients With Moderate to Severe Psoriasis as Measured by [18F]-Fluorodeoxyglucose Positron Emission Tomography-Computed Tomography (FDG-PET/CT): A Pilot Study. *Arch Dermatol* (2011) 147(9):1031–9. doi: 10.1001/archdermatol.2011.119
118. Chi C-C, Wang J, Chen Y-F, Wang S-H, Chen F-L, Tung T-H. Risk of Incident Chronic Kidney Disease and End-Stage Renal Disease in Patients With Psoriasis: A Nationwide Population-Based Cohort Study. *J Dermatol Sci* (2015) 78(3):232–8. doi: 10.1016/j.jdermsci.2015.03.012
119. Chiu HY, Huang HL, Li CH, Yin YJ, Chen HA, Hsu ST, et al. Increased Risk of Glomerulonephritis and Chronic Kidney Disease in Relation to the Severity of Psoriasis, Concomitant Medication, and Comorbidity: A Nationwide Population-Based Cohort Study. *Br J Dermatol* (2015) 173 (1):146–54. doi: 10.1111/bjd.13599
120. Wan J, Wang S, Haynes K, Denburg MR, Shin DB, Gelfand JM. Risk of Moderate to Advanced Kidney Disease in Patients With Psoriasis: Population Based Cohort Study. *BMJ: Br Med J* (2013) 347:f5961. doi: 10.1136/bmj.f5961
121. Dowlatshahi EA, Wakkee M, Arends LR, Nijsten T. The Prevalence and Odds of Depressive Symptoms and Clinical Depression in Psoriasis Patients: A Systematic Review and Meta-Analysis. *J Invest Dermatol* (2014) 134 (6):1542–51. doi: 10.1038/jid.2013.508
122. Olivier C, Robert PD, Daihung DO, UrbÀ G, Catalin MP, Hywel W, et al. The Risk of Depression, Anxiety, and Suicidality in Patients With Psoriasis: A Population-Based Cohort Study. *Arch Dermatol* (2010) 146(8):891–5. doi: 10.1001/archdermatol.2010.186
123. Khalid U, Hansen PR, Gislason GH, Lindhardsen J, Kristensen SL, Winther SA, et al. Psoriasis and New-Onset Diabetes: A Danish Nationwide Cohort Study. *Diabetes Care* (2013) 36(8):2402–7. doi: 10.2337/dc12-2330
124. Armstrong AW, Harskamp CT, Armstrong EJ. Psoriasis and the Risk of Diabetes Mellitus: A Systematic Review and Meta-Analysis. *JAMA Dermatol* (2013) 149(1):84–91. doi: 10.1001/2013.jamadermatol.406
125. Cohen AD, Dreiher J, Shapiro Y, Vidavsky L, Vardy DA, Davidovici B, et al. Psoriasis and Diabetes: A Population-Based Cross-Sectional Study. *J Eur Acad Dermatol Venereol* (2008) 22(5):585–9. doi: 10.1111/j.1468-3083.2008.02636.x
126. Cohen AD, Dreiher J, Birkenfeld S. Psoriasis Associated With Ulcerative Colitis and Crohn's Disease. *J Eur Acad Dermatol Venereol: JEADV* (2009) 23 (5):561–5. doi: 10.1111/j.1468-3083.2008.03031.x
127. Egeberg A, Mallbris L, Warren RB, Bachelez H, Gislason GH, Hansen PR, et al. Association Between Psoriasis and Inflammatory Bowel Disease: A Danish Nationwide Cohort Study. *Br J Dermatol* (2016) 175(3):487–92. doi: 10.1111/bjd.14528

128. Li WQ, Han JL, Chan AT, Qureshi AA. Psoriasis, Psoriatic Arthritis and Increased Risk of Incident Crohn's Disease in US Women. *Ann Rheumatic Dis* (2013) 72(7):1200–5. doi: 10.1136/annrheumdis-2012-202143
129. Brauchli YB, Jick SS, Miret M, Meier CR. Psoriasis and Risk of Incident Cancer: An Inception Cohort Study With a Nested Case-Control Analysis. *J Invest Dermatol* (2009) 129(11):2604–12. doi: 10.1038/jid.2009.113
130. Egeberg A, Thyssen JP, Gislason GH, Skov L. Skin Cancer in Patients With Psoriasis. *J Eur Acad Dermatol Venereol: JEADV* (2016) 30(8):1349–53. doi: 10.1111/jdv.13619
131. Pouplard C, Brenaut E, Horreau C, Barnetche T, Misery L, Richard MA, et al. Risk of Cancer in Psoriasis: A Systematic Review and Meta-Analysis of Epidemiological Studies. *J Eur Acad Dermatol Venereol: JEADV* (2013) 27 Suppl 3:36–46. doi: 10.1111/jdv.12165
132. Langan SM, Seminara NM, Shin DB, Troxel AB, Kimmel SE, Mehta NN, et al. Prevalence of Metabolic Syndrome in Patients With Psoriasis: A Population-Based Study in the United Kingdom. *J Invest Dermatol* (2012) 132(3, Part 1):556–62. doi: 10.1038/jid.2011.365
133. Sommer DM, Jenisch S, Suchan M, Christophers E, Weichenthal M. Increased Prevalence of the Metabolic Syndrome in Patients With Moderate to Severe Psoriasis. *Arch Dermatol Res* (2006) 298(7):321. doi: 10.1007/s00403-006-0703-z
134. Love TJ, Qureshi AA, Karlson EW, Gelfand JM, Choi HK. Prevalence of the Metabolic Syndrome in Psoriasis: Results From the National Health and Nutrition Examination Survey, 2003-2006. *Arch Dermatol* (2011) 147 (4):419–24. doi: 10.1001/archdermatol.2010.370
135. Gisondi P, Targher G, Zoppini G, Girolomoni G. Non-Alcoholic Fatty Liver Disease in Patients With Chronic Plaque Psoriasis. *J Hepatol* (2009) 51 (4):758–64. doi: 10.1016/j.jhep.2009.04.020
136. Candia R, Ruiz A, Torres-Robles R, Chávez-Tapia N, Méndez-Sánchez N, Arrese M. Risk of non-Alcoholic Fatty Liver Disease in Patients With Psoriasis: A Systematic Review and Meta-Analysis. *J Eur Acad Dermatol Venereol: JEADV* (2015) 29(4):656–62. doi: 10.1111/jdv.12847
137. Roberts KK, Cochet AE, Lamb PB, Brown PJ, Battafarano DF, Brunt EM, et al. The Prevalence of NAFLD and NASH Among Patients With Psoriasis in a Tertiary Care Dermatology and Rheumatology Clinic. *Aliment Pharmacol Ther* (2015) 41(3):293–300. doi: 10.1111/apt.13042
138. Cohen AD, Gilutz H, Henkin Y, Zahger D, Shapiro J, Bonneh DY, et al. Psoriasis and the Metabolic Syndrome. *Acta Derm Venereol* (2007) 87 (6):506–9. doi: 10.2340/00015555-0297
139. Cohen AD, Sherf M, Vidavsky L, Vardy DA, Shapiro J, Meyerovitch J. Association Between Psoriasis and the Metabolic Syndrome. A Cross-Sectional Study. *Dermatology* (2008) 216(2):152–5. doi: 10.1159/000111512
140. Tobin A-M, Veale DJ, Fitzgerald O, Rogers S, Collins P, O'Shea D, et al. Cardiovascular Disease and Risk Factors in Patients With Psoriasis and Psoriatic Arthritis. *J Rheumatol* (2010) 37:1386–94. doi: 10.3899/jrheum.090822 jrheum.090822.
141. Fantuzzi G. Adipose Tissue, Adipokines, and Inflammation. *J Allergy Clin Immunol* (2005) 115(5):911–9. doi: 10.1016/j.jaci.2005.02.023
142. Gerdes S, Rostami-Yazdi M, Mrowietz U. Adipokines and Psoriasis. *Exp Dermatol* (2011) 20(2):81–7. doi: 10.1111/j.1600-0625.2010.01210.x
143. Gisondi P, Fostini AC, Fossà I, Girolomoni G, Targher G. Psoriasis and the Metabolic Syndrome. *Clin Dermatol* (2018) 36(1):21–8. doi: 10.1016/j.clindermatol.2017.09.005
144. Takahashi H, Iizuka H. Psoriasis and Metabolic Syndrome. *J Dermatol* (2012) 39(3):212–8. doi: 10.1111/j.1346-8138.2011.01408.x
145. Azfar RS, Gelfand JM. Psoriasis and Metabolic Disease: Epidemiology and Pathophysiology. *Curr Opin Rheumatol* (2008) 20(4):416–22. doi: 10.1097/BOR.0b013e3283031c99
146. Arnett DK, Blumenthal RS, Albert MA, Buroker AB, Goldberger ZD, Hahn EJ, et al. 2019 ACC/AHA Guideline on the Primary Prevention of Cardiovascular Disease: A Report of the American College of Cardiology/American Heart Association Task Force on Clinical Practice Guidelines. *Circulation* (2019) 140(11):e596–646. doi: 10.1161/cir.0000000000000678
147. Gaeta M, Castelvecchio S, Ricci C, Pigatto P, Pellissero G, Cappato R. Role of Psoriasis as Independent Predictor of Cardiovascular Disease: A Meta-Regression Analysis. *Int J Cardiol* (2013) 168(3):2282–8. doi: 10.1016/j.ijcard.2013.01.197
148. Mallbris L, Akre O, Granath F, Yin L, Lindelof B, Ekbom A, et al. Increased Risk for Cardiovascular Mortality in Psoriasis Inpatients But Not in Outpatients. *Eur J Epidemiol* (2004) 19(3):225–30. doi: 10.1023/b:ejep.0000020447.59150.f9
149. Abuabara K, Azfar RS, Shin DB, Neimann AL, Troxel AB, Gelfand JM. Cause-Specific Mortality in Patients With Severe Psoriasis: A Population-Based Cohort Study in the U.K. *Br J Dermatol* (2010) 163(3):586–92. doi: 10.1111/j.1365-2133.2010.09941.x
150. Armstrong EJ, Harskamp CT, Armstrong AW. Psoriasis and Major Adverse Cardiovascular Events: A Systematic Review and Meta-Analysis of Observational Studies. *J Am Heart Assoc* (2013) 2(2):e000062. doi: 10.1161/jaha.113.000062
151. Golia E, Limongelli G, Natale F, Fimiani F, Maddaloni V, Pariggiano I, et al. Inflammation and Cardiovascular Disease: From Pathogenesis to Therapeutic Target. *Curr Atheroscl Rep* (2014) 16(9):435. doi: 10.1007/s11883-014-0435-z
152. Kofler S, Nickel T, Weis M. Role of Cytokines in Cardiovascular Diseases: A Focus on Endothelial Responses to Inflammation. *Clin Sci* (2005) 108 (3):205–13. doi: 10.1042/cs20040174
153. Demetz G, Ott I. The Interface Between Inflammation and Coagulation in Cardiovascular Disease. *Int J Inflammation* (2012) 2012:860301. doi: 10.1155/2012/860301
154. Nagareddy P, Smyth SS. Inflammation and Thrombosis in Cardiovascular Disease. *Curr Opin Hematol* (2013) 20(5):457–63. doi: 10.1097/MOH.0b013e328364219d
155. Marcovina SM, Crea F, Davignon J, Kaski JC, Koenig W, Landmesser U, et al. Biochemical and Bioimaging Markers for Risk Assessment and Diagnosis in Major Cardiovascular Diseases: A Road to Integration of Complementary Diagnostic Tools. *J Internal Med* (2007) 261(3):214–34. doi: 10.1111/j.1365-2796.2006.01734.x
156. Ridker PM, Danielson E, Fonseca FAH, Genest J, Gotto AM, Kastelein JJP, et al. Rosuvastatin to Prevent Vascular Events in Men and Women With Elevated C-Reactive Protein. *New Engl J Med* (2008) 359(21):2195–207. doi: 10.1056/NEJMoa0807646
157. Ridker PM, Everett BM, Thuren T, MacFadyen JG, Chang WH, Ballantyne C, et al. Antiinflammatory Therapy With Canakinumab for Atherosclerotic Disease. *New Engl J Med* (2017) 377(12):1119–31. doi: 10.1056/NEJMoa1707914
158. Szotowski B, Antoniak S, Poller W, Schultheiss HP, Rauch U. Procoagulant Soluble Tissue Factor Is Released From Endothelial Cells in Response to Inflammatory Cytokines. *Circ Res* (2005) 96(12):1233–9. doi: 10.1161/01.RES.0000171805.24799.fa
159. Camerer E, Huang W, Coughlin SR. Tissue Factor- and Factor X-Dependent Activation of Protease-Activated Receptor 2 by Factor VIIa. *Proc Natl Acad Sci USA* (2000) 97(10):5255–60. doi: 10.1073/pnas.97.10.5255
160. Camerer E, Kataoka H, Kahn M, Lease K, Coughlin SR. Genetic Evidence That Protease-Activated Receptors Mediate Factor Xa Signaling in Endothelial Cells. *J Biol Chem* (2002) 277(18):16081–7. doi: 10.1074/jbc.M108555200
161. Vorlova S, Koch M, Manthey HD, Cochain C, Busch M, Chaudhari SM, et al. Coagulation Factor XII Induces Pro-Inflammatory Cytokine Responses in Macrophages and Promotes Atherosclerosis in Mice. *Thromb Haemostasis* (2017) 117(1):176–87. doi: 10.1160/th16-06-0466
162. de Jonge E, Friederich PW, Vlasuk GP, Rote WE, Vroom MB, Levi M, et al. Activation of Coagulation by Administration of Recombinant Factor VIIa Elicits Interleukin 6 (IL-6) and IL-8 Release in Healthy Human Subjects. *Clin Diagn Lab Immunol* (2003) 10(3):495–7. doi: 10.1128/cdli.10.3.495-497.2003
163. Gros A, Ollivier V, Ho-Tin-Noé B. Platelets in Inflammation: Regulation of Leukocyte Activities and Vascular Repair. *Front Immunol* (2014) 5:678. doi: 10.3389/fimmu.2014.00678
164. Raskob GE, Angchaisuksiri P, Blanco AN, Buller H, Gallus A, Hunt BJ, et al. Thrombosis: A Major Contributor to Global Disease Burden. *Arterioscler Thromb Vasc Biol* (2014) 34(11):2363–71. doi: 10.1161/atvbaha.114.304488
165. Lozano R, Naghavi M, Foreman K, Lim S, Shibuya K, Aboyans V, et al. Global and Regional Mortality From 235 Causes of Death for 20 Age Groups in 1990 and 2010: A Systematic Analysis for the Global Burden of Disease Study 2010. *Lancet* (2012) 380(9859):2095–128. doi: 10.1016/S0140-6736(12)61728-0

166. Blann AD, Lip GY. Venous Thromboembolism. *BMJ (Clinical Res ed)* (2006) 332(7535):215–9. doi: 10.1136/bmj.332.7535.215
167. Koupenova M, Kehrel BE, Corkrey HA, Freedman JE. Thrombosis and Platelets: An Update. *Eur Heart J* (2017) 38(11):785–91. doi: 10.1093/eurheartj/ehw550
168. Mackman N. New Insights Into the Mechanisms of Venous Thrombosis. *J Clin Invest* (2012) 122(7):2331–6. doi: 10.1172/jci60229
169. Tanaka T, Narazaki M, Kishimoto T. IL-6 in Inflammation, Immunity, and Disease. *Cold Spring Harb Perspect Biol* (2014) 6(10):a016295–a. doi: 10.1101/cshperspect.a016295
170. Goodman WA, Levine AD, Massari JV, Sugiyama H, McCormick TS, Cooper KD. IL-6 Signaling in Psoriasis Prevents Immune Suppression by Regulatory T Cells. *J Immunol* (2009) 183(5):3170–6. doi: 10.4049/jimmunol.0803721
171. Oliveira P, Cardoso PRG, Lima E, Pereira MC, Duarte ALBP, Pitta I, et al. IL-17a, IL-22, IL-6, and IL-21 Serum Levels in Plaque-Type Psoriasis in Brazilian Patients. *Mediators Inflammation* (2015) 2015:819149. doi: 10.1155/2015/819149
172. Neuner P, Urbanski A, Trautinger F, Möller A, Kirnbauer R, Kapp A, et al. Increased IL-6 Production by Monocytes and Keratinocytes in Patients With Psoriasis. *J Invest Dermatol* (1991) 97(1):27–33. doi: 10.1111/1523-1747.ep12477880
173. van Aken BE, den Heijer M, Bos GM, van Deventer SJ, Reitsma PH. Recurrent Venous Thrombosis and Markers of Inflammation. *Thromb Haemostasis* (2000) 83(4):536–9. doi: 10.1055/s-0037-1613858
174. Reitsma PH, Rosendaal FR. Activation of Innate Immunity in Patients With Venous Thrombosis: The Leiden Thrombophilia Study. *J Thromb Haemost* (2004) 2(4):619–22. doi: 10.1111/j.1538-7836.2004.00689.x
175. Ridker PM, Libby P, MacFadyen JG, Thuren T, Ballantyne C, Fonseca F, et al. Modulation of the Interleukin-6 Signalling Pathway and Incidence Rates of Atherosclerotic Events and All-Cause Mortality: Analyses From the Canakinumab Anti-Inflammatory Thrombosis Outcomes Study (CANTOS). *Eur Heart J* (2018) 39(38):3499–507. doi: 10.1093/eurheartj/ehy310
176. Heinrich PC, Castell JV, Andus T. Interleukin-6 and the Acute Phase Response. *Biochem J* (1990) 265(3):621–36. doi: 10.1042/bj2650621
177. Chen Y, Wang J, Yao Y, Yuan W, Kong M, Lin Y, et al. CRP Regulates the Expression and Activity of Tissue Factor as Well as Tissue Factor Pathway Inhibitor *via* NF-kappaB and ERK 1/2 MAPK Pathway. *FEBS Lett* (2009) 583 (17):2811–8. doi: 10.1016/j.febslet.2009.07.037
178. Zhao Y, Zhou S, Heng CK. Impact of Serum Amyloid A on Tissue Factor and Tissue Factor Pathway Inhibitor Expression and Activity in Endothelial Cells. *Arterioscler Thromb Vasc Biol* (2007) 27(7):1645–50. doi: 10.1161/atvbaha.106.137455
179. Machlus KR, Cardenas JC, Church FC, Wolberg AS. Causal Relationship Between Hyperfibrinogenemia, Thrombosis, and Resistance to Thrombolysis in Mice. *Blood* (2011) 117(18):4953–63. doi: 10.1182/blood-2010-11-316885
180. Marta RF, Goette NP, Lev PR, Chazarreta CD, Pirola CJ, Molinas FC. Normal Platelets Possess the Soluble Form of IL-6 Receptor. *Cytokine* (2005) 29(1):13–7. doi: 10.1016/j.cyto.2004.09.003
181. Marino M, Scuderi F, Ponte E, Maiuri MT, De Cristofaro R, Provenzano C, et al. Novel Path to IL-6 Trans-Signaling Through Thrombin-Induced Soluble IL-6 Receptor Release by Platelets. *J Biol Regul Homeost Agents* (2013) 27(3):841–52.
182. Bernardo A, Ball C, Nolasco L, Moake JF, Dong JF. Effects of Inflammatory Cytokines on the Release and Cleavage of the Endothelial Cell-Derived Ultralarge Von Willebrand Factor Multimers Under Flow. *Blood* (2004) 104 (1):100–6. doi: 10.1182/blood-2004-01-0107
183. Jin W, Dong C. IL-17 Cytokines in Immunity and Inflammation. *Emerg Microbes Infect* (2013) 2(1):1–5. doi: 10.1038/emi.2013.58
184. Kolls JK, Lindén A. Interleukin-17 Family Members and Inflammation. *Immunity* (2004) 21(4):467–76. doi: 10.1016/j.immuni.2004.08.018
185. Onishi RM, Gaffen SL. Interleukin-17 and its Target Genes: Mechanisms of Interleukin-17 Function in Disease. *Immunology* (2010) 129(3):311–21. doi: 10.1111/j.1365-2567.2009.03240.x
186. Kolbinger F, Loesche C, Valentin MA, Jiang X, Cheng Y, Jarvis P, et al. β-Defensin 2 Is a Responsive Biomarker of IL-17A-Driven Skin Pathology in Patients With Psoriasis. *J Allergy Clin Immunol* (2017) 139(3):923–32. doi: 10.1016/j.jaci.2016.06.038
187. Johansen C, Usher PA, Kjellerup RB, Lundsgaard D, Iversen L, Kragballe K. Characterization of the Interleukin-17 Isoforms and Receptors in Lesional Psoriatic Skin. *Br J Dermatol* (2009) 160(2):319–24. doi: 10.1111/j.1365-2133.2008.08902.x
188. de Oliveira PS, Cardoso PR, Lima EV, Pereira MC, Duarte AL, Pitta Ida R, et al. IL-17a, IL-22, IL-6, and IL-21 Serum Levels in Plaque-Type Psoriasis in Brazilian Patients. *Mediators Inflammation* (2015) 2015:819149. doi: 10.1155/2015/819149
189. Simon T, Taleb S, Danchin N, Laurans L, Rousseau B, Cattan S, et al. Circulating Levels of Interleukin-17 and Cardiovascular Outcomes in Patients With Acute Myocardial Infarction. *Eur Heart J* (2013) 34(8):570–7. doi: 10.1093/eurheartj/ehs263
190. Erbel C, Chen L, Bea F, Wangler S, Celik S, Lasitschka F, et al. Inhibition of IL-17a Attenuates Atherosclerotic Lesion Development in ApoE-Deficient Mice. *J Immunol* (2009) 183(12):8167–75. doi: 10.4049/jimmunol.0901126
191. Ding P, Zhang S, Yu M, Feng Y, Long Q, Yang H, et al. IL-17A Promotes the Formation of Deep Vein Thrombosis in a Mouse Model. *Int Immunopharmacol* (2018) 57:132–8. doi: 10.1016/j.intimp.2018.02.006
192. Li Y, Golden JB, Camhi MI, Zhang X, Fritz Y, Diaconu D, et al. Protection From Psoriasis-Related Thrombosis After Inhibition of IL-23 or IL-17a. *J Invest Dermatol* (2018) 138(2):310–5. doi: 10.1016/j.jid.2017.09.021
193. Maione F, Cicala C, Liverani E, Mascolo N, Perretti M, D'Acquisto F. IL-17A Increases ADP-Induced Platelet Aggregation. *Biochem Biophys Res Commun* (2011) 408(4):658–62. doi: 10.1016/j.bbrc.2011.04.080
194. Zhang S, Yuan J, Yu M, Fan H, Guo ZQ, Yang R, et al. IL-17A Facilitates Platelet Function Through the ERK2 Signaling Pathway in Patients With Acute Coronary Syndrome. *PloS One* (2012) 7(7):e40641. doi: 10.1371/journal.pone.0040641
195. Hot A, Lenief V, Miossec P. Combination of IL-17 and TNFalpha Induces a Pro-Inflammatory, Pro-Coagulant and Pro-Thrombotic Phenotype in Human Endothelial Cells. *Ann Rheumatic Dis* (2012) 71(5):768–76. doi: 10.1136/annrheumdis-2011-200468
196. Yuan J, Ding PW, Yu M, Zhang SS, Long Q, Cheng X, et al. IL-17 Induces MPTP Opening Through ERK2 and P53 Signaling Pathway in Human Platelets. *J Huazhong Univ Sci Technol Med Sci = Hua zhong ke ji da xue xue bao Yi xue Ying wen ban = Huazhong keji daxue xuebao Yixue Yingdewen ban* (2015) 35(5):679–83. doi: 10.1007/s11596-015-1489-z
197. Zhu F, Wang Q, Guo C, Wang X, Cao X, Shi Y, et al. IL-17 Induces Apoptosis of Vascular Endothelial Cells: A Potential Mechanism for Human Acute Coronary Syndrome. *Clin Immunol (Orlando Fla)* (2011) 141(2):152–60. doi: 10.1016/j.clim.2011.07.003
198. Hartupee J, Liu C, Novotny M, Li X, Hamilton T. IL-17 Enhances Chemokine Gene Expression Through mRNA Stabilization. *J Immunol* (2007) 179(6):4135–41. doi: 10.4049/jimmunol.179.6.4135
199. Sun D, Novotny M, Bulek K, Liu C, Li X, Hamilton T. Treatment With IL-17 Prolongs the Half-Life of Chemokine CXCL1 mRNA *via* the Adaptor TRAF5 and the Splicing-Regulatory Factor SF2 (ASF). *Nat Immunol* (2011) 12 (9):853–60. doi: 10.1038/ni.2081
200. Maione F, Parisi A, Caiazzo E, Morello S, D'Acquisto F, Mascolo N, et al. Interleukin-17a Exacerbates Ferric Chloride-Induced Arterial Thrombosis in Rat Carotid Artery. *Int J Inflammation* (2014) 2014:247503. doi: 10.1155/2014/247503
201. Zelová H, Hošek J. TNF-α Signalling and Inflammation: Interactions Between Old Acquaintances. *Inflammation Res* (2013) 62(7):641–51. doi: 10.1007/s00011-013-0633-0
202. Baud V, Karin M. Signal Transduction by Tumor Necrosis Factor and its Relatives. *Trends Cell Biol* (2001) 11(9):372–7. doi: 10.1016/s0962-8924(01)02064-5
203. Bonifati C, Ameglio F. Cytokines in Psoriasis. *Int J Dermatol* (1999) 38 (4):241–51. doi: 10.1046/j.1365-4362.1999.00622.x
204. Ettehadi P, Greaves MW, Wallach D, Aderka D, Camp RD. Elevated Tumour Necrosis Factor-Alpha (TNF-Alpha) Biological Activity in Psoriatic Skin Lesions. *Clin Exp Immunol* (1994) 96(1):146–51. doi: 10.1111/j.1365-2249.1994.tb06244.x
205. Kyriakou A, Patsatsi A, Vyzantiadis T-A, Sotiriadis D. Serum Levels of TNF-α, IL-12/23p40, and IL-17 in Plaque Psoriasis and Their Correlation With Disease Severity. *J Immunol Res* (2014) 2014:467541. doi: 10.1155/2014/467541
206. Ridker PM, Rifai N, Pfeffer M, Sacks F, Lepage S, Braunwald E. Elevation of Tumor Necrosis Factor-Alpha and Increased Risk of Recurrent Coronary

Events After Myocardial Infarction. *Circulation* (2000) 101(18):2149–53. doi: 10.1161/01.cir.101.18.2149

207. Kablak-Ziembicka A, Przewlocki T, Sokołowski A, Tracz W, Podolec P. Carotid Intima-Media Thickness, Hs-CRP and TNF-α Are Independently Associated With Cardiovascular Event Risk in Patients With Atherosclerotic Occlusive Disease. *Atherosclerosis* (2011) 214(1):185–90. doi: 10.1016/j.atherosclerosis.2010.10.017
208. Cambien B, Bergmeier W, Saffaripour S, Mitchell HA, Wagner DD. Antithrombotic Activity of TNF-Alpha. *J Clin Invest* (2003) 112(10):1589–96. doi: 10.1172/jci19284
209. Pircher J, Merkle M, Wörnle M, Ribeiro A, Czermak T, Stampnik Y, et al. Prothrombotic Effects of Tumor Necrosis Factor Alpha *In Vivo* Are Amplified by the Absence of TNF-Alpha Receptor Subtype 1 and Require TNF-Alpha Receptor Subtype 2. *Arthritis Res Ther* (2012) 14(5):R225–R. doi: 10.1186/ar4064
210. Pignatelli P, De Biase L, Lenti L, Tocci G, Brunelli A, Cangemi R, et al. Tumor Necrosis Factor-Alpha as Trigger of Platelet Activation in Patients With Heart Failure. *Blood* (2005) 106(6):1992–4. doi: 10.1182/blood-2005-03-1247
211. Pignatelli P, Cangemi R, Celestini A, Carnevale R, Polimeni L, Martini A, et al. Tumour Necrosis Factor Alpha Upregulates Platelet CD40L in Patients With Heart Failure. *Cardiovasc Res* (2008) 78(3):515–22. doi: 10.1093/cvr/cvn040
212. Pignatelli P, Sanguigni V, Lenti L, Ferro D, Finocchi A, Rossi P, et al. Gp91phox-Dependent Expression of Platelet CD40 Ligand. *Circulation* (2004) 110(10):1326–9. doi: 10.1161/01.CIR.0000134963.77201.55
213. Yacoub D, Hachem A, Theoret JF, Gillis MA, Mourad W, Merhi Y. Enhanced Levels of Soluble CD40 Ligand Exacerbate Platelet Aggregation and Thrombus Formation Through a CD40-Dependent Tumor Necrosis Factor Receptor-Associated Factor-2/Rac1/p38 Mitogen-Activated Protein Kinase Signaling Pathway. *Arterioscler Thromb Vasc Biol* (2010) 30(12):2424–33. doi: 10.1161/atvbaha.110.216143
214. Conway EM, Bach R, Rosenberg RD, Konigsberg WH. Tumor Necrosis Factor Enhances Expression of Tissue Factor mRNA in Endothelial Cells. *Thromb Res* (1989) 53(3):231–41. doi: 10.1016/0049-3848(89)90098-4
215. Kirchhofer D, Tschopp TB, Hadváry P, Baumgartner HR. Endothelial Cells Stimulated With Tumor Necrosis Factor-Alpha Express Varying Amounts of Tissue Factor Resulting in Inhomogenous Fibrin Deposition in a Native Blood Flow System. Effects of Thrombin Inhibitors. *J Clin Invest* (1994) 93(5):2073–83. doi: 10.1172/JCI117202
216. Nawroth PP, Stern DM. Modulation of Endothelial Cell Hemostatic Properties by Tumor Necrosis Factor. *J Exp Med* (1986) 163(3):740–5. doi: 10.1084/jem.163.3.740
217. Bussolino F, Camussi G, Baglioni C. Synthesis and Release of Platelet-Activating Factor by Human Vascular Endothelial Cells Treated With Tumor Necrosis Factor or Interleukin 1 Alpha. *J Biol Chem* (1988) 263(24):11856–61. doi: 10.1016/S0021-9258(18)37865-7
218. Camussi G, Bussolino F, Salvidio G, Baglioni C. Tumor Necrosis Factor/Cachectin Stimulates Peritoneal Macrophages, Polymorphonuclear Neutrophils, and Vascular Endothelial Cells to Synthesize and Release Platelet-Activating Factor. *J Exp Med* (1987) 166(5):1390–404. doi: 10.1084/jem.166.5.1390
219. Chignard M, Le Couedic JP, Tence M, Vargaftig BB, Benveniste J. The Role of Platelet-Activating Factor in Platelet Aggregation. *Nature* (1979) 279(5716):799–800. doi: 10.1038/279799a0
220. Camussi G, Tetta C, Baglioni C. The Role of Platelet-Activating Factor in Inflammation. *Clin Immunol Immunopathol* (1990) 57(3):331–8. doi: 10.1016/0090-1229(90)90108-3
221. Conway EM, Rosenberg RD. Tumor Necrosis Factor Suppresses Transcription of the Thrombomodulin Gene in Endothelial Cells. *Mol Cell Biol* (1988) 8(12):5588–92. doi: 10.1128/mcb.8.12.5588
222. Hou B, Eren M, Painter CA, Covington JW, Dixon JD, Schoenhard JA, et al. Tumor Necrosis Factor Alpha Activates the Human Plasminogen Activator Inhibitor-1 Gene Through a Distal Nuclear Factor kappaB Site. *J Biol Chem* (2004) 279(18):18127–36. doi: 10.1074/jbc.M310438200
223. Schleef RR, Bevilacqua MP, Sawdey M, Gimbrone MAJr., Loskutoff DJ. Cytokine Activation of Vascular Endothelium. Effects on Tissue-Type Plasminogen Activator and Type 1 Plasminogen Activator Inhibitor. *J Biol Chem* (1988) 263(12):5797–803. doi: 10.1016/S0021-9258(18)60636-2
224. Aksentijevich M, Lateef SS, Anzenberg P, Dey AK, Mehta NN. Chronic Inflammation, Cardiometabolic Diseases and Effects of Treatment: Psoriasis as a Human Model. *Trends Cardiovasc Med* (2020) 30(8):472–8. doi: 10.1016/j.tcm.2019.11.001

14

Transcription Factor Retinoid-Related Orphan Receptor γt: A Promising Target for the Treatment of Psoriasis

Lipeng Tang[1†], Xiaozhi Yang[2†], Yongxin Liang[2], Hesong Xie[2], Zhenhua Dai[3] and Guangjuan Zheng[1,4*]*

[1] Department of Pharmacology of Traditional Chinese Medicine, The Second Affiliated Hospital of Guangzhou University of Chinese Medicine, Guangzhou, Guangdong, China, [2] School of Bioscience and Bio-Pharmaceutics, Guangdong Pharmaceutical University, Guangzhou, Guangdong, China, [3] Section of Immunology, The Second Affiliated Hospital of Guangzhou University of Chinese Medicine, Guangzhou, Guangdong, China, [4] Department of Pathology, The Second Affiliated Hospital of Guangzhou University of Chinese Medicine, Guangzhou, Guangdong, China

***Correspondence:**
Zhenhua Dai
zdai2009@outlook.com;
Guangjuan Zheng
zhengguangjuan@gzucm.edu.cn

†These authors have contributed equally to this work.

Psoriasis, which is a common chronic inflammatory skin disease, endangers human health and brings about a major economic burden worldwide. To date, treatments for psoriasis remain unsatisfied because of their clinical limitations and various side effects. Thus, developing a safer and more effective therapy for psoriasis is compelling. Previous studies have explicitly shown that psoriasis is an autoimmune disease that is predominantly mediated by T helper 17 (Th17) cells, which express high levels of interleukin-17 (IL-17) in response to interleukin-23 (IL-23). The discovery of the IL-23–Th17–IL-17 axis in the development of psoriasis has led to the paradigm shift of understanding pathogenesis of psoriasis. Although anti-IL-17 antibodies show marked clinical efficacy in treating psoriasis, compared with antibodies targeting IL-17A or IL-17R alone, targeting Th17 cells themselves may have a maximal benefit by affecting multiple proinflammatory cytokines, including IL-17A, IL-17F, IL-22, and granulocyte-macrophage colony-stimulating factor, which likely act synergistically to drive skin inflammation in psoriasis. In this review, we mainly focus on the critical role of Th17 cells in the pathogenesis of psoriasis. Especially, we explore the small molecules that target retinoid-related orphan receptor γt (RORγt), a vital transcription factor for Th17 cells. Given that RORγt is the lineage-defining transcription factor for Th17 cell differentiation, targeting RORγt *via* small molecular inverse agonists may be a promising strategy for the treatment of Th17-mediated psoriasis.

Keywords: autoimmune disorder, psoriasis, T helper 17 cells, retinoid-related orphan receptor γt nuclear receptor, retinoid-related orphan receptor γt inverse agonist

INTRODUCTION

Psoriasis is an autoimmune disease with chronic skin inflammation (1), affecting over 125 million people worldwide (up to 2–4% of the world's population) (2). It is predominantly a skin disease, which can manifest itself as various phenotypes, including plaque-type psoriasis or psoriasis vulgaris, guttate psoriasis, pustular psoriasis such as palmoplantar pustulosis, and erythrodermic psoriasis.

Psoriasis vulgaris, a most common type of psoriasis, is characterized by well-defined areas of erythematous and plaques with overlying silvery scale. The main histopathological changes of psoriasis vulgaris include abnormal cell proliferation, parakeratosis, hyperkeratosis, angiogenesis, and inflammatory cell infiltration (1, 3).

Increasing evidence has shown that comorbid cardiovascular diseases are the leading causes of death among patients with psoriasis (4). In addition, a high prevalence of metabolic syndrome, psychosocial distress or psychiatric disorders, chronic kidney disease, and gastrointestinal disease has been demonstrated in individuals with psoriasis (5, 6). The global financial burden associated with the care of psoriatic patients is substantial and significant (7–10). It was reported that the annual costs for treating psoriasis in USA amounted to approximately $112 billion in 2013 (11). As for individuals, patients with psoriasis would incur a lifetime medical expense for relief of physical symptoms and emotional health (12).

THERAPEUTIC CHALLENGES FOR PSORIASIS

Based on the immunological characteristics of psoriasis, researchers have developed topical treatments, including corticosteroids, vitamin D3 analogs and Victoria A acid, and systemic therapies, including methotrexate and cyclosporine, for psoriasis. In clinic, patients with mild-to-moderate plaque psoriasis are usually treated topically with corticosteroids and vitamin D3 analogs, whereas those with moderate-to-severe psoriasis are systemically treated with methotrexate and cyclosporine (13, 14). However, these treatments exhibit low efficacies, poor tolerability, and various adverse reactions (15) (**Table 1**).

Although the introduction of biological treatments, including tumor necrosis factor (TNF)-α antagonists (Efalizumab), anti-TNF antibody (Adalimumab) (16), IL-12/interleukin-23 (IL-23) antagonists (Ustekinumab) (17), and interleukin-17 (IL-17) antagonists (Secukinumab, Ixekizumab, and Brodalumab) (18, 19), has revolutionized the short-term treatment of moderate-to-severe plaque psoriasis, the long-term use of biological therapies may cause loss of efficacy as well as severe adverse reactions, such as infection, cancer, and hepatic dysfunction (20, 21) (**Table 2**). These clinical side effects of existing treatments strongly suggest that it is still urgent to discover safer and more effective therapeutic drugs for psoriasis.

PATHOGENESIS OF AUTOIMMUNE PSORIASIS

To develop a better, safer, and more effective therapy for psoriasis, it is imperative to understand psoriatic pathogenesis. Previous studies have indicated that psoriasis is a skin disease mainly mediated by dendritic cells and T cells although macrophages, neutrophilic granulocytes, keratinocytes, vascular endothelial cells, and the cutaneous nervous system are involved in its pathogenesis (22, 23).

Epidermis-produced antimicrobial peptide LL-37 (cathelicidin), which acts as a dendritic cell activator, is upregulated in the initial phase of psoriasis (24). LL-37 stimulates dermal plasmacytoid dendritic cells to produce interferon-γ (IFN-γ), which in turn activates myeloid dendritic cells (mDCs) to secrete IL-12 and IL-23. IL-12 promotes the differentiation of Th1 cells, whereas IL-23 enhances T helper 17 (Th17) cell development. Th1 cells secrete more IFN-γ and TNF-α to further stimulate mDCs. In addition, Th17 cells secrete IL-17 to stimulate keratinocytes to over-proliferate, causing psoriasis-like lesions (25). Furthermore, the lesion cells secrete a series of chemokines, attracting more immune cells to inflamed tissue, while the damaged cells are digested by macrophages and produce LL-37, forming a positive feedback path that accelerates the development of psoriasis.

TABLE 1 | Traditional treatment for psoriasis.

Traditional treatments	Molecular mechanisms	Adverse reactions
Corticosteroids	Vascular permeability ↓ Skin edema ↓ Neutrophil infiltration ↓ Cell proliferation ↓	Skin atrophy, hair thinning, hypopigmentation, allergic contact dermatitis
Vitamin D3 analogs	Immune modulation Keratinocyte maturation ↓	Hypercalcemia, urinary calcium concentrations increased, tissue calcification
Victoria A acid	The activity of Th1 and Th17 cells ↓ Keratinocyte differentiation	External medicine: itching and burning sensation and erythema, friction at the erythema Oral administration: dry and exfoliated skin, diffuse baldness, denaturation, and skin adhesion
Methotrexate	Inhibition of the enzyme 5-aminoimidazole-4-carboxamide ribonucleotide transformylase Adenosine ↓ Tumor necrosis factor (TNF) and two nuclear factor κB subunits ↓	Bone marrow toxicity, cirrhosis, nausea, and macrocytic anemia
Cyclosporine	T cell activity ↓	Nephrotoxicity, numerous drug–drug interactions; hypertension, hyperkalemia, increased risk of lymphoma, and squamous cell carcinoma with long-term use
Fumarates	TNF, IL-12, and interleukin-23 production ↓	Gastrointestinal disturbances, flushing, eosinophilia, and proteinuria

TABLE 2 | Biologic therapies for psoriasis.

Biologic therapies	Molecular targets	Adverse reactions
Efalizumab	Tumor necrosis factor (TNF) receptor fusion protein antagonist	Infections, certain malignancies, particularly cutaneous squamous cell carcinoma
Adalimumab	Anti-TNF human monoclonal antibody	Infections and certain malignancies, particularly cutaneous squamous cell carcinoma Serious adverse reactions: active tuberculosis, myocardial infarction, optic neuritis, pancytopenia, lymphoma, etc.
Ustekinumab	Anti-IL-12 and anti-interleukin-23 human monoclonal antibody	Nasopharyngitis, upper respiratory tract infection, headache, diarrhea, muscle pain, dizziness, etc.
Secukinumab	Anti-IL17A human monoclonal antibody	The development of *Candida* infections Special adverse reaction: neutropenia
Ixekizumab	Anti-IL-17A human monoclonal antibody	The development of *Candida* infections
Brodalumab	Anti-IL-17A receptor human monoclonal antibody	The development of *Candida* infections suicidal ideation

Recently, LL-37 has been proved to be a T-cell-reactive autoantigen in psoriasis. LL37-specific CD4+ T cells can produce Th17-related cytokines (26). In summary, these results indicate that psoriasis is an autoimmune disease mediated by dendritic cells and T-cells (**Figure 1**).

THE MAIN ROLE OF PATHOGENIC Th17 CELLS IN PSORIASIS

T helper 17 cells are a distinct subset of T helper cells that mainly produce IL-17A, IL-17F, and IL-22. Mounting evidence shows that there are two subsets of Th17 lineages. A non-pathogenic subset of Th17 cells induced by TGF-β1 and IL-6 has an important role in host defense against specific pathogens by producing IL-17 and IL-10 (27). The production of IL-10 by non-pathogenic Th17 cells restrains Th17 cell-mediated pathology so that they are incapable of promoting autoimmune inflammation. On the other hand, differentiation of highly pathogenic Th17 cells from naïve T cells occurs in the presence of IL-23, IL-6, and TGF-β1 (28, 29). More precisely, exposure to IL-23 diminishes the anti-inflammatory cytokine IL-10 in developing Th17 cells (27). In addition, IL-23 stabilizes and reinforces Th17 phenotypes by increasing expression of IL-23 receptor (30, 31) and endowing Th17 cells with pathogenic effector functions (32–34). These pathogenic Th17 cells contribute to various autoimmune diseases (35, 36).

Psoriasis is primarily characterized as a Th1-driven disease because the levels of Th1 cytokines, such as IFN-γ, TNF-α, and interleukin (IL)-12, are markedly elevated in psoriatic lesions, while there is no such an increase in expression of Th2 cytokines (IL-4, IL-5, and IL-13) (37–39). With the characterization of a distinct subset of Th17 cells, the research field of psoriasis has experienced a major paradigm shift.

Indeed, previous results have confirmed that pathogenic Th17 cells play a central role in the development of psoriasis(40, 41). Pathological or immunohistochemical studies on psoriasis have shown that skin lesions are mainly infiltrated by Th17 cells. In addition, IL-23, which is produced by activated mDCs, drives naïve T cells to develop into pathogenic Th17 cells (42). IL-17, which is predominantly produced by pathogenic Th17 (43), is significantly elevated in patients with psoriasis compared with healthy subjects. Upregulated IL-17 has potent ability to recruit neutrophils (44, 45), to activate T cells, to stimulate fibroblasts (46), and to promote development of multiple lineages of macrophages (47, 48). Moreover, pathogenic Th17-secreted IL-17 induces proliferation of keratinocytes and secretion of antimicrobial peptides, cytokines, and chemokines, which in turn recruit more immune cells to inflamed tissue. This positive feedback loop between Th17 cells and keratinocytes has been proved to contribute to the chronic inflammatory phase of psoriasis (43, 49, 50). Other proinflammatory factors released by pathogenic Th17 cells, such as IL-22, TNF-α, and granulocyte-macrophage colony-stimulating factor (GM-CSF), stimulate keratinocytes to release chemokines, further sustaining the inflammatory cycle to promote the development of psoriasis (51, 52).

RETINOID-RELATED ORPHAN RECEPTOR γt (RORγt): A LINEAGE-DEFINING TRANSCRIPTION FACTOR FOR Th17 CELLS

The differentiation of Th17 cells, similar to that of Th1 and Th2 subsets (53, 54), relies on the action of a lineage-specific transcription factor, identified as the orphan nuclear receptor RORγt (55). RORγt, encoded by RORC2, is an isoform of RORγ that belongs to the NR1F subfamily of orphan receptors, including RORα and RORβ. Previous studies have indicated that RORγt is both necessary and sufficient for Th17 cell differentiation in mouse and human CD4+ T cells. Ivanov et al. reported that T cells lacking RORγt ($Rorc^{-/-}$) failed to differentiate into Th17 cells even under Th17-polarizing culture conditions, while over-expression of Rorc in naïve CD4+ T cells was sufficient to accelerate the expression of Th17-related cytokines and chemokines, including IL-17A, IL-17F, IL-22, IL-26, CCR6, and CCL20. Moreover, mice lacking RORγt were much less susceptible to experimental autoimmune encephalomyelitis (EAE), and CD4+ splenocytes from those mice could not induce the disease (55). A similarly crucial role for RORγt in human Th17 cells was also demonstrated (56). IL-6 and IL-23 signals strongly phosphorylated and dimerized signal transducer and activator of transcription 3 (STAT3), resulting in enhanced expression and nuclear translocation of RORγt,

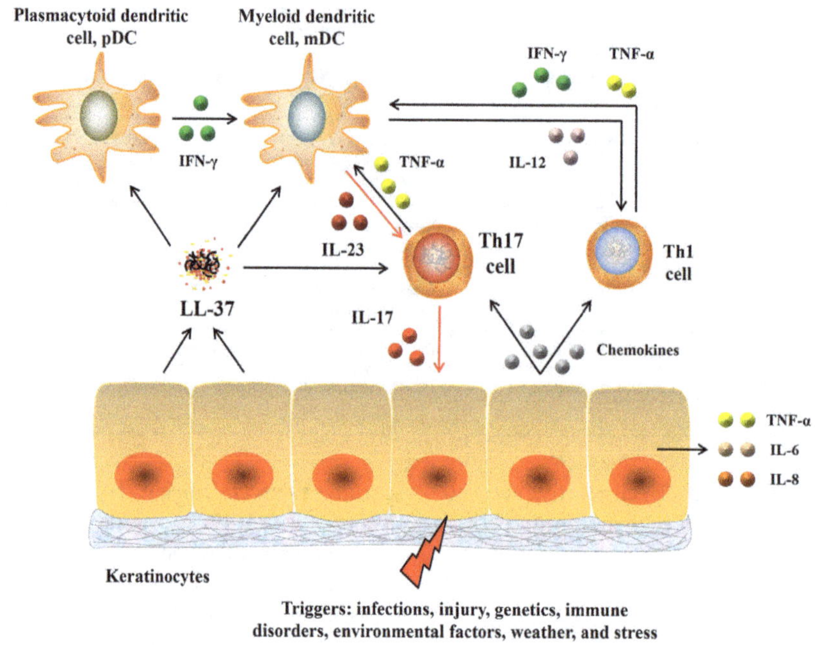

FIGURE 1 | Pathogenesis of psoriasis. Upon activation, keratinocytes secrete LL-37 that in turn activates dendritic cells, which then produce IL-23 and IL-12. IL-23 induces differentiation of naive T cells into Th17 cells that then overproduce IL-17 and IL-22. IL-17 activates keratinocytes, promotes epidermal hyperplasia and recruits proinflammatory cells, resulting in a positive proinflammatory feedback that accelerates the development of psoriasis. Moreover, IL-12 produced by dondritic cells also promotes the differentiation of Th1 cells that in turn produce Th1 cytokines, including IFN-γ. Abbreviations: IL, interleukin; TNF, tumor necrosis factor; IFN-γ, interferon-γ; Th17, T helper 17; IL-23, interleukin-23; IL-17, interleukin-17.

which then promoted Th17 responses by activating Th17 gene promoters, including Il17a, Il17f, Il22, Il26, Il23r, Csf-2, Ccr6, and Ccl20. In addition, IL-23 signaling-induced transcription factor Blimp-1 enhanced pathogenic Th17 function by co-localizes RORγt and STAT-3 at *Il17a, Il23r,* and *Csf-2* enhancer sites (34, 57, 58) (**Figure 2**). Interestingly, neither IL-23 nor IL-6 alone was sufficient to effectively generate Th17 cells (59). Nevertheless, either IL-23 or IL-6 induced IL-17 production by naïve precursors in the presence of IL-1β rather than TGF-β. T-bet + RORγt + Th17 cells were generated without TGF-β and were pathogenic in an EAE animal model, indicating an alternative pathway for Th17 differentiation (59).

Taken together, previous studies have confirmed an essential role of RORγt in the differentiation of pathogenic Th17 cells. Given that pathogenic Th17 cells play such a pivotal role in the pathogenesis of psoriasis, targeting Th17 cells, especially *via* blocking RORγt, may be a good option for treating psoriasis. In addition, RORγt might be a uniquely tractable drug target by virtue of being a nuclear receptor. Therefore, RORγt can be an attractive pharmacologic target for the treatment of Th17-mediated autoimmune diseases, including psoriasis.

SMALL MOLECULES TARGETING RORγt

Retinoid-related orphan receptor γt contains identical DNA-binding domain and ligand-binding domain (LBD). Like other nuclear receptors, the binding of ligands to the region LBD causes a conformational change, which results in recruiting transcriptional co-activators as well as activating transcriptional activity.

Since RORγt receptor was initially identified as an orphan receptor, its endogenous ligands attracted more attention at first. Previous studies have revealed that several oxysterols are endogenous modulators of RORγt activity with high-affinity. For example, 7-oxygenated sterols function as high-affinity ligands for RORγt *via* directly binding their LBDs, modulating co-activator binding, and suppressing the transcriptional activity of the receptors (60). In addition, 24S-hydroxycholestrol acts as an inverse agonist that suppresses the transcriptional activity of RORγt (61).

To develop potent synthetic RORγt ligands that selectively suppress pathogenic effector functions of Th17 cells, researchers have used many strategies to screen for potentially regulatory drug candidates, as described below.

Digoxin, the cardiotonic glycoside extracted mainly from *Digitalis lanata*, has been identified as a specific inhibitor of RORγ transcriptional activity without affecting other nuclear hormone receptors, including human androgen receptor (AR) and liver X receptor α (62). It specifically inhibits IL-17 production by Th17 cells. Moreover, it is effective in attenuating EAE in mice and decreasing the disease severity in a rat model of arthritis (62–64). However, it is toxic for human cells at high doses and may cause some adverse reactions, including arrhythmia, nausea, vomiting, blurred vision, diarrhea, depression, and even lethargy. Further studies have shown that derivatives of digoxin, such as Dig(dhd) 20,22-dihydrodigoxin-21,23-diol, and Dig(sal) digoxin-21-salicylidene, specifically inhibit the differentiation of Th17 cells in

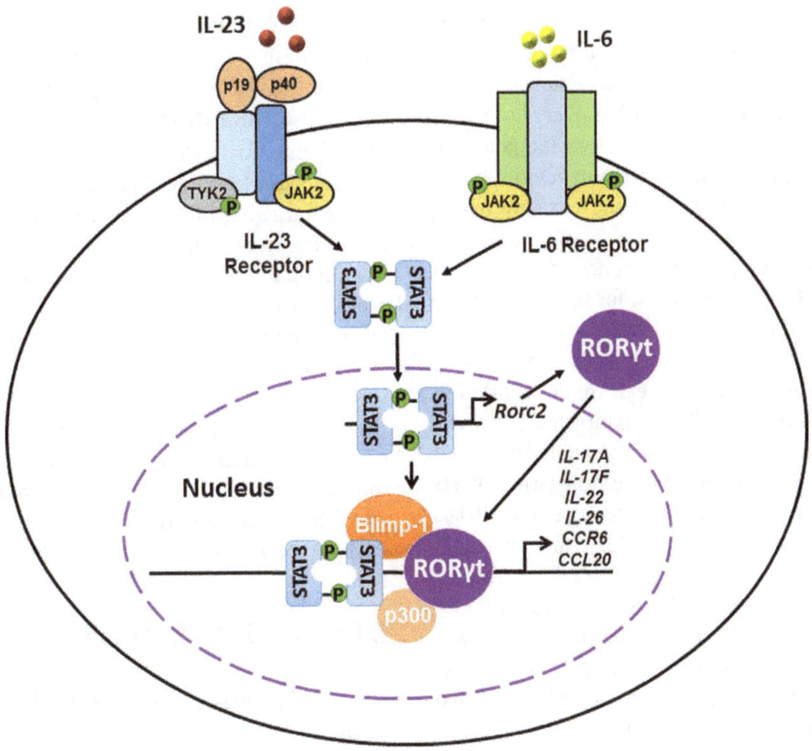

FIGURE 2 | Interplays of interleukin-23 (IL-23), IL-6, signal transducer and activator of transcription 3 (STAT3), and retinoid-related orphan receptor γt (RORγt) in the differentiation of pathogenic T helper 17 (Th17) cells. IL-23 and IL-6 signals activate the JAK–STAT signaling pathway, inducing a strong phosphorylation and dimerization of STAT3. STAT3 homodimers induce the expression and nuclear translocation of RORγt, which in turn promotes Th17 responses by activating Th17 gene promoters, including *Il17a*, *Il17f*, *Il22*, *Il26*, *Il23r*, *Csf-2*, *Ccr6*, and *Ccl20*. In addition, IL-23 signaling-induced transcription factor Blimp-1 enhances pathogenic Th17 function by co-localizes RORγt and STAT-3 at *Il17a*, *Il23r*, and *Csf-2* enhancer sites.

human CD4+ T cells without significant toxicity (62), indicating that nontoxic derivatives of digoxin may be utilized as chemical templates for the development of RORγt negative regulators.

SR1001, a derivative of liver X receptor agonist, is capable of suppressing the transcriptional activity of RORα and RORγ (65). It is a high-affinity synthetic ligand that can bind the LBD of RORα and RORγ, resulting in inhibition of murine Th17 cell differentiation and IL-17 expression by inducing conformational changes that in turn suppress the receptors' transcriptional activity. Thence, SR1001 might be an attractive lead compound for drug development to treat Th17-mediated autoimmune diseases, such as psoriasis as well as RORα- and RORγ-mediated metabolic diseases (66, 67).

SR2211, a derivative of SR1001, only binds the LBD of RORγ and inhibits the transcriptional activity of RORγ without affecting RORα function (68). In addition, SR2211 suppresses the intracellular expression of IL-17 and has potential utility for the treatment of inflammatory diseases, such as experimental arthritis (69, 70). SR2211 has been shown to diminish genome-wide AR binding, H3K27ac abundance and expression of the AR target gene networks, and it could serve as a potential drug for the treatment of castration-resistant prostate cancer (71).

Ursolic acid (UA), a small molecule present in medicinal herbs such as *Prunella vulgaris* L., effectively inhibits the function of RORγt, resulting in greatly reduced IL-17 expression in both developing and differentiated Th17 cells (72, 73). However, UA also has other cellular targets, including the liver kinase B1–AMP-activated protein kinase (74), the NFE2 related factor 2 (75), nuclear factor-κB (76), and STAT3 pathway (77, 78), suggesting that it is not RORγt-specific *in vivo*.

TMP920, which can displace RORγt from its target loci, suppresses Th17 cell differentiation and Th17 signature gene expression (79). Based on TMP920, additional inverse agonists are developed, including TMP778, which exhibits an increase in potency and specificity. It predominantly affects RORγt transcription without removing DNA binding (79). Interestingly, the diastereomer of TMP778 or TMP776 displays no inverse agonist activity against RORγt. In experiments *in vivo*, TMP778 suppresses imiquimod-induced cutaneous inflammation and attenuates EAE. Furthermore, TMP778 also reduces expression of Th17-signature genes in cells isolated from the blood and skin of psoriatic patients (80).

Other RORγt inverse agonists have also been discovered. Using a scaffold hybridization strategy, a series of carbazole carboxamides are found to be potent RORγt inverse agonists (81). In addition, MG 2778, a cyclopenta[a]phenanthrene derivative, is identified as a lead compound for developing synthetic steroidal inverse agonists of RORγt (82). Furthermore, TAK-828F, a potent and selective RORγt inverse agonist, strongly inhibits Tc17 and Th17 cell differentiation from naive T cells and memory CD4+

T cells without affecting Th1 cell differentiation (83). In another study, Barbay et al. have identified 6-substituted quinolines as modulators of RORγt using a RORγt-driven cell-based reporter assay. They have further elucidated the interaction between 6-substituted quinolones and RORγt in an X-ray crystal structure (84). Moreover, A213, a potent and selective antagonist of RORγt, is found to inhibit Th17 cell differentiation *in vitro*. It also attenuates psoriatic skin lesion in two different mouse models by suppressing IL-17 production (85).

Taken together, previous studies have implicated a potential therapeutic application of RORγt antagonist for the treatment of Th17-mediated diseases, including psoriasis. Especially, targeting RORγt for the treatment of cutaneous inflammatory disorders may afford additional therapeutic benefits over existing modalities, in which only one Th17 cytokine such as IL-17A is targeted. However, the small molecules targeting RORγt could generate unwanted or unexpected results given that they may exert off-target effects *in vivo*. Those molecules must undergo rigorous clinical trials prior to a clinical application to carefully evaluate their potential side effects. In addition, other types of immune cells, including type 3 innate lymphoid cells, $CD8^+$ IL-17-producing (Tc17) cells, γδT, and even Treg cells, may also express RORγt. Target RORγt could affect these cells as well. Thus, strategies targeting RORγt in Th17 cells are preferred so that we can attenuate Th17-mediated inflammation while limiting potential side effects.

SUMMARY AND OUTLOOK

Since there are many limitations of traditional and biological treatments for psoriasis, it is important to develop more effective and safer therapies of psoriasis. The finding of RORγt/Th17/IL-17 signaling pathway has provided further insights into the pathogenesis of psoriasis. Compared with antibodies targeting IL-17A or IL-17R alone, targeting Th17 cells themselves might benefit psoriatic patients to a greatest extent by impacting multiple proinflammatory cytokines (IL-17A, IL-17F, IL-22, and GM-CSF) that are likely to act synergistically to drive psoriatic inflammation. Hence, targeting RORγt *via* small molecule inverse agonists is a promising strategy for treating psoriasis *via* suppressing Th17 cell differentiation. Furthermore, small molecules disrupting RORγt are also expected to be safer than global immunosuppressive agents, such as cyclosporine. However, there are several challenges that need to be overcome. Researchers should generate safer and more potent compounds. Moreover, rigorous clinical studies are needed to assess their actual clinical efficacy and side effects since they could generate off-target effects. In conclusion, given the importance of Th17 cells and their proinflammatory cytokines in the pathogenesis of psoriasis, targeting RORγt seems to be a promising approach to treating psoriasis effectively and perhaps safely.

ETHICS STATEMENT

The epidemiological data were cited without any commercial or financial uses.

AUTHOR CONTRIBUTIONS

LT and XY wrote the manuscript; YL and HX searched the literature; ZD and GZ edited the paper.

REFERENCES

1. Boehncke W, Schön MP. Psoriasis. *Lancet* (2015) 386(9997):983–94. doi:10.1016/S0140-6736(14)61909-7
2. Kaufman BP, Alexis AF. Psoriasis in skin of color: insights into the epidemiology, clinical presentation, genetics, quality-of-life impact, and treatment of psoriasis in non-white racial/ethnic groups. *Am J Clin Dermatol* (2017) 19(3):405–23. doi:10.1007/s40257-017-0332-7
3. Griffiths CE, Barker JN. Pathogenesis and clinical features of psoriasis. *Lancet* (2007) 370(9583):263–71. doi:10.1016/S0140-6736(07)61128-3
4. Puig L. Cardiometabolic comorbidities in psoriasis and psoriatic arthritis. *Int J Mol Sci* (2018) 19:58. doi:10.3390/ijms19010058
5. Oliveira MDFS, Rocha BDO, Duarte GV. Psoriasis: classical and emerging comorbidities. *An Bras Dermatol* (2015) 90:9–20. doi:10.1590/abd1806-4841.20153038
6. Dominguez PL, Han J, Li T, Ascherio A, Qureshi AA. Depression and the risk of psoriasis in US women. *J Eur Acad Dermatol Venereol* (2013) 27:1163–7. doi:10.1111/j.1468-3083.2012.04703.x
7. Al SS, Foster SA, Goldblum OM, Malatestinic WN, Zhu B, Shi N, et al. Healthcare costs in psoriasis and psoriasis sub-groups over time following psoriasis diagnosis. *J Med Econ* (2017) 20:982–90. doi:10.1080/13696998.2017.1345749
8. Hay RJ, Johns NE, Williams HC, Bolliger IW, Dellavalle RP, Margolis DJ, et al. The global burden of skin disease in 2010: an analysis of the prevalence and impact of skin conditions. *J Invest Dermatol* (2014) 134:1527–34. doi:10.1038/jid.2013.446
9. Brezinski EA, Dhillon JS, Armstrong AW. Economic burden of psoriasis in the United States: a systematic review. *JAMA Dermatol* (2015) 151:651–8. doi:10.1001/jamadermatol.2014.3593
10. Goff KL, Karimkhani C, Boyers LN, Weinstock MA, Lott JP, Hay RJ, et al. The global burden of psoriatic skin disease. *Br J Dermatol* (2015) 172:1665–8. doi:10.1111/bjd.13715
11. Feldman SR, Tian H, Gilloteau I, Mollon P, Shu M. Economic burden of comorbidities in psoriasis patients in the United States: results from a retrospective U.S. database. *BMC Health Serv Res* (2017) 17(1):337. doi:10.1186/s12913-017-2278-0
12. Hawro T, Zalewska A, Hawro M, Kaszuba A, Królikowska M, Maurer M. Impact of psoriasis severity on family income and quality of life. *J Eur Acad Dermatol Venereol* (2015) 29:438–43. doi:10.1111/jdv.12572
13. Menter A, Korman NJ, Elmets CA, Feldman SR, Gelfand JM, Gordon KB, et al. Guidelines of care for the management of psoriasis and psoriatic arthritis: section 4. Guidelines of care for the management and treatment of psoriasis with traditional systemic agents. *J Am Acad Dermatol* (2009) 61:451–85. doi:10.1016/j.jaad.2009.03.027
14. Greb JE, Goldminz AM, Elder JT, Lebwohl MG, Gladman DD, Wu JJ, et al. Psoriasis. *Nat Rev Dis Primers* (2016) 2:16082. doi:10.1038/nrdp.2016.82
15. Descalzo MA, Carretero G, Ferrandiz C, Rivera R, Dauden E, Gomez-Garcia FJ, et al. Change over time in the rates of adverse events in patients receiving systemic therapy for psoriasis: a cohort study. *J Am Acad Dermatol* (2018) 78(4):798–800. doi:10.1016/j.jaad.2017.10.051
16. Lee EB, Amin M, Egeberg A, Wu JJ. Treatment changes in patients with psoriasis on etanercept or adalimumab: a retrospective chart review. *J Dermatolog Treat* (2018) 6:1–2. doi:10.1080/09546634.2018.1443198
17. Mugheddu C, Atzori L, Del Piano M, Lappi A, Pau M, Murgia S, et al. Successful ustekinumab treatment of noninfectious uveitis and concomitant severe psoriatic arthritis and plaque psoriasis. *Dermatol Ther* (2017) 30:e12527. doi:10.1111/dth.12527
18. Sekhon S, Jeon C, Nakamura M, Yan D, Afifi L, Bhutani T, et al. Clinical

utility of ixekizumab in the treatment of moderate-to-severe plaque psoriasis. *Psoriasis* (2017) 7:65–72. doi:10.2147/PTT.S129792
19. Rothstein B, Gottlieb A. Secukinumab for treating plaque psoriasis. *Expert Opin Biol Ther* (2016) 16:119–28. doi:10.1517/14712598.2016.1121986
20. Belinchón I, Ramos JM, Carretero G, Ferrándiz C, Rivera R, Daudén E, et al. Adverse events associated with discontinuation of the biologics/classic systemic treatments for moderate-to-severe plaque psoriasis: data from the Spanish Biologics Registry, Biobadaderm. *J Eur Acad Dermatol Venereol* (2017) 31:1700–8. doi:10.1111/jdv.14314
21. Lockwood SJ, Prens LM, Kimball AB. Adverse reactions to biologics in psoriasis. *Curr Probl Dermatol* (2018) 53:1–14. doi:10.1159/000478072
22. Diani M, Altomare G, Reali E. T cell responses in psoriasis and psoriatic arthritis. *Autoimmun Rev* (2015) 14:286–92. doi:10.1016/j.autrev.2014.11.012
23. Kim T, Kim DS, Kim H, Lee M. The pathophysiological role of dendritic cell subsets in psoriasis. *BMB Rep* (2014) 47:60–8. doi:10.5483/BMBRep.2014.47.2.014
24. Frohm M, Agerberth B, Ahangari G, Ståhle-Bäckdahl M, Lidén S, Wigzell H, et al. The expression of the gene coding for the antibacterial peptide LL-37 is induced in human keratinocytes during inflammatory disorders. *J Biol Chem* (1997) 272:15258–63. doi:10.1074/jbc.272.24.15258
25. Ogawa E, Sato Y, Minagawa A, Okuyama R. Pathogenesis of psoriasis and development of treatment. *J Dermatol* (2018) 45(3):264–72. doi:10.1111/1346-8138.14139
26. Lande R, Botti E, Jandus C, Dojcinovic D, Fanelli G, Conrad C, et al. The antimicrobial peptide LL37 is a T-cell autoantigen in psoriasis. *Nat Commun* (2014) 5:5621. doi:10.1038/ncomms6621
27. McGeachy MJ, Bak-Jensen KS, Chen Y, Tato CM, Blumenschein W, McClanahan T, et al. TGF-beta and IL-6 drive the production of IL-17 and IL-10 by T cells and restrain T(H)-17 cell-mediated pathology. *Nat Immunol* (2007) 8:1390–7. doi:10.1038/ni1539
28. Lee Y, Awasthi A, Yosef N, Quintana FJ, Xiao S, Peters A, et al. Induction and molecular signature of pathogenic TH17 cells. *Nat Immunol* (2012) 13:991–9. doi:10.1038/ni.2416
29. Wu C, Yosef N, Thalhamer T, Zhu C, Xiao S, Kishi Y, et al. Induction of pathogenic TH17 cells by inducible salt-sensing kinase SGK1. *Nature* (2013) 496:513–7. doi:10.1038/nature11984
30. Langrish CL, Chen Y, Blumenschein WM, Mattson J, Basham B, Sedgwick JD, et al. IL-23 drives a pathogenic T cell population that induces autoimmune inflammation. *J Exp Med* (2005) 201:233–40. doi:10.1084/jem.20041257
31. Chen Z, Tato CM, Muul L, Laurence A, O'Shea JJ. Distinct regulation of interleukin-17 in human T helper lymphocytes. *Arthritis Rheum* (2007) 56: 2936–46. doi:10.1002/art.22866
32. Park H, Li Z, Yang XO, Chang SH, Nurieva R, Wang Y, et al. A distinct lineage of CD4 T cells regulates tissue inflammation by producing interleukin 17. *Nat Immunol* (2005) 6:1133–41. doi:10.1038/ni1261
33. Zheng Y, Danilenko DM, Valdez P, Kasman I, Eastham-Anderson J, Wu J, et al. Interleukin-22, a TH17 cytokine, mediates IL-23-induced dermal inflammation and acanthosis. *Nature* (2007) 445(7128):648–51. doi:10.1038/nature05505
34. Jain R, Chen Y, Kanno Y, Joyce-Shaikh B, Vahedi G, Hirahara K, et al. Interleukin-23-induced transcription factor Blimp-1 promotes pathogenicity of T helper 17 cells. *Immunity* (2016) 44:131–42. doi:10.1016/j.immuni.2015.11.009
35. Puwipirom H, Hirankarn N, Sodsai P, Avihingsanon Y, Wongpiyabovorn J, Palaga T. Increased interleukin-23 receptor(+) T cells in peripheral blood mononuclear cells of patients with systemic lupus erythematosus. *Arthritis Res Ther* (2010) 12:R215. doi:10.1186/ar3194
36. Martin BN, Wang C, Zhang C, Kang Z, Gulen MF, Zepp JA, et al. T cell-intrinsic ASC critically promotes TH17-mediated experimental autoimmune encephalomyelitis. *Nat Immunol* (2016) 17:583–92. doi:10.1038/ni.3389
37. Nestle FO, Turka LA, Nickoloff BJ. Characterization of dermal dendritic cells in psoriasis. Autostimulation of T lymphocytes and induction of Th1 type cytokines. *J Clin Invest* (1994) 94:202–9. doi:10.1172/JCI117308
38. Schlaak JF, Buslau M, Jochum W, Hermann E, Girndt M, Gallati H, et al. T cells involved in psoriasis vulgaris belong to the Th1 subset. *J Invest Dermatol* (1994) 102:145–9. doi:10.1111/1523-1747.ep12371752
39. Austin LM, Ozawa M, Kikuchi T, Walters IB, Krueger JG. The majority of epidermal T cells in psoriasis vulgaris lesions can produce type 1 cytokines, interferon-γ, interleukin-2, and tumor necrosis factor-α, defining TC1 (cytotoxic T lymphocyte) and TH1 effector populations: a type 1 differentiation bias is also measured in circulating blood T cells in psoriatic patients. *J Invest Dermatol* (1999) 113:752–9.
40. Harden JL, Krueger JG, Bowcock AM. The immunogenetics of psoriasis: a comprehensive review. *J Autoimmun* (2015) 64:66–73. doi:10.1016/j.jaut.2015.07.008
41. Marinoni B, Ceribelli A, Massarotti MS, Selmi C. The Th17 axis in psoriatic disease: pathogenetic and therapeutic implications. *Auto Immun Highlights* (2014) 5:9–19. doi:10.1007/s13317-013-0057-4
42. Boutet M, Nerviani A, Gallo Afflitto G, Pitzalis C. Role of the IL-23/IL-17 axis in psoriasis and psoriatic arthritis: the clinical importance of its divergence in skin and joints. *Int J Mol Sci* (2018) 19:530. doi:10.3390/ijms19020530
43. Couderc E, Morel F, Levillain P, Buffière-Morgado A, Camus M, Paquier C, et al. Interleukin-17A-induced production of acute serum amyloid A by keratinocytes contributes to psoriasis pathogenesis. *PLoS One* (2017) 12:e181486. doi:10.1371/journal.pone.0181486
44. Reich K, Papp KA, Matheson RT, Tu JH, Bissonnette R, Bourcier M, et al. Evidence that a neutrophil-keratinocyte crosstalk is an early target of IL-17A inhibition in psoriasis. *Exp Dermatol* (2015) 24:529–35. doi:10.1111/exd.12710
45. Keijsers RR, Hendriks AGM, Van Erp PEJ, Van Cranenbroek B, Van De Kerkhof PCM, Koenen HJPM, et al. In vivo induction of cutaneous inflammation results in the accumulation of extracellular trap-forming neutrophils expressing RORγt and IL-17. *J Invest Dermatol* (2014) 134:1276--1284. doi:10.1038/jid.2013.526
46. Schirmer C, Klein C, von Bergen M, Simon JC, Saalbach A. Human fibroblasts support the expansion of IL-17-producing T cells via up-regulation of IL-23 production by dendritic cells. *Blood* (2010) 116:1715–25. doi:10.1182/blood-2010-01-263509
47. Zhang J, Lin Y, Li C, Zhang X, Cheng L, Dai L, et al. IL-35 decelerates the inflammatory process by regulating inflammatory cytokine secretion and M1/M2 macrophage ratio in psoriasis. *J Immunol* (2016) 197:2131–44. doi:10.4049/jimmunol.1600446
48. Lorthois I, Asselineau D, Seyler N, Pouliot R. Contribution of in vivo and organotypic 3D models to understanding the role of macrophages and neutrophils in the pathogenesis of psoriasis. *Mediators Inflamm* (2017) 2017:7215072. doi:10.1155/2017/7215072
49. Senra L, Stalder R, Alvarez MD, Chizzolini C, Boehncke WH, Brembilla NC. Keratinocyte-derived IL-17E contributes to inflammation in psoriasis. *J Invest Dermatol* (2016) 136:1970–80. doi:10.1016/j.jid.2016.06.009
50. Pfaff CM, Marquardt Y, Fietkau K, Baron JM, Lüscher B. The psoriasis-associated IL-17A induces and cooperates with IL-36 cytokines to control keratinocyte differentiation and function. *Sci Rep* (2017) 7(1):15631. doi:10.1038/s41598-017-15892-7
51. Schäkel K, Schön MP, Ghoreschi K. Pathogenesis of psoriasis. *Hautarzt* (2016) 67:422–31. doi:10.1007/s00105-016-3800-8
52. Eberle FC, Bruck J, Holstein J, Hirahara K, Ghoreschi K. Recent advances in understanding psoriasis. *F1000Res* (2016) 5. doi:10.12688/f1000research.7927.1
53. Zheng W, Flavell RA. The transcription factor GATA-3 is necessary and sufficient for Th2 cytokine gene expression in CD4 T cells. *Cell* (1997) 89: 587–96. doi:10.1016/S0092-8674(00)80240-8
54. Szabo SJ, Kim ST, Costa GL, Zhang X, Fathman CG, Glimcher LH. A novel transcription factor, T-bet, directs Th1 lineage commitment. *Cell* (2000) 100:655–69. doi:10.1016/S0092-8674(00)80702-3
55. Ivanov II, McKenzie BS, Zhou L, Tadokoro CE, Lepelley A, Lafaille JJ, et al. The orphan nuclear receptor RORgammat directs the differentiation program of proinflammatory IL-17+ T helper cells. *Cell* (2006) 126:1121–33. doi:10.1016/j.cell.2006.07.035
56. Annunziato F, Cosmi L, Santarlasci V, Maggi L, Liotta F, Mazzinghi B, et al. Phenotypic and functional features of human Th17 cells. *J Exp Med* (2007) 204:1849–61. doi:10.1084/jem.20070663
57. Calautti E, Avalle L, Poli V. Psoriasis: a STAT3-centric view. *Int J Mol Sci* (2018) 19:171. doi:10.3390/ijms19010171
58. McGeachy MJ, Chen Y, Tato CM, Laurence A, Joyce-Shaikh B, Blumenschein WM, et al. The interleukin 23 receptor is essential for the terminal differentiation of interleukin 17-producing effector T helper cells in vivo. *Nat Immunol* (2009) 10:314–24. doi:10.1038/ni.1698

59. Ghoreschi K, Laurence A, Yang XP, Tato CM, McGeachy MJ, Konkel JE, et al. Generation of pathogenic T(H)17 cells in the absence of TGF-β signaling. *Nature* (2010) 467:967–71. doi:10.1038/nature09447
60. Wang Y, Kumar N, Solt LA, Richardson TI, Helvering LM, Crumbley C, et al. Modulation of retinoic acid receptor-related orphan receptor α and γ activity by 7-oxygenated sterol ligands. *J Biol Chem* (2010) 285:5013–25. doi:10.1074/jbc.M109.080614
61. Wang Y, Kumar N, Crumbley C, Griffin PR, Burris TP. A second class of nuclear receptors for oxysterols: regulation of RORα and RORγ activity by 24S-hydroxycholesterol (cerebrosterol). *Biochim Biophys Acta* (2010) 1801: 917–23. doi:10.1016/j.bbalip.2010.02.012
62. Huh JR, Leung MWL, Huang P, Ryan DA, Krout MR, Malapaka RRV, et al. Digoxin and its derivatives suppress TH17 cell differentiation by antagonizing RORγt activity. *Nature* (2011) 472:486–90. doi:10.1038/nature09978
63. Lee J, Baek S, Lee J, Lee J, Lee D, Park M, et al. Digoxin ameliorates autoimmune arthritis via suppression of Th17 differentiation. *Int Immunopharmacol* (2015) 26:103–11. doi:10.1016/j.intimp.2015.03.017
64. Fujita-Sato S, Ito S, Isobe T, Ohyama T, Wakabayashi K, Morishita K, et al. Structural basis of digoxin that antagonizes RORγt receptor activity and suppresses Th17 cell differentiation and interleukin (IL)-17 production. *J Biol Chem* (2011) 286:31409–17. doi:10.1074/jbc.M111.254003
65. Solt LA, Kumar N, Nuhant P, Wang Y, Lauer JL, Liu J, et al. Suppression of TH17 differentiation and autoimmunity by a synthetic ROR ligand. *Nature* (2011) 472:491–4. doi:10.1038/nature10075
66. Beurel E, Harrington LE, Jope RS. Inflammatory T helper 17 cells promote depression-like behavior in mice. *Biol Psychiatry* (2013) 73:622–30. doi:10.1016/j.biopsych.2012.09.021
67. Solt LA, Banerjee S, Campbell S, Kamenecka TM, Burris TP. ROR inverse agonist suppresses insulitis and prevents hyperglycemia in a mouse model of type 1 diabetes. *Endocrinology* (2015) 156:869–81. doi:10.1210/en.2014-1677
68. Kumar N, Lyda B, Chang MR, Lauer JL, Solt LA, Burris TP, et al. Identification of SR2211: a potent synthetic RORγ-selective modulator. *ACS Chem Biol* (2012) 7:672–7. doi:10.1021/cb200496y
69. Chang MR, Lyda B, Kamenecka TM, Griffin PR. Pharmacologic repression of retinoic acid receptor-related orphan nuclear receptor γ is therapeutic in the collagen-induced arthritis experimental model. *Arthritis Rheumatol* (2014) 66:579–88. doi:10.1002/art.38272
70. Lin H, Song P, Zhao Y, Xue L, Liu Y, Chu C. Targeting Th17 cells with small molecules and small interference RNA. *Mediators Inflamm* (2015) 2015:290657. doi:10.1155/2015/290657
71. Wang J, Zou JX, Xue X, Cai D, Zhang Y, Duan Z, et al. ROR-γ drives androgen receptor expression and represents a therapeutic target in castration-resistant prostate cancer. *Nat Med* (2016) 22:488–96. doi:10.1038/nm0616-692b
72. Baek S, Lee J, Lee D, Park M, Lee J, Kwok S, et al. Ursolic acid ameliorates autoimmune arthritis via suppression of Th17 and B cell differentiation. *Acta Pharmacol Sin* (2014) 35:1177–87. doi:10.1038/aps.2014.58
73. Xu T, Wang X, Zhong B, Nurieva RI, Ding S, Dong C. Ursolic acid suppresses interleukin-17 (IL-17) production by selectively antagonizing the function of RORγt protein. *J Biol Chem* (2011) 286:22707–10. doi:10.1074/jbc.C111.250407
74. He Y, Li Y, Zhao T, Wang Y, Sun C. Ursolic acid inhibits adipogenesis in 3T3-L1 adipocytes through LKB1/AMPK pathway. *PLoS One* (2013) 8:e70135. doi:10.1371/journal.pone.0070135
75. Li L, Zhang X, Cui L, Wang L, Liu H, Ji H, et al. Ursolic acid promotes the neuroprotection by activating Nrf2 pathway after cerebral ischemia in mice. *Brain Res* (2013) 1497:32–9. doi:10.1016/j.brainres.2012.12.032
76. You HJ, Choi CY, Kim JY, Park SJ, Hahm KS, Jeong HG. Ursolic acid enhances nitric oxide and tumor necrosis factor-alpha production via nuclear factor-kappaB activation in the resting macrophages. *FEBS Lett* (2001) 509:156–60. doi:10.1016/S0014-5793(01)03161-1
77. Lin J, Chen Y, Wei L, Shen A, Sferra TJ, Hong Z, et al. Ursolic acid promotes colorectal cancer cell apoptosis and inhibits cell proliferation via modulation of multiple signaling pathways. *Int J Oncol* (2013) 43:1235–43. doi:10.3892/ijo.2013.2040
78. Pathak AK, Bhutani M, Nair AS, Ahn KS, Chakraborty A, Kadara H, et al. Ursolic acid inhibits STAT3 activation pathway leading to suppression of proliferation and chemosensitization of human multiple myeloma cells. *Mol Cancer Res* (2007) 5:943–55. doi:10.1158/1541-7786.MCR-06-0348
79. Xiao S, Yosef N, Yang J, Wang Y, Zhou L, Zhu C, et al. Small-molecule RORγ antagonists inhibit T helper 17 cell transcriptional network by divergent mechanisms. *Immunity* (2014) 40:477–89. doi:10.1016/j.immuni.2014.04.004
80. Skepner J, Ramesh R, Trocha M, Schmidt D, Baloglu E, Lobera M, et al. Pharmacologic inhibition of RORγ regulates Th17 signature gene expression and suppresses cutaneous inflammation in vivo. *J Immunol* (2014) 192:2564–75. doi:10.4049/jimmunol.1302190
81. Huang Y, Yu M, Sun N, Tang T, Yu F, Song X, et al. Discovery of carbazole carboxamides as novel RORγt inverse agonists. *Eur J Med Chem* (2018) 148: 465–76. doi:10.1016/j.ejmech.2018.02.050
82. Dal Prà M, Carta D, Szabadkai G, Suman M, Frión-Herrera Y, Paccagnella N, et al. Targeting RORs nuclear receptors by novel synthetic steroidal inverse agonists for autoimmune disorders. *Bioorg Med Chem* (2018) 26(8):1686–704. doi:10.1016/j.bmc.2018.02.018
83. Shibata A, Uga K, Sato T, Sagara M, Igaki K, Nakamura Y, et al. Pharmacological inhibitory profile of TAK-828F, a potent and selective orally available RORγt inverse agonist. *Biochem Pharmacol* (2018) 150:35–45. doi:10.1016/j.bcp.2018.01.023
84. Barbay JK, Cummings MD, Abad M, Castro G, Kreutter KD, Kummer DA, et al. 6-Substituted quinolines as RORgammat inverse agonists. *Bioorg Med Chem Lett* (2017) 27(23):5277–83. doi:10.1016/j.bmcl.2017.10.027
85. Takaishi M, Ishizaki M, Suzuki K, Isobe T, Shimozato T, Sano S. Oral administration of a novel RORγt antagonist attenuates psoriasis-like skin lesion of two independent mouse models through neutralization of IL-17. *J Dermatol Sci* (2017) 85:12–9. doi:10.1016/j.jdermsci.2016.10.001

15

Anti-LL37 Antibodies are Present in Psoriatic Arthritis (PsA) Patients: New Biomarkers in PsA

Loredana Frasca[1*†], Raffaella Palazzo[1], Maria S. Chimenti[2], Stefano Alivernini[3,4], Barbara Tolusso[3], Laura Bui[5], Elisabetta Botti[6], Alessandro Giunta[6], Luca Bianchi[6], Luca Petricca[3], Simone E. Auteri[7], Francesca Spadaro[8], Giulia L. Fonti[2], Mario Falchi[9], Antonella Evangelista[5], Barbara Marinari[6], Immacolata Pietraforte[10], Francesca R. Spinelli[7], Tania Colasanti[7], Cristiano Alessandri[7], Fabrizio Conti[7], Elisa Gremese[3,4], Antonio Costanzo[11], Guido Valesini[7], Roberto Perricone[2] and Roberto Lande[1*†]

[1] Istituto Superiore di Sanità, National Center for Drug Research and Evaluation, Rome, Italy, [2] Rheumatology, Allergology and Clinical Immunology, University of Rome Tor Vergata, Rome, Italy, [3] Division of Rheumatology, Fondazione Policlinico Universitario A. Gemelli, IRCCS, Rome, Italy, [4] Division of Rheumatology, Università Cattolica del Sacro Cuore, Rome, Italy, [5] Institute of Pathology, Fondazione Policlinico Universitario A. Gemelli, Rome, Italy, [6] Dermatology Unit, Department of Systems Medicine, University of Rome Tor Vergata, Rome, Italy, [7] Rheumatology Unit, Department of Internal Medicine and Medical Specialties, Sapienza University of Rome, Rome, Italy, [8] Confocal Microscopy Unit, Core Facilities, Istituto Superiore di Sanità, Rome, Italy, [9] National AIDS Center, Istituto Superiore di Sanità, Rome, Italy, [10] Department of Oncology and Molecular Medicine, Istituto Superiore di Sanità, Rome, Italy, [11] Skin Pathology Lab, Humanitas Clinical and Research Center, Milan, Italy

***Correspondence:**
Loredana Frasca
Loredana.frasca@iss.it
Roberto Lande
roberto.lande@iss.it

†These authors jointly supervised this study

Psoriatic arthritis (PsA) is a chronic inflammatory arthritis associated with psoriasis. A third of psoriatic patients develop PsA *via* unknown mechanisms. No reliable diagnostic markers are available for PsA, or prognostic biomarkers for PsA development in psoriasis. We previously uncovered a pro-inflammatory role for cathelicidin LL37 in lesional psoriasis skin. LL37 binds nucleic acids and stimulates plasmacytoid/myeloid dendritic cells (pDC, mDCs) to secrete type I interferon (IFN-I) and pro-inflammatory factors. LL37 becomes an autoantigen for psoriatic Th1-Th17/CD8 T cells. Anti-LL37 antibodies were detected in systemic lupus erythematosus, an autoimmune disease characterized by neutrophil-extracellular-traps release (NETosis) in target organs. LL37 can be substrate of irreversible post-translational modifications, citrullination or carbamylation, linked to neutrophil activity. Here we analyzed inflammatory factors, included LL37, in PsA and psoriasis plasma and PsA synovial fluids (SF)/biopsies. We show that LL37 (as a product of infiltrating neutrophils) and autoantibodies to LL37 are elevated in PsA, but not OA SF. Anti-LL37 antibodies correlate with clinical inflammatory markers. Anti-carbamylated/citrullinated-LL37 antibodies are present in PsA SF/plasma and, at lower extent, in psoriasis plasma, but not in controls. Plasma anti-carbamylated-LL37 antibodies correlate with PsA (DAS44) but not psoriasis (PASI) disease activity. Ectopic lymphoid structures, and deposition of immunoglobulin-(Ig)G-complexes (IC) co-localizing with infiltrating neutrophils, are observed in PsA and not OA synovial tissues (ST). Activated complement (C5a, C9), GM-CSF and IFN I are up-regulated in PsA and not OA synovia and in PsA and psoriasis plasma but not in HD. C9 and GM-CSF levels in PsA SF correlate with clinical inflammatory markers and DAS44 (C9) and with anti-carbamylated/citrullinated-LL37 antibodies (GM-CSF and IFN-I). Thus, we uncover a role for LL37 as a novel PsA autoantibody target and correlation studies suggest participation of anti-LL37 antibodies to PsA pathogenesis. Notably, plasma antibodies to carbamylated-LL37, which correlate with DAS44, suggest their use as new disease activity markers. GM-CSF and complement C5a and C9 elevation may be responsible for autoantigens release by neutrophils and their modification, fueling inflammation and autoreactivity establishment. Finally, targeting GM-CSF, C5a, C9 can be beneficial in PsA.

Keywords: Psoriatic arthritis, psoriasis, LL37, autoantibodies complement, neutrophils

INTRODUCTION

Psoriasis is a systemic inflammatory and autoimmune skin disease of unclear etiology affecting 1–3% of individuals worldwide (1). Red and scaly plaques caused by the hyperproliferation of skin epithelial cells characterize plaque psoriasis, the most common form (1). Notably, up to 30% of psoriasis patients develop Psoriatic arthritis (PsA) (2), a type of spondyloarthritis characterized by enthesitis, dactylitis peripheral arthritis and axial involvement. Diagnostic criteria of PsA are primarily clinical and based on the Classification Criteria for Psoriatic Arthritis (CASPAR) and include evidence of psoriasis, absence of rheumatoid arthritis (AR), and the exclusion of other seronegative arthritis (3). Thus, no reliable serological markers are available to identify PsA, as for RA. Histologically, PsA is characterized by lining layer hyperplasia, innate immune cell activation, T and B-lymphocytes infiltrated synovial tissues, and synovial angiogenesis (4). As for RA, a role of B cells and autoantibodies has been suggested in the pathogenesis of PsA (5). Indeed, although the presence of rheumatoid factor (RF) and anti-citrullinated peptide antibodies (ACPA) are characteristic of RA, and uncommon in PsA (6), the detection of ectopic lymphoid structures in PsA synovia (7) suggests production of antibodies against local autoantigens. Notably, anti-carbamylated peptide autoantibodies (anti-CarP Abs) have been recently identified not only in RA (8), but also PsA plasma (9). Currently, no reliable diagnostic biomarkers distinguish PsA from psoriasis and no prognostic markers are available to predict the development of PsA in psoriasis patients.

Cationic antimicrobial peptides (AMP) including the cathelicidin LL37 are aberrantly produced by psoriatic keratinocytes and released by degranulating neutrophils or during neutrophil extracellular trap formation (NETosis) (10–12). LL37 has the ability to bind nucleic acids and induce the production of pro-inflammatory cytokines and type I interferon (IFN-I), by plasmacytoid dendritic cells (pDCs) and myeloid dendritic cells (mDCs) via TLR7/8/9 triggering (13, 14). Moreover, LL37 has been recognized as self-antigen for psoriatic autoreactive T-cells that are detected in circulation or in lesional skin (15). Both CD4 and CD8 T lymphocytes respond to LL37 and LL37-specific CD4 T cells belong to Th1/Th17 sub-populations. Interestingly, in a systemic autoimmune disease such as systemic lupus erythematosus (SLE), where LL37-DNA complexes are highly released during NETosis, LL37 becomes the target of pathogenic autoantibodies (12, 16). Although neutrophils can infiltrate psoriatic skin (17), and a study suggests that NETosis is possibly occurring in skin lesions (18), whether LL37 becomes the target of autoantibodies in psoriasis patients has not been investigated. Notably, there are few reports that show expression of LL37 in inflamed synovia (19). However, whether and how LL37 plays a role as autoantigen in PsA is still unknown.

In this picture, with the idea to: (1) identify the pathogenic players in PsA, (2) discriminate the immunological pathways that are in common or are distinct between psoriasis and PsA, and (3) identify new disease activity markers for PsA, we have investigated the presence of LL37 and related autoantibodies in PsA and psoriasis patients and analyzed their correlations with clinical parameters and inflammatory factors.

RESULTS

LL37 and Autoantibodies to LL37 Are Present in PsA Synovia

In order to investigate the putative role of LL37 in PsA, we firstly analyzed whether LL37 was measurable in the synovial compartments. As shown in **Figure 1A**, higher levels of LL37 were detected in the synovial fluids (SF) of PsA (median: 0.153, IQR: 0.114) compared to control osteo-arthritis (OA) patients (median: 0.1, IQR: 0.036), $p = 0.031$, by ELISA assay. Laser scanner confocal microscopy of synovial biopsies from patients affected by early PsA showed a consistent staining for LL37, coupled to high staining for myeloperoxidase (MPO), the typical marker of neutrophils, in the lining and sub-lining areas of the synovial membranes (**Figure 1B**). This suggested that LL37 was present in PsA synovial tissues (ST) as the product of neutrophils, although a contribution of other cells might not be excluded. In contrast, only occasionally neutrophils and LL37 positivity were detectable in control OA synovia (**Figure 1B**). Neutrophil-derived antimicrobial peptides, including LL37, have been shown to become target of circulating autoantibodies in SLE patients (12, 16) and, to date, one study reported ectopic lymphoid tissues in PsA synovia (7). Thus we assessed the presence of anti-LL37 antibodies in SF of PsA and control OA patients. Although the antibody levels did not reach a statistical significance between PsA (median: 0.348, IQR: 0.233) and OA SF (median: 0.26, IQR: 0.126), $p = 0.28$, by setting a cut-off (as in **Figure 1A**) we found that autoantibodies to LL37 were present in 7 out of 19 PsA SF (37%) (**Figure 2**).

It is reported that LL37 can become a substrate for post-translational modifications such as citrullination and carbamylation (20, 21). Of note, carbamylated proteins can be the

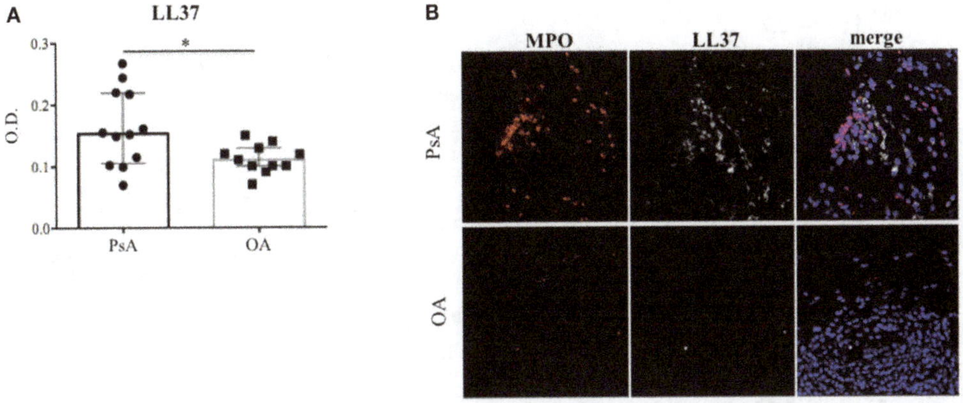

FIGURE 1 | LL37 is expressed in synovial compartment of PsA. **(A)** LL37 was measured by ELISA in synovial fluids of PsA ($N = 12$) and control OA patients ($N = 11$), and LL37 levels are shown as median with Interquartile Range (IQR). P-value is calculated by two-tailed Mann-Whitney U test $^*p < 0.05$. **(B)** Confocal microscopy images of synovial tissues of PsA and OA patients stained for myeloperoxidase (MPO; red), LL37 (gray) (original magnification 63x). For PsA, 1 representative staining of 7 patients is shown. For OA, 1 representative staining of 4 patients is shown.

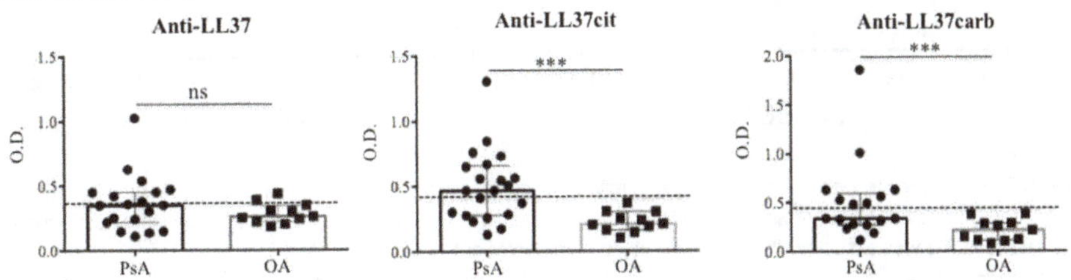

FIGURE 2 | Anti-LL37 antibodies are present in synovial fluids of PsA. Synovial fluids of PsA and OA ($N = 11$) patients were analyzed by ELISA for the presence of anti-LL37 (PsA, $N = 19$), anti-LL37cit (PsA, $N = 21$) and anti-LL37carb (PsA, $N = 17$). Antibody levels are shown as median with Interquartile Range (IQR). *P*-value is calculated by two-tailed Mann-Whitney U test, $^{***}p < 0.0001$. The mean+2 SD (standard deviation) of OA antibody reactivity to native LL37 or modified LL37 was used as cut-off (dotted line).

targets of autoantibodies in PsA (9). In this context, we wondered whether we could also detect antibody reactivity toward either citrullinated (LL37cit) or carbamylated (LL37carb) LL37 or both in PsA SF.

Interestingly, anti-LL37cit antibodies were higher in PsA SF (median: 0.464, IQR: 0.379; 12 out of 21: 57%) than in OA SF (median: 0.207, IQR: 0.14), $p = 0.0008$; similarly, anti-LL37carb antibodies were higher in PsA SF (median: 0.335, IQR: 0.321; 8 out of 17: 47%) than in OA SF (median: 0.214, IQR: 0.174), $p = 0.004$, (**Figure 2**). Of note, there was no significant correlation between anti-LL37 antibody reactivity to native and either citrullinated or carbamylated LL37, suggesting that anti-LL37cit and anti-LL37carb antibody reactivity is probably not due to cross-reactivity but is likely specifically directed toward modified LL37. This indicates that pathways of protein modification are likely to be activated in PsA synovia. Next, we investigated possible correlation between anti-LL37-autoantibody reactivity and clinical parameters such as inflammatory markers and disease activity (DAS44). We found that levels of anti-LL37 antibodies to native protein correlated with C-reactive protein (CRP), erythrocyte sedimentation rate (ESR), swollen joints and DAS44 (**Figure 3**). In contrast, no significant correlation was observed between the same clinical data and antibodies to LL37cit or LL37carb. Altogether, these results suggest that LL37 can become an autoantigen in PsA and the antibody response to LL37 in SF may represent a marker of inflammation and disease activity.

Anti-LL37 Autoantibodies Are Detected in Circulation of PsA and Psoriasis Patients

In order to establish whether the presence of anti-LL37 antibody reactivity was a local phenomenon or whether the same reactivity was systemically detectable, we assessed plasma of PsA, psoriasis and control healthy donors (HD), for antibodies to native LL37, LL37cit, and LL37carb by ELISA. Anti-LL37 antibody reactivity to the unmodified peptide was below the cut-off both in PsA and psoriasis (not shown). However, anti-LL37cit antibodies were higher in PsA plasma (median: 0.544, IQR: 0.495; 11 out of 29: 32%) than in HD plasma (median: 0.394; IQR: 0.16), $p = 0.007$. Anti-LL37carb antibodies were higher in PsA (median: 0.66, IQR: 0.439; 18 out of 32: 52%) than in HD plasma (median: 0.158, IQR: 0.099), $p = 0.0001$ (**Figure 4A**). No statistical significance was observed between anti-LL37cit plasma levels of PsA vs. psoriasis plasma (median: 0.49, IQR: 0.478), $p = 0.3$. In contrast, the

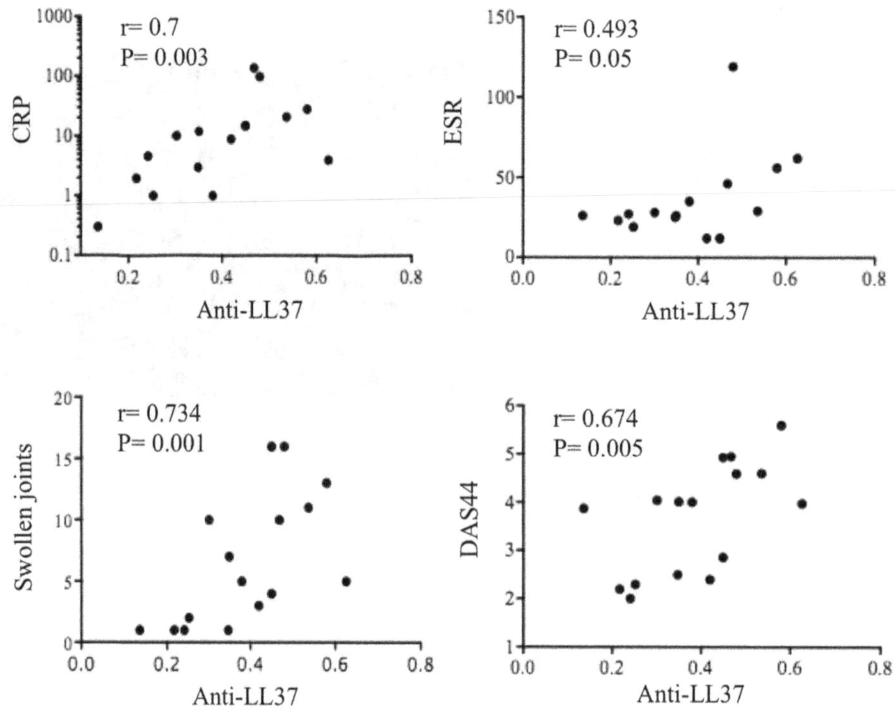

FIGURE 3 | Anti-LL37 levels in SF PsA correlate with disease activity and inflammation markers. SF PsA levels of anti-LL37 Abs ($N = 16$) measured by ELISA as shown in **Figure 2** were correlated with Disease Activity Score (DAS44), C reactive Protein (CRP), Eritrocyte Sedimentation Rate (ESR) and number of swollen joints. The correlation between the two variables was assessed by Spearman correlation coefficient.

anti-LL37carb levels of PsA plasma were significantly higher also when compared to psoriasis plasma (median: 0.43, IQR: 0.47), $p = 0.02$. By setting a cut-off we found that 5 out of 17 (29%) psoriasis patients were positive for anti-LL37cit or anti-LL37carb antibody reactivity (**Figure 4A**). However, levels of anti-LL37cit of psoriasis plasma were not significantly higher compared to HD plasma ($p = 0.15$); in contrast, levels of anti-LL37carb antibodies of psoriasis plasma were significantly higher compared to levels of HD plasma ($p = 0.0001$). Moreover, we observed a significant positive correlation between plasma anti-LL37carb antibodies and disease activity (DAS44) in PsA (**Figure 4B**), in line with recent evidences reporting presence of antibodies to carbamylated proteins in plasma of PsA patients (9). No correlations were apparent between plasma anti-LL37carb or anti-LL37cit antibodies and clinical inflammatory parameters in PsA. Antibody reactivity to LL37cit and LL37carb did not show any correlation with psoriasis activity score index (PASI) in psoriasis patients. These data suggest that measurement of serum levels of anti-LL37carb, but not anti-LL37cit antibodies, may be used as a marker of disease activity in PsA and not in psoriasis.

PsA Synovia Show IgG-Immune Complex Deposition

The deposition of immune complexes (IC) in inflamed tissues is a pathogenic mechanism described in various autoimmune diseases (22, 23). The presence of autoantibodies in synovial fluids and plasma of PsA patients prompted us to investigate the deposition of IgG-IC in ST of PsA, and in OA as control, by confocal microscopy. We visualized the presence of IC in ST of PsA (**Figure 5**) but not of control OA patients (not shown). Interestingly, some of the IC^{+}-synovial cells were infiltrating neutrophils, as demonstrated by a consistent co-localization of IgG and LL37 staining in cells with the typical polymorfo-nuclear shape (**Figure 5,** inset). IgG staining was detectable also in LL37-negative cells, probably macrophages and/or fibroblasts. These results indicate that IgG are detectable in ST of early PsA patients and that they may represent deposit of immune complexes in PsA synovia; these IgG seemed to include ANCA-like antibodies, suggesting that, among the various antibody specificities, anti-LL37 antibodies may be present and target neutrophils.

Ectopic Germinal Center-Like Structures Are Detected in Synovia of Early PsA

Ectopic lymphoid structures resembling germinal centers have been characterized in chronically inflamed tissues in RA and their presence was associated with an antigen driven B cell response (24–27). To date, only one study addressed the presence of ectopic lymphoid structures in PsA ST (7). We addressed whether lymphoid-like structures might develop in PsA ST already at early disease stage and tried to more finely characterize them: we selected PsA patients with early stage of psoriatic arthritis and naïve to any disease modifying anti-rheumatic drugs (DMARD). We analyzed, by immunohistochemistry (IHC), the presence of infiltrating T and B lymphocytes and presence of

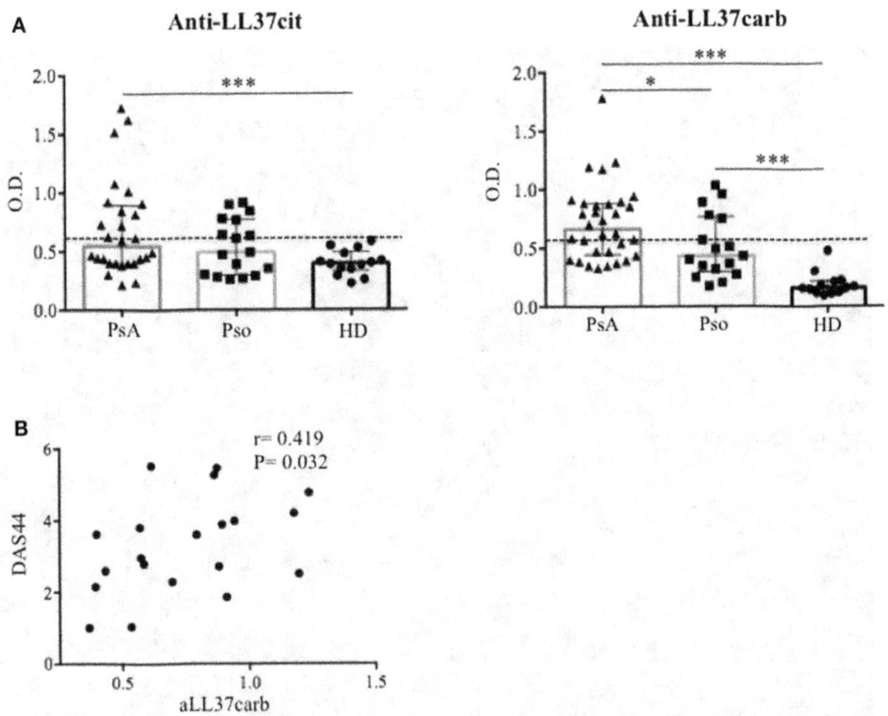

FIGURE 4 | Autoantibody reactivity to citrullinated and carbamylated LL37 in plasma of PsA and Pso patients. **(A)** Levels of anti-LL37cit ($N = 29$) and anti-LL37carb ($N = 32$) were measured in plasma of PsA, Pso (without PsA, $N = 17$) and healthy donors (HD, $N = 14$) by ELISA. Antibody levels are shown as median with Interquartile Range (IQR). *P*-value is calculated by two-tailed Mann-Whitney U test, $^*p < 0.05$, $^{***}p < 0.0001$. The mean of HD antibody reactivity+2 SD was used as cut-off (dotted line). **(B)** Levels of PsA anti-LL37carb were correlated with Disease Activity Score (DAS44) by Spearman correlation coefficient and the significant *P* value by two-tailed Mann-Whitney U test.

$CD21^+$ or $CD23^+$ follicular dendritic cells (FDC), together with the expression of the activation/proliferation marker Ki67 and Bcl6, the latter expressed by GC B cells and involved in the development of $CD4^+$ T-follicular helper cells during the GC reaction [Tfh; (28–30)]. As shown in **Figure 6**, we observed the presence of $CD3^+$ T cells and $CD20^+$ B cells aggregates in the ST of early naïve PsA that were associated to $CD21^+$ and $CD23^+$ FDC. The presence of a lower staining for $CD23^+$ cells as compared to that for $CD21^+$ cells appears in line with other works reporting that the complement receptor CD21 represents a more stable phenotypic marker of FDC (31, 32). Moreover, we found a wide expression of the cell proliferation marker Ki67 and presence of $Bcl6^+$ cells located in the T and B cell aggregates. Altogether these data indicate the presence of organized extra-nodal lymphoid structures in PsA synovia and suggest that such structures can develop at very early stages of disease. Indeed, anti-LL37 antibody reactivity was detectable in PsA synovial fluids and plasma of individuals with early stage disease.

Activated Complement And GM-CSF Are Present in PsA Synovial Compartments and in Circulation

The complement system is activated at tissue site where there is antibody deposition, as described in systemic lupus erythematosus (SLE) and RA (33, 34). Complement C5a has been described either as a potent granulocyte chemoattractant (35) or as a priming factor for neutrophil degranulation (36). Moreover C5a, in the presence of GM-CSF, activates neutrophils to undergo NETosis accompanied by release of granules (37). Other complement members, such as C5b-C9, are involved in the activation of citrullination pathways. This is mediated by the peptidyl arginine deiminase (PAD) activation via Ca^{++} influx, following formation of the Membrane Attack Complex (MAC) that induces pore formation in leukocytes (38). Since we observed presence of IgG in the PsA synovial compartment and antibody reactivity to both native and citrullinated LL37, we assessed the content of C5a, C9, and GM-CSF in SF of PsA and control OA patients and, for comparison, in plasma of PsA and psoriasis patients.

As shown in **Figure 7A**, we found a significantly higher concentration of C5a in PsA SF (median: 3590, IQR: 2234) as compared to OA SF (median: 2426, IQR: 1065), $p = 0.007$; C9 was also higher in PsA SF (median: 4727, IQR: 1665) than OA SF (median: 2884, IQR: 2399), $p = 0.001$. GM-CSF was up-regulated in PsA SF (median: 94.45, IQR: 187) as compared to OA SF (median: 1.79, IQR: 13.21), $p = 0.001$. Moreover, C5a in PsA plasma was higher (median: 24309, IQR: 13863) than in HD plasma (median: 16107, IQR: 17310), $p = 0.013$; C9 in PsA plasma was higher (median: 18542, IQR: 7425) than in HD (median: 11292, IQR: 6023), $p = 0.0009$; GM-CSF in PsA plasma was

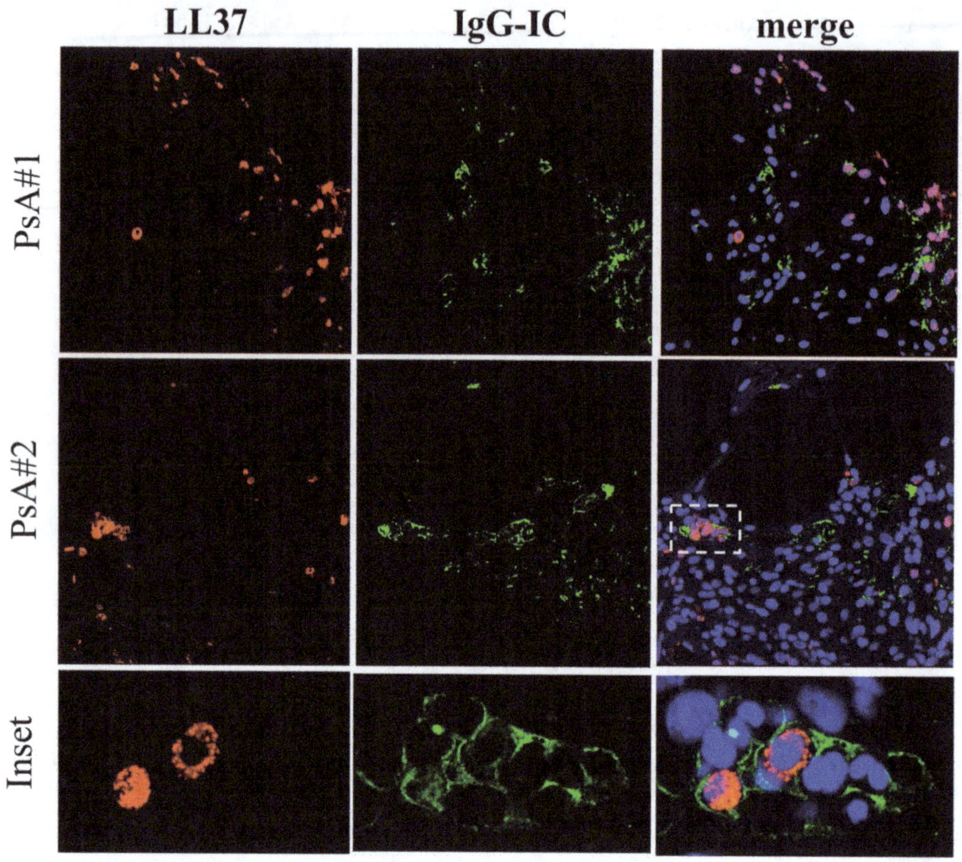

FIGURE 5 | IgG-immune complexes deposition and colocalization with neutrophil-derived LL37 in synovia of PsA. Confocal microscopy images of synovial tissues of two PsA patients stained for LL37 (red), IgG-IC (green) (original magnification, 63x). The dotted white line in PsA#2 indicates the inset of the corresponding picture of the bottom panel. Data are representative of 7 PsA patients.

higher (median: 2.79, IQR: 29.87) than in HD plasma (median: 2.79, IQR: 0), $p = 0.001$ (**Figure 7B**). Of note, the same factors were elevated in the plasma of psoriasis patients. Indeed, the concentration of C5a (median: 19741, IQR: 17432), $p = 0.05$, C9 (median: 21526, IQR: 17432), $p = 0.0001$ and GM-CSF (median: 2.79, IQR: 0), $p = 0.05$, were higher in psoriasis as compared to HD plasma, although the elevation of GM-CSF and C5a were at the limit of the statistical significance (**Figure 7B**). By comparing PsA plasma to psoriasis plasma, only C9 levels were significantly higher in psoriasis than in PsA, $p = 0.02$. C9 levels in synovial fluids, but not in plasma, strongly correlated with disease activity (DAS44; $r = 0.773$, $P = 0.001$; $N = 16$) and various inflammatory parameters: CRP ($r = 0.734$, $P = 0.008$), swollen joints ($r = 0.726$, $P = 0.01$) and tender joints ($r = 0.729$, $P = 0.009$). GM-CSF levels correlated with both anti-LL37cit and anti-LL37carb antibodies in PsA plasma (**Figure 8B**) and with anti-LL37carb (but not with anti-LL37cit) in PsA SF (**Figure 8A**). Moreover, GM-CSF correlated with C5a in PsA plasma (**Figure 8B**). Finally, C5a levels significantly correlated with both anti-LL37cit and anti-LL37carb antibodies in plasma (**Figure 9**), and showed a correlation with DAS44 in PsA, although this correlation was at the limit of the statistical significance ($P = 0.05$; **Figure 9**). Of note, we observed no correlation between circulating C9 or C5a levels and PASI in psoriasis patients. In line with the presence of C9 in PsA SF, we have visualized an abundant presence of C9 in ST of PsA as compared to OA patients by confocal microscopy (**Figure 10**). C9 staining partially colocalized with neutrophils (**Figure 10**).

These results and the relative correlation analyses suggest a participation of activated complement and GM-CSF to antibody reactivity development in PsA and suggest a link between presence of these factors and posttranslational modification of self-proteins in PsA (namely citrullination and, in particular, carbamylation).

An IFN-I Signature Is Present in SF of PsA Patients

Given that immune complexes can induce IFNα (13–15) and an IFN-I signature is present in several immune mediated diseases (SLE, RA), we assessed the presence of IFNα in the synovial compartment of PsA and OA patients.

IFNα was measurable by ELISA assay in 8 out of 20 (35%) PsA SF (median: 1.7, IQR: 63.5) and not in OA SF (median: 1.5, IQR: 0), $p = 0.0001$ (**Figure 11A**). To confirm this, we

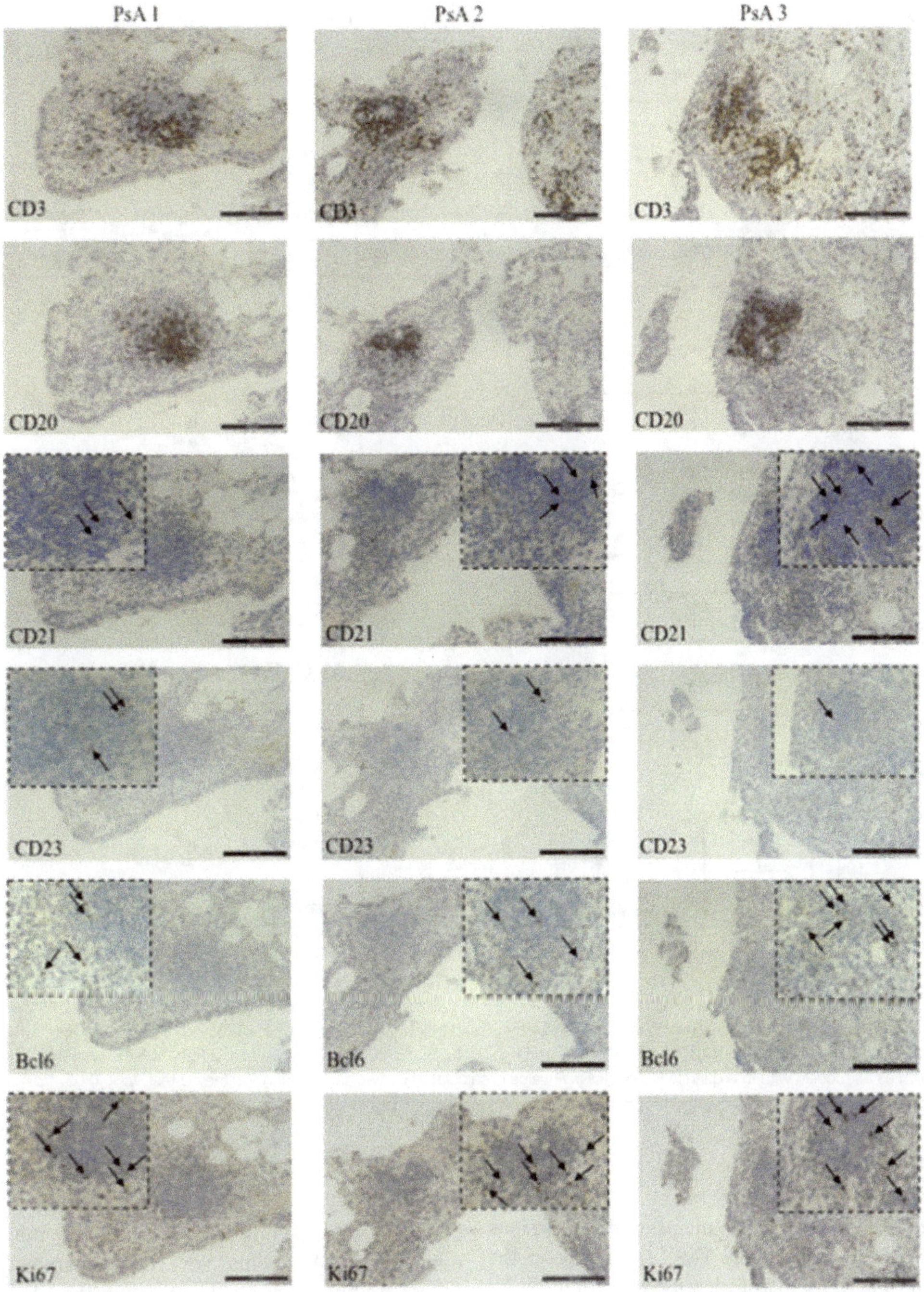

FIGURE 6 | Germinal Center-like structures in synovial tissues of PsA patients. IHC for CD3, CD20, CD21, CD23, Bcl6, and Ki67 (all DAB, brown) of synovial tissue from three early, naive to DMARDs treatment PsA patients (original magnification, 20x). The black arrows indicate a positive staining for CD21, CD23, Ki67, and Bcl6. The dotted black line indicates the insert of the corresponding picture at 40x magnification.

stained PsA and OA ST with a specific surrogate marker of local IFN-I production, the protein MxA (39, 40). MxA staining was extensively found in all PsA ST analyzed (**Figure 11B**), but not in OA ST. MxA staining was distributed either on neutrophils or other unidentified cell types. Although MxA was in part distributed in the vicinity of LL37, the levels of SF IFNα did not correlate with LL37 or anti-LL37 antibodies, with disease activity and/or clinical inflammation markers.

Altogether these findings suggest IFN-I pathways are activated in PsA synovia, and, since ST analyzed by confocal microscopy belong to early diagnosed PsA, an IFN-I signature can represent an early event in disease onset.

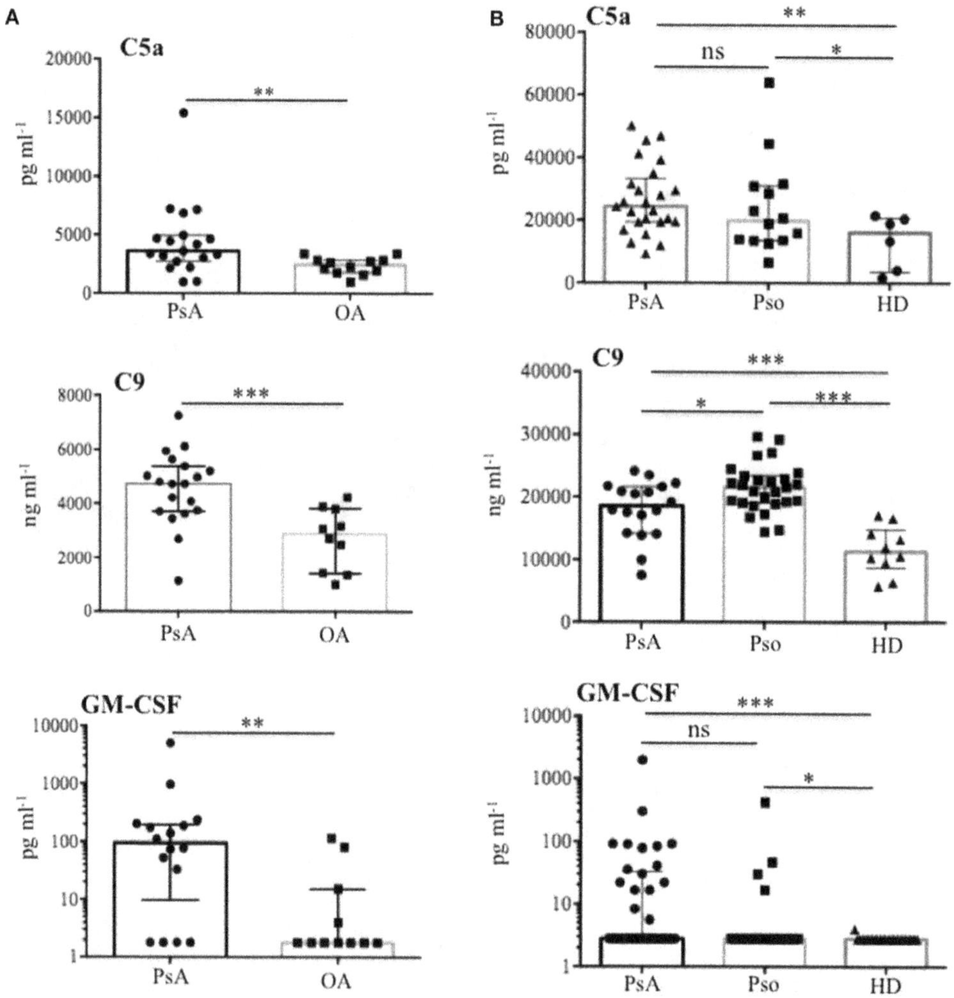

FIGURE 7 | Complement C5a, C9, and GM-CSF in SF and plasma of PsA and Pso patients. **(A)** Content of C5a ($N = 19$), C9 ($N = 19$), and GM-CSF ($N = 21$) were measured by ELISA in SF of PsA and OA ($N = 12$). P-value is calculated by two-tailed Mann-Whitney U test, $^*p < 0.05$, $^{**}p < 0.01$, $^{***}p < 0.0001$. **(B)** Plasma levels of C5a in PsA ($N = 25$) and Pso (without PsA, $N = 14$), PsA C9 ($N = 18$), and Pso ($N = 25$), PsA GM-CSF ($N = 25$) and Pso ($N = 16$) were assessed by ELISA. All data in **(A)** and **(B)** are shown as as median with Interquartile Range (IQR). P-value is calculated by two-tailed Mann-Whitney U test, $^*p < 0.05$, $^{**}p < 0.01$, $^{***}p < 0.001$.

DISCUSSION

PsA develops in 20–30% of psoriasis patients, and skin lesions of psoriasis develop 5–10 years before PsA (41). However the mechanisms linking psoriasis to the development of PsA are still elusive. More generally, no reliable serological markers are available for PsA diagnosis as compared to RA, and PsA pathogenesis is not elucidated.

Results of this study suggest novel factors, some of which are also implicated in psoriasis pathogenesis (13, 15, 36), included the antimicrobial peptide LL37, that seem at work in the pathogenesis of PsA and are potential biomarkers of inflammation/disease status. First of all, we found that LL37 is highly up regulated in SF of PsA patients as compared to control OA. A previous study showed the presence of mRNA for LL37 in inflamed synovial membranes, however analysis of the protein on PsA synovial tissues and fluids were not addressed (42). We found that LL37 is abundantly expressed in PsA ST by confocal microscopy. Since the ST included in the present study belong to very early (<8 months from disease diagnosis) PsA patients, naïve to any pharmacological treatment, these findings indicate an early up regulation of LL37 in PsA ST. Second, we show for the first time that LL37 becomes the target of autoantibodies, representing a novel autoantigen in PsA which sustains the idea of PsA as an autoimmune disease (9). Of note, these anti-LL37 antibodies have been found in synovia and plasma of patients with a very early disease (disease duration between 3 and 10 months) suggesting the development of autoimmunity as an early event. Noteworthy, the patient cohort analyzed in this study includes mainly early PsA patients, in that the mean of disease duration is 11 months. Most intriguing, the presence of autoantibodies to native LL37 in SF well correlates with several inflammatory makers (CRP, ESR, swollen joints count) and disease activity (DAS44) in the

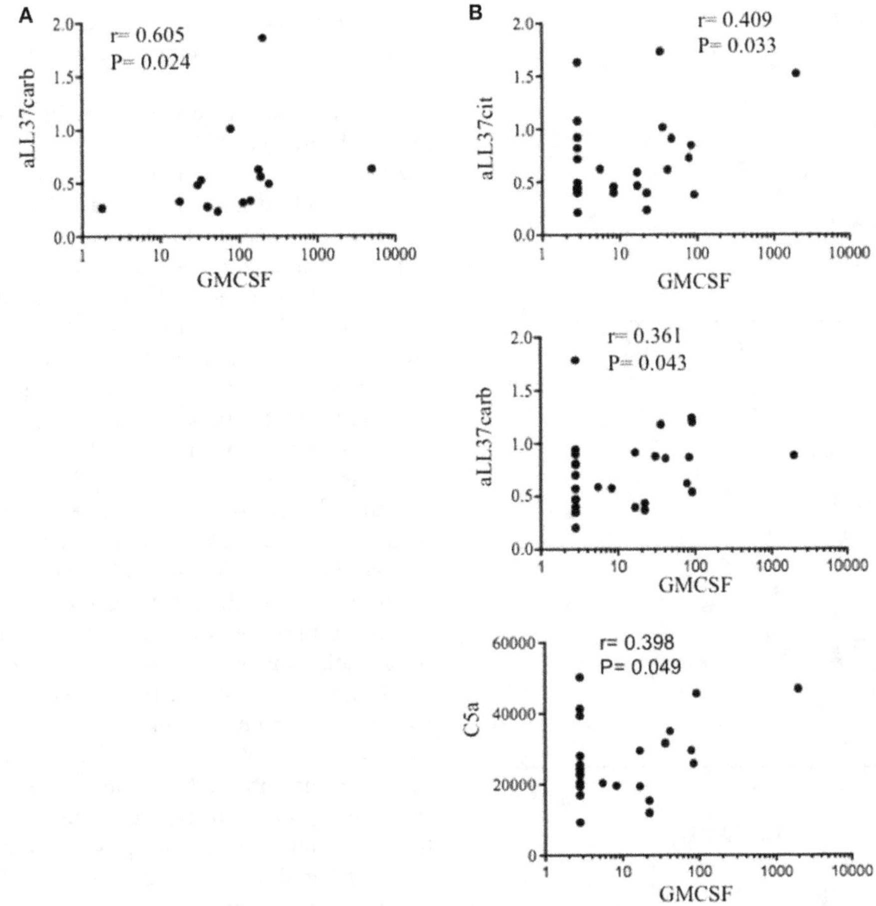

FIGURE 8 | GM-CSF correlates with complement and anti-LL37 antibodies in PsA. **(A)** Spearman correlation analysis was performed between levels of GM-CSF and anti-LL37carb in SF PsA ($N = 17$). **(B)** Spearman correlation analysis between GM-CSF and C5a, anti-LL37cit, and anti-LL37carb in plasma of PsA patients ($N = 23$).

patients analyzed, suggesting a pathogenic role of anti-LL37 antibodies in PsA. These observations fit with the detection of extra-nodal germinal centers (GC)-like structures in PsA ST, which shows that these lymphoid ectopic structures are present in early and naïve ST of PsA. This suggests that the production of autoantibodies occurring at early stages may start as a local phenomenon. Indeed, we visualized for the first time the presence of rare FDC (CD21^{+} and CD23^{+} cells) together with evidences of cell proliferation (Ki67^{+} cells) and markers of both GC B cells and follicular T helper cells (Bcl6^{+} cells), which suggests that these ectopic lymphoid aggregates can be functional in early PsA. Extranodal lymphoid structures have been identified in other autoimmune or chronic inflammatory diseases such as RA, Sjogren's syndrome, autoimmune thyroid disease, multiple sclerosis or chronic infections (32, 43–45). In these structures lymphocytes are organized and aggregated to form B cell follicles and T cell areas. The functional activity of GC is dependent on the presence of a network of FDC, which retain antigens on their membranes in the form of IC leading to B cell maturation (46). In addition, we show that early synovia also present tissue IgG-IC deposition. Interestingly, IgG staining by confocal microscopy shows co-localization with LL37 in tissue infiltrating neutrophils. These findings suggest an important role of neutrophils as a source of local autoantigens in PsA and may indicate these cells as the target of autoantibody aggression. Neutrophils deliver the content of their granules by degranulation and/or NETosis, phenomena favored by C5a and/or GM-CSF (47, 48) stimulation. Our data show the abundant presence of these factors in SF and also in circulation of PsA patients. Thus C5a and GM-CSF can initiate PsA pathogenesis by attracting and activating neutrophils to deliver their factors by degranulation or in the form of NET (37, 49). NET release of LL37 has been described in SLE where anti-LL37 antibodies are indeed generated (12). Neutrophils have been indicated as a source of autoantigens also in RA (50, 51). The suggestion that C5a and GM-CSF play a role in pathogenic pathways that ultimately lead to autoimmunity via neutrophil activation is supported by the fact that GM-CSF levels in the synovial compartments correlate with autoantibody reactivity. This correlation has been found, in particular, with the presence of anti-LL37 antibodies that react to the post-translational modified versions of LL37 (LL37cit and LL37carb),

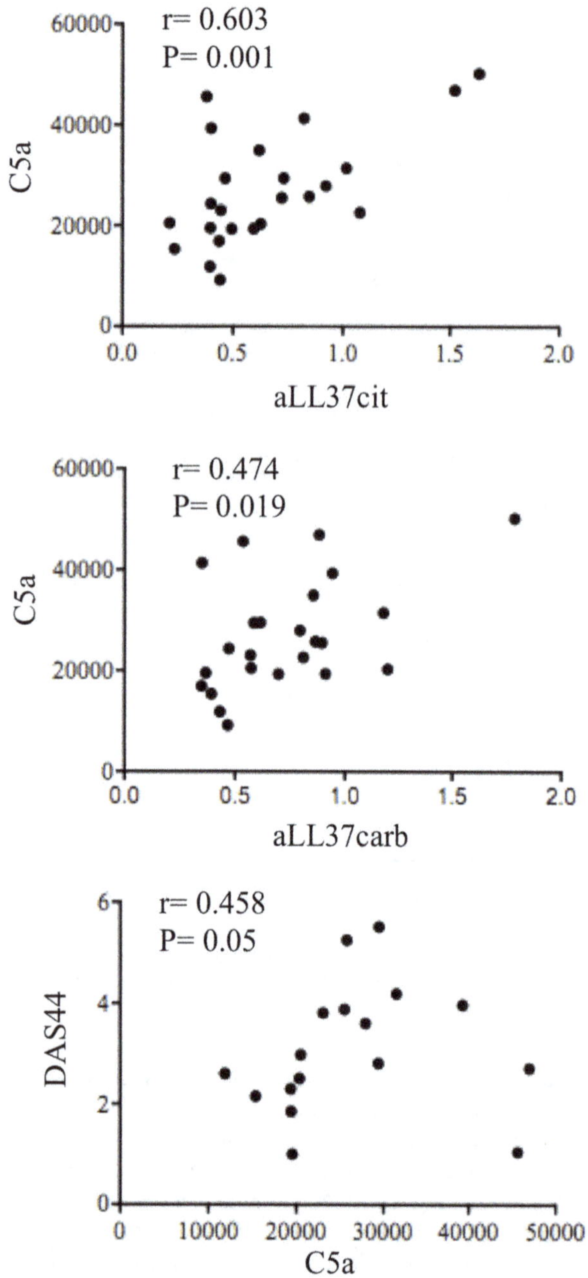

FIGURE 9 | Circulating C5a correlates with anti-LL37 antibodies and disease activity. Spearman correlation analysis was performed between levels of C5a with anti-LL37cit ($N = 24$), anti-LL37carb ($N = 24$) and DAS44 in plasma of PsA ($N = 17$).

whereas a good correlation has been also found between anti-native LL37 antibodies and inflammatory parameters in SF. The reason for this discrepancy is unclear at present, and we are not able to explain it completely. However, it is possible that the determination of reactivity to the native or modified LL37 forms may depend on the specific affinity of the tested autoantibodies, as well from the LL37 preparations used in the assay. Crucial can be their degree of citrullination or carbamylation that is high (see Methods) and may not exactly reflect degree of such modifications *in vivo*. Indeed, LL37 carbamylation and citrullination have been observed *in vitro* and not *in vivo* so far (20, 21).

However, the detected reactivity to both citrullinated and carbamylated LL37 is intriguing and deserves further investigation to understand whether reactivity to the modified LL37 is really distinct from reactivity to the native peptide and the site where this autoreactivity is firstly generated. An important finding is that anti-LL37 antibodies were below the detection limit in PsA circulation, whereas antibodies to modified LL37 were consistent, which is difficult to explain. However, the observation that a percentage of PsA patients respond to carbamylated LL37 and, most importantly, that the magnitude of the antibody reactivity significantly correlates with disease activity (DAS44), suggests to use this immunological parameter as a disease marker in PsA, distinct from psoriasis. Indeed, although also psoriasis patients show antibody reactivity to LL37carb, psoriasis activity index (PASI) did not correlate with this type of antibodies, and levels of anti-LL37carb in psoriasis is significantly lower than that observed in PsA plasma. Our data also support previous findings that PsA patients have high levels of circulating antibodies recognizing carbamylated proteins (9).

The importance of post-translational modification of LL37 in PsA in breaking immunological tolerance to native LL37 is not clarified by our data. However, the fact that antibody reactivity against an autoantigen that is the substrate of both citrullination and carbamylation (20, 21) is induced, reinforces the assumption that neutrophils are crucial player. Indeed, we found strong neutrophil infiltrate in ST of PsA, with abundant presence of MPO, whose activity is strictly connected to production of cyanate (52), which, in turn, favors carbamylation of self-proteins during neutrophilic inflammation. Citrullination is another self-protein modification classically ascribed to neutrophils activity, namely NETosis (50). Although it is matter of debate whether citrullination always occur during NETosis, it is also possible to hypothesize that hypercitrullination phenomena may occur due to MAC activation (38). In this regards, our data show a high presence of activated complement in PsA and C9 detection in tissues. Thus, out data suggest that anti-neutrophil cytoplasmic (ANCA)-like antibodies, such as anti-native LL37, can deposit in ST early during the disease course, where they target neutrophils and activate complement: we assume that abundant neutrophil proteins are released and undergo citrullination and/or carbamylation. This phenomenon activates specific autoantibodies, included anti-LL37 antibodies reacting to the modified antigen, which amplifies a pathogenic pernicious loop. The action of LL37 antibodies can also favor the activation of an IFN-I signature in tissues via TLR7/8/9, as shown in SLE (12), given the binding capacity of LL37 for self-nucleic acids. Cells other than pDCs can also contribute the IFN-I signature observed in PsA synovial, via this mechanism. Moreover, some kind of NETosis (included live NETosis; 37, 39) is likely to occur in PsA (our unpublished observations) as in RA (38), and this may also explain the IFN-signature that we have observed (MxA staining in synovial tissues). Levels of IFNα were also elevated in some PsA SF, although IFNα did not correlate with

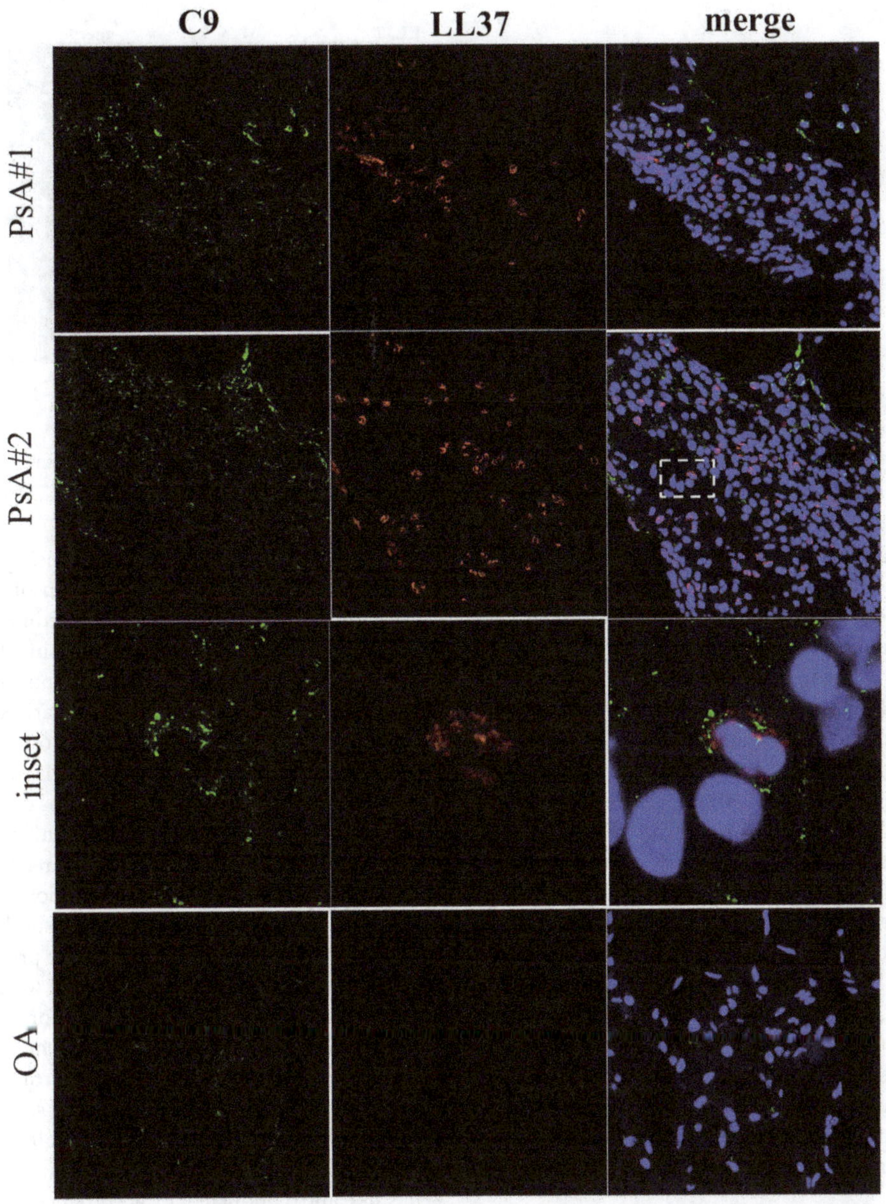

FIGURE 10 | C9 staining in synovial tissues of PsA. Confocal microscopy images of synovial tissues of two PsA and one OA patients stained for LL37 (red) and C9 (green) (original magnification, 63x). The dotted white line in PsA#2 indicates the inset of the corresponding picture of the lower panel. Data are representative of 7 PsA patients and 4 OA subjects.

autoantibodies or disease activity. However, this finding lead us to speculate that, in PsA, IFN-I and NET may directly favor the generation of autoantibodies, at least in memory B cells (16).

Finally, our data showing the presence of complement component C9 in ST and peripheral blood of PsA patients are intriguing, since levels of C9, especially in SF, strongly correlate with all disease parameters (clinically relevant inflammatory parameters and disease activity, as DAS44). Thus, these data lend support to the hypothesis that complement activation is an important player in PsA, and its targeting may be beneficial (53).

In conclusion, the data of the present study shed light on possible new players/mechanisms in PsA pathogenesis (LL37, anti-LL37 antibodies, NETosis, self-protein modifications) while reinforcing involvement of previously suspect players (activated complement, carbamylation, GM-CSF) in the disease. We report that, (i) LL37 behaves as a novel B cell autoantigen in PsA, also in its modified form (LL37cit and LL37carb), (ii) pathways of protein carbamylation and citrullination are likely activated in PsA, (iii) degranulating/netting neutrophils are players in the release of the autoantigens (for instance LL37), under the effect of inflammatory factors, such as GM-CSF and C5a. IgG-immune

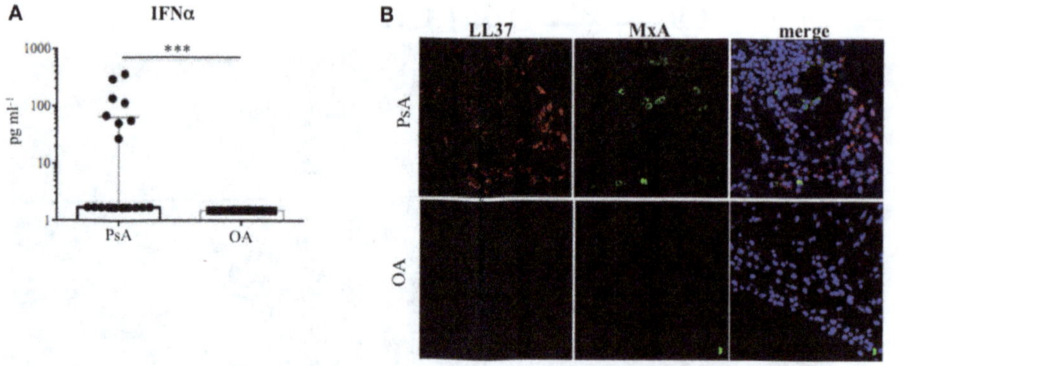

FIGURE 11 | Type I IFN in the synovial compartment of PsA. **(A)** IFNa was measured by ELISA in SF of PsA ($N = 20$) and OA ($N = 12$) subjects. Data are shown as median with Interquartile Range (IQR). *P*-value is calculated by two-tailed Mann-Whitney U test ***$p < 0.001$. **(B)** Confocal microscopy images of synovial tissues of one PsA and one OA patient stained for LL37 (red) and MxA (green) (original magnification, 63x). Data are representative of 7 PsA patients and 4 OA subjects.

complexes formation and their deposition in PsA ST can fuel this vicious circle and also induce an IFN-I signature (12). Since we have shown through our study that some of the characteristics found in PsA are present also in psoriasis patients without PsA (circulating complement, anti-LL37carb antibodies, GM-CSF), longitudinal follow-up of psoriasis patients with antibody reactivity to LL37 and higher complement and GM-CSF levels may be highly informative about the evolution of psoriasis into a more systemic inflammation that eventually develop to PsA. This may allow the identification of prognostic biomarkers for PsA development in psoriasis patients. Finally, almost all patients with PsA have psoriasis and we have shown that LL37 is a CD4 and CD8 T cell autoantigen in at least 46% of psoriasis patients (15). LL37-specific-T cells and their Th1/Th17 secretion pattern correlate with PASI (15). Approximately, the same percentage of PsA patients show CD4 and CD8 T cells proliferating to LL37, which is reasonable (our unpublished data). Whether these PsA T cells exhibit a different phenotype (cytokines secreted, homing receptors and/or T-helper cells markers) that may explain the development of PsA in psoriasis-affected patients in comparison to psoriasis-only patients is under investigation.

MATERIALS AND METHODS

Study Population

The study included thirty-two Caucasian patients 18 years old or older, rheumatoid factor and ACPA negative, affected by PsA according to the CASPAR classification criteria for Psoriatic Arthritis, and recruited from the Rheumatology Unit of the University of Rome Tor Vergata, Sapienza University of Rome, and the Institute of Rheumatology of Fondazione Policlinico Universitario A. Gemelli IRCCS - Catholic University of the Sacred Hearth of Rome.

Patients were treated with csDMARDs (conventional synthetic Disease-Modifying Anti-Rheumatic drugs) in 43% (14/32) and with bDMARDs (biological-DMARDs) in 12% (4/32). Joint disease activity was measured with the number of tender and swollen joint, the pain-VAS (visual analogue scale) and the GH (global health) and by using the Disease Activity Score 44 (DAS44) with the evaluation of the CRP (C-Reactive Protein) and of the erythrocyte sedimentation rate (ESR). Skin disease activity was assessed using PASI (Psoriasis Area Severity Index). Clinical and demographic data of PsA, Pso, and osteoarthritis (OA) subjects are summarized in **Table 1**. Chronic plaque psoriasis diagnosis was based on a confirmed diagnosis for at least 6 months before. Criteria of exclusion: pustular, erythrodermic, and/or arthritis form of psoriasis; history of drug-induced psoriasis; clinically significant flare of psoriasis during 12 weeks prior; concurrent or recent use of any biologic or systemic therapy; received non-biologic systemic psoriasis therapy or phototherapy (including psoralen and ultraviolet A, PUVA), ultraviolet B (UVB) within the previous 4 weeks; or had topical treatment within the previous 2 weeks prior.

Age- and sex-matched healthy donors (HD; $N = 14$) served as normal control (none of them exhibited psoriatic skin or joint symptoms) and were obtained from Blood Center of the Policlinico Umberto I, Roma. Age- and sex-matched OA patients ($N = 12$) served as disease control (**Table 1**).

The study was carried out according to the Declaration of Helsinki and conducted in accordance with the International Conference on Harmonisation Good Clinical Practice Guidelines. The study protocols were approved by ethic committee of the University of Rome Tor Vergata, Catholic University of the Sacred Hearth of Rome and Sapienza University of Rome. All patients provided written informed consent before participating in any study-related activities.

Reagents and Carbamylation

LL37 peptide was purchased from Proteogenix (F); citrullinated-LL37 (LL37cit), citrullinated at all five arginin position, was from Anawa. Carbamylation of LL37 (LL37carb) was obtained by incubating LL37 with 1M potassium cyanate (Sigma Aldrich) at 4°C for 3 days, followed by extensive dialysis against PBS as described (54). To verify the carbamylation reaction, a dot-blot assay was performed. Briefly, LL37carb were spotted onto a nitrocellulose membrane (GE Healthcare Life Sciences). After

TABLE 1 | Data are expressed as mean ± standard deviation unless otherwise specified; range of possible values are indicated in square brackets.

Demographic and clinical data	PsA patients (n = 32)	PsO patients (n = 24)	OA patients (n = 12)
Male sex (N/%)	19 (59)	11 (13)	7 (58)
Age (years)	54.3 ± 11.9	51.1 ± 12.1	45.7 ± 15.7
Pso (N/%)	22 (69)		
PsA disease duration (months)	11 ± 5	0 (0)	
Pso disease duration (months)	20 ± 10	15.3 ± 10	
ESR (mm/h)	16.6 ± 10,1		
CRP (mg/dl)	1.6 ± 2.2	2.2 ± 2.6	
N. of tender joints	7.2 ± 9.1		
N. of swollen joints	5.4 ± 3.7		
Pain VAS	4.75 ± 6.69		
GH	4.6± 2.3		
DAS44	2.41 ± 16.1		
PASI	3.4 ± 2.1	14.6 ± 7.2	
ACPA positivity	0 (0)		
IgM/IgA-RF positivity	0 (0)		
csDMARDs (N/%)	14 (43)	22 (91.6)	
bDMARDs (N/%)	4 (12)	15 (62.5)	

PsA, Psoriatic Arthritis; Pso, Psoriasis; OA, Osteoarthritis; DAS44, Disease Activity Score 44; ESR, erythrocyte sedimentation rate; CRP, C-reactive protein; ACPA, Anti-Citrullinated Peptide Antibodies; RF, Rheumatoid Factor; VAS, visual analoghe scale; GH, global health; csDMARDs, conventional synthetic Disease-modifying antirheumatic drugs; bDMARDs, biological Disease-modifying antirheumatic drugs.

blocking in PBS containing 0.05% Tween 20 (PBS Tween) and 5% non-fat dry milk, the membrane was incubated with a polyclonal anti-carbamyl-lysine antibody (Cell Biolabs, Inc., San Diego, CA, USA) and anti-LL37, O/N at 4°C. The next day, after washings with PBS Tween, peroxidase-conjugated goat anti-rabbit IgG (BioRad Laboratories, Richmond, CA, USA) were used as second antibodies and the reactions were developed with 3-3′ diaminobenzidine (Sigma Aldrich).

Antibodies against LL37, (Mab137), was provided by the Antibody Facility of University of Geneva (CMU; CH). Rabbit polyclonal anti-LL37 was from Innovagen. Both were used for immunofluorescence staining in parallel with appropriate control antibodies.

Human Samples

Synovial fluids (SF) were collected from active knee PsA and age- and sex-matched patients with knee osteoarthritis (OA). Exclusion criteria for SF analysis were local intra-articular corticosteroid injection within 5 weeks before SF aspiration. SF was collected via joint aspiration in association with therapeutic arthrocentesis. Approximately 2–4 ml of SF was collected in sodium heparin-coated Vacutainer^{TM} tubes (Becton-Dickinson); samples contaminated with blood were discarded. Immediately after collection, samples were centrifuged at 1,000g for 15 min at 4°C, and the resulting supernatants were stored at −80°C. Plasma from PsA, psoriasis and HD subjects were collected following standard protocol and stored at −80°C. Synovial tissues were collected from Consecutive patients fulfilling the classification criteria for Psoriatic Arthritis [PsA; (55)] undergoing ultrasound guided synovial minimally invasive tissue biopsy following the published protocol using a 14G needle (Precisa 1410-HS Hospital Service Spa, Italy) (56). Once collected ST specimens were fixed in 10% neutral-buffered formalin and embedded in paraffin for Immunohistochemistry (IHC) or immunofluorescence staining.

Immunohistochemistry (IHC)

Synovial tissue (ST) sections were stained with IgG1 mouse anti-human monoclonal antibody for CD20 (clone L26; at 1.2 μg/ml) or IgG1 mouse anti-human monoclonal antibody for CD3 (clone LN 10; at 1.0 μg/ml) or IgG2a mouse anti-human monoclonal antibody for CD21 (clone 2G9; at 0.34 μg/ml), IgG1 mouse anti-human monoclonal antibody for CD23 (clone 1B12; at 1 μg/ml), IgG1 mouse anti-human monoclonal antibody for Ki67 (clone K2; at 1.2 μg/ml), or IgG2b mouse anti-human monoclonal antibody for Bcl6 (clone LN22; at 1 μg/ml) (all from Leica Biosystem, Newcastle, UK) by immunostainer BOND MAX III (Leica, Newcastle, UK). IHC for CD20, CD3, CD21, CD23, Ki67, and Bcl6 was performed as follows: 3-μm-thick sections were prepared from formalin-fixed paraffin-embedded tissue blocks and were dried in a 60°C oven for 30 min. The sections were placed in a Bond Max Automated Immunohistochemistry Vision Biosystem (Leica Microsystems GmbH, Wetzlar, Germany) according to the following protocol: firstly, tissues were deparaffinized and pre-treated with the Epitope Retrieval Solution 1 (CITRATE buffer) or Solution 2 (EDTA-buffer) at 98°C for 10 min according to the manufacturer's instructions. After washing, peroxidase blocking was carried out for 10 min using the Bond Polymer Refine Detection Kit DC9800 (Leica Microsystems GmbH). Tissues were again washed and then incubated with the primary antibody for 30 min. Subsequently, tissues were incubated with polymer for 10 min and developed with DAB-Chromogen and finally counterstained with hematoxylin (57).

Confocal Microscopy

Three-μm-thick sections in paraffin of human PsA and OA synovia were stained after deparaffination in xilene (5 min, two times), followed by passages in: absolute ethanol (3 min), 95% ethanol in water (3 min), 80% ethanol in water (3 min), 70% ethanol in water, and antigen retrival (5 min at 95°C in 10 mM sodium citrate, pH 6.0). Slides were saturated with blocking buffer (PBS, 0.05% tween 20, 4% BSA) for 1 hour at room temperature. Specimens were stained with a polyclonal rabbit anti-LL37 (Innovagen), rabbit anti-MPO (Abcam), mouse anti-MxA (Novus Bio), monoclonal mouse anti-LL37 (Mab137), polyclonal rabbit anti-human C9 (ATLAS). The following antibodies were used: donkey anti-rabbit IgG AlexaFluor-568 or-647, anti-mouse AlexaFluor-647 and an anti-goat AlexaFluor-488 (Abcam). After washing, slides were mounted in Prolong Gold anti-fade media containing a DNA dye (DAPI) (Molecular Probes). CLSM observations were performed with a Leica

TCS SP2 AOBS apparatus, using a 63x/1.40 NA oil objective. Acquisition of images was performed by a Leica confocal software 2.6 (Leica, Germany).

ELISA

Anti-LL37 antibodies against LL37, LL37cit and LL37carb, were measured by ELISA as previously described (12). Briefly, 96-well flat-bottom plates are coated with 2 μg ml^{-1} of LL37, citrullinated-LL37 or carbamylated-LL37 in carbonate buffer (0.1M $NaHCO_3$, pH 9.6) overnight and washed five times with 0.1% Tween-20 in PBS. This washing buffer was used for washing at all steps. The blocking buffer containing 4% Bovine serum albumin (BSA, Sigma) in PBS was used for at least 1 h (or overnight) to saturate unspecific binding sites. After washing, plasma were diluted 1:100 in PBS 4% BSA followed by 1 hour incubation with a horseradish peroxidase—conjugated goat anti-human IgG (Sigma-Aldrich) diluted 1:5,000 in PBS. Synovial fluids were diluted 1:20. The color was developed with 3,3′, 5,5′-tetramethylbenzidine (TMB) substrate (Sigma-Aldrich). The reaction was stopped by adding 50 μl of 2N H_2SO_4 and absorbance determined at 450 nm with a reference wavelength of 540 nm. The cut-off (for both LL37 and related antibodies) was identified by calculating the mean of controls (HD or OA) and by adding 2 standard deviations of the mean: cut-off = mean (HD or OA)+2SD.

To detect IFNα and GM-CSF, plasma and SF were diluted 1:5 and measured by ELISA from MabTech, accordingly to the manufacturer protocol. Plasma and SF content of complement C5a was measured by ELISA from MyBioSource (USA) according to the manufacturer protocol. C9 in plasma and SF was measured by ELISA from Biomatik (USA) according to the manufacturer protocol. LL37 levels of plasma and SF were measured by the Human antibacterial peptide LL37 ELISA Kit (Cusabio, China).

Statistical Analysis

Data were expressed as medians with Interquartile Range (IQR). Differences between median values were determined by two-tailed Mann-Whitney U test ($*p < 0.05$; $**p < 0.01$; $***p < 0.001$). Correlation analyses were performed by Spearman rank-correlation test. The cut-off value was determined by using the mean + 2SD (Standard Deviation) of the control subjects (HD or OA). Statistical analysis was performed by using GraphPad Prism software version 6 (San Diego, CA, USA).

AUTHOR CONTRIBUTIONS

LF conceived the research with RL, directed and supervised the research with the RL, performed staining of tissue biopsies for confocal microscopy, analyzed and interpreted the data, performed statistical analyses, wrote the manuscript. RaP performed most ELISA experiments and helped with statistical analysis. MC, GF, RoP delivered the clinical ethical and patient-related aspect of the project and provided clinical samples (plasma and SF). SA, BT, LP, EG delivered the clinical ethical and patient-related aspect of the project and obtained clinical samples (plasma, SF and ST biopsies). LaB, AE performed immunohistochemistry on ST. EB, AG, LuB, BM delivered the clinical ethical and patient-related aspect of the project and obtained clinical samples of psoriasis patients and patients' data (plasma). SEA provided patients samples and clinical data, performed ELISA. FS acquired and analyzed most confocal microscopy images. MF acquired some confocal images. IP processed blood samples of HD and patients. FRS, CA, FC, GV delivered the clinical ethical and patient-related aspect of the project and obtained clinical samples and patients data (plasma, SF). TC performed protein carbamylation. AC delivered the clinical ethical and patient-related aspect of the project and obtained clinical samples of psoriasis patients and clinical data (plasma). RL conceived the research with LF, directed and supervised the research with the LF, performed analysis of confocal microscopy, performed ELISA, analyzed and interpreted the data, performed statistical analyses, wrote the manuscript.

ACKNOWLEDGMENTS

This work was supported by a Fondazione Roma research grant (NCDS-2013-00000318) to RL, AC, LF (Italy) and, in part, by the Carlos et Elsie De Reuter Foundation 2015-2016 (CH) to LF and Ernst and Lucie Schmidheiny Foundation 2015-2016 (CH) to LF.

REFERENCES

1. Nestle FO, Kaplan DH, Barker J. Psoriasis. *N Engl J Med.* (2009) 361:496–509. doi: 10.1056/NEJMra0804595
2. Ritchlin CT, Colbert RA, Gladman D. Psoriatic Arthritis. *N Engl J Med.* (2017) 376:957–70. doi: 10.1056/NEJMra1505557
3. Lubrano E, Cantini F, Costanzo A, Girolomoni G, Prignano F, Olivieri I. et al. Measuring psoriatic disease in clinical practice. An expert opinion position paper. *Autoimmun Rev.* (2015) 14:864–74. doi: 10.1016/j.autrev.2015.05.010
4. Cafaro G, McInnes IB. Psoriatic arthritis: tissue-directed inflammation? *Clin Rheumatol.* (2018) 37:859–68. doi: 10.1007/s10067-018-4012-7
5. Conigliaro P, Triggianese P, Perricone C, Chimenti MS, Di Muzio G, Ballanti E, et al. Restoration of peripheral blood natural killer and B cell levels in patients affected by rheumatoid and psoriatic arthritis during etanercept treatment. *Clin Exp Immunol.* (2014) 177:234–43. doi: 10.1111/cei.12335
6. Sakkas LI, Bogdanos DP, Katsiari C, Platsoucas CD. Anto-citrullinated peptides as autoantigens in rheumatoid arthritis-relevance to treatment. *Autoimmun Rev.* (2014) 13:1114–20. doi: 10.1016/j.autrev.2014.08.012
7. Canete JD, Santiago B, Cantaert T, Sanmartì R, Palacin A, Celis R, et al. Ectopic lymphoid neogenesis in psoriatic arthritis. *Ann Rheum Dis.* (2007) 66:720–26. doi: 10.1136/ard.2006.062042
8. Brink M, Verheul MK, Ronnelid J, Berglin E, Holmdahl R, Toes RE, et al. Anti-carbamylated protein antibodies in the pre-symptomatic phase of theumatoid arthritis, their relationship with multiple anti-citrul line peptide antibodies and association with radiological damage. *Arthritis Res Ther.* (2015) 17:25. doi: 10.1186/s13075-015-0536-2
9. Chimenti MS, Triggianese P, Nuccetelli M, Terracciano C, Crisanti A, Guarino MD, et al. Auto-reactions, autoimmunity and psoriatic arthritis. *Autoimmun Rev.* (2015) 14:1142–46. doi: 10.1016/j.autrev.2015.08.003
10. Dorschner RA, Pestonjamasp VK, Tamakuwala S, Ohtake T, Rudisill J, Nizet V, et al. Cutaneous injury induces the release of cathelicidin anti-microbial

peptides active against group A Streptococcus. *J Invest Dermatol.* (2001) 117:91–7. doi: 10.1046/j.1523-1747.2001.01340.x

11. Heliborn JD, Nilsson MF, Kratz G, Weber G, Sorensen O, Borregard N, et al. The cathelicidin anti-microbial peptide LL-37 is involved in re-epithelialization of human skin wounds and is lacking in chronic ulcer epithelium. *J Invest Dermatol.* (2003) 120:379–89. doi: 10.1046/j.1523-1747.2003.12069
12. Lande R, Ganguly D, Facchinetti V, Frasca L, Conrad C, Gregorio J, et al. Neutrophils activate palsmacytoid dendritic cells by releasing self-DNA-peptide complexes in systemic lupus erythematosus. *Sci Transl Med.* (2011) 3:73ra19. doi: 10.1126/scitranslmed.3001180
13. Lande R, Gregorio J, Facchinetti V, Chatterjee B, Wang YH, Homey B, et al. Plasmacytoid dendritic cells sense self-DNA coupled with antimicrobial peptide. *Nature* (2007) 449:564–9. doi: 10.1038/nature06116
14. Ganguly D, Chamilos G, Lande R, Gregorio J, Meller S, Facchinetti V, et al. Self-RNA-antimicrobial peptide complexes activate human dendritic cells through TLR7 and TLR8. *J Exp Med.* (2009) 206:1983–94. doi: 10.1084/jem.20090480
15. Lande R, Botti E, Jandus C, Dojcinovic D, Fanelli G, Conrad C, et al. The antimicrobial peptide LL37 is a T-cell autoantigen in psoriasis. *Nat Commun.* (2014) 5:5621. doi: 10.1038/ncomms6621
16. Gestermann N, Di Domizio J, Lande R, Demaria O, Frasca L, Feldmeyer L, et al. Netting neutrophils activate autoreactive B cells in Lupus. *J Immunol.* (2018) 200:3364–71. doi: 10.4049/jimmunol.1700778
17. Kruithof E, Baeten D, De Rycke L, Vandooren B, Foell D, Roth J, et al. Synovial histopathology of psoriatic arthritis, both oligo- and polyarticular, resembles spondyloarthropathy more than it does rheumatoid arthritis. *Arthritis Res Ther.* (2005) 7:R569–80. doi: 10.1186/ar1698
18. Lin AM, Rubin CJ, Khandpur R, Wang JY, Riblett M, Yalavarthi S, et al. Mast cells and neutrophils release IL-17 through extracellular traps formation in psoriasis. *J Immunol.* (2011) 187:490–500. doi: 10.4049/jimmunol.1100123
19. Biekarre H, Harder J, Cuthbert R, Emery P, Leuschner I, Mrowietz J, et al. Differential expression of antimicrobial peptides in psoriasis and psoriatic arthritis as a novel contributory mechanism for skin and joint disease heterogeneity. *Scand J Rheumatol.* (2016) 45:188–96. doi: 10.3109/03009742.2015.1091497
20. Kilsgard O, Andersson P, Malmsten M, Nordin SL, Linge HM, Eliasson M, et al. Peptidylarginine deiminases present in the airways during tobacco smoking and inflammation can citrullinate the host defense peptide LL-37, resulting in altered activities. *Am J Respir Cell Mol Biol.* (2012) 46:240–8. doi: 10.1165/rcmb.2010-0500OC
21. Koro C, Hellvard A, Delaleu N, Binder V, Scavenius C, Bergum B, et al. Carbamylated LL-37 as a modulator of the immune response. *Innate Immun.* (2016) 22:218–29. doi: 10.1177/1753425916631404
22. Seelen MA, Daha MR. The role of complement in autoimmune renal disease. *Autoimmunity* (2006) 39:411–5. doi: 10.1080/08916930600739688
23. Okroj M, Heinegard D, Holmdahl R, Blom AM. Rheumatoid arthritis and the complement system. *Ann Med.* (2007) 39:517–30. doi: 10.1080/07853890701477546
24. Takemura S, Klimiuk PA, Braun A, Goronzy JJ, Weyand CM. T cell activation in synovium is B cell dependent. *J Immunol.* (2001) 167:4710–8. doi: 10.4049/jimmunol.167.8.4710
25. Randen I, Mellbye OJ, Forre O, Natvig JB. The identification of germinal centres and follicular dendritic cell networks in rheumatoid synovial tissue. *Scand J Immunol.* (1995) 41:481–6. doi: 10.1111/j.1365-3083.1995.tb03596.x
26. Humby F, Bombardieri M, Manzo A, Kelly S, Blades MC, Kirkham B, et al. Ectopic lymphoid structures support ongoing production of class-switched autoantibodies in rheumatoid synovium. *PLoS Med.* (2009) 6:e1. doi: 10.1371/journal.pmed.0060001
27. Kurowska-Stolarska M, Alivernini S, Melchor EG, Elmesmari A, Tolusso B, Tange C, et al. MicroRNA-34a dependent regulation of AXL controls the activation of dendritic cells in inflammatory arthritis. *Nat Commun.* (2017) 22:15877. doi: 10.1038/ncomms15877
28. Okada T, Moriyama S, Kitana M. Differentiation of germinal center B cells and follicular helper T cells as viewed by tracking Bcl6 expression. *Immunol Rev.* (2012) 247:120–32. doi: 10.1111/j.1600-065X.2012.01120.x
29. Johnston RJ, Poholek AC, DiToro D, Yusuf I, Eto D, Barnett B, et al. Bcl6 and Blimp-1 are reciprocal and antagonistic regulators of T follicular helper cell differentiation. *Science* (2009) 325:1006–10. doi: 10.1126/science.1175870
30. Yu D, Rao S, Tsai LM, Lee SK, He Y, Sutcliffe EL, et al. The transcriptional repressor Bcl-6 directs T follicular helper cell lineage commitment. *Immunity* (2009) 31:457–68. doi: 10.1016/j.immunity.2009.07.002
31. Rezk SA, Nathwani BN, Zhao X, Weiss LM. Follicular dendritic cells: origin, function, and different disease-associated patterns. *Hum Pathol.* (2013) 44:937–50. doi: 10.1016/j.humpath.2012.10.005
32. Jonsson MV, Skarstein K. Follicular dendritic cells confirm lymphoid organization in the minor salivary glands of primary Sjogren's syndrome. *J Oral Pathol Med.* (2008) 37:515–21. doi: 10.1111/j.1600-0714.2008.00674.x
33. Jose PJ, Moss IK, Maini RN, Williams TJ. Measurement of the chemotactic complement fragment C5a in rheumatoid synovial fluids by radioimmunoassay: role of C5a in the acute inflammatory phase. *Ann Rheum Dis.* (1990) 49:747–52. doi: 10.1136/ard.49.10.747
34. Trouw LA, Pickering MC, Blom AM. The complement system as a potential therapeutic target in rheumatic disease. *Nat Rev Rheumatol.* (2017) 13:538–47. doi: 10.1038/nrrheum.2017.125
35. Manthey HD, Woodruff TM, Taylor SM, Monk PN. Complement component 5a (C5a). *Int J Biochem Cell Biol.* (2009) 41:2114–7. doi: 10.1016/j.biocel.2009.04.005
36. Sadik CD, Miyabe Y, Sezin T, Luster AD. The critical role of C5a as an initiator of neutrophil-mediated autoimmune inflammation of the joint and skin. *Semin Immunol.* (2018) 37:21–9. doi: 10.1016/j.smim.2018.03.002
37. Stojkov D, Amini P, Oberson K, Sokollik C, Duppenthaler A, Simon HU, et al. ROS and glutathionylation balance cytoskeletal dynamics in neutrophil extracellular trap formation. *J Cell Biol.* (2017) 16:4073–90. doi: 10.1083/jcb.201611168
38. Romero V, Fert-Bober J, Nigrovic PA, Darrah E, Haque UJ, Lee DM, et al. Immune-mediated pore-forming pathways induce cellular hypercitrullination and generate citrullinated autoantigens in rheumatoid arthritis. *Sci Tranls Med.* (2013) 5:209ra150. doi: 10.1126/scitranslmed.3006869
39. Vermi W, Bonecchi R, facchetti F, Bianchi D, Sozzani S, Festa S, et al. Recruitment of immature plasmacytoid dendritic cells (plasmacytoid monocytes) and myeloid dendritic cells in primary cutaneous melanomas. *J Pathol.* (2003) 200:255. doi: 10.1002/path.1344
40. Lande R, Giacomini E, Serafini B, Rosicarelli B, Sebastiani GD, Minisola G, et al. Characterization and recruitment of plasmacytoid dendritic cells in synovial fluids and tissue of patients with chronic inflammatory arthritis. *J Immunol.* (2004) 173:2815–24. doi: 10.4049/jimmunol-173.4.2815
41. Gladman DD, Mease Pj, Krueger G, van der Heidje DM, Antoni C, Helliwell PS, et al. Outcome measures in psoriatic arthritis. *J Rheumatol.* (2005) 32:2262–9.
42. Paulsen F, Pufe T, Conradi L, Varoga D, Tsokos M, Papendieck J, et al. Antimicrobial peptides are expressed and produced in healthy and inflamed synovial membranes. *J Pathol.* (2002) 198:369–77. doi: 10.1002/path.1224
43. Armengol MP, Juan M, Lucas-Martin A, Fernandez-Figuera MT, Jaraquemada D, Gallart T, et al. Thyroid autoimmune disease: demonstration of thyroid antigen-specific B cells and recombination-activating gene expression in chemokine-containing active intrathyroidal germinal centers. *Am J Pathol.* (2001) 159:861–73. doi: 10.1016/S0002-9440(10)61762-2
44. Weyand CM, Goronzy JJ. Ectopic germinal center formation in rheumatoid synovitis. *Ann NY Acad Sci.* (2003) 987:140–9. doi: 10.1111/j.1749-6632.2003.tb06042.x
45. Aloisi F, Pujol-Borrel R. Lymphoid neogenesis in chronic inflammatory diseases. *Nat Rev Immunol.* (2006) 6:205–17. doi: 10.1038/nri1786
46. Park CS, Choi YS. How do follicular dendritic cells interact intimately with B cells in the germinal centre? *Immunology* (2005) 114:2–10. doi: 10.1111/j.1365-2567.2004.02075.x
47. Denk S, Taylor RP, Wiegner R, Cook EM, Lindorfer MA, Pfeiffer K, et al. Complement C5a-induced changes in neutrophil morphology during inflammation. *Scand J Immunol.* (2017) 86:143–55. doi: 10.1111/sji.12580
48. Van Pelt LJ, Huisman MV, Weening RS, von dem Borne AE, Roos D, van Oers RH. A single dose of granulocyte-macrophage colony-stimulating factor induces systemic interleukin-8 and neutrophil activation in healthy volunteers. *Blood* (1996) 87:5305–13.

49. Yousefi S, Mihalache C, Kozlowski E, Schmid I, Simon HU. Viable neutrophil release mitochondrial DNA to form neutrophil extracellular traps. *Cell Death Differ.* (2009) 16:1438–44. doi: 10.1038/cdd.2009.96
50. Khandpur R, Carmona-Rivera C, Vivekanandan-Girl A, Gizinski A, Yalavarthi S, Knight JS, et al. NETs are a source of citrullinated autoantigens and stimulate inflammatory responses in rheumatoid arthritis. *Sci Transl Med.* (2013) 5:178ra40. doi: 10.1126/scitranslmed.3005580
51. Sur Chowdhury C, Giaglis S, Walker UA, Buser A, Hahn S, Hasler P. Enhanced neutrophil extracellular trap generation in rheumatoid arthritis: analysis of underlying signal transduction pathways and potential diagnostic utility. *Arthritis Res Ther.* (2014) 13:R122. doi: 10.1186/ar4579
52. Delanghe S, Delanghe JR, Speeckaert R, Van Biesen W, Speeckaert MM. Mechanism and consequences of carbamoylation. *Nat Rev Nephrol.* (2017) 13:580–93. doi: 10.1038/nrneph.2017.103
53. Woodruff TM, Nandakumarb KS, Tedesco F. Inhibiting the C5–C5a receptor axis. *Mol Immunol.* (2011) 48:1631–42. doi: 10.1016/j.molimm.2011.04.014
54. Shi J, Knevel R, Suwannalai P, van der Linden MP, Janssen GM, van Veelen PA, et al. Autoantibodies recognizing carbamylated proteins are present in sera of patients with rheumatoid arthritis and predict joint damage. *Proc Natl Acad Sci USA.* (2011) 108:17327–7. doi: 10.1073/pnas.1114465108
55. Taylor W, Gladman D, Helliwell P, Marchesoni A, Mease P, Mielants H. Classification criteria for psoriatic arthritis. Development of new criteria from a large international study. *Arthritis Rheumatol.* (2006) 54:2665–73. doi: 10.1002/art.21972
56. Van de Sande MG, Gerlag DM, Lodde BM, van Baarsen LG, et al. Evaluating anti-rheumatic treatments using synovial biopsy: a recommendation for standardisation to be used in clinical trials. *Ann Rheum Dis.* (2011) 70:423–27. doi: 10.1136/ard.2010.139550
57. Alivernini S, Tolusso B, Petricca L, Bui L, Di Sante G, Peluso G, et al. Synovial features of patients with rheumatoid arthritis and psoriatic arthritis in clinical and ultrasound remission differ under anti-TNF therapy: a clue to interpret different chances of relapse after clinical remission? *Ann Rheum Dis.* (2017) 76:1228–36. doi: 10.1136/annrheumdis-2016-210424

16

Gamma Delta T Cells and their Pathogenic Role in Psoriasis

Cong Qi[1,2], *Yazhuo Wang*[1,2], *Ping Li*[1,2] *and Jingxia Zhao*[1,2*]

[1] *Beijing Hospital of Traditional Chinese Medicine, Capital Medical University, Beijing, China,*
[2] *Beijing Key Laboratory of Clinic and Basic Research with Traditional Chinese Medicine on Psoriasis, Beijing Institute of Traditional Chinese Medicine, Beijing, China*

***Correspondence:**
Jingxia Zhao
zhaojingxia@bjzhongyi.com

γδT cells are an unconventional population of T lymphocytes that play an indispensable role in host defense, immune surveillance, and homeostasis of the immune system. They display unique developmental, distributional, and functional patterns and rapidly respond to various insults and contribute to diverse diseases. Although γδT cells make up only a small portion of the total T cell pool, emerging evidence suggest that aberrantly activated γδT cells may play a role in the pathogenesis of psoriasis. Dermal γδT cells are the major IL-17-producing cells in the skin that respond to IL-23 stimulation. Furthermore, γδT cells exhibit memory-cell-like characteristics that mediate repeated episodes of psoriatic inflammation. This review discusses the differentiation, development, distribution, and biological function of γδT cells and the mechanisms by which they contribute to psoriasis. Potential therapeutic approaches targeting these cells in psoriasis have also been detailed.

Keywords: psoriasis, γδT, IL-17, skin inflammation, biological function

INTRODUCTION

Gamma delta T cells (γδ T cells) are T cells that have a distinctive T-cell receptor (TCR) on their surface. Most T cells are αβ (alpha beta) T cells with TCR composed of two glycoprotein chains called α (alpha) and β (beta) TCR chains. In contrast, gamma delta (γδ) T cells have a TCR that is made up of one γ (gamma) chain and one δ (delta) chain (1). This group of T cells is usually less common than αβ T cells, but significantly enriched in mucosal and epithelial sites, such as the skin and respiratory, digestive, and reproductive tracts. γδT cells are major histocompatibility complex (MHC)-unrestricted innate-like lymphocytes with more unique antigen receptors compared to αβT cells (2). They produce cytokines such as IL-17/IFN-γ/IL-22 (3–5). Although they constitute a small portion of the total T cell pool, γδT cells bridge the innate and adaptive immune system and contribute to various physiological and pathological processes (2). Relative to αβT cells, γδT cells have been less studied and characterized. It is becoming clear that γδT cells are heterogeneous populations of cells with multifunctional capacities in repairing host tissue (6), pathogen clearance (7), tumor surveillance (8, 9), and proinflammatory effects (10).

Psoriasis is a chronic inflammatory skin disease with an autoimmune component and a strong genetic basis. Plaque psoriasis is characterized by well-defined, raised, chronic erythematous plaques with silver patches observed commonly in the elbows, knees, scalp, umbilicus, and lumbar area (11–13). The worldwide reported prevalence of psoriasis ranges from 0.09% to 11.43% and results in a severe economic burden to patients and a significant challenge to public health (14, 15). Multiple comorbidities and other autoimmune disorders have been correlated with psoriasis, which includes arthritis, cardiovascular disease, obesity, diabetes mellitus, and inflammatory bowel disease, indicate common cellular mediators that drive the pathogenesis of these diseases (16). Increasing evidence has demonstrated that aberrantly activated γδT cells may direct the pathogenesis of autoimmune disorders, such as psoriasis (17–19). To understand what they do in psoriasis, it is important to understand their the differentiation, development, distribution, and biological function.

In this review, we expound on the properties of γδT cells and review the effects of γδT cells in psoriasis. We hope that this review provides insights into its pathogenesis, especially in disease recurrence, and sheds light on potentially novel therapies targeting γδ T cell function.

DIFFERENTIATION AND DEVELOPMENT OF γδT CELLS IN THE THYMUS

γδT cells were first discovered and reported 30 years ago during the manufacture of antibodies using the *TCRγ* gene sequence (20). αβT and γδT cell lineages originate from common T precursor cells that lack CD4 and CD8 coreceptors (CD4-CD8-), also known as double-negative (DN) thymocytes. Based on their differential CD44 and CD25 expression, DN cells can be further subdivided into DN1 (CD44+CD25-), DN2 (CD44+CD25+), DN3 (CD44-CD25+), and DN4 (CD44-CD25-) stages, as indicated in **Figure 1**. Clonal assays for determining DNT cell progenitors permit the identification of the branch-point of αβT and γδT cell lineages at the late DN2 to DN3 developmental stages (21, 22). DN3 is the critical selection stage that determines the fate of γδ or αβ cell lineages (22). Rearrangements at the *Tcrd*, *Tcrg*, and *Tcrb* loci are initiated at the DN2 stage, and αβ and γδ lineage divergence occur at the DN3 stage (23, 24). Successful rearrangement of the TCRβ chain is achieved with the assembly of the constant pTα and CD3 subunits to form the pre-TCR complex. Commitment to the αβT cell lineage and differentiation of DN3 cells into DN4 (CD44-CD25-) cells transpires in a ligand-independent manner. This process is termed β-selection and is a checkpoint for the generation of a functional TCRβ chain (25, 26). TCRγ and δ chains rearrange during the DN stages and express γδTCR/CD3 on the plasma membrane. 'γδ selection' is associated with increased extracellular signal-related kinase 1/2(ERK1/2) phosphorylation and early growth response gene (Egr) protein expression. Ectopic expression of Egr proteins promotes the selection of the γδ T cells. Inhibitor of DNA binding 3 (Id3) is an essential target by which Egr proteins regulate αβ/γδ lineages (26–29).

What determines cell fate specification and differentiation from precursors to αβT or γδT lineage? Two models have been proposed, an instructive model and a stochastic model. In the instructive model, pre-TCR or γδ TCR signaling intensities decide the fate of αβT/γδT cell lineage (30). The instructive model is based on several lines of evidence showing that the strong TCR signals are inclined to γδT cells, while the relatively weak TCR signals are inclined to generate abundant αβT lineage cells (27, 31, 32). The stronger signals that promote adoption of the γδ-fate involve activation of the ERK-Egr-Id3 pathway (29, 33). Sang-Yun et al. demonstrated that ERK signaling promotes γδT cell maturation. ERK signaling that promotes γδT cell fate depends not only on conventional substrate targeting through the D-domain but also through an alternate mode of ERK action mediated by its DBP. This induces molecular effectors responsible for the execution of ERK-mediated developmental outcomes post-transcriptionally (34). E proteins are helix-loop-helix transcription factors that bind DNA at E-box motifs (CANNTG). It acts as a downstream focal point for TCR and plays an essential role in thymocyte development (35). Strong TCR signals could selectively restrain αβT cell development by phenocopying E protein insufficiency and increasing ERK activation. This induces early growth response (EGR1, EGR3) transcription factors and targets DNA-binding inhibitors (ID3). ID3 has been shown to interact with and suppress E protein targets (33, 36, 37).

Under stochastic conditions, other signals dominate this differentiation before TCR expression, hence pre-committing cell fate and allowing them to mature further. Increasing evidence has presented that progenitor T cells are heterogeneous in their developmental potential prior to TCR gene rearrangement. Their development potential has been associated with IL-7R expression (pre-T cells) and was independent of TCR-mediated signals (30). High mobility group box transcription factor 13 (Sox13) that modulate Wnt/TCF1 signaling has also been reported to regulate the T cell-fate decision process, while Sox13 expression has been shown to promote γδT cell development and restrain αβT cell development (38, 39). Nevertheless, γδT cell development has been observed in Sox13-deficient mice, suggesting that it is dispensable for γδT cell development. This is contrary to what has been suggested in the stochastic model (38).

DISTRIBUTION OF γδT

Human γδT Cells

Humans γδT cells can be distinguished based on δ chain expression, which includes the Vδ1, Vδ2, and Vδ3 subtypes (40) (**Table 1**). Vδ1 cells are mainly found in the gut epithelium, skin, spleen, and liver, and are involved in maintaining epithelial tissue integrity. They constitute approximately 30% of the γδT cells in the peripheral blood (PB). Typically, the Vδ1 chain is associated with different VγI family members (Vγ2/3/4/5/8/9) (41–43). Vδ1 cells exert their effector function through TCR recognition of stress molecules on epithelial cells. Furthermore, Vδ1 cells express natural killer receptors (NKG2C, NKG2D, NKp30), Toll-like receptors, CD8, and the β-glucan receptor, dectin-1 (44–48). Activated Vδ1T cells release IL-10, IL-2, IL-4, IL-17, IFN-γ, TNF-α, and chemokines (CCL3, CCL4, and CCL5). Vδ1T cells play an essential role in maintaining barrier tissue integrity and establishing antiviral immunity (49–51). Studies have demonstrated that Vδ1 cells are involved in

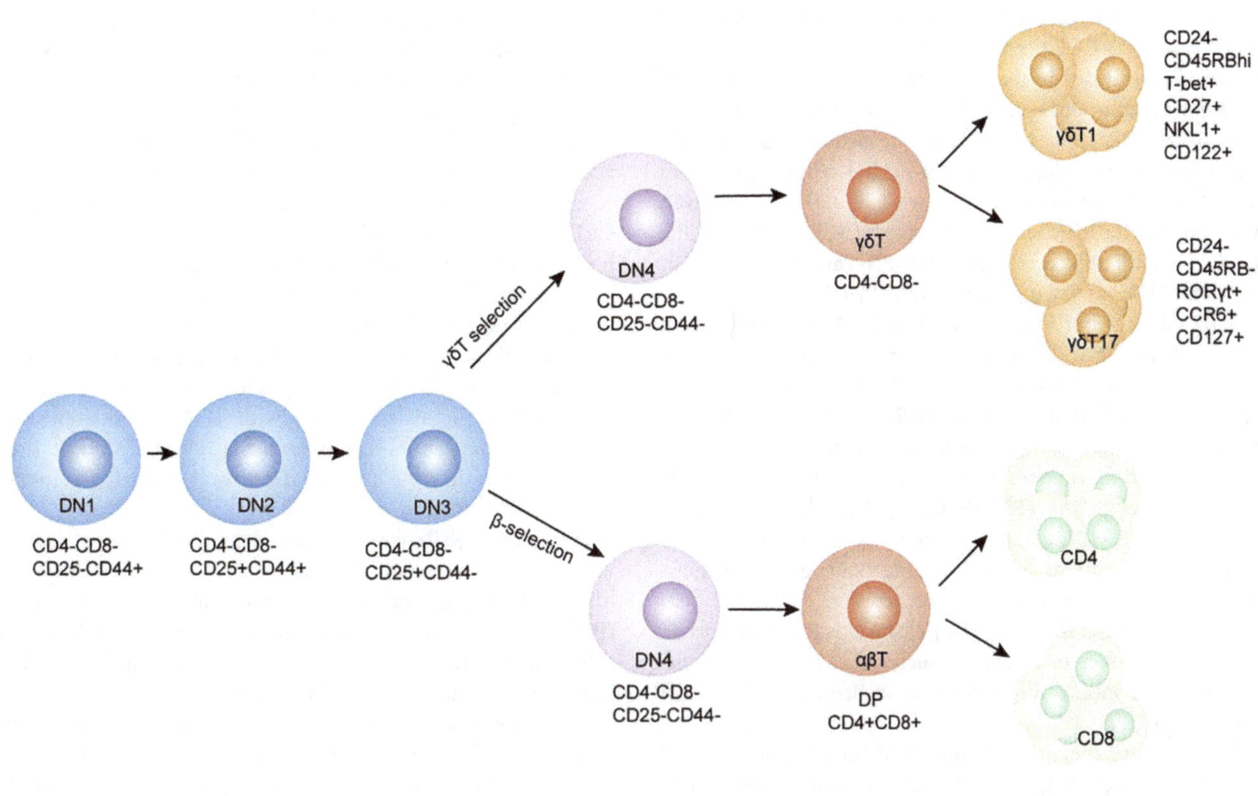

FIGURE 1 | Schematic depicting the development of γδ and αβ T cells in the thymus. γδ and αβ cells develop from the same ancestral DN (CD4-CD8-) cells. Lineage changes in γδ and αβ cells mainly occur at the DN3 stage. Cell surface markers and transcription factors of the cells have been labeled alongside.

several diseases, such as malaria (52, 53), human immune deficiency virus (HIV) (54, 55), cytomegalovirus (CMV) (56), inflammatory bowel disease, and Crohn's disease by exerting their cytotoxic effects and secreting cytokines (57). Notably, activated Vδ1T cells recognize B7-H6 *via* NKp30. B7-H6 is a B7 family member exclusively expressed on tumor cells and is involved in the antitumor effect (58).

Vδ2T cells are primarily distributed in the blood and the lymphoid system and are the main subset found in healthy humans. It accounts for 50%–90% of the γδT cell population in peripheral blood (59). Vδ2T cells are divided into the innate-like (Vγ9+) and adaptive (Vγ9-) subsets, with the majority of Vδ2T cells being Vδ2Vγ9+T cells (60). Vδ2Vγ9+T cells are responsive to cytokines, such as CCR1, CCR2, CCR5, and CXCR6 ligands and IL-12, and produce proinflammatory factors, such as IFN-γ, TNF-α, IL-17, IL-21, and IL-24 (61, 62). Vδ2Vγ9+T cells can be divided into naive γδT (CD45RA+CD27+Vδ2Vγ9+), central memory γδT (TCM, CD45RA-CD27+Vδ2Vγ9), effector memory γδT (TEM, CD45RA-CD27-Vδ2 Vγ9+), and CD45RA+ effector memory γδT (TEMRA, CD45RA+CD27-Vδ2Vγ9+) based on their surface

TABLE 1 | Characteristics of human and murine γδT cell subsets.

	Classify	Common pairs	Tissue resident	Production of cytokines
Human	Vδ1	$V\gamma2^+/3^+/4^+/5^+/8^+/9^+$	gut, skin, liver PB (peripheral blood)	IL-10,IL-2,IL-4,IL-17,IFN-γ, TNF-α
	Vδ2	$V\gamma9^-/9^+$	PB, skin	IFN-γ,TNF-α,IL-17,IL-21,IL-24
	Vδ3	$V\gamma2^+/3^+/4^+$	PB, liver	IL-10,IL-4,IL-17,IFN-γ,TNF-α
Murine	Vγ1	Vγ6.3/6.4	skin, lung, colon, liver, PB	IL-4,IFN-γ
	Vγ2	Vδ4	skin, lung, colon, liver, PB	IL-17
	Vγ3	Vδ1	skin	?
	Vγ4	Vδ4	skin, lung, colon, liver, PB, joint	IL-17,IFN-γ
	Vγ5	Vδ1	skin, liver	IL-17,IFN-γ
	Vγ6	Vδ1	genital tract, togue, lung, colon, skin, adipose tissue	IL-17,IFN-γ,IL-22
	Vγ7	Vδ4/5/6	IEL (Intraepithelial lymphocytes)	IFN-γ

Heilig and Tonegawa nomenclature used for classification.

expression of CD45RA and CD27. Naive γδT cells comprise of the Vδ2Vγ9+T cell subset in the lymph nodes and express CCR7 and CD62L. However, CCR2, CCR5, CCR6, and CXCR3 are only expressed and activated in the presence of high concentrations of isopentenyl pyrophosphate (IPP) but do not produce IFN-γ. CM cells express CCR7 and CD62L and are activated at low IPP concentrations and produce some IFN-γ. TEM cells are present in the blood and inflammatory sites and are CCR7-CD62L-. However, they are positive for the chemokine receptors CCR2, CCR5, CCR6, and CXCR3. TEM cells secrete abundant IFN-γ and tumor necrosis factor-alpha (TNF-a) when activated with IPP+IL-2. TEMRA cells are CCR7-CD62L- but express CCR5 and CXCR3, and have a cytotoxic effect. TEMRA cells also secrete abundant perforin, granulysin, and N-a-benzyloxycarbonyl-L-lysine thiobenzyl ester (BLT)-esterase, but do not produce IFN-γ. In addition, they are terminally differentiated and are no longer able to respond to TCR stimulation, and have poor proliferative ability (63–66). Vδ2 specifically recognizes (E)-4-hydroxy-3-methyl-but-2-enyl pyrophosphate (HMB-PP) and isopentenyl pyrophosphate (IPP) and rapidly respond to exogenous infections or endogenous transformed cells (67, 68). Furthermore, activated Vδ2Vγ9+T cells acquire antigen-presenting cell (APC) characteristics and display a strong ability to secrete cytokines, such as Th1/Th2/Th17-type cytokines. These induce the maturation of dendritic cells (DCs) into APCs (69–71).

Vδ3T cells are the smallest subsets of the peripheral blood lymphocytes, accounting for 0.2% of circulating cells. They express CD56, NKG2D, CD28, HLA-DR, CD161, and T cell activation marker CD69, but not CD25, NKG2A, or NKG2C (72). Vδ3T cells are abundant in the liver and gut and are involved in chronic viral infections and leukemia (73, 74). Expanded Vδ3T cells only recognize CD1d and release Th1, Th2, and Th17 cytokines to induce the maturation of dendritic cells into APCs. They do not recognize CD1a, CD1b, or CD1c (72). Vδ3 T cells and B cells reciprocally regulate the expression of maturation markers, CD40, CD86, and HLA-DR, and promote IgM release by B cells (75).

Interestingly, Vδ4, Vδ6, Vδ7, and Vδ8 T cells have been observed in the PB of lymphoma patients, however, their roles are yet to be deciphered (76).

Murine γδ T Cells

Murine γδT cells can be distinguished based on their γ chain expression. Two nomenclature methods have been commonly reported in the literature, i.e., the Heilig and Tonegawa, and the Garman classification (77, 78). This review uses the Heilig and Tonegawa nomenclature and is used for the Vγ1–Vγ7 subtypes (79) (**Table 1**).

The development of the γδT subsets begins during the fetal period. First are the Vγ5+cells that are produced between embryonic day13 (E13) to approximately E17, followed by Vγ6+ cells from E14 to around birth, and the last are the Vγ1+, Vγ2+, and Vγ4+ cells from E16 onward (25, 80, 81). Vγ5+ cells, also known as dendritic epidermal T cells (DETCs), are involved in innate body barrier defense. The increased expression of sphingosine-1-phosphate receptor 1 (S1P1), E and P selectin ligands, and chemokines CCR10 and CCR4 in mature Vγ5+ cells, and the decreased expression of CCR6, CCR9, CCR7, and CD62L allow the egression of Vγ5+ cells from the thymus to the epidermis (82, 83). In normal healthy skin, DETC secretes IL-15 and IGF-1 to maintain skin homeostasis and promote wound healing (84, 85). After skin trauma, DETCs undergo morphological changes accompanied by the upregulation of the activation marker, CD69. It then releases soluble factors that regulate various aspects of tissue repair (85). DETCs produce CCL3 and CCL4 chemokines that are important for macrophage homing. Furthermore, DETCs promotes macrophage recruitment by regulating hyaluronan production through DETC-derived keratinocyte growth factor (KGF) (86, 87). Vγ5+Vδ1+cells produce IFN-γ by activating the Egr3-mediated pathway while suppressing the γδT cell lineage factor, Sox13, and the RORγt transcription factor associated with IL-17 production (39). However, some studies have shown that DETCs produce IL-17, promote keratinocyte proliferation, and participate in skin inflammation (88).

The second γδT subsets produced are the Vγ6 cells. They pair with the Vδ1 subsets of γδ TCR (Vγ6Jγ1 and Vδ1Dδ2Jδ2) and migrate to the genital tract, tongue, lungs, peritoneal cavity (PEC), dermis, colon, and adipose tissues (89). Vγ6+Vδ1+ γδT cells that produce IL-17 and other effector molecules drive inflammation and tumor cell proliferation (90).

Typically, Vγ1+, Vγ2+, and Vγ4+ cells migrate to the dermis, lungs, colon, liver, and peripheral lymphoid organs (91). Both Vγ1+ and Vγ4+ cells can secrete IFN-γ, TNF-a, TGF-β, and IL-10 upon activation. However, Vγ1+γδT cells are predisposed to produced IL-4 and IL-5, while Vγ4+γδT cells preferentially produce IL-17 (92). Vγ1+γδT cells occur mainly in the form of Vγ1Vδ6.3/6.4 TCR cells and secrete IL-4 and IFN-γ (93). Upon acute infection with Coxsackievirus B3 (CVB3), Vγ1+γδT cells are the early and primary producers of IL-4 and play a protective role in CVB3 myocarditis (94). Vγ4+ γδT cells express high levels of Rorc, Sox13, Scart, Bclaf1, and Atf2 and secrete abundant levels of IL-17A and IL-17F (92) (95). IL-17A-producing Vγ4+γδT cells also express high levels of CCR6 on their surface and are chemoattracted by CCL20 that are secreted by keratinocytes to inflammatory sites, which in turn facilitates keratinocytes to secrete IL-1β and IL-23 (96). In addition, IL-17 secreted by Vγ4+γδT cells inhibits the production of IGF-1, thereby delaying skin wound healing (84, 97). Studies have shown that Vγ2+ T cells recruit neutrophils and aggravate liver fibrosis by secreting IL-17A (98, 99). It has also been demonstrated that Vγ7+T cells are the main components of the murine intestinal intraepithelial T cell compartment. Consequently, the selective maturation and expansion of Vγ7+T cells are driven by both Btnl1 and Btnl6 (100).

BIOLOGICAL EFFECTS OF γδT CELLS

γδT cells have strong plasticity and secrete different cytokines and chemokines. They exhibit diverse functions similar to Th1, Th2, Tregs, and Th17 cells in different microenvironments (2).

Some γδ T cells generate growth factors such as VEGF, FGF-2, and IGF-1, suggesting that these cells have the capacity to maintain epithelial integrity and wound repair (101). Nonetheless, some γδ T cells have been reported to induce the production of antimicrobial peptides, including β-defensin 2, S100A7, and S100A8 in keratinocytes to exert a protective function in local epithelial defense (101). γδT cells secrete interleukin-10 (IL-10), control CD8+ T cell expansion, and regulate and reduce TNF-a secretion by activated CD8+ T cells (102). The role of IL-17-producing γδT cells has been investigated in various models of infection and autoimmunity (103, 104). IL-17-producing γδT cells robustly direct the recruitment of neutrophils and monocytes to increase the inflammatory response.

γδ T cells are involved in the regulation of macrophage homeostasis and recruitment. In patients suffering from listeriosis (a serious infection caused by the germ Listeria monocytogenes), γδT cells play a critical role in neutrophil replacement by producing chemokines such as macrophage chemoattractant protein1 (MCP-1) (105). Additional evidence has shown that γδT cells facilitate differentiation of the monocyte/macrophage lineage. Remarkably, monocytes differentiate into inflammatory macrophages during bacterial infections but fail to undergo maturation in mice lacking γδT cells (106). In contrast, the role of Vγ4 has been demonstrated to enhance macrophage activity and the production of specific pro-inflammatory and immunoregulatory cytokines by macrophages. Different subsets of γδT cells have opposing roles in macrophage homeostasis, indicating the complexity and plasticity of γδT cells (107). γδT cells present antigens to αβT cells, while Vδ2+ T cells display characteristics similar to professional APCs. Once activated, these cells efficiently process and present antigens and prime co-stimulatory signals for potent induction of αβT cell proliferation and differentiation (108). Receptors associated with DC, such as antigen presentation molecules (MHC class II), co-stimulatory receptors (CD40, CD80, and CD86), maturation markers (CD83), and adhesion receptors (CD11a, CD11b, CD11c, CD18, CD50, and CD54) have been found to be expressed on the surface of activated γδT cells (109, 110).

Activated γδT cells exhibit a broad range of cytotoxic activity, especially against a wide variety of tumor cells that utilize death receptor/ligand (Fas/Fas-ligand)-dependent and perforin/granzyme or granulysin-dependent pathways. Exogenous IL-18 promotes the expansion of γδT cells in human peripheral blood mononuclear cells (PBMCs) stimulated by Zoledronate (Zol) and IL-2 (109). The expansion of γδT cells is inhibited by neutralizing anti-IL-18 receptor antibodies, indicating that IL-18 efficiently promotes the expansion of γδT cells with potent antitumor activity (110). Furthermore, studies have shown that γδT cells directly kill activated hepatic stellate cells (HSCs) and increase NK cell-mediated cytotoxicity against activated HSCs in liver fibrosis (10).

γδT cells are highly efficient in promoting B cell maturation and producing IgM, IgG, and IgA antibodies. Vδ2Vγ9 T cells express IL-21R on their surface, which is enhanced upon HMB-PP induced irritation (111, 112). Activated Vδ2Vγ9T cells express CXCL13, CXCR5, and ICOS and upregulate the expression of B cell surface markers CD25, CD69, CD40, and CD86. This suggests that CXCR5+ Vδ2Vγ9 T cells are a distinct memory T cell subset with B cell helper function (111, 113).

γδT IN PSORIASIS

Dysregulation of the immune system and T cell activation has been well demonstrated to play an essential role in psoriasis development. Several studies have attributed T cell function in the skin to αβT cells, while γδT cells have been often overlooked. IFN-γ-producing T helper (Th) 1 cells were initially thought to be primary drivers of psoriasis. However, substantial clinical and basic research findings in the past decade have proved that the interleukin (IL)-23/Th17 axis plays an important role in the pathogenesis of psoriasis (114, 115). Psoriatic inflammation was found to be impaired in IL-23- and IL-17-deficient mice, thereby confirming the involvement of the IL-23/IL-17 axis (116, 117). Th17 cells and their downstream effector molecules, including IL-17A, IL-17F, IL-22, and tumor necrosis factor (TNF-α), were found to be increased in the sera and psoriatic skin lesion (118). Recently, Th17 cells were found not to be the primary source of these pathogenic cytokines in psoriasis. Instead, IL-17A, IL-17F, and IL-22 were found to be produced by γδT cells (115). Injecting IL-23 into the skin of mice or applying a topical dose of imiquimod cream (5%) induced a typical psoriasis-like phenotype, i.e., epidermal thickness, erythema, and inflammation. These two models were demonstrated to mimic psoriasis-like inflammation and have been used to evaluate the efficacy of different treatment methods (119). Epidermal hyperplasia and inflammation response induced by IL-23/IMQ was observed to be significantly reduced in T cell receptor δ deficient ($Tcrd^{-/-}$) mice, however, no significant changes were observed in T cell receptor β deficient $Tcrb^{-/-}$ mice (120). In addition, Cai et al. demonstrated that upon IL-23 stimulation, IL-17 produced in $Tcrd^{-/-}$ mice was significantly lower compared to WT or $Tcra^{-/-}$ mice (121). These data further suggested that dermal γδT cells were the major IL-17-producing cells in the skin in response to IL-23 stimulation.

The production of IL-17 by dermal γδ T cells requires endogenous IL-1β (121). Mechanistically, IL-1β activates the mammalian target of rapamycin (mTOR) signaling pathway *via* IL-1R-MyD88, whereas IL-23 activates the STAT3 pathway. Transcription factor IRF-4 links the IL-1R and IL-23R pathways to induce enhanced IL-17 production in dermal γδ T cells (122). Both Vγ4 and Vγ6 dermal T cells produce IL-17, however, dermal Vγ4 T cells expand and produce significantly more IL-17 compared to Vγ6 (123). Dermal Vγ4 and Vγ6T cells have different effector signaling requirements. Dermal Vγ4 T cell proliferation and IL-17 production are dependent on STAT3, whereas dermal Vγ6 T cells may be activated through the STAT3-independent RelA/NF-kB pathway (122). Thus, dermal Vγ4 T cells appear to have a critical role in IMQ-induced psoriasis-like dermatitis (123).

Dermal γδT cells constitutively express IL-23R, IL-17R, RORγt, and the chemokine receptors CCR1, CCR2, CCR4, CCR5, CCR6,

CXCR3, and CXCR4 (120, 121). CCL20, which is a unique CCR6 ligand, mediates skin infiltration of IL-17-producing γδT-cells and DCs. Numerous studies have shown that CCL20/CCR6 regulates T migration from the dermis to the epidermis, promotes neutrophil aggregation, and exacerbates inflammation (124). In IL-23-injected WT mice, CCL20 was highly upregulated with numerous CCR6+γδT cells observed in the epidermis (125). Anti-CCL20-neutralizing antibodies or engineered CCL20 variants with minimal chemotactic activity prevented the infiltration of IL-17-producing γδT-cell into the skin of IL-23-injected mice. This lead to IL-17 and IL-22 downregulation, blocked γδT cell recruitment to the epidermis, and reduced psoriasiform dermatitis (126, 127). In CCR6-knockout (KO) mice, γδT cells failed to migrate and accumulate in the epidermis after IL-23 treatment. Keratinocytes secrete CCL20, bind and activate CCR6, and regulate the migration of γδT cell subsets into the skin. This suggests the potential relevance of CCR6/CCL20 as a therapeutic target for psoriasis (126, 128, 129).

Psoriasis recurs frequently and relapse occurs in the same area after treatment discontinuation. Hence, recurrent psoriasis is a major problem that needs to be solved. TNF-a, IL-12/23, and IL-17 inhibitors have been shown to exhibit potent and rapid therapeutic efficacy (130, 131). However, these biological agents have been associated with several adverse events, the most common being susceptibility to infections (130). In addition to infections, biological inhibitors have been associated with demyelinating diseases, nasopharyngitis, upper respiratory infection, headaches, lupus, or lupus-like syndromes, mucocutaneous candidiasis, mild neutropenia, and new-onset or worsening of heart failure. The long-term safety concerns and high cost hamper the extensive use of these agents (130, 132, 133).

Psoriasis relapses around the original lesion area suggest these manifestations have an "immune memory." Adaptive immune responses by memory T cells are not limited to foreign antigens, and relapses in autoimmune diseases are typically driven by auto-aggressive memory lymphocytes. There have been published reports regarding the adaptive-type memory responses in γδT cells. The response of human Vγ9Vδ2+ T cells to phospho-antigens is increased after initial *Mycobacterium bovis* BCG vaccinations (134). In macaques, a memory-type response and rapid expansion of Vγ9Vδ2 T cells have been observed after a secondary challenge with *Bacillus Calmette-Guerin* (135). Mouse "memory-like" Vγ6+ γδT cells were found to be retained for more than five months in the mesenteric lymph nodes after *Listeria monocytogenes* infection (136).

Memory-like γδT has been seen in psoriasiform mouse model, IL-17A-producing Vγ2Vδ4+ T cells initially derive from the neonatal thymus where they are instructed with tissue tropism. These Vγ2Vδ4+ T cells were phenotypically memory-like with a CD44hi CD62Llo CD27- expression pattern (137). After exposure to IMQ, Vγ4+γδT17 cells in the skin have been shown to rapidly expand in the draining lymph nodes (LNs) and then release from the LNs. They then migrate *via* the action of the chemokine, CCR2, to accumulate at sites of both inflamed and uninflamed skin in a S1P1-dependent manner. This in turn exacerbates the inflammatory response and recruitment of neutrophils. They have also been shown to migrate *via* the blood and persist in normal skin and peripheral LNs for a minimum of three months. Importantly, when subjected to the same second challenge at a distant skin site, memory-like Vγ4+γδT17 cells expand at a faster rate and produce more IL-17 compared to that after exposure to the first challenge, leading to a rapid and severe skin inflammatory response (19) (**Figure 2**). Sensitized mice showed elevated skin inflammation, significant cell proliferation, and IL-17 production by Vγ4+γδT cells upon IMQ challenge. Adoptive transfer experiments have confirmed that memory-like Vγ4+γδT17 cells respond rapidly, and their memory drives their involvement in the psoriasis recurrence (19, 138, 139).

γδT cells are rarely found in healthy human skin (140), however, they are easily generated from the skin of psoriatic patients. γδT cells have different adhesion properties compared to αβT cell subsets (141). A higher frequency of sequence sharing of the γ-chain has been found in psoriatic lesions from different individuals compared to those without psoriasis, suggesting that although the T cell response in psoriasis is highly polyclonal, particular γδT cell subsets could be associated with this disease (142). Following study demonstrated that an increased level of Vγ9Vδ2 T cells was present in psoriatic skin compared to healthy controls, while a significant reduction in Vγ9Vδ2 cells was observed in the blood of psoriasis patients. The number of circulating Vγ9Vδ2 T cells returned to normal levels after successful psoriasis-targeted treatment. These findings demonstrated the redistribution of Vγ9Vδ2 T cells from the blood to the skin of psoriasis patients (101). The recruitment of specific monoclonal population of γδT cells to psoriatic skin suggests local expression or modification of a cognate TCR ligand that is recognized by this population of memory-like γδT cells (143). Consistently, Zheng group found the higher expression of Vγ9 in psoriasis lesion than that in healthy individuals, indicating that Vγ9 γδT cells may be the main pathogenic cell (144). Additionally, Vγ9Vδ2 T cells have been shown to produce psoriasis-relevant cytokines, such as IFN-γ, TNF-α, and IL-17A and chemokines such as IL-8, CCL3, CCL4, CCL5, and CCR6. These cytokines and chemokines are responsible for recruiting crucial immune effector cells to the skin to activate keratinocytes (63, 145).

TARGETING γδT CELLS FOR PSORIASIS THERAPY

The important role of dermal immobilized γδT cells in the pathogenesis of psoriasis has been elucidated in the past years. Hence, dermal γδT cells and their associated molecules have become attractive targets for drug development. Adiponectin, a metabolic mediator of insulin sensitivity, plays a crucial role in metabolic regulation and inflammatory/anti-inflammatory processes. Studies have demonstrated that in psoriasiform skin, inflammation, and infiltration of dermal γδT cells producing IL-17 were significantly enhanced in the absence of adiponectin. The negative regulation of adiponectin on IL-17 production from dermal γδT cells is mainly mediated through AdipoR1. This

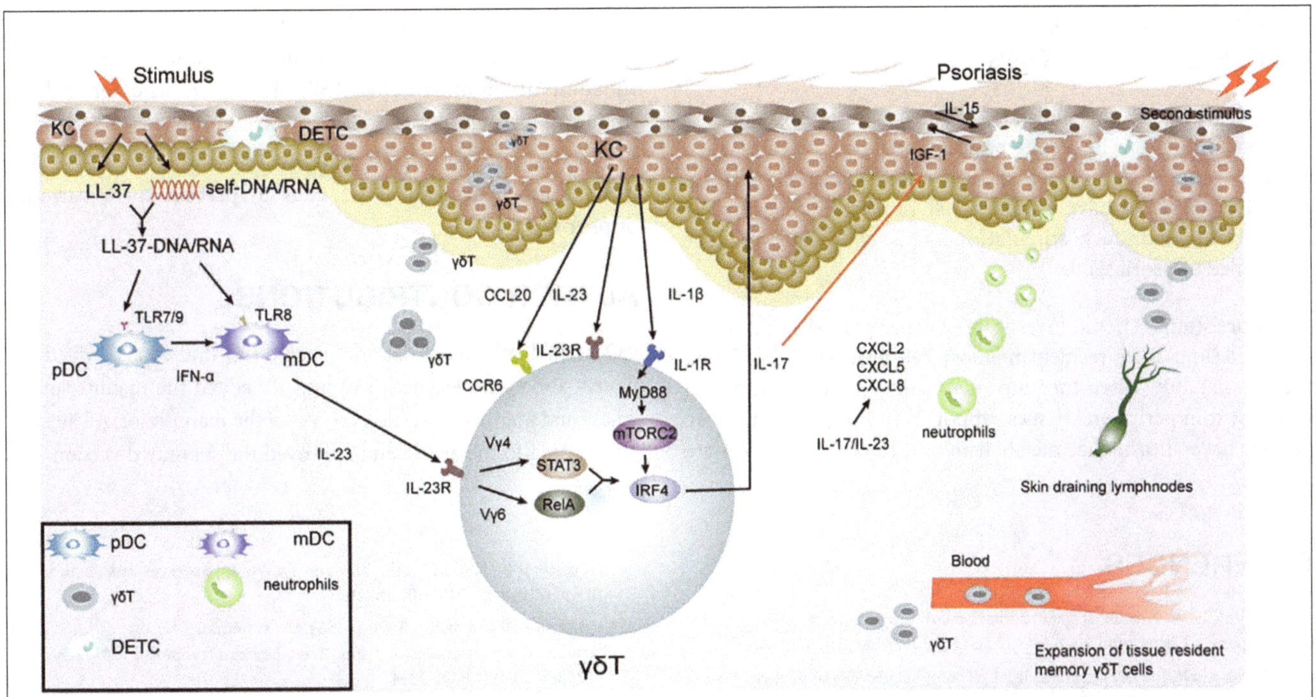

FIGURE 2 | Role of γδT cells in the immune pathogenesis of psoriasis. Keratinocytes in the epidermis undergo apoptosis, necrosis, or death when exposed to certain external stimulation. With the release of cell contents, such as DNA and RNA, keratinocytes release antimicrobial peptides, such as LL-37. LL-37 binds with DNA and RNA to form a complex, promote immature DC activation, and secrete IFN-γ/IL-23 through the TLR7/8/9 pathway. IL-23 activates RORγt+γδT cells to secrete IL-17. γδT cell-derived IL-17 directly inhibits IGF-1 production in DETCs by increasing epidermal IL-23/IL-1β expression. During excessive keratinocyte proliferation, the secretion of TNF-α and chemokine ligand 20 (CCL20) increases, which consequently recruits CCR6+γδT cells to the inflammatory site of the epidermis. IL-17 cytokines produced by γδT cells potently upregulate the chemokine, CCL20, in keratinocytes, which chemoattracts IL-17A-producing CCR6+ immune cells to the inflamed site, thus forming a positive feedback loop. Il-23/IL-17 also promotes the recruitment of neutrophils to inflammatory sites, leading to excessive proliferation of the stratum corneum to form psoriatic inflammatory lesions. γδT cells have memory properties and can migrate rapidly to inflammatory sites through the blood and skin when subjected to a secondary stimulation. This consequently gives rise to severe inflammatory manifestations.

suggests that increasing adiponectin levels may be effective for improving psoriasis as well as metabolic disorders (146, 147). BTLA belongs to the immunoglobulin superfamily and has been reported to play a role in the homeostasis of γδT cells/ILCs in lymphoid tissues and controls the production of IL-17 in mature lymph node γδT cells. BTLA-deficient animal models have been shown to have a dysregulated proportion of inflammatory γδT cells and were susceptible to psoriasis and severe skin inflammation. BTLA agonism was found to limit the progression of these phenotypes. Activation of BTLA may restore the balance of γδT cell subsets to control autoimmune pathogenesis (148, 149). The agonistic anti-BTLA antibody (clone 6A6) was demonstrated to suppress γδT cell expansion and IL-17 production within the lymph nodes and skin induced by IMQ (149, 150). Thus, BTLA may be a potential target for the treatment of psoriasis. Dermal γδT cells constitutively express CCR6. CCR6KO or anti-CCL20 monoclonal antibodies administered to mice resulted in a decline in psoriatic dermatitis in IL-23-induced skin inflammation mouse models. This demonstrates that CCL20, together with its receptor, CCR6, are potential targets for the treatment of psoriasis (129, 151). CCL20 S64C is a CCL20 variant that binds to CCR6 and inhibits CCR6-mediated T cell migration. Previous studies have shown that CCL20 S64C alleviates the inflammatory response in psoriasis-like models induced by IL-23, and have been associated with reduced accumulation of CCR6+ IL-17-producing γδT cells in the epidermis (127). FTY720 is an FDA-approved immunomodulatory drug for the treatment of multiple sclerosis. It reduces lymphocyte egress from lymphoid tissues by inhibiting the sphingosine-1 phosphate receptor (S1PR). FTY720 inhibits the migration of Vγ4+VγT4+ T17 cells from the lymph nodes to the skin, suggesting its potential as a treatment for psoriasis (152). Indirubin (IR) is a bisindole compound extracted from the leaves of the Chinese herb *Indigo naturalis*. It has been demonstrated to alleviate IMQ-induced psoriasis-like dermatitis by primarily reducing the inflammatory responses mediated by IL-17 A-producing γδT cells through Jak3/Stat3 activation (153). Dashlkhumbe et al. reported a newly formulated methotrexate (MTX, a chemical conjugate of MTX with a cell-permeable peptide) for the treatment of psoriasis. Topically applied skin-penetrating (SP)-MTX reduced the psoriasiform skin phenomenon and epidermal thickness by reducing CD11c+, CD4+, and IL-17-producing γδT cell-containing infiltrate of immune cells in the skin (154).

CONCLUSIONS AND FUTURE DIRECTIONS

Psoriasis has a complex and varied pathogenesis. During disease development, γδT cells secrete proinflammatory cytokines, such as IL-17 and IFN-γ, which induce and aggravate psoriasis. Notably, γδT cells have memory cell properties that rapidly respond to secondary stimulation. This contributes to the recurrence of psoriasis.

Future studies should investigate whether γδT cells that reside in skin lesions have resident memory cell properties, how long they persist, how often they turn over, and what environmental niches within peripheral tissues support their long-term survival. Studies have shown that metabolism and immune function are tightly linked (155, 156). Nutrient availability and cellular metabolism tightly control the differentiation, survival, and function of immune cells (157). However, whether cellular metabolism regulates γδT fate decisions remains to be deciphered. Additional studies are necessary to identify the mechanisms that reduce γδT cells to prevent the recurrence of psoriasis.

AUTHOR CONTRIBUTIONS

CQ drafted and edited the manuscript. CQ drafted and edited the figures and figure legends. YW and PL edited the manuscript. JZ edited and approved the final version of the manuscript. All authors contributed to the article and approved the submitted version.

REFERENCES

1. Holtmeier W, Kabelitz D. gammadelta T cells link innate and adaptive immune responses. *Chem Immunol Allergy* (2005) 86:151–83. doi: 10.1159/000086659
2. Lu H, Li DJ, Jin LP. gammadeltaT Cells and Related Diseases. *Am J Reprod Immunol* (2016) 75:609–18. doi: 10.1111/aji.12495
3. Ness-Schwickerath KJ, Morita CT. Regulation and function of IL-17A- and IL-22-producing gammadelta T cells. *Cell Mol Life Sci* (2011) 68:2371–90. doi: 10.1007/s00018-011-0700-z
4. Reinhardt A, Prinz I. Whodunit? The Contribution of Interleukin (IL)-17/IL-22-Producing gammadelta T Cells, alphabeta T Cells, and Innate Lymphoid Cells to the Pathogenesis of Spondyloarthritis. *Front Immunol* (2018) 9:885. doi: 10.3389/fimmu.2018.00885
5. Raverdeau M, Cunningham SP, Harmon C, Lynch L. gammadelta T cells in cancer: a small population of lymphocytes with big implications. *Clin Transl Immunol* (2019) 8:e01080. doi: 10.1002/cti2.1080
6. Xu P, Fu X, Xiao N, Guo Y, Pei Q, Peng Y, et al. Involvements of gammadeltaT Lymphocytes in Acute and Chronic Skin Wound Repair. *Inflammation* (2017) 40:1416–27. doi: 10.1007/s10753-017-0585-6
7. Zhang S, Kan X, Li Y, Li P, Zhang C, Li G, et al. Deficiency of gammadeltaT cells protects against abdominal aortic aneurysms by regulating phosphoinositide 3-kinase/AKT signaling. *J Vasc Surg* (2018) 67:899–908.e1. doi: 10.1016/j.jvs.2016.03.474
8. Girard P, Charles J, Cluzel C, Degeorges E, Manches O, Plumas J, et al. The features of circulating and tumor-infiltrating gammadelta T cells in melanoma patients display critical perturbations with prognostic impact on clinical outcome. *Oncoimmunology* (2019) 8:1601483. doi: 10.1080/2162402X.2019.1601483
9. Kierkels GJJ, Scheper W, Meringa AD, Johanna I, Beringer DX, Janssen A, et al. Identification of a tumor-specific allo-HLA-restricted gammadeltaTCR. *Blood Adv* (2019) 3:2870–82. doi: 10.1182/bloodadvances.2019032409
10. Liu M, Hu Y, Yuan Y, Tian Z, Zhang C. gammadeltaT Cells Suppress Liver Fibrosis via Strong Cytolysis and Enhanced NK Cell-Mediated Cytotoxicity Against Hepatic Stellate Cells. *Front Immunol* (2019) 10:477. doi: 10.3389/fimmu.2019.00477
11. Schadler ED, Ortel B, Mehlis SL. Biologics for the primary care physician: Review and treatment of psoriasis. *Dis Mon* (2019) 65:51–90. doi: 10.1016/j.disamonth.2018.06.001
12. Arnone M, Takahashi MDF, Carvalho AVE, Bernardo WM, Bressan AL, Ramos AMC, et al. Diagnostic and therapeutic guidelines for plaque psoriasis - Brazilian Society of Dermatology. *Bras Dermatol* (2019) 94:76–107. doi: 10.1590/abd1806-4841.2019940211
13. Lee EB, Wu KK, Lee MP, Bhutani T, Wu JJ. Psoriasis risk factors and triggers. *Cutis* (2018) 102:18–20.
14. Michalek IM, Loring B, John SM. A systematic review of worldwide epidemiology of psoriasis. *J Eur Acad Dermatol Venereol* (2017) 31:205–12. doi: 10.1111/jdv.13854
15. Boehncke WH, Schon MP. Psoriasis. *Lancet* (2015) 386:983–94. doi: 10.1016/S0140-6736(14)61909-7
16. Hawkes JE, Chan TC, Krueger JG. Psoriasis pathogenesis and the development of novel targeted immune therapies. *J Allergy Clin Immunol* (2017) 140:645–53. doi: 10.1016/j.jaci.2017.07.004
17. Mo WX, Yin SS, Chen H, Zhang X. Amino-bisphosphonates, gammadeltaT cells, and their roles in Rheumatoid Arthritis. *Ann Rheum Dis* (2018) 77:e58. doi: 10.1136/annrheumdis-2017-212569
18. Ma H, Yuan Y, Zhao L, Ye Z, Xu J, Li M, et al. Association of gammadelta T Cell Compartment Size to Disease Activity and Response to Therapy in SLE. *PLoS One* (2016) 11:e0157772. doi: 10.1371/journal.pone.0157772
19. Ramirez-Valle F, Gray EE, Cyster JG. Inflammation induces dermal Vgamma4+ gammadeltaT17 memory-like cells that travel to distant skin and accelerate secondary IL-17-driven responses. *Proc Natl Acad Sci U S A* (2015) 112:8046–51. doi: 10.1073/pnas.1508990112
20. Brenner MB, McLean J, Dialynas DP, Strominger JL, Smith JA, Owen FL, et al. Identification of a putative second T-cell receptor. *Nature* (1986) 322:145–9. doi: 10.1038/322145a0
21. Zhang X, Dong X, Wang H, Li J, Yang B, Zhang J, et al. FADD regulates thymocyte development at the beta-selection checkpoint by modulating Notch signaling. *Cell Death Dis* (2014) 5:e1273. doi: 10.1038/cddis.2014.198
22. Michie AM, Zuniga-Pflucker JC. Regulation of thymocyte differentiation: pre-TCR signals and beta-selection. *Semin Immunol* (2002) 14:311–23. doi: 10.1016/S1044-5323(02)00064-7
23. Fahl SP, Coffey F, Wiest DL. Origins of gammadelta T cell effector subsets: a riddle wrapped in an enigma. *J Immunol* (2014) 193:4289–94. doi: 10.4049/jimmunol.1401813
24. Livak F, Tourigny M, Schatz DG, Petrie HT. Characterization of TCR gene rearrangements during adult murine T cell development. *J Immunol* (1999) 162:2575–80.
25. Muro R, Takayanagi H, Nitta T. T cell receptor signaling for gammadeltaT cell development. *Inflammation Regener* (2019) 39:6. doi: 10.1186/s41232-019-0095-z
26. Chann AS, Russell SM. An integrated transcriptional switch at the beta-selection checkpoint determines T cell survival, development and leukaemogenesis. *Biochem Soc Trans* (2019) 47:1077–89. doi: 10.1042/BST20180414

27. Haks MC, Lefebvre JM, Lauritsen JP, Carleton M, Rhodes M, Miyazaki T, et al. Attenuation of gammadeltaTCR signaling efficiently diverts thymocytes to the alphabeta lineage. *Immunity* (2005) 22:595–606. doi: 10.1016/j.immuni.2005.04.003
28. Taghon T, Yui MA, Pant R, Diamond RA, Rothenberg EV. Developmental and molecular characterization of emerging beta- and gammadelta-selected pre-T cells in the adult mouse thymus. *Immunity* (2006) 24:53–64. doi: 10.1016/j.immuni.2005.11.012
29. Carpenter AC, Bosselut R. Decision checkpoints in the thymus. *Nat Immunol* (2010) 11:666–73. doi: 10.1038/ni.1887
30. Kang J, Volkmann A, Raulet DH. Evidence that gammadelta versus alphabeta T cell fate determination is initiated independently of T cell receptor signaling. *J Exp Med* (2001) 193:689–98. doi: 10.1084/jem.193.6.689
31. Kreslavsky T, Garbe AI, Krueger A, von Boehmer H. T cell receptor-instructed alphabeta versus gammadelta lineage commitment revealed by single-cell analysis. *J Exp Med* (2008) 205:1173–86. doi: 10.1084/jem.20072425
32. Zarin P, Wong GW, Mohtashami M, Wiest DL, Zuniga-Pflucker JC. Enforcement of gammadelta-lineage commitment by the pre-T-cell receptor in precursors with weak gammadelta-TCR signals. *Proc Natl Acad Sci U S A* (2014) 111:5658–63. doi: 10.1073/pnas.1312872111
33. Lauritsen JP, Wong GW, Lee SY, Lefebvre JM, Ciofani M, Rhodes M, et al. Marked induction of the helix-loop-helix protein Id3 promotes the gammadelta T cell fate and renders their functional maturation Notch independent. *Immunity* (2009) 31:565–75. doi: 10.1016/j.immuni.2009.07.010
34. Lee SY, Coffey F, Fahl SP, Peri S, Rhodes M, Cai KQ, et al. Noncanonical mode of ERK action controls alternative alphabeta and gammadelta T cell lineage fates. *Immunity* (2014) 41:934–46. doi: 10.1016/j.immuni.2014.10.021
35. Engel I, Murre C. The function of E- and Id proteins in lymphocyte development. *Nat Rev Immunol* (2001) 1:193–9. doi: 10.1038/35105060
36. Ciofani M, Zuniga-Pflucker JC. Determining gammadelta versus alphass T cell development. *Nat Rev Immunol* (2010) 10:657–63. doi: 10.1038/nri2820
37. Zarin P, Chen EL, In TS, Anderson MK, Zuniga-Pflucker JC. Gamma delta T-cell differentiation and effector function programming, TCR signal strength, when and how much? *Cell Immunol* (2015) 296:70–5. doi: 10.1016/j.cellimm.2015.03.007
38. Melichar HJ, Narayan K, Der SD, Hiraoka Y, Gardiol N, Jeannet G, et al. Regulation of gammadelta versus alphabeta T lymphocyte differentiation by the transcription factor SOX13. *Science* (2007) 315:230–3. doi: 10.1126/science.1135344
39. Turchinovich G, Hayday AC. Skint-1 identifies a common molecular mechanism for the development of interferon-gamma-secreting versus interleukin-17-secreting gammadelta T cells. *Immunity* (2011) 35:59–68. doi: 10.1016/j.immuni.2011.04.018
40. Fichtner AS, Ravens S, Prinz I. Human gammadelta TCR Repertoires in Health and Disease. *Cells* (2020) 9:800. doi: 10.3390/cells9040800
41. Bonneville M, O'Brien RL, Born WK. Gammadelta T cell effector functions: a blend of innate programming and acquired plasticity. *Nat Rev Immunol* (2010) 10:467–78. doi: 10.1038/nri2781
42. Wesch D, Hinz T, Kabelitz D. Analysis of the TCR Vgamma repertoire in healthy donors and HIV-1-infected individuals. *Int Immunol* (1998) 10:1067–75. doi: 10.1093/intimm/10.8.1067
43. Davey MS, Willcox CR, Joyce SP, Ladell K, Kasatskaya SA, McLaren JE, et al. Clonal selection in the human Vdelta1 T cell repertoire indicates gammadelta TCR-dependent adaptive immune surveillance. *Nat Commun* (2017) 8:14760. doi: 10.1038/ncomms14760
44. Maher CO, Dunne K, Comerford R, O'Dea S, Loy A, Woo J, et al. Candida albicans stimulates IL-23 release by human dendritic cells and downstream IL-17 secretion by Vdelta1 T cells. *J Immunol* (2015) 194:5953–60. doi: 10.4049/jimmunol.1403066
45. Fausther-Bovendo H, Wauquier N, Cherfils-Vicini J, Cremer I, Debre P, Vieillard V. NKG2C is a major triggering receptor involved in the V[delta]1 T cell-mediated cytotoxicity against HIV-infected CD4 T cells. *AIDS* (2008) 22:217–26. doi: 10.1097/QAD.0b013e3282f46e7c
46. Wesch D, Peters C, Oberg HH, Pietschmann K, Kabelitz D. Modulation of gammadelta T cell responses by TLR ligands. *Cell Mol Life Sci* (2011) 68:2357–70. doi: 10.1007/s00018-011-0699-1
47. Hudspeth K, Fogli M, Correia DV, Mikulak J, Roberto A, Della Bella S, et al. Engagement of NKp30 on Vdelta1 T cells induces the production of CCL3, CCL4, and CCL5 and suppresses HIV-1 replication. *Blood* (2012) 119:4013–6. doi: 10.1182/blood-2011-11-390153
48. Kuroda H, Saito H, Ikeguchi M. Decreased number and reduced NKG2D expression of Vdelta1 gammadelta T cells are involved in the impaired function of Vdelta1 gammadelta T cells in the tissue of gastric cancer. *Gastric Cancer* (2012) 15:433–9. doi: 10.1007/s10120-011-0138-x
49. Mao Y, Yin S, Zhang J, Hu Y, Huang B, Cui L, et al. A new effect of IL-4 on human gammadelta T cells: promoting regulatory Vdelta1 T cells via IL-10 production and inhibiting function of Vdelta2 T cells. *Cell Mol Immunol* (2016) 13:217–28. doi: 10.1038/cmi.2015.07
50. Chabab G, Barjon C, Abdellaoui N, Salvador-Prince L, Dejou C, Michaud HA, et al. Identification of a regulatory Vdelta1 gamma delta T cell subpopulation expressing CD73 in human breast cancer. *J Leukoc Biol* (2020) 107:1057–67. doi: 10.1002/JLB.3MA0420-278RR
51. Singh AK, Novakova L, Axelsson M, Malmestrom C, Zetterberg H, Lycke J, et al. High Interferon-gamma Uniquely in Vdelta1 T Cells Correlates with Markers of Inflammation and Axonal Damage in Early Multiple Sclerosis. *Front Immunol* (2017) 8:260. doi: 10.3389/fimmu.2017.00260
52. Hviid L, Smith-Togobo C, Willcox BE. Human Vdelta1(+) T Cells in the Immune Response to Plasmodium falciparum Infection. *Front Immunol* (2019) 10:259. doi: 10.3389/fimmu.2019.00259
53. Rutishauser T, Lepore M, Di Blasi D, Dangy JP, Abdulla S, Jongo S, et al. Activation of TCR Vdelta1(+) and Vdelta1(-)Vdelta2(-) gammadelta T Cells upon Controlled Infection with Plasmodium falciparum in Tanzanian Volunteers. *J Immunol* (2020) 204:180–91. doi: 10.4049/jimmunol.1900669
54. Dunne PJ, Maher CO, Freeley M, Dunne K, Petrasca A, Orikiiriza J, et al. CD3epsilon Expression Defines Functionally Distinct Subsets of Vdelta1 T Cells in Patients With Human Immunodeficiency Virus Infection. *Front Immunol* (2018) 9:940. doi: 10.3389/fimmu.2018.00940
55. Pauza CD, Poonia B, Li H, Cairo C, Chaudhry S. gammadelta T Cells in HIV Disease: Past, Present, and Future. *Front Immunol* (2014) 5:687. doi: 10.3389/fimmu.2014.00687
56. Knight A, Arnouk H, Britt W, Gillespie GY, Cloud GA, Harkins L, et al. CMV-independent lysis of glioblastoma by ex vivo expanded/activated Vdelta1+ gammadelta T cells. *PLoS One* (2013) 8:e68729. doi: 10.1371/journal.pone.0068729
57. Lo Presti E, Di Mitri R, Mocciaro F, Di Stefano AB, Scibetta N, Unti E, et al. Characterization of gammadelta T Cells in Intestinal Mucosa From Patients With Early-Onset or Long-Standing Inflammatory Bowel Disease and Their Correlation With Clinical Status. *J Crohns Colitis* (2019) 13:873–83. doi: 10.1093/ecco-jcc/jjz015
58. Correia DV, Fogli M, Hudspeth K, da Silva MG, Mavilio D, Silva-Santos B. Differentiation of human peripheral blood Vdelta1+ T cells expressing the natural cytotoxicity receptor NKp30 for recognition of lymphoid leukemia cells. *Blood* (2011) 118:992–1001. doi: 10.1182/blood-2011-02-339135
59. Dimova T, Brouwer M, Gosselin F, Tassignon J, Leo O, Donner C, et al. Effector Vgamma9Vdelta2 T cells dominate the human fetal gammadelta T-cell repertoire. *Proc Natl Acad Sci U S A* (2015) 112:E556–65. doi: 10.1073/pnas.1412058112
60. Davey MS, Willcox CR, Hunter S, Kasatskaya SA, Remmerswaal EBM, Salim M, et al. The human Vdelta2(+) T-cell compartment comprises distinct innate-like Vgamma9(+) and adaptive Vgamma9(-) subsets. *Nat Commun* (2018) 9:1760. doi: 10.1038/s41467-018-04076-0
61. Kress E, Hedges JF, Jutila MA. Distinct gene expression in human Vdelta1 and Vdelta2 gammadelta T cells following non-TCR agonist stimulation. *Mol Immunol* (2006) 43:2002–11. doi: 10.1016/j.molimm.2005.11.011
62. Moens E, Brouwer M, Dimova T, Goldman M, Willems F, Vermijlen D. IL-23R and TCR signaling drives the generation of neonatal Vgamma9Vdelta2 T cells expressing high levels of cytotoxic mediators and producing IFN-gamma and IL-17. *J Leukoc Biol* (2011) 89:743–52. doi: 10.1189/jlb.0910501
63. Pang DJ, Neves JF, Sumaria N, Pennington DJ. Understanding the complexity of gammadelta T-cell subsets in mouse and human. *Immunology* (2012) 136:283–90. doi: 10.1111/j.1365-2567.2012.03582.x
64. Caccamo N, Meraviglia S, Ferlazzo V, Angelini D, Borsellino G, Poccia F, et al. Differential requirements for antigen or homeostatic cytokines for proliferation and differentiation of human Vgamma9Vdelta2 naive, memory and effector T cell subsets. *Eur J Immunol* (2005) 35:1764–72. doi: 10.1002/eji.200525983

65. Dieli F, Poccia F, Lipp M, Sireci G, Caccamo N, Di Sano C, et al. Differentiation of effector/memory Vdelta2 T cells and migratory routes in lymph nodes or inflammatory sites. *J Exp Med* (2003) 198:391–7. doi: 10.1084/jem.20030235
66. De Rosa SC, Andrus JP, Perfetto SP, Mantovani JJ, Herzenberg LA, Herzenberg LA, et al. Ontogeny of gamma delta T cells in humans. *J Immunol* (2004) 172:1637–45. doi: 10.4049/jimmunol.172.3.1637
67. Hintz M, Reichenberg A, Altincicek B, Bahr U, Gschwind RM, Kollas AK, et al. Identification of (E)-4-hydroxy-3-methyl-but-2-enyl pyrophosphate as a major activator for human gammadelta T cells in Escherichia coli. *FEBS Lett* (2001) 509:317–22. doi: 10.1016/S0014-5793(01)03191-X
68. Wang H, Sarikonda G, Puan KJ, Tanaka Y, Feng J, Giner JL, et al. Indirect stimulation of human Vgamma2Vdelta2 T cells through alterations in isoprenoid metabolism. *J Immunol* (2011) 187:5099–113. doi: 10.4049/jimmunol.1002697
69. Dunne MR, Mangan BA, Madrigal-Estebas L, Doherty DG. Preferential Th1 cytokine profile of phosphoantigen-stimulated human Vgamma9Vdelta2 T cells. *Mediators Inflamm* (2010) 2010:704941. doi: 10.1155/2010/704941
70. Petrasca A, Doherty DG. Human Vdelta2(+) gammadelta T Cells Differentially Induce Maturation, Cytokine Production, and Alloreactive T Cell Stimulation by Dendritic Cells and B Cells. *Front Immunol* (2014) 5:650. doi: 10.3389/fimmu.2014.00650
71. Devilder MC, Maillet S, Bouyge-Moreau I, Donnadieu E, Bonneville M, Scotet E. Potentiation of antigen-stimulated V gamma 9V delta 2 T cell cytokine production by immature dendritic cells (DC) and reciprocal effect on DC maturation. *J Immunol* (2006) 176:1386–93. doi: 10.4049/jimmunol.176.3.1386
72. Mangan BA, Dunne MR, O'Reilly VP, Dunne PJ, Exley MA, O'Shea D, et al. Cutting edge: CD1d restriction and Th1/Th2/Th17 cytokine secretion by human Vdelta3 T cells. *J Immunol* (2013) 191:30–4. doi: 10.4049/jimmunol.1300121
73. Kenna T, Golden-Mason L, Norris S, Hegarty JE, O'Farrelly C, Doherty DG. Distinct subpopulations of gamma delta T cells are present in normal and tumor-bearing human liver. *Clin Immunol* (2004) 113:56–63. doi: 10.1016/j.clim.2004.05.003
74. Dunne MR, Elliott L, Hussey S, Mahmud N, Kelly J, Doherty DG, et al. Persistent changes in circulating and intestinal gammadelta T cell subsets, invariant natural killer T cells and mucosal-associated invariant T cells in children and adults with coeliac disease. *PLoS One* (2013) 8:e76008. doi: 10.1371/journal.pone.0076008
75. Petrasca A, Melo AM, Breen EP, Doherty DG. Human Vdelta3(+) gammadelta T cells induce maturation and IgM secretion by B cells. *Immunol Lett* (2018) 196:126–34. doi: 10.1016/j.imlet.2018.02.002
76. Wang L, Xu M, Wang C, Zhu L, Hu J, Chen S, et al. The feature of distribution and clonality of TCR gamma/delta subfamilies T cells in patients with B-cell non-Hodgkin lymphoma. *J Immunol Res* (2014) 2014:241246. doi: 10.1155/2014/241246
77. Heilig JS, Tonegawa S. Diversity of murine gamma genes and expression in fetal and adult T lymphocytes. *Nature* (1986) 322:836–40. doi: 10.1038/322836a0
78. Garman RD, Doherty PJ, Raulet DH. Diversity, rearrangement, and expression of murine T cell gamma genes. *Cell* (1986) 45:733–42. doi: 10.1016/0092-8674(86)90787-7
79. Munoz-Ruiz M, Sumaria N, Pennington DJ, Silva-Santos B. Thymic Determinants of gammadelta T Cell Differentiation. *Trends Immunol* (2017) 38:336–44. doi: 10.1016/j.it.2017.01.007
80. Prinz I, Silva-Santos B, Pennington DJ. Functional development of gammadelta T cells. *Eur J Immunol* (2013) 43:1988–94. doi: 10.1002/eji.201343759
81. Carding SR, Egan PJ. Gammadelta T cells: functional plasticity and heterogeneity. *Nat Rev Immunol* (2002) 2:336–45. doi: 10.1038/nri797
82. Jiang X, Campbell JJ, Kupper TS. Embryonic trafficking of gammadelta T cells to skin is dependent on E/P selectin ligands and CCR4. *Proc Natl Acad Sci U S A* (2010) 107:7443–8. doi: 10.1073/pnas.0912943107
83. Nakamura K, White AJ, Parnell SM, Lane PJ, Jenkinson EJ, Jenkinson WE, et al. Differential requirement for CCR4 in the maintenance but not establishment of the invariant Vgamma5(+) dendritic epidermal T-cell pool. *PLoS One* (2013) 8:e74019. doi: 10.1371/journal.pone.0074019
84. Li Y, Wu J, Luo G, He W. Functions of Vgamma4 T Cells and Dendritic Epidermal T Cells on Skin Wound Healing. *Front Immunol* (2018) 9:1099. doi: 10.3389/fimmu.2018.01099
85. Havran WL, Jameson JM. Epidermal T cells and wound healing. *J Immunol* (2010) 184:5423–8. doi: 10.4049/jimmunol.0902733
86. Jameson JM, Cauvi G, Sharp LL, Witherden DA, Havran WL. Gammadelta T cell-induced hyaluronan production by epithelial cells regulates inflammation. *J Exp Med* (2005) 201:1269–79. doi: 10.1084/jem.20042057
87. Ramirez K, Witherden DA, Havran WL. All hands on DE(T)C: Epithelial-resident gammadelta T cells respond to tissue injury. *Cell Immunol* (2015) 296:57–61. doi: 10.1016/j.cellimm.2015.04.003
88. Nielsen MM, Lovato P, MacLeod AS, Witherden DA, Skov L, Dyring-Andersen B, et al. IL-1beta-dependent activation of dendritic epidermal T cells in contact hypersensitivity. *J Immunol* (2014) 192:2975–83. doi: 10.4049/jimmunol.1301689
89. Hatano S, Tun X, Noguchi N, Yue D, Yamada H, Sun X, et al. Development of a new monoclonal antibody specific to mouse Vgamma6 chain. *Life Sci Alliance* (2019) 2. doi: 10.26508/lsa.201900363
90. Jin C, Lagoudas GK, Zhao C, Bullman S, Bhutkar A, Hu B, et al. Commensal Microbiota Promote Lung Cancer Development via gammadelta T Cells. *Cell* (2019) 176:998–1013.e16. doi: 10.1016/j.cell.2018.12.040
91. Buus TB, Schmidt JD, Bonefeld CM, Geisler C, Lauritsen JP. Development of interleukin-17-producing Vgamma2+ gammadelta T cells is reduced by ICOS signaling in the thymus. *Oncotarget* (2016) 7:19341–54. doi: 10.18632/oncotarget.8464
92. Dong P, Zhang S, Cai M, Kang N, Hu Y, Cui L, et al. Global characterization of differential gene expression profiles in mouse Vgamma1+ and Vgamma4+ gammadelta T cells. *PLoS One* (2014) 9:e112964. doi: 10.1371/journal.pone.0112964
93. Pereira P, Berthault C, Burlen-Defranoux O, Boucontet L. Critical role of TCR specificity in the development of Vgamma1Vdelta6.3+ innate NKTgammadelta cells. *J Immunol* (2013) 191:1716–23. doi: 10.4049/jimmunol.1203168
94. Wan F, Yan K, Xu D, Qian Q, Liu H, Li M, et al. Vgamma1(+)gammadeltaT, early cardiac infiltrated innate population dominantly producing IL-4, protect mice against CVB3 myocarditis by modulating IFNgamma(+) T response. *Mol Immunol* (2017) 81:16–25. doi: 10.1016/j.molimm.2016.11.006
95. Papotto PH, Ribot JC, Silva-Santos B. IL-17(+) gammadelta T cells as kick-starters of inflammation. *Nat Immunol* (2017) 18:604–11. doi: 10.1038/ni.3726
96. Li Y, Huang Z, Yan R, Liu M, Bai Y, Liang G, et al. Vgamma4 gammadelta T Cells Provide an Early Source of IL-17A and Accelerate Skin Graft Rejection. *J Invest Dermatol* (2017) 137:2513–22. doi: 10.1016/j.jid.2017.03.043
97. Li Y, Wang Y, Zhou L, Liu M, Liang G, Yan R, et al. Vgamma4 T Cells Inhibit the Pro-healing Functions of Dendritic Epidermal T Cells to Delay Skin Wound Closure Through IL-17A. *Front Immunol* (2018) 9:240. doi: 10.3389/fimmu.2018.00240
98. Spidale NA, Sylvia K, Narayan K, Miu B, Frascoli M, Melichar HJ, et al. Interleukin-17-Producing gammadelta T Cells Originate from SOX13(+) Progenitors that Are Independent of gammadeltaTCR Signaling. *Immunity* (2018) 49:857–72.e5. doi: 10.1016/j.immuni.2018.09.010
99. Zheng L, Hu Y, Wang Y, Huang X, Xu Y, Shen Y, et al. Recruitment of Neutrophils Mediated by Vgamma2 gammadelta T Cells Deteriorates Liver Fibrosis Induced by Schistosoma japonicum Infection in C57BL/6 Mice. *Infect Immun* (2017) 85. doi: 10.1128/IAI.01020-16
100. Di Marco Barros R, Roberts NA, Dart RJ, Vantourout P, Jandke A, Nussbaumer O, et al. Epithelia Use Butyrophilin-like Molecules to Shape Organ-Specific gammadelta T Cell Compartments. *Cell* (2016) 167:203–18.e17. doi: 10.1016/j.cell.2016.08.030
101. Laggner U, Di Meglio P, Perera GK, Hundhausen C, Lacy KE, Ali N, et al. Identification of a novel proinflammatory human skin-homing Vgamma9Vdelta2 T cell subset with a potential role in psoriasis. *J Immunol* (2011) 187:2783–93. doi: 10.4049/jimmunol.1100804
102. Rhodes KA, Andrew EM, Newton DJ, Tramonti D, Carding SR. A subset of IL-10-producing gammadelta T cells protect the liver from Listeria-elicited, CD8(+) T cell-mediated injury. *Eur J Immunol* (2008) 38:2274–83. doi: 10.1002/eji.200838354
103. Patil RS, Bhat SA, Dar AA, Chiplunkar SV. The Jekyll and Hyde story of IL17-Producing gammadeltaT Cells. *Front Immunol* (2015) 6:37. doi: 10.3389/fimmu.2015.00037

104. Palomino-Segura M, Latino I, Farsakoglu Y, Gonzalez SF. Early production of IL-17A by gammadelta T cells in the trachea promotes viral clearance during influenza infection in mice. *Eur J Immunol* (2020) 50:97–109. doi: 10.1002/eji.201948157
105. DiTirro J, Rhoades ER, Roberts AD, Burke JM, Mukasa A, Cooper AM, et al. Disruption of the cellular inflammatory response to Listeria monocytogenes infection in mice with disruptions in targeted genes. *Infect Immun* (1998) 66:2284–9. doi: 10.1128/IAI.66.5.2284-2289.1998
106. Skeen MJ, Freeman MM, Ziegler HK. Changes in peritoneal myeloid populations and their proinflammatory cytokine expression during infection with Listeria monocytogenes are altered in the absence of gamma/delta T cells. *J Leukoc Biol* (2004) 76:104–15. doi: 10.1189/jlb.1103574
107. Tramonti D, Andrew EM, Rhodes K, Newton DJ, Carding SR. Evidence for the opposing roles of different gamma delta T cell subsets in macrophage homeostasis. *Eur J Immunol* (2006) 36:1729–38. doi: 10.1002/eji.200635959
108. Brandes M, Willimann K, Moser B. Professional antigen-presentation function by human gammadelta T Cells. *Science* (2005) 309:264–8. doi: 10.1126/science.1110267
109. D'Asaro M, La Mendola C, Di Liberto D, Orlando V, Todaro M, Spina M, et al. V gamma 9V delta 2 T lymphocytes efficiently recognize and kill zoledronate-sensitized, imatinib-sensitive, and imatinib-resistant chronic myelogenous leukemia cells. *J Immunol* (2010) 184:3260–8. doi: 10.4049/jimmunol.0903454
110. Li W, Kubo S, Okuda A, Yamamoto H, Ueda H, Tanaka T, et al. Effect of IL-18 on expansion of gammadelta T cells stimulated by zoledronate and IL-2. *J Immunother* (2010) 33:287–96. doi: 10.1097/CJI.0b013e3181c80ffa
111. Bansal RR, Mackay CR, Moser B, Eberl M. IL-21 enhances the potential of human gammadelta T cells to provide B-cell help. *Eur J Immunol* (2012) 42:110–9. doi: 10.1002/eji.201142017
112. Wu K, Zhao H, Xiu Y, Li Z, Zhao J, Xie S, et al. IL-21-mediated expansion of Vgamma9Vdelta2 T cells is limited by the Tim-3 pathway. *Int Immunopharmacol* (2019) 69:136–42. doi: 10.1016/j.intimp.2019.01.027
113. Caccamo N, Battistini L, Bonneville M, Poccia F, Fournie JJ, Meraviglia S, et al. CXCR5 identifies a subset of Vgamma9Vdelta2 T cells which secrete IL-4 and IL-10 and help B cells for antibody production. *J Immunol* (2006) 177:5290–5. doi: 10.4049/jimmunol.177.8.5290
114. Hawkes JE, Yan BY, Chan TC, Krueger JG. Discovery of the IL-23/IL-17 Signaling Pathway and the Treatment of Psoriasis. *J Immunol* (2018) 201:1605–13. doi: 10.4049/jimmunol.1800013
115. Ogawa E, Sato Y, Minagawa A, Okuyama R. Pathogenesis of psoriasis and development of treatment. *J Dermatol* (2018) 45:264–72. doi: 10.1111/1346-8138.14139
116. Rizzo HL, Kagami S, Phillips KG, Kurtz SE, Jacques SL, Blauvelt A. IL-23-mediated psoriasis-like epidermal hyperplasia is dependent on IL-17A. *J Immunol* (2011) 186:1495–502. doi: 10.4049/jimmunol.1001001
117. Tortola L, Rosenwald E, Abel B, Blumberg H, Schafer M, Coyle AJ, et al. Psoriasiform dermatitis is driven by IL-36-mediated DC-keratinocyte crosstalk. *J Clin Invest* (2012) 122:3965–76. doi: 10.1172/JCI63451
118. Brembilla NC, Senra L, Boehncke WH. The IL-17 Family of Cytokines in Psoriasis: IL-17A and Beyond. *Front Immunol* (2018) 9:1682. doi: 10.3389/fimmu.2018.01682
119. Singh TP, Zhang HH, Hwang ST, Farber JM. IL-23- and Imiquimod-Induced Models of Experimental Psoriasis in Mice. *Curr Protoc Immunol* (2019) 125:e71. doi: 10.1002/cpim.71
120. Pantelyushin S, Haak S, Ingold B, Kulig P, Heppner FL, Navarini AA, et al. Rorgammat+ innate lymphocytes and gammadelta T cells initiate psoriasiform plaque formation in mice. *J Clin Invest* (2012) 122:2252–6. doi: 10.1172/JCI61862
121. Cai Y, Shen X, Ding C, Qi C, Li K, Li X, et al. Pivotal role of dermal IL-17-producing gammadelta T cells in skin inflammation. *Immunity* (2011) 35:596–610. doi: 10.1016/j.immuni.2011.08.001
122. Cai Y, Xue F, Qin H, Chen X, Liu N, Fleming C, et al. Differential Roles of the mTOR-STAT3 Signaling in Dermal gammadelta T Cell Effector Function in Skin Inflammation. *Cell Rep* (2019) 27:3034–48.e5. doi: 10.1016/j.celrep.2019.05.019
123. Cai Y, Xue F, Fleming C, Yang J, Ding C, Ma Y, et al. Differential developmental requirement and peripheral regulation for dermal Vgamma4 and Vgamma6T17 cells in health and inflammation. *Nat Commun* (2014) 5:3986. doi: 10.1038/ncomms4986
124. Katayama H. Development of psoriasis by continuous neutrophil infiltration into the epidermis. *Exp Dermatol* (2018) 27:1084–91. doi: 10.1111/exd.13746
125. Mabuchi T, Takekoshi T, Hwang ST. Epidermal CCR6+ gammadelta T cells are major producers of IL-22 and IL-17 in a murine model of psoriasiform dermatitis. *J Immunol* (2011) 187:5026–31. doi: 10.4049/jimmunol.1101817
126. Mabuchi T, Singh TP, Takekoshi T, Jia GF, Wu X, Kao MC, et al. CCR6 is required for epidermal trafficking of gammadelta-T cells in an IL-23-induced model of psoriasiform dermatitis. *J Invest Dermatol* (2013) 133:164–71. doi: 10.1038/jid.2012.260
127. Getschman AE, Imai Y, Larsen O, Peterson FC, Wu X, Rosenkilde MM, et al. Protein engineering of the chemokine CCL20 prevents psoriasiform dermatitis in an IL-23-dependent murine model. *Proc Natl Acad Sci U S A* (2017) 114:12460–5. doi: 10.1073/pnas.1704958114
128. Hedrick MN, Lonsdorf AS, Hwang ST, Farber JM. CCR6 as a possible therapeutic target in psoriasis. *Expert Opin Ther Targets* (2010) 14:911–22. doi: 10.1517/14728222.2010.504716
129. Furue K, Ito T, Tsuji G, Nakahara T, Furue M. The CCL20 and CCR6 axis in psoriasis. *Scand J Immunol* (2020) 91:e12846. doi: 10.1111/sji.12846
130. Gisondi P, Geat D, Pizzolato M, Girolomoni G. State of the art and pharmacological pipeline of biologics for chronic plaque psoriasis. *Curr Opin Pharmacol* (2019) 46:90–9. doi: 10.1016/j.coph.2019.05.007
131. Sbidian E, Chaimani A, Afach S, Doney L, Dressler C, Hua C, et al. Systemic pharmacological treatments for chronic plaque psoriasis: a network meta-analysis. *Cochrane Database Syst Rev* (2020) 1:CD011535. doi: 10.1002/14651858.CD011535.pub3
132. Conrad C, Gilliet M. Psoriasis: from Pathogenesis to Targeted Therapies. *Clin Rev Allergy Immunol* (2018) 54:102–13. doi: 10.1007/s12016-018-8668-1
133. Mrowietz U, Barker J, Boehncke WH, Iversen L, Kirby B, Naldi L, et al. Clinical use of dimethyl fumarate in moderate-to-severe plaque-type psoriasis: a European expert consensus. *J Eur Acad Dermatol Venereol* (2018) 32(Suppl 3):3–14. doi: 10.1111/jdv.15218
134. Dieli F, Sireci G, Di Sano C, Romano A, Titone L, Di Carlo P, et al. Ligand-specific alphabeta and gammadelta T cell responses in childhood tuberculosis. *J Infect Dis* (2000) 181:294–301. doi: 10.1086/315180
135. Pitard V, Roumanes D, Lafarge X, Couzi L, Garrigue I, Lafon ME, et al. Long-term expansion of effector/memory Vdelta2-gammadelta T cells is a specific blood signature of CMV infection. *Blood* (2008) 112:1317–24. doi: 10.1182/blood-2008-01-136713
136. Sheridan BS, Romagnoli PA, Pham QM, Fu HH, Alonzo F,3, Schubert WD, et al. gammadelta T cells exhibit multifunctional and protective memory in intestinal tissues. *Immunity* (2013) 39:184–95. doi: 10.1016/j.immuni.2013.06.015
137. Khairallah C, Chu TH, Sheridan BS. Tissue Adaptations of Memory and Tissue-Resident Gamma Delta T Cells. *Front Immunol* (2018) 9:2636. doi: 10.3389/fimmu.2018.02636
138. Zhu R, Cai X, Zhou C, Li Y, Zhang X, Li Y, et al. Dermal Vgamma4(+)T cells enhance the IMQ-induced psoriasis-like skin inflammatidon in re-challenged mice. *Am J Transl Res* (2017) 9:5347–60.
139. Hartwig T, Pantelyushin S, Croxford AL, Kulig P, Becher B. Dermal IL-17-producing gammadelta T cells establish long-lived memory in the skin. *Eur J Immunol* (2015) 45:3022–33. doi: 10.1002/eji.201545883
140. Holtmeier W, Pfander M, Hennemann A, Zollner TM, Kaufmann R, Caspary WF. The TCR-delta repertoire in normal human skin is restricted and distinct from the TCR-delta repertoire in the peripheral blood. *J Invest Dermatol* (2001) 116:275–80. doi: 10.1046/j.1523-1747.2001.01250.x
141. de Boer OJ, Verhagen CE, Visser A, Bos JD, Das PK. Cellular interactions and adhesion molecules in psoriatic skin. *Acta Derm Venereol Suppl (Stockh)* (1994) 186:15–8.
142. Harden JL, Hamm D, Gulati N, Lowes MA, Krueger JG. Deep Sequencing of the T-cell Receptor Repertoire Demonstrates Polyclonal T-cell Infiltrates in Psoriasis. *F1000Res* (2015) 4:460. doi: 10.12688/f1000research.6756.1
143. Lalor SJ, McLoughlin RM. Memory gammadelta T Cells-Newly Appreciated Protagonists in Infection and Immunity. *Trends Immunol* (2016) 37:690–702. doi: 10.1016/j.it.2016.07.006
144. Liu JT, Xue F, Li X, Shi RF, Zheng J. Preliminary Study of T Cell Receptor Vγ Gene Usage of γδT Cells in Psoriatic Skin Lesions. *Chin J Dermatovenereol* (2012) 26:571–4.
145. Ness-Schwickerath KJ, Jin C, Morita CT. Cytokine requirements for the differentiation and expansion of IL-17A- and IL-22-producing human

Vgamma2Vdelta2 T cells. *J Immunol* (2010) 184:7268–80. doi: 10.4049/jimmunol.1000600

146. Ruan H, Dong LQ. Adiponectin signaling and function in insulin target tissues. *J Mol Cell Biol* (2016) 8:101–9. doi: 10.1093/jmcb/mjw014
147. Shibata S, Tada Y, Hau CS, Mitsui A, Kamata M, Asano Y, et al. Adiponectin regulates psoriasiform skin inflammation by suppressing IL-17 production from gammadelta-T cells. *Nat Commun* (2015) 6:7687. doi: 10.1038/ncomms8687
148. Bekiaris V, Sedy JR, Macauley MG, Rhode-Kurnow A, Ware CF. The inhibitory receptor BTLA controls gammadelta T cell homeostasis and inflammatory responses. *Immunity* (2013) 39:1082–94. doi: 10.1016/j.immuni.2013.10.017
149. Youssef RM, El-Ramly AZ, Hussien MF, Shoukry NM, Amr K. Expression of B and T lymphocyte attenuator, retinoid-related orphan receptor gamma-isoform-t and interleukin 7 in psoriasis vulgaris. *Australas J Dermatol* (2019) 60:e132–7. doi: 10.1111/ajd.12965
150. Hurchla MA, Sedy JR, Gavrieli M, Drake CG, Murphy TL, Murphy KM, et al. B and T lymphocyte attenuator exhibits structural and expression polymorphisms and is highly Induced in anergic CD4+ T cells. *J Immunol* (2005) 174:3377–85. doi: 10.4049/jimmunol.174.6.3377
151. Cochez PM, Michiels C, Hendrickx E, Dauguet N, Warnier G, Renauld JC, et al. Ccr6 Is Dispensable for the Development of Skin Lesions Induced by Imiquimod despite its Effect on Epidermal Homing of IL-22-Producing Cells. *J Invest Dermatol* (2017) 137:1094–103. doi: 10.1016/j.jid.2016.12.023
152. Maeda Y, Seki N, Kataoka H, Takemoto K, Utsumi H, Fukunari A, et al. IL-17-Producing Vgamma4+ gammadelta T Cells Require Sphingosine 1-Phosphate Receptor 1 for Their Egress from the Lymph Nodes under Homeostatic and Inflammatory Conditions. *J Immunol* (2015) 195:1408–16. doi: 10.4049/jimmunol.1500599
153. Xie XJ, Di TT, Wang Y, Wang MX, Meng YJ, Lin Y, et al. Indirubin ameliorates imiquimod-induced psoriasis-like skin lesions in mice by inhibiting inflammatory responses mediated by IL-17A-producing gammadelta T cells. *Mol Immunol* (2018) 101:386–95. doi: 10.1016/j.molimm.2018.07.011
154. Byamba D, Kim DY, Kim DS, Kim TG, Jee H, Kim SH, et al. Skin-penetrating methotrexate alleviates imiquimod-induced psoriasiform dermatitis via decreasing IL-17-producing gamma delta T cells. *Exp Dermatol* (2014) 23:492–6. doi: 10.1111/exd.12448
155. Buck MD, Sowell RT, Kaech SM, Pearce EL. Metabolic Instruction of Immunity. *Cell* (2017) 169:570–86. doi: 10.1016/j.cell.2017.04.004
156. Shehata HM, Murphy AJ, Lee MKS, Gardiner CM, Crowe SM, Sanjabi S, et al. Sugar or Fat?-Metabolic Requirements for Immunity to Viral Infections. *Front Immunol* (2017) 8:1311. doi: 10.3389/fimmu.2017.01311
157. Dimeloe S, Burgener AV, Grahlert J, Hess C. T-cell metabolism governing activation, proliferation and differentiation; a modular view. *Immunology* (2017) 150:35–44. doi: 10.1111/imm.12655

17

CLA+ T Cell Response to Microbes in Psoriasis

*Carmen De Jesús-Gil[1], Ester Ruiz-Romeu[1], Marta Ferran[2,3], Anca Chiriac[4,5,6], Gustavo Deza[2,3], Péter Hóllo[7], Antonio Celada[8], Ramon M. Pujol[2,3] and Luis F. Santamaria-Babí[1]**

[1] *Translational Immunology, Department of Cellular Biology, Physiology and Immunology, Faculty of Biology, Universitat de Barcelona, Barcelona, Spain,* [2] *Department of Dermatology, Hospital del Mar.Barcelona, Barcelona, Spain,* [3] *IMIM (Hospital del Mar Medical Research Institute), Barcelona, Spain,* [4] *Nicolina Medical Center, Department of Dermatology, Iasi, Romania,* [5] *Apollonia University, Iasi, Romania,* [6] *"P.Poni" Institute of Macromolecular Chemistry, Romanian Academy, Iasi, Romania,* [7] *Department of Dermatovenerology and Oncodermatology, Semmelweis Egyetem, Budapest, Hungary,* [8] *Macrophage Biology, Department of Cellular Biology, Physiology and Immunology, Faculty of Biology, Universitat de Barcelona, Barcelona, Spain*

***Correspondence:**
Luis F. Santamaria-Babí
luis.santamaria@ub.edu

Streptococcus pyogenes throat infection is a clinically relevant trigger of both guttate and chronic plaque psoriasis, and it provides an ideal context in which to study the pathogenesis of these diseases using an antigen-dependent approach. Circulating cutaneous lymphocyte-associated antigen (CLA) positive (+) memory T cells are a subset of peripheral lymphocytes whose phenotype and function are related to immunological mechanisms in the skin. These cells are considered peripheral biomarkers of T-cell-mediated skin diseases. The coculture of autologous epidermal cells with CLA+ T cells from psoriasis patients activated by *S. pyogenes* allows the reproduction of the *ex vivo* initial molecular events that occur during psoriatic lesion formation. With cooperation of autologous epidermal cells, *S. pyogenes* selectively activates CLA+ T cells both in guttate and plaque psoriasis, inducing key mediators, including an IL-17 response. Here, we explore potential new mechanisms of psoriasis development including the influence of HLA-Cw6 on *S. pyogenes* CLA+ T cell activation in guttate psoriasis, the relevance of IL-9 on microbe induced IL-17 response in guttate and plaque psoriasis, and novel effector functions of *Candida albicans*. This review will summarize recent knowledge of psoriatic mechanisms elicited by microbes that have been studied through an innovative translational perspective based on CLA+ T cell-mediated cutaneous immune response.

Keywords: psoriasis, cutaneous lymphocyte-associated antigen, homing, *Candida albicans*, *Streptococcus pyogenes*

INTRODUCTION

Molecular studies of psoriasis lesions and patients have allowed translational research to generate potent and novel therapies (1). However, our understanding of the influence of environmental factors on the psoriatic cutaneous immune response is still limited (1). Several microorganisms, including bacteria, fungi, and viruses, have been postulated to be potential triggers and/or exacerbating factors of psoriasis (2). Bacterial genome DNA sequencing in psoriasis is an area of great interest, some microorganisms have been identified but their functional relevance for psoriasis is still to be determined. Psoriasis can be classified as early or late onset (3). The former is associated with the HLA-Cw6 allele, streptococcal throat infection, and a higher tendency to be generalized

(4, 5). Interestingly, patients with this type often present a more intense inflammatory lymphocytic infiltrate and are more likely to receive biological therapy (6). All these observations suggest that the presentation of psoriasis is associated with the present bacterial infection. *Streptococcus pyogenes* throat infection is a well-characterized infectious trigger of gutatte psoriasis (GP) and chronic plaque psoriasis (CPP). More than 60 years ago, it was reported that two-third of GP patients present an acute sore throat 12 weeks before the skin eruption (7). Similarly, CPP can also be triggered by *S. pyogenes* throat infections (8), and interestingly, CPP patients have a higher incidence of recurrent sore throats compared with controls (9, 10). The presence of *S. pyogenes* has been detected in the blood of both GP and CPP patients (11). In addition, tonsillectomy can be a useful therapeutic intervention in CPP patients with a history of streptococcal-associated exacerbations (12). It has been proposed that psoriasis tonsillar CLA$^+$ T cells (13) activated by streptococcal antigens migrate to the skin where they react to antigens that share sequence homology with the streptococcal proteins (14). However, other microbes may also participate in psoriasis. Fungal cutaneous infections caused by *Candida albicans* have been associated with exacerbation of the disease and a higher frequency of intestinal *C. albicans* isolation in psoriasis patients than controls has been reported (2), although the mechanisms involved in *C. albicans*-induced psoriasis remain poorly characterized.

Interestingly, microbes such as *C. albicans* induce type I interferon response and, type I interferon production by plasmacytoid dendritic cells in skin has been stated to be an important trigger for psoriasis development (15). However, clinical efficacy blocking antibodies against IFN-α have not shown clinical efficacy in psoriasis (16), rising questions about the translational relevance of this mechanism.

In this review, we cover the current state of the art in psoriasis immunopathogenic mechanisms brought out by disease-related microorganisms, such as *S. pyogenes* or *C. albicans*. We focus on cutaneous immune response mediated by CLA$^+$ T cells and how these microbes affect T cell activation and production of clinically relevant cytokines.

CIRCULATING CLA$^+$ T CELLS AND THE STUDY OF THE CUTANEOUS IMMUNE SYSTEM

The immune responses of T cells during cutaneous chronic inflammation in psoriasis involve a subset of memory T lymphocytes that can be distinguished from other memory T cells by the surface expression of the cutaneous lymphocyte-associated antigen (CLA) antigen. This antigen is a cell surface carbohydrate that allows the identification of memory T cells that belong to the cutaneous immune system. CLA is an adhesion molecule expressed by 15% of circulating T cells in humans, and by most (>90%) skin-infiltrating T cells, contrary to other inflamed organs (17). In addition to several ligands for chemokine receptors (CCR10, CCR4, CCR6, and CCR8), CLA binds to E-selectin and together with the interaction between the very late antigen-4/vascular cell adhesion protein-1 and lymphocyte function-associated antigen-1/intercellular adhesion molecule-1, forms a code bar system enabling skin lymphoid infiltration (18). The relevance of circulating CLA$^+$ T cells in the cutaneous immune response lies not only in the skin-seeking capacity of these cells but also in their functional relation to the immune response that occurs in inflamed cutaneous lesions. This feature is derived from the recirculating capacity of these cells between skin lesion and blood during cutaneous inflammation (18, 19). The antigen-specific response and phenotype of circulating CLA$^+$ T cells has been studied in many human skin conditions. CLA$^+$ T cells respond to antigens, allergens, or superantigens involved in disease by triggering T cell-mediated skin diseases, such as psoriasis, atopic dermatitis, and contact dermatitis (18). Furthermore, the phenotype and function of these cells are related to the clinical status of the patient, thereby explaining why circulating CLA$^+$ T cells are considered peripheral cell biomarkers of T cell-mediated cutaneous disease in humans (18). Using CLA$^+$ T cells from psoriasis patients and healthy controls, our group explores the influence of microbes on cutaneous immune response in psoriasis.

CLA$^+$ T CELL ACTIVATION BY *S. pyogenes* IN PSORIASIS INDUCES IL-17 AND IL-9 RESPONSES

Studying the antigen-specific immune response of CLA$^+$ T cells induced by clinically relevant triggers of psoriasis may allow the identification of the translational mechanisms involved in psoriasis. The stimulation of autologous coculture CLA$^+$ T cells and epidermal cells with *S. pyogenes* leads to an inflammatory immune response that shows the hallmarks of psoriasis. By contrast, the same stimulation of CLA$^-$ cells from the same patient or cultures using CLA$^+$/CLA$^-$ T cells from healthy controls does not have this effect (20). The CLA$^+$ T cell response in this model is related to the clinical response of patients in terms of anti-streptolysin O levels, PASI, and duration of flare in GP (21), and to anti-streptolysin O in CPP (20). This activation is determined by the presence of autologous epidermal cells (lesional/non-lesional) and MHC class I and class II presentation. Supernatants of *S. pyogenes*-activated cocultures of CLA$^+$ T cells and epidermal cells induce epidermal hyperplasia upon intradermal injection in mouse skin (20). IL-17A and IL-17F production is probably the most relevant effect of *S. pyogenes* on CLA$^+$ T cells in psoriasis. The influence of *S. pyogenes* through the response of these cells and the relevance of IL-17 production in GP have been extensively studied (21). In HLA-Cw6$^+$ patients whose GP flare is associated with a pharyngitis episode, the Th17-associated response is greater than that exerted by samples from GP patients not associated with pharyngitis. In fact, significantly higher levels of IL-17A, IL-17F, and even IL-6, which participates in Th17-differentiation, were found (21). Thus, the observed response of psoriasis memory T cells to *S. pyogenes* seems to be restricted to CLA$^+$ T cells, leading to IL-17 production. This cytokine is a key driver of psoriasis, and its neutralization in patients, or receptor blockade improves the skin condition (1).

The cytokine IL-9 is involved in chronic inflammation and has recently been associated with psoriasis (22, 23). We have demonstrated how *S. pyogenes* preferentially induces IL-9 production during the coculture of autologous CLA$^+$ T cells and epidermal cells in psoriasis but not in healthy controls. IL-9 is produced in the same culture conditions in which IL-17A and IL-17F are detected in a time-dependent manner. IL-9 production is dependent on MHC class I and class II presentation, and it preferentially prolongs CLA$^+$ T cell survival. Higher amounts of IL-9 were detected in psoriasis patients than in healthy controls, but no differences were observed between GP and CPP patients (24). IL-9 has been associated with increased IL-17A production in an animal model of psoriasis (23). Since *S. pyogenes* induces both IL-9 and IL-17A, we examined the interaction between these two cytokines in CLA$^+$ T cells. To this end, we blocked IL-9 function using a neutralizing. A 50% reduction in IL-17A production, but not IFN-γ, was found when was IL-9 was neutralized in CLA$^+$ cells activated by *S. pyogenes*.

Our studies have shown that, in CPP patients without clinical evidence of *S. pyogenes* infection, only CLA$^+$ T cells respond to this microbe in comparison to healthy controls. This observation indicates that psoriasis patients present an adaptive immune response to *S. pyogenes* through IL-17A, IL-17F, IL-9, and IFN-γ production (20, 21, 24) and suggests that *S. pyogenes* modulates the response of the CLA$^+$ T cells that maintain psoriatic lesions, i.e., pyogenes infection has been describe to participate in CPP infection, since higher levels of IgG against *S. pyogenes* proteins are detected in psoriasis patients in comparison to healthy controls (25). Some studies have reported the presence of the genera *Streptococcus* in normal and psoriatic skin (26) and the isolation of *S. pyogenes* in the skin of GP patients (4), probably leading to cutaneous immunization and a CLA$^+$ T cell-restricted response in psoriasis.

CLA$^+$ T CELL RESPONSE TO *C. albicans* IN PSORIASIS

The cutaneous adaptive immune response to *C. albicans* infection is mediated by a Th17 profile since Th17 cells are essential for anti-fungal barrier immunity (27). Patients with Th17 deficiencies have an increased susceptibility to candidiasis (28), and CD45RA$^+$ human T cells may lead to an increase in the number of IL-17 and IFN-γ-producing cells (29). Cutaneous candidal infections have been reported in association with psoriasis exacerbation (30); however, the mechanisms by which *C. albicans* induces psoriasis are poorly understood (2). In psoriasis, *C. albicans*-derived superantigens may induce an expansion of lymphocytes expressing the T-cell receptor variable region beta 5.1 (31). Like in the case of *S. pyogenes*, CLA$^+$ T cells, together with autologous epidermal cells, preferentially respond to *C. albicans* extract by inducing IL-9, IL-17A, and IFN-γ production in psoriasis. This response appears to be restricted to CLA$^+$CD4$^+$ memory T cells since CD4-depleted CLA$^+$ memory T cells do not respond to this microorganism in a coculture model with psoriasis cells (24). These results are in line with the expected immune response to *C. albicans* in the skin. However, the observed preferential response of CLA$^+$ T cells in psoriasis suggests an adaptive immune response to *C. albicans*, underlying its importance as a relevant antigen likely to be involved in triggering the disease.

INFLUENCE OF *S. pyogenes* AND *C. albicans* ON IL-17 ADAPTIVE IMMUNE RESPONSE IN PSORIASIS

The precise mechanisms by which environmental factors trigger psoriasis are not well understood (1). Biological therapies have revealed the clinical relevance of the IL-23/IL-17 axis in this skin disease. Thus, environmental factors that contribute to fueling the IL-23/IL-17 response may induce the condition. The observation that CLA$^+$ T cells in psoriasis patients respond to skin *S. pyogenes* and *C. albicans* extracts indicates a relationship between memory T cells and environmental microbes. Such preferential sensitization to these microorganisms in psoriasis can be either at the tonsillar level in psoriasis through the abnormal generation of CLA$^+$ T cells or at the skin level, since the presence of both *S. pyogenes* and *C. albicans* in psoriatic lesions (13). The CLA$^+$ T cell response to these microbes is based on IL-17A, IL-17F, IL-9, and IFN-γ production. This response indicates that these skin-homing cells will migrate to psoriatic lesions and thus that they may be involved in the local inflammatory response. IL-17A and IL-17F are clinically validated mediators of psoriasis. *S. pyogenes*-driven IL-9 production through CLA$^+$ T cells supports IL-17A production in human lymphocytes, since *in vitro* neutralization of IL-9 reduces IL-17A production by 50% (24).

A current model of IL-17 production in psoriasis considers that some autoantigens, such as LL-37 and ADAMTS-like protein 5, would activate T17 cells (32), initiating the immune circuit of the psoriasis pathogenetic mechanism in the disease. Also, IL-23 production by inflammatory dendritic cells favors the generation and maintenance of the T17 phenotype in psoriasis. Interestingly, regarding the possible interplay between *C. albicans* and *S. pyogenes* and the IL-23/Th17 axis, it has been recently shown that *C. albicans* stimulates dendritic cells to release IL-23 (33). There is a complex interplay between these two microbes and CLA$^+$ T cells in psoriasis; however, the influence of microbes in psoriasis may be more complex that originally believed since microbiota studies demonstrate the presence of a range of microorganisms in psoriatic lesions (34). The functional relevance of these microorganisms for the disease has not been determined (35).

In summary, the observations made to date suggest that circulating CLA$^+$ T cells in psoriasis patients produce increased amounts of IL-17A, IL-17F, and IL-9, in comparison to healthy controls, when activated by *S. pyogenes* (**Figure 1**). Interestingly, the response to *C. albicans* is restricted mainly to CLA$^+$ T cells in cocultures with autologous epidermal cells in psoriasis with a similar cytokine profile. Psoriatic lesions produce several chemokines to attract skin-seeking CLA$^+$ T cells (21) with IL-17 capacity to the skin with potential to induce IL-17-dependent autoantigens and promote and maintain lesion activity. The study of the cutaneous immune response of CLA$^+$ T cells allows us to gain insight into how environmental factors, such microbes, shape psoriasis inflammation.

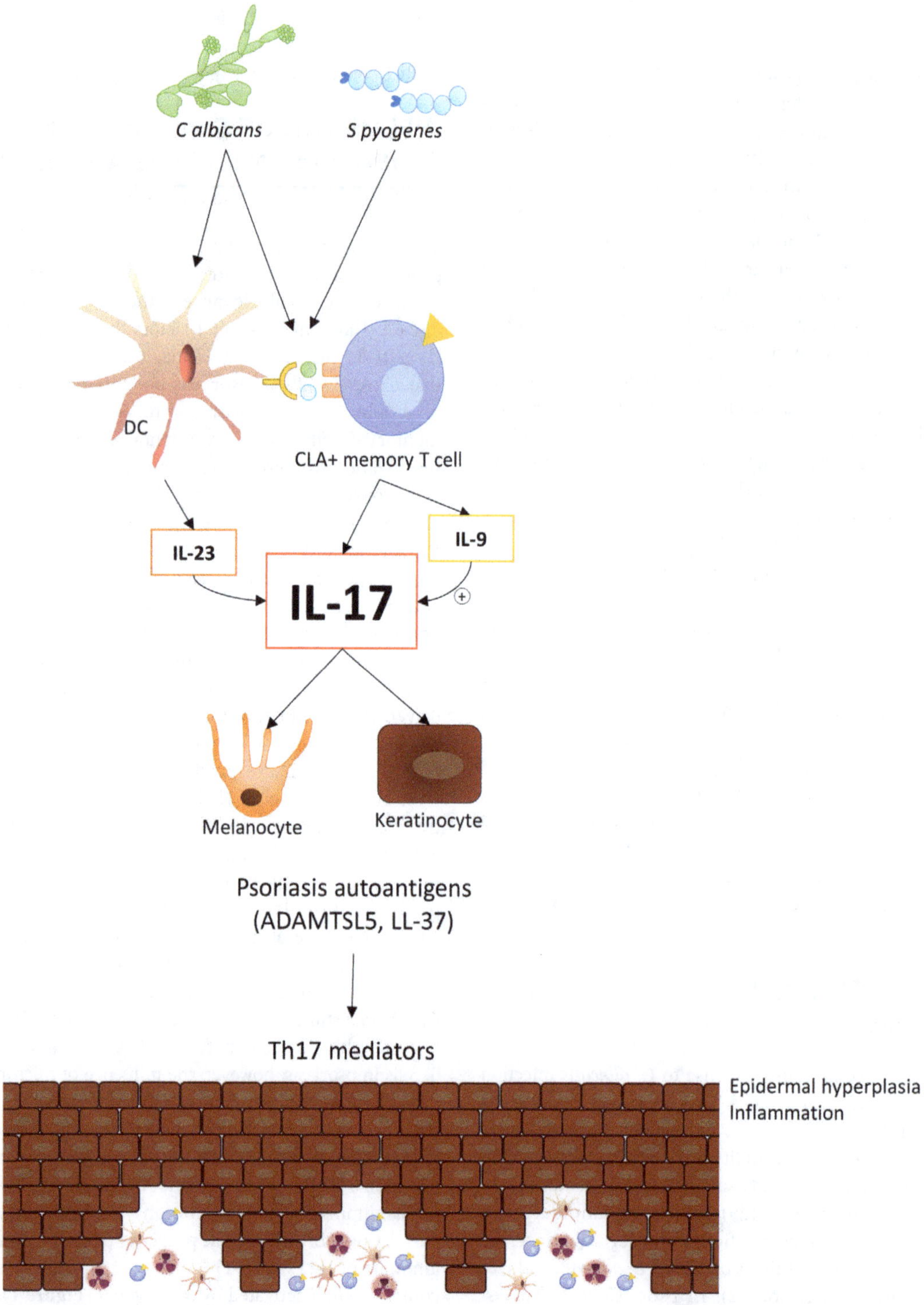

FIGURE 1 | *Candida albicans* and *Streptococcus pyogenes* induce IL-17 response in circulating CLA+ T cells in psoriasis, thereby indicating an established adaptive immune response to these microorganisms in this disease. Upon migration to cutaneous lesions, these cells react with those microbes and locally trigger IL-17 and IL-9 production, which will contribute to inducing psoriasis autoantigens.

AUTHOR CONTRIBUTIONS

All authors listed have made a substantial, direct, and intellectual contribution to the work and approved it for publication. LFSB conceived the ideas and together drafted the manuscript. All authors revised and approved the final version of the manuscript.

REFERENCES

1. Hawkes JE, Chan TC, Krueger JG. Psoriasis pathogenesis and the development of novel targeted immune therapies. *J Allergy Clin Immunol* (2017) 140:645–53. doi:10.1016/j.jaci.2017.07.004
2. Fry L, Baker BS. Triggering psoriasis: the role of infections and medications. *Clin Dermatol* (2007) 25:606–15. doi: 10.1016/j.clindermatol.2007.08.015
3. Henseler T, Christophers E. Psoriasis of early and late onset: characterization of two types of psoriasis vulgaris. *J Am Acad Dermatol* (1985) 13:450–6. doi:10.1016/S0190-9622(85)70188-0
4. Mallbris L, Larsson P, Bergqvist S, Vingard E, Granath F, Stahle M. Psoriasis phenotype at disease onset: clinical characterization of 400 adult cases. *J Invest Dermatol* (2005) 124:499–504. doi:10.1111/j.0022-202X.2004.23611.x
5. Mallbris L, Wolk K, Sanchez F, Stahle M. HLA-Cw*0602 associates with a twofold higher prevalence of positive streptococcal throat swab at the onset of psoriasis: a case control study. *BMC Dermatol* (2009) 9:5. doi:10.1186/1471-5945-9-5
6. Theodorakopoulou E, Yiu ZZ, Bundy C, Chularojanamontri L, Gittins M, Jamieson LA, et al. Early- and late-onset psoriasis: a cross-sectional clinical and immunocytochemical investigation. *Br J Dermatol* (2016) 175:1038–44. doi:10.1111/bjd.14886
7. Norrlind R. The significance of infections in the origination of psoriasis. *Acta Rheumatol Scand* (1955) 1:135–44. doi:10.3109/03009745509164855
8. Tervaert WC, Esseveld H. A study of the incidence of haemolytic streptococci in the throat in patients with psoriasis vulgaris, with reference to their role in the pathogenesis of this disease. *Dermatologica* (1970) 140:282–90. doi:10.1159/000252565
9. Wardrop P, Weller R, Marais J, Kavanagh G. Tonsillitis and chronic psoriasis. *Clin Otolaryngol Allied Sci* (1998) 23:67–8. doi:10.1046/j.1365-2273.1998.00084.x
10. Gudjonsson JE, Thorarinsson AM, Sigurgeirsson B, Kristinsson KG, Valdimarsson H. Streptococcal throat infections and exacerbation of chronic plaque psoriasis: a prospective study. *Br J Dermatol* (2003) 149:530–4. doi:10.1046/j.1365-2133.2003.05552.x
11. Munz OH, Sela S, Baker BS, Griffiths CE, Powles AV, Fry L. Evidence for the presence of bacteria in the blood of psoriasis patients. *Arch Dermatol Res* (2010) 302:495–8. doi:10.1007/s00403-010-1065-0
12. Thorleifsdottir RH, Sigurdardottir SL, Sigurgeirsson B, Olafsson JH, Sigurdsson MI, Petersen H, et al. Patient-reported outcomes and clinical response in patients with moderate-to-severe plaque psoriasis treated with tonsillectomy: a randomized controlled trial. *Acta Derm Venereol* (2017) 97:340–5. doi:10.2340/00015555-2562
13. Sigurdardottir SL, Thorleifsdottir RH, Valdimarsson H, Johnston A. The association of sore throat and psoriasis might be explained by histologically distinctive tonsils and increased expression of skin-homing molecules by tonsil T cells. *Clin Exp Immunol* (2013) 174:139–51. doi:10.1111/cei.12153
14. Valdimarsson H, Thorleifsdottir RH, Sigurdardottir SL, Gudjonsson JE, Johnston A. Psoriasis – as an autoimmune disease caused by molecular mimicry. *Trends Immunol* (2009) 30:494–501. doi:10.1016/j.it.2009.07.008
15. Nestle FO, Conrad C, Tun-Kyi A, Homey B, Gombert M, Boyman O, et al. Plasmacytoid predendritic cells initiate psoriasis through interferon-alpha production. *J Exp Med* (2005) 202:135–43. doi:10.1084/jem.20050500
16. Bissonnette R, Papp K, Maari C, Yao Y, Robbie G, White WI, et al. A randomized, double-blind, placebo-controlled, phase I study of MEDI-545, an anti-interferon-alfa monoclonal antibody, in subjects with chronic psoriasis. *J Am Acad Dermatol* (2010) 62:427–36. doi:10.1016/j.jaad.2009.05.042
17. Picker LJ, Michie SA, Rott LS, Butcher EC. A unique phenotype of skin-associated lymphocytes in humans. Preferential expression of the HECA-452 epitope by benign and malignant T cells at cutaneous sites. *Am J Pathol* (1990) 136:1053–68.
18. Ferran M, Romeu ER, Rincon C, Sagrista M, Gimenez Arnau AM, Celada A, et al. Circulating CLA+ T lymphocytes as peripheral cell biomarkers in T-cell-mediated skin diseases. *Exp Dermatol* (2013) 22:439–42. doi:10.1111/exd.12154
19. Czarnowicki T, Santamaria-Babi LF, Guttman-Yassky E. Circulating CLA(+) T cells in atopic dermatitis and their possible role as peripheral biomarkers. *Allergy* (2017) 72:366–72. doi:10.1111/all.13080
20. Ferran M, Galvan AB, Rincon C, Romeu ER, Sacrista M, Barboza E, et al. *Streptococcus* induces circulating CLA(+) memory T-cell-dependent epidermal cell activation in psoriasis. *J Invest Dermatol* (2013) 133:999–1007. doi:10.1038/jid.2012.418
21. Ruiz-Romeu E, Ferran M, Sagrista M, Gomez J, Gimenez-Arnau A, Herszenyi K, et al. *Streptococcus pyogenes*-induced cutaneous lymphocyte antigen-positive T cell-dependent epidermal cell activation triggers TH17 responses in patients with guttate psoriasis. *J Allergy Clin Immunol* (2016) 138:491–9. doi:10.1016/j.jaci.2016.02.008
22. Schlapbach C, Gehad A, Yang C, Watanabe R, Guenova E, Teague JE, et al. Human TH9 cells are skin-tropic and have autocrine and paracrine proinflammatory capacity. *Sci Transl Med* (2014) 6:219ra8. doi:10.1126/scitranslmed.3007828
23. Singh TP, Schon MP, Wallbrecht K, Gruber-Wackernagel A, Wang XJ, Wolf P. Involvement of IL-9 in Th17-associated inflammation and angiogenesis of psoriasis. *PLoS One* (2013) 8:e51752. doi:10.1371/journal.pone.0051752
24. Ruiz-Romeu E, Ferran M, de Jesus-Gil C, Garcia P, Sagrista M, Casanova JM, et al. Microbe-dependent induction of IL-9 by CLA(+) T cells in psoriasis and relationship with IL-17A. *J Invest Dermatol* (2018) 138:580–7. doi:10.1016/j.jid.2017.08.048
25. El-Rachkidy RG, Hales JM, Freestone PP, Young HS, Griffiths CE, Camp RD. Increased blood levels of IgG reactive with secreted Streptococcus pyogenes proteins in chronic plaque psoriasi. *J Invest Dermatol* (2007) 127:1337–42. doi:10.1038/sj.jid.5700744
26. Fahlen A, Engstrand L, Baker BS, Powles A, Fry L. Comparison of bacterial microbiota in skin biopsies from normal and psoriatic skin. *Arch Dermatol Res* (2012) 304:15–22. doi:10.1007/s00403-011-1189-x
27. Kashem SW, Kaplan DH. Skin immunity to *Candida albicans*. *Trends Immunol* (2016) 37:440–50. doi:10.1016/j.it.2016.04.007
28. de Beaucoudrey L, Puel A, Filipe-Santos O, Cobat A, Ghandil P, Chrabieh M, et al. Mutations in STAT3 and IL12RB1 impair the development of human IL-17-producing T cells. *J Exp Med* (2008) 205:1543–50. doi:10.1084/jem.20080321
29. Becattini S, Latorre D, Mele F, Foglierini M, De GC, Cassotta A, et al. T cell immunity. Functional heterogeneity of human memory CD4(+) T cell clones primed by pathogens or vaccines. *Science* (2015) 347:400–6. doi:10.1126/science.1260668
30. Leung DY, Walsh P, Giorno R, Norris DA. A potential role for superantigens in the pathogenesis of psoriasis. *J Invest Dermatol* (1993) 100:225–8. doi:10.1111/1523-1747.ep12468941
31. Walsh P, Norris DA, Abe J, Martin DK, Giorno R, Leung DY. *Candida albicans* induces selective expansion of human T lymphocytes expressing the T-cell receptor variable region V beta 5.1. *J Dermatol Sci* (1996) 12:140–6. doi:10.1016/0923-1811(95)00473-4
32. Kim J, Krueger JG. Highly effective new treatments for psoriasis target the IL-23/type 17 T cell autoimmune axis. *Annu Rev Med* (2017) 68:255–69. doi:10.1146/annurev-med-042915-103905
33. Maher CO, Dunne K, Comerford R, O'Dea S, Loy A, Woo J, et al. *Candida albicans* stimulates IL-23 release by human dendritic cells and downstream IL-17 secretion by Vdelta1 T cells. *J Immunol* (2015) 194:5953–60. doi:10.4049/jimmunol.1403066
34. Gao Z, Tseng CH, Strober BE, Pei Z, Blaser MJ. Substantial alterations of the cutaneous bacterial biota in psoriatic lesions. *PLoS One* (2008) 3:e2719. doi:10.1371/journal.pone.0002719
35. Langan EA, Griffiths CEM, Solbach W, Knobloch JK, Zillikens D, Thaci D. The role of the microbiome in psoriasis: moving from disease description to treatment selection? *Br J Dermatol* (2018) 178(5):1020–7. doi:10.1111/bjd.16081

18

The IL-17 Family of Cytokines in Psoriasis: IL-17A and Beyond

Nicolo Costantino Brembilla[1]*, Luisa Senra[1] and Wolf-Henning Boehncke[1,2]

[1] Department of Pathology and Immunology, Faculty of Medicine, University of Geneva, Geneva, Switzerland,
[2] Division of Dermatology and Venereology, Geneva University Hospitals, Geneva, Switzerland

****Correspondence:***
Nicolo Costantino Brembilla
nicolo.brembilla@unige.ch

Psoriasis is a frequent chronic inflammatory skin disease, nowadays considered a major global health problem. Several new drugs, targeting the IL-23/IL-17A pathway, have been recently licensed or are in clinical development. These therapies represent a major improvement of the way in which psoriasis is managed, since they show an unprecedented efficacy on skin symptoms of psoriasis. This has been made possible, thanks to an increasingly more accurate pathogenic view of psoriasis. Today, the belief that Th17 cells mediate psoriasis is moving to the concept of psoriasis as an IL-17A-driven disease. New questions arise at the horizon, given that IL-17A is part of a newly described family of cytokines, which has five distinct homologous: IL-17B, IL-17C, IL-17D, IL-17E, also known as IL-25 and IL-17F. IL-17 family cytokines elicit similar effects in target cells, but simultaneously trigger different and sometimes opposite functions in a tissue-specific manner. This is complicated by the fact that IL-17 cytokines show a high capacity of synergisms with other inflammatory stimuli. In this review, we will summarize the current knowledge around the cytokines belonging to the IL-17 family in relation to skin inflammation in general and psoriasis in particular, and discuss possible clinical implications. A comprehensive understanding of the different roles played by the IL-17 cytokines is crucial to appreciate current and developing therapies and to allow an effective pathogenesis- and mechanisms-driven drug design.

Keywords: psoriasis, IL-17 family, IL-25, IL-17E, interleukin, comorbidities, Th17 cells, IL-17A

INTRODUCTION

Psoriasis is a frequent, chronic, non-communicable inflammatory skin disease, for which there is no clear cause or cure. Psoriasis affects people of all countries and of all ages. The disease manifests as well-defined, red, scaly plaques, appearing with a chronic-recurrent course at preferential sites such as elbows, knees, and scalp. Individuals with psoriasis are at an increased risk of developing other chronic and serious diseases, including psoriatic arthritis, metabolic syndrome, cardiovascular diseases, and depression (1–3). The negative impact of psoriasis on people's lives can be immense. Disfiguration and disability are common aspects experienced by patients, who are in addition challenged by emotional and social burden caused by psoriasis stigmatization. In 2014, the Executive Board of the Word Health Organization became spokesman of more than 100 million people affected worldwide, approving a resolution to raise awareness of psoriasis as a major global health problem (4).

Psoriatic hallmark features include profound modification of the epidermis, such as hyperproliferation and altered differentiation of keratinocytes, concurrent with the presence of a prominent inflammatory infiltrate and neo-angiogenesis. T cells, along with innate immune cells, are thought to produce a key effector cytokine, IL-17A, which then triggers the epidermal modification (1). The emergence of a detailed pathogenic concept in the last decade has fueled the development of targeted therapies. Thus, treatments have moved from broad immunosuppression to interference with T cells and the IL-23/IL-17 pathway, and nowadays to downstream effector molecules such as IL-17A and its cell targets (5).

IL-17A was initially thought to be a "unique" cytokine, exclusively produced by T cells in psoriasis. To date, it is evident that many other cells contribute to the bulk of IL-17A found in the diseased skin, and that many isoforms of IL-17 may participate to psoriasis. These data open a new scenario for innovative therapeutic interventions, as our knowledge of the pathophysiology of psoriasis becomes more precise. This review will briefly debate the role of IL-17A as key effector molecule, retracing the key discoveries that led to the current understanding of psoriasis as an IL-17A driven disease. This will lead to an in-depth discussion of the IL-17 family of cytokines and the contribution of IL-17 isoforms other than IL-17A to psoriasis manifestations in the skin and its comorbidities. Finally, the clinical implications will be addressed.

PSORIASIS: AN IL-17A-DRIVEN DISEASE

In the 1960, psoriasis was thought to be a primary disease of the epidermis caused by hyperproliferative keratinocytes. The involvement of the immune system became apparent only in the 1980, when lymphocyte-targeted therapies were proven to be an effective way to treat the disease (6, 7). The pathogenesis of psoriasis was initially proposed to rely on Th1 responses, based on the identification of elevated expression of Th1 cytokines, such as IFNγ, TNFα, and IL-12, in the lesion (8). In the wake of these results, a monoclonal antibody (ustekinumab) designed to block the p40 subunit of IL-12, key factor in Th1 cell commitment, was developed. This antibody showed the highest therapeutical efficacy ever observed at that time. Concomitant to ustekinumab generation, a second cytokine, named IL-23, was found to contain the identical p40 subunit (9). The "unwanted" blockade of this latter cytokine turned out to be the more relevant mechanism of action in the context of treating psoriasis.

In the mid 2000s, IL-23 was shown to induce the production of IL-17 by activated T lymphocytes, later named Th17 cells (10, 11). These cells, which express RORγt as master transcription factor, have limited inherent pathogenicity and promote mucosal defense, whereas exposure to IL-23 turns them into autoimmune-associated inflammatory cells (12). The involvement of IL-23 in psoriasis was supported by its ability to induce psoriasiform characteristics in a preclinical model of intradermal administration (13); a phenotype linked to the infiltration of IL-22- and IL-17A-producing T cells (14). Th17 cells became thus the center of extensive research, and the hallmark cytokine IL-17A was identified as a novel key effector pathogenic factor in psoriasis.

Genome-wide association studies also confirm the role of the immune system in the pathogenesis of psoriasis, with the HLA-Cw6 allele accounting for almost 50% of the disease heritability. Variations in loci containing genes involved in the IL-23/Th17 signaling are frequently observed and suggest the particular involvement of Th17 cells: these include genes upstream of the IL-17 expression, such as IL-23R and IL-12B, or downstream the IL-17 receptor, such as STAT3 and Act1 (15). No variants in the IL-17A gene itself was shown to predispose to psoriasis so far, whereas the IL-17RA allele rs4819554 was recently associated with risk of developing psoriasis in a Spanish cohort (16).

The central role of IL-17A in the pathophysiology of psoriasis has recently been reviewed elsewhere (17) and will only be briefly described here. IL-17A mainly acts on non-hematopoietic cells, particularly epithelial cells, and consistently participates in protective immunity at boundary tissues. With regard to the skin, IL-17A leads to increased proliferation and aberrant differentiation of keratinocytes (18) and contributes to skin barrier disruption by downregulating the expression of molecules involved in keratinocyte differentiation, such as fillagrin (19). In addition, IL-17A participates in generating and amplifying the inflammatory network by promoting the release of antimicrobial peptides and proinflammatory cytokines/chemokines (20, 21). The factors induced by IL-17A are poised toward the activation of a neutrophil/Th17 cell-dependent immune response. These include IL-8, a potent neutrophil chemoattractant; G-CSF, a survival factor for neutrophils; CCL20 that favors Th17 cell recruitment; and the key Th17 polarizing cytokines IL-1β and IL-6. In addition, IL-17A directly contributes to leukocyte migration and tissue remodeling by promoting the secretion of metalloproteases. To note, IL-17A synergizes with and potentiates the effects of many other inflammatory mediators, possibly *via* stabilization of target mRNA. IL-10 and IL-1 family members, as well as type-I cytokines, such as TNFα, are the most relevant factors in this regard (22–24). The genes synergistically upregulated by TNFα and IL-17A in keratinocytes were shown to mimic the gene signature observed in the lesional skin, underling the importance of these integrative responses (23). Similarly, IL-17A, together with TNF and IL-22, were reported to upregulate the expression of the IL-1 like family member IL-36, which in turn was found to augment the function of Th17 cytokines, revealing the existence of a feedback loop between Th17 and IL-36 cytokines (24). These cytokine networks may also be of particular importance to distinguish different forms of psoriasis: inactivating mutation of the IL36RN gene, which encodes the IL-36 receptor antagonist, have been particularly associated with generalized pustular psoriasis (25). The importance of IL-17A and its interaction with other cytokines has also extensively been proved in murine models of psoriasiform inflammation, through the use of deficient mice and in neutralizing experiments. Finally, the first biologics following ustekinumab that entered the market of anti-psoriatics were specific anti IL-17A antibodies, namely secukinumab and ixekizumab (26, 27). Stressing the importance of IL-17A, these therapies represent the most effective approach to treat psoriasis so far.

The effects of IL-17A are not limited to keratinocytes and encompass several other cells, including endothelial cells, fibroblasts, chondrocytes, and synovial cells. IL-17A is clearly of major importance also in the context of psoriasis-associated comorbidity, namely, psoriatic arthritis and cardiovascular disease/atherosclerosis, as highlighted elsewhere (28, 29) and summarized in **Table 1**.

TABLE 1 | Overview of the role exerted by IL-17A in inflammation.

Skin inflammation - *Human/patient data*: IL-17A is increased in several skin disorders, including psoriasis, atopic dermatitis as well as neutrophilic, granulomatous, and bullous skin diseases (30) - *Animal models*: IL-17A contributes to skin inflammation in multiple models of cutaneous inflammation, including IMQ application and K5hTGFβ1 transgenic mice (17).
Joint inflammation - *Human/patient data*: IL-17A is expressed in the synovium of RA and PsA patients and promotes bone-destructive cytokine production and bone resorption *in vitro* (28) - *Animal models*: IL-17A contributes to the immune-inflammatory events in CIA and other models of arthritis (28)
Gut inflammation - *Human/patient data*: IL17A expression is increased in inflammatory bowel disease, while neutralization of IL-17A has no effect or rather exacerbate CD (31). - *Animal models*: IL-17A neutralization exacerbates symptoms in DSS and CD4+ t cell transfer model of colitis, while reduced pathology in an IL-10-deficient colitogenic model. IL-17A has important roles in preserving the intestinal epithelial barrier in DSS mice (32, 33)
CNS - *Human/patient data:* IL-17A levels are increased in MS lesions and peripheral blood (34) - *Animal models:* IL-17A plays an important role in EAE (35)
Cardiovascular disease - *Human/patient data*: IL-17A/Th17 cells are increased in patients with acute coronary syndrome and correlate with systemic inflammation markers (36) - *Animal models*: IL-17A inhibition results in the reduction of the size of atherosclerotic plaques in apoE deficient mice (37)

CNS, central nervous system; IMQ, imiquimod; RA, rheumatoid arthritis; CIA, collagen-induced arthritis; CD, Crohn's disease; DSS, dextran-sulfate sodium; MS, multiple sclerosis; EAE, experimental autoimmune encephalomyelitis.

The current view of the pathogenesis of psoriasis relies thus on pathogenic Th17 cells, which arise following an unknown trigger in genetically predisposed individuals as result of the production of Th17 polarizing cytokines by myeloid cells. The antimicrobial peptide LL37, in complex with nucleic acids released by dying cells, has been proposed as a possible autoantigen driving the activation of cutaneous plasmacytoid and myeloid DCs (38). Th17 cells would travel back to the skin, where they directly activate keratinocytes *via* the release of effector cytokines, among which IL-17A is the most important. Activated keratinocytes proliferate in an abnormal manner and release further inflammatory mediators and chemokines amplifying the inflammatory response (1).

Recent findings provide new evidence that is slightly but definitely changing the paradigmatic view of the pathogenesis of psoriasis: from Th17- to IL-17A-driven disease (**Figure 1**). Reich and colleagues demonstrated that a single dose of the anti-IL-17A antibody secukinumab resulted in skin normalization as soon as 2 weeks after injection, a finding paralleled by disappearance of IL-17A + neutrophils but not T cells (39). Meanwhile, many immune cells other than Th17 lymphocytes, globally called "Type 17" cells, were reported to release IL-17A. Many of them are thymus dependent, including adaptive and natural Th17 cells, T CD8 cells, γδ T cells, and invariant NKT (iNKT) cells; others are rather thymus independent, such as group 3 innate lymphoid cells (ILC), mast cells, and neutrophils (12, 40, 41). Th17 cells, with the exception of tissue-resident memory cells, reside in lymphoid organs in steady state and drain peripheral tissues only in inflammatory situations. Conversely, the other cells are found at the periphery, particularly at mucosal and skin tissues, thus representing a potential immediate source of IL-17A. Of interest, in lesional psoriatic skin, at least from a histological point of view, IL-17A + T cells are sparse, while the bulk of IL-17A-expressing cells is represented by neutrophils and mast cells (42, 43). Whether being still debated, neutrophils and mast cells appear to actively synthetize IL-17A in the skin, and release IL-17A, at least in part, *via* extracellular trap formation (40, 42). The abovementioned subsets express RORγt and the IL-23R, and require IL-23 for their effective activation (12). This might explain why targeting specifically IL-23 through blockade of the p19 subunits represents a promising therapeutic option, even in a scenario dominated by anti-IL-17A treatments (44). IL-17A production can, however, also occur in both γδ and iNKT cells independently of IL-23 (45, 46).

The idea that psoriasis is purely a Th17 cell-dependent disease is thus replaced by the concept of psoriasis as an IL-17A-driven disease (**Figure 1**). This further evolution of the pathogenic concept opens new questions, which will likely allow a better understanding of the disease and a rational drug design. One of these questions is whether IL-17A has "homologous" cytokines, which would be simultaneously produced, and which might substitute for or synergize with IL-17A, or affect sites other than the skin such as the joints. In the next sections, we will thus discuss the IL-17 family of cytokines and its implication in psoriatic skin inflammation.

AN OVERVIEW OF THE IL-17 FAMILY OF CYTOKINES

IL-17A, originally termed CTLA-8, was cloned in 1993 from a rodent-activated T cell hybridoma (47). Its amino acid sequence is unusual for a cytokine, being 58% identical to the open reading frame of the T cell-tropic gammaherpesvirus *Herpesvirus samiri* (48). In the early 2000s, genomic sequencing led to the identification of several proteins structurally related to IL-17A: IL-17B, IL-17C, IL-17D, IL-17E (also called IL-25) and IL-17F. Together, these cytokines are known as the IL-17 family. IL-17F shares the highest homology with IL-17A (55%) and is often co-expressed with IL-17A (49). IL-17B, IL-17D, and IL-17C sequences overlap from 29 to 23% with IL-17A, while IL-17E appears to be the most divergent member of the family, sharing only 16% sequence homology. The members of the IL-17 family exert their functions as disulfide-linked homodimers, with a molecular weight of the monomer ranging from 17 to 21 kDa. As an exception to the rule, IL-17A and IL-17F can also form heterodimers.

History repeated itself for the IL-17 receptor. Discovered in 1995, the IL-17R did not fall into any previously known class of receptors (48). Later, it was discovered the existence of five homologous subunits, namely IL-17RA to IL-17RE, which

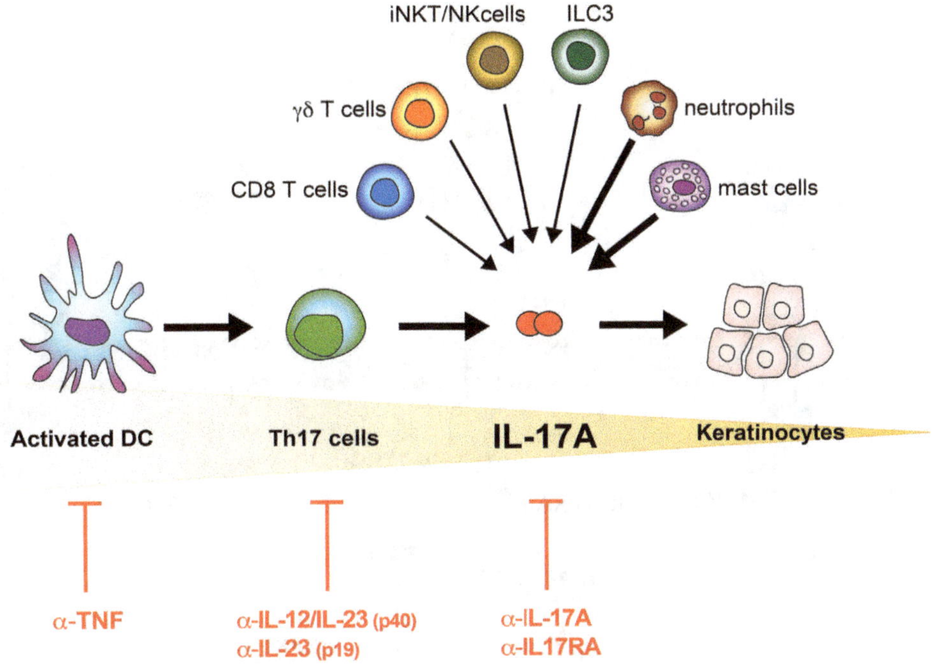

FIGURE 1 | IL-17A in the pathogenesis of psoriasis. Schematic representation of the increasingly accurate selection of therapeutic targets in psoriasis. The cells possibly contributing to the bulk of IL-17A in lesional psoriatic skin are shown. Bolded arrows indicate higher contribution to IL-17A production in psoriatic lesional skin.

together are now classified as a new class of receptors: the IL-17R family. All IL-17 cytokines signal *via* a heterodimeric receptor composed by a different combination of these subunits (**Figure 2**). IL-17A homodimers, IL-17F homodimers, and IL-17A/F heterodimers bind to the same receptor complex, comprising IL-17RA and IL-17RC subunits. IL-17RA is also the co-receptor used by two additional IL-17 family members, associated to IL-17RB mediates IL-17E signaling, bound to IL-17RE transduces signals by IL-17C. All subunits of the IL-17R family exhibit a broad expression pattern, with IL-17RA being ubiquitous (50).

All receptor subunits are single transmembrane chains sharing unique properties. The extracellular region of the IL-17R family members contains two fibronectin III-like (FN) domains, which mediate protein–protein interactions and ligand binding. The cytoplasmic region, at the C-terminus, contains a conserved sequence known as SEFIR (similar expression of fibroblast growth factor genes and IL-17Rs) domain. This region, which helped defining the IL-17 family as a new receptor class, is related to the TIR (toll/interleukin-1 receptor) domain found in IL-1 and toll-like receptor family. While having many features in common with the signaling induced by these innate receptors, the IL-17R-induced pathway has notable differences (12, 51). The study of the interaction of IL-17A with its receptor has generated many insights in that regard, as briefly described below and extensively discussed elsewhere (51, 52). The most striking difference is the unique usage of a cytoplasmic protein, called Act1, which also contains a SEFIR domain. Upon ligand binding, this molecule is engaged to the IL-17R complex through homotypic SEFIR interactions to mediate downstream events (53). Recruitment of Act1 represents a hallmark of IL-17 signaling, an event not shared by any other known class of receptors. Act-1 activates several independent signaling pathways operating as a docking station for different TRAF proteins. Upon recruitment of TRAF6 and its ubiquitination (Act1 may indeed function as E3 ubiquitin ligase), a cascade of molecular interactions is turned on, leading to the phosphorylation and consequent proteasomal degradation of IκB, ultimately allowing the nuclear translocation of NFκB and the activation of NFκB targeted genes (54–56). Although less clear mechanistically, TRAF6 has been also linked to the activation of MAPK pathways, including ERK, p38, and JNK, and C/EBP molecules (51). By recruiting TRAF2/5, Act-1 favors the sequestration of RNA decay factor, such as SF2 (57), as well as the activation of RNA-binding proteins as, such HuR (58), which results in increased mRNA stability of target genes. Thus, the signaling pathways downstream the IL-17A receptor may induce at least two distinct events: *de novo* inflammatory gene transcription and stabilization of target mRNA (**Figure 2**). Whether the other members of the IL-17 family similarly activate these pathways is unknown, but highly probable.

One peculiarity of IL-17s is that they are not strong inducers of signaling when acting in an isolated manner. Early reports have shown the implication of NFκB in mediating the pro-inflammatory role of IL-17A in fibroblasts and synoviocytes. However, IL-17A resulted to be far less potent than other inflammatory molecules, such as TNF. Nevertheless, IL-17A is an extremely powerful inducer of inflammation due to its capacity to

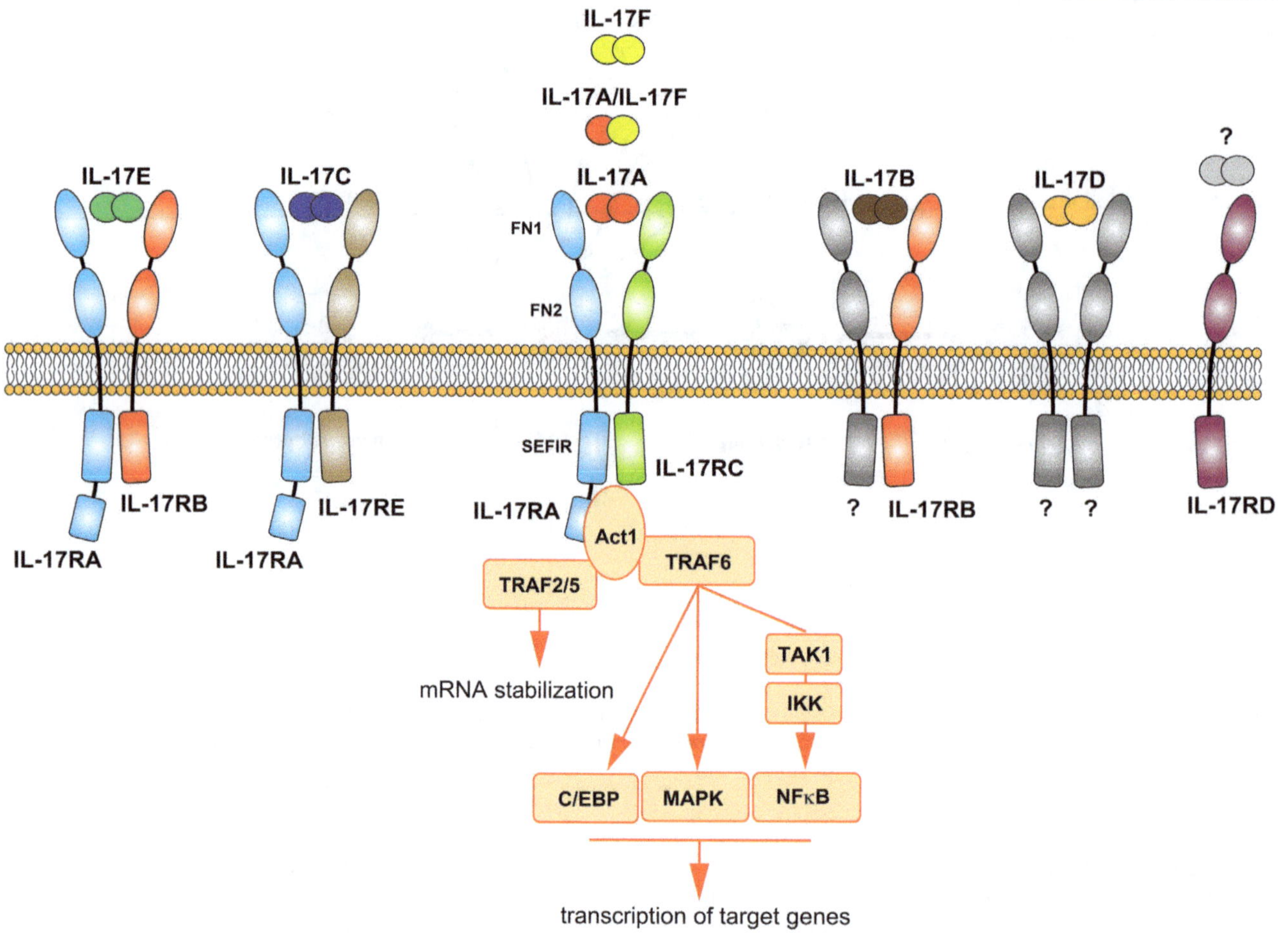

FIGURE 2 | The IL-17 family of cytokines. Schematic representation of the different IL-17 cytokines and their receptors. The main signaling events downstream the activation of the IL-17A receptor are summarized.

synergistically act with other stimuli. In the case of TNF, IL-17A helps stabilizing the mRNA of the TNF-activated genes, which are inherently unstable, leading to a great amplification of TNF effects (59, 60). Therefore, even though in isolated experimental conditions, IL-17A does not appear to be potent, its physiological impact *in vivo* could be profound. An additional feature of the IL-17 family is that IL-17 cytokines might regulate several genes in a tissue-specific fashion. For instance, IL-17A was shown to induce the production of occludin specifically in the gut, where it helps maintaining the intestinal barrier integrity (46), or favor the release of kallikrein 1 by renal epithelial cells, conferring protection against candidiasis (61).

High capacity of synergy and tissue-specific functions are features shared by several members of the IL-17 family. As shown below, a considerable functional overlap, as well as main differences, characterizes the members of the IL-17 family. The following section will describe the contribution of each IL-17 family member to psoriasis, while especially focusing on isoforms other than IL-17A, as this latter has recently extensively been reviewed elsewhere (17).

IL-17s IN PSORIASIS: BEYOND IL-17A

IL-17F

IL-17F, discovered in 2001 on chromosome 6p12 (the same locus as IL-17A!), is the most homologous cytokine to IL-17A and signals *via* a receptor composed by the IL-17RA and IL-17RC subunits (again, the same used by IL-17A). IL-17F levels are elevated in sera and lesional psoriatic skin compared to non-lesional tissue (62, 63). Despite that, no specific polymorphisms in the IL-17F gene have so far been associated with psoriasis susceptibility, although the IL-17F polymorphism rs763780 was linked to a better response to anti-TNF therapy (64). IL-17F is also increased in sera of atopic dermatitis patients and positively correlates with higher clinical score (65). Additional evidence of the involvement of IL-17F in psoriatic inflammation comes from experiments in mice models. Indeed, IL-17F together with IL-17A and IL-22, are rapidly induced upon imiquimod application, as result of infiltration of γδ T cells and RORγt + innate lymphocytes. Of interest, IL-17F$^{-/-}$ mice show a higher disease resistance than IL-17A$^{-/-}$ mice (66, 67).

Both IL-17A and IL-17F are expressed by the same immune cell types, including Th17 cells, γδ T cells and ILC3. Human *IL17A* and *IL17F* genes are found in the same locus and are genetically co-regulated, thus it is not surprising that these cytokines are often co-expressed (49). IL-23 participates in IL-17A and IL-17F co-production in Th17 cells (10). As mentioned earlier, IL-17A and IL-17F can be secreted as homodimers or IL-17A/IL-17F heterodimers. IL-17F has been shown to stimulate *in vitro* a qualitative similar pattern of genes than IL-17A, although being generally weaker, with IL-17A/IL-17F heterodimers having an intermediate potency (52). However, this is not always true, either in cell- and target-specific situations or because of synergism with other inflammatory mediators. Thus, IL-17F was shown to be more potent than IL-17A, or even TNF, to induce IL-8 and IL-6 production in normal human epidermal keratinocytes (68, 69). Or, though less potent in absolute terms, IL-17F was shown to be almost as potent as IL-17A when combined with TNF in RA synoviocytes (60, 70). Moreover, IL-17A and IL-17F have been shown to synergistically act, since their dual neutralization leads to greater downregulation of inflammatory mediators than IL-17A blockade alone in skin and joint fibroblasts (71).

With respect to their similar functions, both cytokines are needed for effective responses against mucoepithelial bacterial infections and synergistically cooperate to protect the host from fungal infections (72, 73). Consistently, inborn errors of IL-17F, as well as of IL-17RA or ACT1, display chronic mucocutaneous candidiasis (74). Candida infections are also a common adverse event observed upon anti-IL-17A or anti-IL-17RA-targeted therapies. Whether bi-specific antibodies blocking both IL-17A and IL-17F have an increased risk of Candidiasis is not yet known. Despite having similar, and sometimes even synergistic actions *in vitro*, knock-out experiments in mice revealed also diverse roles of IL-17A and IL-17F in complex *in vivo* inflammatory settings. This might well reflect tissue-specific functions and the capacity of IL-17 cytokines to synergize with other inflammatory mediators. IL-17F, at difference to IL-17A, is not required in several T-cell-dependent autoimmune diseases in mice, while being pathogenic in DSS colitis model and in acute allergic responses in the lung (72, 75–78). Nevertheless, IL-17F gene expression is increased in human active Crohn's disease (CD) and multiple sclerosis (79, 80). Finally, IL-17F was associated with increased susceptibility in many forms of human cancer, while playing rather a protective role in colon tumorigenesis in mice (81). **Table 2** shows an overview of the role of IL-17F in inflammation.

In summary, IL-17F acts in a similar manner as IL-17A, although being generally weaker. IL-17F might contribute to skin manifestations and comorbidities of psoriasis in a tissue-specific fashion. The function of IL-17F may become prominent in complex cytokine milieus, and preclinical data suggest that it might be pathogenic in both joint and gut inflammation.

TABLE 2 | Overview of the role exerted by IL-17F in inflammation.

Skin inflammation - *Human/patient data*: IL-17F is increased in psoriatic lesional skin. Elevated levels of IL-17F are found in sera from psoriatic and atopic dermatitis patients (62, 63, 65). - *Animal models*: IL-17F contributes to skin inflammation induced by IMQ application (66, 67).
Joint inflammation - *Human/patient data*: IL-17F is expressed in the synovial tissue from RA patients and contributes to human chronic joint inflammation *in vitro* and *in vivo* (62, 70, 71) - *Animal models*: IL-17F is increased in CIA (78), while playing only marginal roles on CIA and arthritis in Il1rn$^{-/-}$ mice (72, 74).
Gut inflammation - *Human/patient data*: IL17F gene expression is increased in active CD (80) - *Animal models*: IL-17F contributes to experimental induced colitis (76, 82)
CNS - *Human/patient data:* IL-17F mRNA is increased in mononuclear cells from MS patients (79) - *Animal models*: Neutralization of IL-17F (alone) does not prevent the development of EAE (77)
Cardiovascular disease - Not investigated yet

CNS, central nervous system; IMQ, imiquimod; RA, rheumatoid arthritis; CIA, collagen-induced arthritis; CD, Crohn's disease; MS, multiple sclerosis; EAE, experimental autoimmune encephalomyelitis.

TABLE 3 | Overview of the role exerted by IL-17B in inflammation.

Skin inflammation - *Human/patient data*: IL-17B mRNA levels are decreased in lesional psoriatic skin (62)
Joint inflammation - *Human/patient data*: IL-17B is expressed in RA and OA synovia, and RA pannus (83, 84). - *Animal models*: IL-17B contributes to the exacerbation of inflammatory arthritis in CIA model (78)
Gut inflammation - *Human/patient data*: IL-17B is expressed in the intestine and stomach, unknown function (85, 86)
CNS - *Human/patient data*: IL-17B is localized to the neuronal cell bodies and axons in humans. IL-17B gene maps to a region associated with a rare autosomal recessive form of Charcot–Marie–Tooth demyelinating disease (86). - *Animal models*: IL-17B is expressed by neurons of the cerebral cortex and the adjacent hippocampal (H) layer (86).
Cardiovascular disease - Not yet investigated

CNS, central nervous system; RA, rheumatoid arthritis; OA, osteoarthritis; CIA, collagen-induced arthritis.

IL-17B and IL-17D

Transcripts of IL-17B and IL-17D are decreased in psoriatic lesional skin when compared to non-lesional tissue (62). For that reason, they have not been studied in detail in the context of psoriasis. It is, however, relevant to briefly review their reported functions, as clinical targeting of IL-17 signaling molecules might also affect the functions of these isoforms. The roles exerted by IL-17B and IL-17D in inflammation are summarized in **Tables 3** and **4**, respectively.

IL-17B, discovered in 2000 on chromosome 5q32, is secreted as non-covalent dimer, and signals *via* a still unknown receptor

TABLE 4 | Overview of the role exerted by IL-17D in inflammation.

Skin inflammation - *Human/patient data*: IL-17D mRNA levels are decreased in lesional psoriatic skin, unknown function (62)
Joint inflammation - *Human/patient data*: IL-17D is expressed in the rheumatoid nodule, unknown function (83)
Gut inflammation - Not yet investigated
CNS - *Human/patient data*: IL-17D is expressed in the brain, unknown function (87)
Cardiovascular disease - *Human/patient data*: IL-17D is expressed in the heart, unknown function (87)

CNS, central nervous system.

containing the subunit IL-17RB. This latter is shared with the IL-17E receptor (12). Regarding the cells producing IL-17B, information is punctual. Activated T cells do not produce IL-17B, while IL-17B was found to be expressed in neutrophils, germinal center B cells, neurons and stromal cells, and gut epithelium (88). In terms of function, high expression of IL-17B was mainly linked to poor prognosis in cancer; such as breast and gastric cancer (88) Besides that, IL-17B could play a pathogenic role in the joint (78, 83, 84). IL-17B is overexpressed in the inflammatory cartilage of the collagen-induced arthritis mouse model, where it induces the production of IL-8 and the recruitment of neutrophils. Consistently, neutralizing antibodies targeting IL-17B ameliorates signs and symptoms in this model (78). Thus, while not being involved in skin manifestation of psoriasis, IL-17B was shown to play an important role in the pathogenesis of inflammatory arthritis in preclinical models (78, 84, 89).

IL-17D, cloned in 2002 and mapping to chromosome 13q12, is the cytokine most recently added to the IL-17 family. IL-17D is most homologous to IL-17B, with 27% identity. It is secreted as disulfide-linked homodimer and signals *via* a still unknown receptor. IL-17D is found in a variety of tissues, including skeletal muscle, brain, adipose, heart, lung, and pancreas, while is poorly expressed by activated immune cells, such as lymphocytes and monocytes (87). IL-17D levels have been reported increased in rheumatoid nodules (83). Although not directly stimulating immune cells, IL-17D has been shown to modulate the production of cytokines by endothelial cells. Similar to other members of the family, these include pro-inflammatory cytokines such as IL-6, IL-8, and GM-CSF. Despite that, IL-17D demonstrates an inhibitory effect on hematopoiesis of myeloid progenitors cells *in vitro* (87). In addition, IL-17D plays a role in the control of viral infections and cancer, as IL-17D deficiency predisposes animals to these conditions (90).

Taken together, the knowledge around IL-17B and IL-17D is still limited. Overall, these isoforms induce pro-inflammatory responses in non-immune cells, leading to regulation of tumor or joint immunity, at least in the case of IL-17B. The reason of their reduced expression in psoriasis remains unknown and awaits further investigation.

IL-17C

IL-17C was cloned at the same time as IL-17B in 2000. It maps to chromosome 16q24 and signals *via* a receptor composed by IL-17RA/IL-17RE subunits (85). IL17C shows only 23% homology with IL-17A, and unlike IL-17A, is expressed mainly by epithelial cells rather than immune cells. Much evidence links IL-17C to skin inflammation. Importantly, IL-17C is overexpressed in lesional skin of psoriatic (91, 92) and atopic dermatitis patients (93). IL-17C is secreted by epithelial cells *in vitro* in response to inflammatory stimuli, such as TNF and TLRs (91, 94, 95). Epithelial cells of the skin and the gut are also main targets of IL-17C, which acts in an autocrine manner to induce a pattern of genes similar to those induced by IL-17A, including pro-inflammatory cytokines, chemokines, and antimicrobial peptides (92, 96, 97). Similar to IL-17A, IL-17C was shown to synergize with TNF in this respect (92).

Experiments in mice confirmed that IL-17C participates in skin inflammation. Intradermal injection of IL-17C leads to epidermal thickening (96). In addition, IL-17C is upregulated in murine psoriasiform dermatitis (62, 92, 93), and IL-17C-deficient mice develop milder skin inflammation upon imiquimod application (96, 98). Conversely, selective overexpression of IL-17C in murine epidermis results in marked psoriasiform dermatitis (92). Finally, antibody-dependent blockade of IL-17C inhibited cutaneous inflammation in the IL-23-induced psoriasis model and in AD-like inflammation in mice (93).

Studies in mice also corroborate some clinical evidence obtained with targeted antibody therapies. In this respect, TNF-alpha blocking therapies result in early decrease of IL-17C levels in patients (91). The same neutralizing strategy led to an amelioration of the psoriasiform phenotype in IL-17C transgenic mice (92), pointing toward a possible role of the TNF/IL-17C axis in psoriasis. Despite this evidence, IL-17C was shown to be upregulated in paradoxical psoriasis upon anti-TNF therapy in patients presenting inflammatory bowel disease (IBD), in a mechanisms depended on IL-36γ (99). Paradoxical psoriasis onset in RA patients has also been reported after IL-6 inhibition. Similarly, genetic ablation of IL-6 leads to an increased psoriasiform phenotype in an IL-17C transgenic mouse model. This suggests that in absence of IL-6, compensatory mechanisms may occur resulting in exacerbation of disease (100).

Outside the skin, IL-17C promotes protective antimicrobial responses in the gut (96, 97, 101) and participates in mucosal responses to *Citrobacter rodentium* (97). Mice lacking IL-17C exhibited exacerbated DSS-induced colitis and IL-17C was shown to induce the production of occludin, participating in the establishment of intestinal barrier functions (101). On the other hand, IL-17C is found overexpressed in tissue from IBD patients (102, 103). In addition, IL-17C was implicated in pathogenic responses in the joints, leading to the exacerbation of arthritis induced by collagen in the mouse (78). Of interest, IL-17C was found upregulated in rheumatoid nodules and in extract from synovial fluid mononuclear cells of RA patients (83, 104). Despite its action at epithelial surface, IL-17C was shown to potentiate Th17 cell responses in EAE model (105) and to act in a pro-atherogenic manner in transgenic IL-17C mice (106, 107). With regards to cancer, IL-17C is upregulated in several forms of cancer, including colorectal and lung cancer, and was consistently shown to contribute to enhanced tumorigenesis in mice models (108). An overview of the role of IL-17C in inflammation is reported in **Table 5**.

Taken together, IL-17C appears to have much in common with the most widely studied members of the family: IL-17A and IL-17F. Synergizing with TNF, IL-17C potentiates protective antibacterial immune responses at epithelial surfaces, including the gut and the skin. Its overexpression is linked to skin conditions such as psoriasis. Similar to IL-17F, preclinical data in mice suggest that IL-17C might be pathogenic in joint disease while being protective in gut inflammation.

IL-17E (Also Known as IL-25)

Cloned in 2001, IL-17E maps to chromosome 14q11 and signals via a heterodimeric receptor complex composed of IL-17RB (also known as IL-25R) and IL-17RA (52) (**Table 6**). IL-17E is more commonly known as IL-25. As for other members of the IL-17 family, IL-17E is secreted as a disulfide-linked homodimer (50), while sharing only 16% sequence homology with IL-17A. This makes IL-17E the most divergent cytokine of the family. IL-17E is produced by many cell types: including epithelial cells, endothelial cells and several immune cells, such as T cells, macrophages, type-2 myeloid cells, DC, eosinophils and ILC2s (109, 110).

Several observations argue for a possible role of IL-17E in the skin. IL-17E is upregulated in the lesional tissue of several skin inflammatory disorders: atopic dermatitis (111–113), psoriasis (43, 111, 114), and, recently, contact dermatitis (115). The precise role of IL-17E in skin inflammation may well be disease-specific. In atopic dermatitis, IL-17E is reported to negatively affect the level of the barrier protein fillagrin and to favor the loss of epidermal barrier function (111, 112). In addition, IL-17E-stimulated ILC2 cells were reported to play important roles in the regulation of skin inflammation in a mouse atopic dermatitis model (123). In psoriasis, we have found that IL-17E, produced by epidermal keratinocytes in the lesional skin, activates dermal macrophages to produce inflammatory cytokines, including TNF, and neutrophil chemokines, such as IL-8. Of note, IL-17E expression in lesional psoriatic skin correlated with the number of neutrophils, while negatively correlating with the number of T cells, suggesting that IL-17E may play a role in the chemoattraction of innate immune cells in the skin (43). These data are consistent with experiments *in vitro*, in which IL-17E has been shown to promote the expression of pro-inflammatory cytokines such as IL-8, CCL-5, and GM-CS, by human dermal and lung fibroblasts, and kidney cells (32, 78, 124, 125). The fact that a single nucleotide polymorphism (rs79877597) in the IL-17E gene associates with more severe disease and the presence of psoriatic arthritis further suggests that IL-17E may be pathogenic in psoriasis (16). In addition, improved symptoms after phototherapy was shown to correlate with a decrease in IL-17E serum levels in one patient presenting high steady-state levels of this cytokine (126). In contact dermatitis, IL-17E was shown to stimulate IL-1β production by DC, leading to enhanced Th17-, but not Th2 cell-, mediated inflammation (115).

The abovementioned results are puzzling, because the current belief depicts IL-17E as a Th2 cytokine, or a cytokine favoring Type 2 responses. IL-17E was originally reported to be expressed by Th2-polarized CD4$^+$ T cells (127). Later, other immune cells were found to respond to IL-17E by producing Th2 cytokines, and transgenic overexpression or systemic administration of IL-17E in mice results in eosinophilia in addition to neutrophilia, increased production of Th2 cytokines and pathological changes in the lungs and digestive tract. These included the presence of immune infiltrates, increased mucus production, and epithelial cell hyperplasia (128, 129). IL-17E was found to induce Th2 cell

TABLE 5 | Overview of the role exerted by IL-17C in inflammation.

Skin inflammation - *Human/patient data*: IL-17C is increased in lesional psoriatic and atopic dermatitis skin (62, 91–93) - *Animal models*: IL-17C contributes to skin inflammation induced by IMQ application and IL-23-injection (93, 96, 98). IL-17C overexpression in keratinoctes induces psoriasiform dermatitis (92).
Joint inflammation - *Human/patient data*: IL-17C is expressed in the rheumatoid nodule (83) and by synovial fluid mononuclear cells of RA patients (104) - *Animal models*: IL-17C contributes to the exacerbation of inflammatory arthritis in CIA model (78)
Gut inflammation - *Human/patient data*: IL-17C expression is enhanced in the intestinal tissues from active IBD patients (102, 103) - *Animal models*: IL-17C participates in mucosal responses to *Citrobacter rodentium*, promotes intestinal barrier functions, and protects from DSS-induced colitis (96, 97, 101)
CNS - *Animal models*: IL-17C potentiates Th17 cell responses in EAE (105)
Cardiovascular disease - *Animal models*: IL-17C plays a pro-atherogenic role (106). IL-17C induced skin inflammation (K5-IL17C model) is associated with faster arterial thrombotic occlusion (107)

CNS, central nervous system; IMQ, imiquimod; RA, rheumatoid arthritis; CIA, collagen-induced arthritis; IBD, inflammatory bowel disease; DSS, dextran-sulfate sodium; EAE, experimental autoimmune encephalomyelitis.

TABLE 6 | Overview of the role exerted by IL-17E in inflammation.

Skin inflammation - *Human/patient data*: IL-17E is increased in the lesional skin of psoriasis, atopic dermatitis, and contact dermatitis (43, 111–115)
Joint inflammation - *Human/patient data*: IL-17E is increased in the serum and synovial fluid of RA patients (116, 117) - *Animal models*: IL-17E attenuates CIA development (117)
Gut inflammation - *Human/patient data*: IL-17E is downregulated in patients with IBD (118) - *Animal models:* 17E was found to either ameliorate or aggravate colitis in mice depending on model (118, 119)
CNS - *Animal models*: IL-17E suppresses Th17 immune responses in EAE (120)
Cardiovascular disease - *Animal models*: IL-17E inhibits atherosclerosis development (121, 122)

CNS, central nervous system; RA, rheumatoid arthritis; CIA, collagen-induced arthritis; IBD, inflammatory bowel disease; EAE, experimental autoimmune encephalomyelitis.

differentiation and activation (110), being thus crucial in host immune responses to nematode infections (130) and the development of allergic airway inflammation (131). Furthermore, IL-17E was shown to suppress Th17-mediated autoimmune diseases in mice, such as EAE and rheumatoid arthritis, mainly by skewing the immune system toward a Th2 response (120). In the gut, IL-17E may play both anti- and pro-inflammatory roles depending on the type of inflammation that is present (118). Moreover, IL-17E has been shown to inhibit atherosclerosis development in mice (121).

In summary, IL-17E is essential for protection against parasites and plays critical roles in Th2-mediated diseases (such as allergic asthma). In addition, it may limit Th17 cell responses, at least in mouse models of EAE and colitis. On the other hand, IL-17E is pathogenic in skin diseases, where it may function in « opposite » fashion and rather favor Th17 responses and recruitment of neutrophils. Thus, IL-17E effects appear to be highly tissue-specific.

CLINICAL IMPLICATIONS

Neutralization of IL-17A (secukinumab and ixekizumab) or the receptor subunit IL17RA (brodalumab) *via* monoclonal antibodies represents a highly effective approach to treat psoriasis (26, 27, 132). Blockade of IL-17RA also results in the inhibition of an array of members of the IL-17 family: namely IL-17A, IL-17F, IL-17C, and IL-17E. In addition to these licensed drugs, several other molecules targeting multiple IL-17 family members [IL-17A and IL-17F in the case of bimekizumab (71)], or the IL-17 pathway (either upstream, i.e., IL-23, or downstream signaling molecules) are in clinical development (133). Thus, a better knowledge of the structure of the IL-17 family and the function of their members with respect to inflammation is critical.

Although direct comparative trials have not been performed yet, indirect evidence suggests that IL-17RA inhibition may be superior to IL-17A inhibition, at least with respect to a greater likelihood of achieving PASI 100 and PASI 90 (134). Consistently, IL-17A, IL-17F, IL-17C, and IL-17E (all signaling *via* IL-17RA) have similar pro-inflammatory functions in the skin and have shown to play a pathogenic role in psoriatic skin manifestations. However, these same cytokines have also been reported to have non-redundant functions outside the skin, at least in the mouse. Thus, IL-17E has a protective role in CNS inflammation (120) and participates in protective responses against parasites in the intestine (130, 135, 136); and IL-17F and IL-17C are important for antibacterial immunity at epithelial surfaces (72, 73, 96, 97, 101). It remains to be addressed whether these tissue-specific functions exist in man too, and whether neutralization of several IL-17 cytokines might generate unwanted side effects outside the skin.

The possibility of inhibiting more than one IL-17 family member at a time could, however, reveal to be promising, as shown in the case of bimekizumab, a bi-specific anti-IL-17A and anti-IL-17F antibody (71, 137). While having a similar efficacy in the skin compared to IL-17A inhibition, this approach seems to perform better at the level of the joints, though larger trials have still to confirm this initial observation. This is consistent with a pathogenic role of IL-17F in joint inflammation, as observed in the mouse. Since IL-17C also participates in joint damage in mouse models of arthritis (133), it remains to be addressed whether its inhibition could be advantageous. On the other hand, both IL-17F and IL-17C are protective in murine gut inflammation (76, 96, 97, 101, 138). Whether a higher risk of intestinal inflammation due to IL-17F or IL-17C inhibition exists is unknown.

In summary, IL-17 family cytokines may elicit similar effects in target cells, but simultaneously may have very different (and sometimes opposite) functions in a tissue-specific manner. In addition, IL-17 cytokines have a great capacity of synergism, and their potency could be highly augmented by the cytokine milieu found at the inflamed site. These properties of the IL-17 family have direct clinical implications, as blocking more than one cytokine is a strategy currently under evaluation. A more comprehensive understanding of the mechanisms orchestrating the tissue-specific functions of the IL-17 family members in humans, and the relationship (causal or effector) existing among the different members of the family is required for a more rational drug design.

AUTHOR CONTRIBUTIONS

NB and W-HB defined the content of the manuscript, contributed to literature search and manuscript writing. LS contributed to literature search and manuscript writing. NB created graphical illustrations. All authors approved the final version of the manuscript.

REFERENCES

1. Boehncke WH, Schon MP. Psoriasis. *Lancet* (2015) 386(9997):983–94. doi:10.1016/S0140-6736(14)61909-7
2. Schon MP, Boehncke WH. Psoriasis. *N Engl J Med* (2005) 352(18):1899–912. doi:10.1056/NEJMra041320
3. Dauden E, Castaneda S, Suarez C, Garcia-Campayo J, Blasco AJ, Aguilar MD, et al. Clinical practice guideline for an integrated approach to comorbidity in patients with psoriasis. *J Eur Acad Dermatol Venereol* (2013) 27(11): 1387–404. doi:10.1111/jdv.12024
4. WHO. *World Psoriasis wdocument EB133.R2, Agenda Item 6.2. May 30.* (2013). http://apps.who.int/gb/ebwha/pdf_files/EB133/B133_R2-en.pdf
5. Lynde CW, Poulin Y, Vender R, Bourcier M, Khalil S. Interleukin 17A: toward a new understanding of psoriasis pathogenesis. *J Am Acad Dermatol* (2014) 71(1):141–50. doi:10.1016/j.jaad.2013.12.036
6. Ellis CN, Gorsulowsky DC, Hamilton TA, Billings JK, Brown MD, Headington JT, et al. Cyclosporine improves psoriasis in a double-blind study. *JAMA* (1986) 256(22):3110–6. doi:10.1001/jama.256.22.3110
7. Gottlieb SL, Gilleaudeau P, Johnson R, Estes L, Woodworth TG, Gottlieb AB, et al. Response of psoriasis to a lymphocyte-selective toxin (DAB389IL-2)

suggests a primary immune, but not keratinocyte, pathogenic basis. *Nat Med* (1995) 1(5):442–7. doi:10.1038/nm0595-442

8. Chamian F, Krueger JG. Psoriasis vulgaris: an interplay of T lymphocytes, dendritic cells, and inflammatory cytokines in pathogenesis. *Curr Opin Rheumatol* (2004) 16(4):331–7. doi:10.1097/01.bor.0000129715.35024.50
9. Oppmann B, Lesley R, Blom B, Timans JC, Xu Y, Hunte B, et al. Novel p19 protein engages IL-12p40 to form a cytokine, IL-23, with biological activities similar as well as distinct from IL-12. *Immunity* (2000) 13(5):715–25. doi:10.1016/S1074-7613(00)00070-4
10. Aggarwal S, Ghilardi N, Xie MH, de Sauvage FJ, Gurney AL. Interleukin-23 promotes a distinct CD4 T cell activation state characterized by the production of interleukin-17. *J Biol Chem* (2003) 278(3):1910–4. doi:10.1074/jbc.M207577200
11. Langrish CL, Chen Y, Blumenschein WM, Mattson J, Basham B, Sedgwick JD, et al. IL-23 drives a pathogenic T cell population that induces autoimmune inflammation. *J Exp Med* (2005) 201(2):233–40. doi:10.1084/jem.20041257
12. Gaffen SL, Jain R, Garg AV, Cua DJ. The IL-23-IL-17 immune axis: from mechanisms to therapeutic testing. *Nat Rev Immunol* (2014) 14(9):585–600. doi:10.1038/nri3707
13. Chan JR, Blumenschein W, Murphy E, Diveu C, Wiekowski M, Abbondanzo S, et al. IL-23 stimulates epidermal hyperplasia via TNF and IL-20R2-dependent mechanisms with implications for psoriasis pathogenesis. *J Exp Med* (2006) 203(12):2577–87. doi:10.1084/jem.20060244
14. Hedrick MN, Lonsdorf AS, Shirakawa AK, Richard Lee CC, Liao F, Singh SP, et al. CCR6 is required for IL-23-induced psoriasis-like inflammation in mice. *J Clin Invest* (2009) 119(8):2317–29. doi:10.1172/JCI37378
15. Ray-Jones H, Eyre S, Barton A, Warren RB. One SNP at a time: moving beyond GWAS in psoriasis. *J Invest Dermatol* (2016) 136(3):567–73. doi:10.1016/j.jid.2015.11.025
16. Batalla A, Coto E, Gonzalez-Lara L, Gonzalez-Fernandez D, Gomez J, Aranguren TF, et al. Association between single nucleotide polymorphisms IL17RA rs4819554 and IL17E rs79877597 and psoriasis in a Spanish cohort. *J Dermatol Sci* (2015) 80(2):111–5. doi:10.1016/j.jdermsci.2015.06.011
17. Martin DA, Towne JE, Kricorian G, Klekotka P, Gudjonsson JE, Krueger JG, et al. The emerging role of IL-17 in the pathogenesis of psoriasis: preclinical and clinical findings. *J Invest Dermatol* (2013) 133(1):17–26. doi:10.1038/jid.2012.194
18. Lai Y, Li D, Li C, Muehleisen B, Radek KA, Park HJ, et al. The antimicrobial protein REG3A regulates keratinocyte proliferation and differentiation after skin injury. *Immunity* (2012) 37(1):74–84. doi:10.1016/j.immuni.2012.04.010
19. Gutowska-Owsiak D, Schaupp AL, Salimi M, Selvakumar TA, McPherson T, Taylor S, et al. IL-17 downregulates filaggrin and affects keratinocyte expression of genes associated with cellular adhesion. *Exp Dermatol* (2012) 21(2):104–10. doi:10.1111/j.1600-0625.2011.01412.x
20. Nograles KE, Zaba LC, Guttman-Yassky E, Fuentes-Duculan J, Suarez-Farinas M, Cardinale I, et al. Th17 cytokines interleukin (IL)-17 and IL-22 modulate distinct inflammatory and keratinocyte-response pathways. *Br J Dermatol* (2008) 159(5):1092–102. doi:10.1111/j.1365-2133.2008.08769.x
21. Liang SC, Tan XY, Luxenberg DP, Karim R, Dunussi-Joannopoulos K, Collins M, et al. Interleukin (IL)-22 and IL-17 are coexpressed by Th17 cells and cooperatively enhance expression of antimicrobial peptides. *J Exp Med* (2006) 203(10):2271–9. doi:10.1084/jem.20061308
22. Eyerich K, Dimartino V, Cavani A. IL-17 and IL-22 in immunity: driving protection and pathology. *Eur J Immunol* (2017) 47(4):607–14. doi:10.1002/eji.201646723
23. Chiricozzi A, Guttman-Yassky E, Suarez-Farinas M, Nograles KE, Tian S, Cardinale I, et al. Integrative responses to IL-17 and TNF-alpha in human keratinocytes account for key inflammatory pathogenic circuits in psoriasis. *J Invest Dermatol* (2011) 131(3):677–87. doi:10.1038/jid.2010.340
24. Carrier Y, Ma HL, Ramon HE, Napierata L, Small C, O'Toole M, et al. Inter-regulation of Th17 cytokines and the IL-36 cytokines in vitro and in vivo: implications in psoriasis pathogenesis. *J Invest Dermatol* (2011) 131(12):2428–37. doi:10.1038/jid.2011.234
25. Capon F. IL36RN mutations in generalized pustular psoriasis: just the tip of the iceberg? *J Invest Dermatol* (2013) 133(11):2503–4. doi:10.1038/jid.2013.361
26. Griffiths CE, Reich K, Lebwohl M, van de Kerkhof P, Paul C, Menter A, et al. Comparison of ixekizumab with etanercept or placebo in moderate-to-severe psoriasis (UNCOVER-2 and UNCOVER-3): results from two phase 3 randomised trials. *Lancet* (2015) 386(9993):541–51. doi:10.1016/S0140-6736(15)60125-8
27. Papp KA, Langley RG, Sigurgeirsson B, Abe M, Baker DR, Konno P, et al. Efficacy and safety of secukinumab in the treatment of moderate-to-severe plaque psoriasis: a randomized, double-blind, placebo-controlled phase II dose-ranging study. *Br J Dermatol* (2013) 168(2):412–21. doi:10.1111/bjd.12110
28. Kirkham BW, Kavanaugh A, Reich K. Interleukin-17A: a unique pathway in immune-mediated diseases: psoriasis, psoriatic arthritis and rheumatoid arthritis. *Immunology* (2014) 141(2):133–42. doi:10.1111/imm.12142
29. Boehncke WH. Systemic inflammation and cardiovascular comorbidity in psoriasis patients: causes and consequences. *Front Immunol* (2018) 9:579. doi:10.3389/fimmu.2018.00579
30. Speeckaert R, Lambert J, Grine L, Van Gele M, De Schepper S, van Geel N. The many faces of interleukin-17 in inflammatory skin diseases. *Br J Dermatol* (2016) 175(5):892–901. doi:10.1111/bjd.14703
31. Hueber W, Sands BE, Lewitzky S, Vandemeulebroecke M, Reinisch W, Higgins PD, et al. Secukinumab, a human anti-IL-17A monoclonal antibody, for moderate to severe Crohn's disease: unexpected results of a randomised, double-blind placebo-controlled trial. *Gut* (2012) 61(12):1693–700. doi:10.1136/gutjnl-2011-301668
32. Lee J, Ho WH, Maruoka M, Corpuz RT, Baldwin DT, Foster JS, et al. IL-17E, a novel proinflammatory ligand for the IL-17 receptor homolog IL-17Rh1. *J Biol Chem* (2001) 276(2):1660–4. doi:10.1074/jbc.M008289200
33. Whibley N, Gaffen SL. Gut-busters: IL-17 Ain't Afraid of No IL-23. *Immunity* (2015) 43(4):620–2. doi:10.1016/j.immuni.2015.10.001
34. Tzartos JS, Friese MA, Craner MJ, Palace J, Newcombe J, Esiri MM, et al. Interleukin-17 production in central nervous system-infiltrating T cells and glial cells is associated with active disease in multiple sclerosis. *Am J Pathol* (2008) 172(1):146–55. doi:10.2353/ajpath.2008.070690
35. Komiyama Y, Nakae S, Matsuki T, Nambu A, Ishigame H, Kakuta S, et al. IL-17 plays an important role in the development of experimental autoimmune encephalomyelitis. *J Immunol* (2006) 177(1):566–73. doi:10.4049/jimmunol.177.1.566
36. Cheng X, Yu X, Ding YJ, Fu QQ, Xie JJ, Tang TT, et al. The Th17/Treg imbalance in patients with acute coronary syndrome. *Clin Immunol* (2008) 127(1):89–97. doi:10.1016/j.clim.2008.01.009
37. Erbel C, Chen L, Bea F, Wangler S, Celik S, Lasitschka F, et al. Inhibition of IL-17A attenuates atherosclerotic lesion development in apoE-deficient mice. *J Immunol* (2009) 183(12):8167–75. doi:10.4049/jimmunol.0901126
38. Ganguly D, Chamilos G, Lande R, Gregorio J, Meller S, Facchinetti V, et al. Self-RNA-antimicrobial peptide complexes activate human dendritic cells through TLR7 and TLR8. *J Exp Med* (2009) 206(9):1983–94. doi:10.1084/jem.20090480
39. Reich K, Papp KA, Matheson RT, Tu JH, Bissonnette R, Bourcier M, et al. Evidence that a neutrophil-keratinocyte crosstalk is an early target of IL-17A inhibition in psoriasis. *Exp Dermatol* (2015) 24(7):529–35. doi:10.1111/exd.12710
40. Brembilla NC, Stalder R, Senra L, Bohencke WH. IL-17A localizes in the exocytic compartment of mast cells in psoriatic skin. *Br J Dermatol* (2017) 177(5):1458–60. doi:10.1111/bjd.15358
41. Keijsers RR, Hendriks AG, van Erp PE, van Cranenbroek B, van de Kerkhof PC, Koenen HJ, et al. In vivo induction of cutaneous inflammation results in the accumulation of extracellular trap-forming neutrophils expressing RORgammat and IL-17. *J Invest Dermatol* (2014) 134(5):1276–84. doi:10.1038/jid.2013.526
42. Lin AM, Rubin CJ, Khandpur R, Wang JY, Riblett M, Yalavarthi S, et al. Mast cells and neutrophils release IL-17 through extracellular trap formation in psoriasis. *J Immunol* (2011) 187(1):490–500. doi:10.4049/jimmunol.1100123
43. Senra L, Stalder R, Alvarez Martinez D, Chizzolini C, Boehncke WH, Brembilla NC. Keratinocyte-derived IL-17E contributes to inflammation in psoriasis. *J Invest Dermatol* (2016) 136(10):1970–80. doi:10.1016/j.jid.2016.06.009
44. Hawkes JE, Chan TC, Krueger JG. Psoriasis pathogenesis and the development of novel targeted immune therapies. *J Allergy Clin Immunol* (2017) 140(3):645–53. doi:10.1016/j.jaci.2017.07.004
45. Yoshiga Y, Goto D, Segawa S, Ohnishi Y, Matsumoto I, Ito S, et al. Invariant NKT cells produce IL-17 through IL-23-dependent and -independent

pathways with potential modulation of Th17 response in collagen-induced arthritis. *Int J Mol Med* (2008) 22(3):369–74. doi:10.3892/ijmm_00000032
46. Lee JS, Tato CM, Joyce-Shaikh B, Gulen MF, Cayatte C, Chen Y, et al. Interleukin-23-independent IL-17 production regulates intestinal epithelial permeability. *Immunity* (2015) 43(4):727–38. doi:10.1016/j.immuni.2015.09.003
47. Rouvier E, Luciani MF, Mattei MG, Denizot F, Golstein P. CTLA-8, cloned from an activated T cell, bearing AU-rich messenger RNA instability sequences, and homologous to a herpesvirus saimiri gene. *J Immunol* (1993) 150(12):5445–56.
48. Yao Z, Fanslow WC, Seldin MF, Rousseau AM, Painter SL, Comeau MR, et al. *Herpesvirus Saimiri* encodes a new cytokine, IL-17, which binds to a novel cytokine receptor. *Immunity* (1995) 3(6):811–21. doi:10.1016/1074-7613(95)90070-5
49. Akimzhanov AM, Yang XO, Dong C. Chromatin remodeling of interleukin-17 (IL-17)-IL-17F cytokine gene locus during inflammatory helper T cell differentiation. *J Biol Chem* (2007) 282(9):5969–72. doi:10.1074/jbc.C600322200
50. Gaffen SL. Recent advances in the IL-17 cytokine family. *Curr Opin Immunol* (2011) 23(5):613–9. doi:10.1016/j.coi.2011.07.006
51. Amatya N, Garg AV, Gaffen SL. IL-17 signaling: the Yin and the Yang. *Trends Immunol* (2017) 38(5):310–22. doi:10.1016/j.it.2017.01.006
52. Gaffen SL. Structure and signalling in the IL-17 receptor family. *Nat Rev Immunol* (2009) 9(8):556–67. doi:10.1038/nri2586
53. Chang SH, Park H, Dong C. Act1 adaptor protein is an immediate and essential signaling component of interleukin-17 receptor. *J Biol Chem* (2006) 281(47):35603–7. doi:10.1074/jbc.C600256200
54. Liu C, Qian W, Qian Y, Giltiay NV, Lu Y, Swaidani S, et al. Act1, a U-box E3 ubiquitin ligase for IL-17 signaling. *Sci Signal* (2009) 2(92):ra63. doi:10.1126/scisignal.2000382
55. Schwandner R, Yamaguchi K, Cao Z. Requirement of tumor necrosis factor receptor-associated factor (TRAF)6 in interleukin 17 signal transduction. *J Exp Med* (2000) 191(7):1233–40. doi:10.1084/jem.191.7.1233
56. Song X, Qian Y. The activation and regulation of IL-17 receptor mediated signaling. *Cytokine* (2013) 62(2):175–82. doi:10.1016/j.cyto.2013.03.014
57. Sun D, Novotny M, Bulek K, Liu C, Li X, Hamilton T. Treatment with IL-17 prolongs the half-life of chemokine CXCL1 mRNA via the adaptor TRAF5 and the splicing-regulatory factor SF2 (ASF). *Nat Immunol* (2011) 12(9):853–60. doi:10.1038/ni.2081
58. Herjan T, Yao P, Qian W, Li X, Liu C, Bulek K, et al. HuR is required for IL-17-induced Act1-mediated CXCL1 and CXCL5 mRNA stabilization. *J Immunol* (2013) 191(2):640–9. doi:10.4049/jimmunol.1203315
59. Hartupee J, Liu C, Novotny M, Li X, Hamilton T. IL-17 enhances chemokine gene expression through mRNA stabilization. *J Immunol* (2007) 179(6):4135–41. doi:10.4049/jimmunol.179.6.4135
60. Hot A, Miossec P. Effects of interleukin (IL)-17A and IL-17F in human rheumatoid arthritis synoviocytes. *Ann Rheum Dis* (2011) 70(5):727–32. doi:10.1136/ard.2010.143768
61. Ramani K, Garg AV, Jawale CV, Conti HR, Whibley N, Jackson EK, et al. The Kallikrein-Kinin system: a novel mediator of IL-17-driven anti-*Candida* immunity in the kidney. *PLoS Pathog* (2016) 12(11):e1005952. doi:10.1371/journal.ppat.1005952
62. Johansen C, Usher PA, Kjellerup RB, Lundsgaard D, Iversen L, Kragballe K. Characterization of the interleukin-17 isoforms and receptors in lesional psoriatic skin. *Br J Dermatol* (2009) 160(2):319–24. doi:10.1111/j.1365-2133.2008.08902.x
63. Soderstrom C, Berstein G, Zhang W, Valdez H, Fitz L, Kuhn M, et al. Ultra-sensitive measurement of IL-17A and IL-17F in psoriasis patient serum and skin. *AAPS J* (2017) 19(4):1218–22. doi:10.1208/s12248-017-0094-4
64. Prieto-Perez R, Solano-Lopez G, Cabaleiro T, Roman M, Ochoa D, Talegon M, et al. The polymorphism rs763780 in the IL-17F gene is associated with response to biological drugs in patients with psoriasis. *Pharmacogenomics* (2015) 16(15):1723–31. doi:10.2217/pgs.15.107
65. Park YA, Kim YH, Sol IS, Yoon SH, Hong JY, Kim MN, et al. Relationship between serum interleukin-17F level and severity of atopic dermatitis in children. *Pediatr Allergy Immunol Pulmonol* (2015) 28(2):112–6. doi:10.1089/ped.2014.0482
66. Pantelyushin S, Haak S, Ingold B, Kulig P, Heppner FL, Navarini AA, et al. Rorgammat+ innate lymphocytes and gammadelta T cells initiate psoriasiform plaque formation in mice. *J Clin Invest* (2012) 122(6):2252–6. doi:10.1172/JCI61862
67. van der Fits L, Mourits S, Voerman JS, Kant M, Boon L, Laman JD, et al. Imiquimod-induced psoriasis-like skin inflammation in mice is mediated via the IL-23/IL-17 axis. *J Immunol* (2009) 182(9):5836–45. doi:10.4049/jimmunol.0802999
68. Watanabe H, Kawaguchi M, Fujishima S, Ogura M, Matsukura S, Takeuchi H, et al. Functional characterization of IL-17F as a selective neutrophil attractant in psoriasis. *J Invest Dermatol* (2009) 129(3):650–6. doi:10.1038/jid.2008.294
69. Fujishima S, Watanabe H, Kawaguchi M, Suzuki T, Matsukura S, Homma T, et al. Involvement of IL-17F via the induction of IL-6 in psoriasis. *Arch Dermatol Res* (2010) 302(7):499–505. doi:10.1007/s00403-010-1033-8
70. Zrioual S, Ecochard R, Tournadre A, Lenief V, Cazalis MA, Miossec P. Genome-wide comparison between IL-17A- and IL-17F-induced effects in human rheumatoid arthritis synoviocytes. *J Immunol* (2009) 182(5):3112–20. doi:10.4049/jimmunol.0801967
71. Glatt S, Baeten D, Baker T, Griffiths M, Ionescu L, Lawson ADG, et al. Dual IL-17A and IL-17F neutralisation by bimekizumab in psoriatic arthritis: evidence from preclinical experiments and a randomised placebo-controlled clinical trial that IL-17F contributes to human chronic tissue inflammation. *Ann Rheum Dis* (2018) 77(4):523–32. doi:10.1136/annrheumdis-2017-212127
72. Ishigame H, Kakuta S, Nagai T, Kadoki M, Nambu A, Komiyama Y, et al. Differential roles of interleukin-17A and -17F in host defense against mucoepithelial bacterial infection and allergic responses. *Immunity* (2009) 30(1):108–19. doi:10.1016/j.immuni.2008.11.009
73. Whibley N, Tritto E, Traggiai E, Kolbinger F, Moulin P, Brees D, et al. Antibody blockade of IL-17 family cytokines in immunity to acute murine oral mucosal candidiasis. *J Leukoc Biol* (2016) 99(6):1153–64. doi:10.1189/jlb.4A0915-428R
74. Boisson B, Wang C, Pedergnana V, Wu L, Cypowyj S, Rybojad M, et al. An ACT1 mutation selectively abolishes interleukin-17 responses in humans with chronic mucocutaneous candidiasis. *Immunity* (2013) 39(4):676–86. doi:10.1016/j.immuni.2013.09.002
75. Sarkar S, Justa S, Brucks M, Endres J, Fox DA, Zhou X, et al. Interleukin (IL)-17A, F and AF in inflammation: a study in collagen-induced arthritis and rheumatoid arthritis. *Clin Exp Immunol* (2014) 177(3):652–61. doi:10.1111/cei.12376
76. Yang XO, Chang SH, Park H, Nurieva R, Shah B, Acero L, et al. Regulation of inflammatory responses by IL-17F. *J Exp Med* (2008) 205(5):1063–75. doi:10.1084/jem.20071978
77. Haak S, Croxford AL, Kreymborg K, Heppner FL, Pouly S, Becher B, et al. IL-17A and IL-17F do not contribute vitally to autoimmune neuro-inflammation in mice. *J Clin Invest* (2009) 119(1):61–9. doi:10.1172/JCI35997
78. Yamaguchi Y, Fujio K, Shoda H, Okamoto A, Tsuno NH, Takahashi K, et al. IL-17B and IL-17C are associated with TNF-alpha production and contribute to the exacerbation of inflammatory arthritis. *J Immunol* (2007) 179(10):7128–36. doi:10.4049/jimmunol.179.10.7128
79. Babaloo Z, Babaie F, Farhoodi M, Aliparasti MR, Baradaran B, Almasi S, et al. Interleukin-17A and interleukin-17F mRNA expression in peripheral blood mononuclear cells of patients with multiple sclerosis. *Iran J Immunol* (2010) 7(4):202–9.
80. Seiderer J, Elben I, Diegelmann J, Glas J, Stallhofer J, Tillack C, et al. Role of the novel Th17 cytokine IL-17F in inflammatory bowel disease (IBD): upregulated colonic IL-17F expression in active Crohn's disease and analysis of the IL17F p.His161Arg polymorphism in IBD. *Inflamm Bowel Dis* (2008) 14(4):437–45. doi:10.1002/ibd.20339
81. Tong Z, Yang XO, Yan H, Liu W, Niu X, Shi Y, et al. A protective role by interleukin-17F in colon tumorigenesis. *PLoS One* (2012) 7(4):e34959. doi:10.1371/journal.pone.0034959
82. Wedebye Schmidt EG, Larsen HL, Kristensen NN, Poulsen SS, Lynge Pedersen AM, Claesson MH, et al. TH17 cell induction and effects of IL-17A and IL-17F blockade in experimental colitis. *Inflamm Bowel Dis* (2013) 19(8):1567–76. doi:10.1097/MIB.0b013e318286fa1c
83. Stamp LK, Easson A, Lehnigk U, Highton J, Hessian PA. Different T cell subsets in the nodule and synovial membrane: absence of interleukin-17A in rheumatoid nodules. *Arthritis Rheum* (2008) 58(6):1601–8. doi:10.1002/art.23455

84. Kouri VP, Olkkonen J, Ainola M, Li TF, Bjorkman L, Konttinen YT, et al. Neutrophils produce interleukin-17B in rheumatoid synovial tissue. *Rheumatology (Oxford)* (2014) 53(1):39–47. doi:10.1093/rheumatology/ket309
85. Li H, Chen J, Huang A, Stinson J, Heldens S, Foster J, et al. Cloning and characterization of IL-17B and IL-17C, two new members of the IL-17 cytokine family. *Proc Natl Acad Sci U S A* (2000) 97(2):773–8. doi:10.1073/pnas.97.2.773
86. Moore EE, Presnell S, Garrigues U, Guilbot A, LeGuern E, Smith D, et al. Expression of IL-17B in neurons and evaluation of its possible role in the chromosome 5q-linked form of Charcot-Marie-Tooth disease. *Neuromuscul Disord* (2002) 12(2):141–50. doi:10.1016/S0960-8966(01)00250-4
87. Starnes T, Broxmeyer HE, Robertson MJ, Hromas R. Cutting edge: IL-17D, a novel member of the IL-17 family, stimulates cytokine production and inhibits hemopoiesis. *J Immunol* (2002) 169(2):642–6. doi:10.4049/jimmunol.169.2.642
88. Bie Q, Jin C, Zhang B, Dong H. IL-17B: a new area of study in the IL-17 family. *Mol Immunol* (2017) 90:50–6. doi:10.1016/j.molimm.2017.07.004
89. Kokubu T, Haudenschild DR, Moseley TA, Rose L, Reddi AH. Immunolocalization of IL-17A, IL-17B, and their receptors in chondrocytes during fracture healing. *J Histochem Cytochem* (2008) 56(2):89–95. doi:10.1369/jhc.7A7223.2007
90. Seelige R, Washington A Jr, Bui JD. The ancient cytokine IL-17D is regulated by Nrf2 and mediates tumor and virus surveillance. *Cytokine* (2017) 91:10–2. doi:10.1016/j.cyto.2016.11.017
91. Johansen C, Vinter H, Soegaard-Madsen L, Olsen LR, Steiniche T, Iversen L, et al. Preferential inhibition of the mRNA expression of p38 mitogen-activated protein kinase regulated cytokines in psoriatic skin by anti-TNFalpha therapy. *Br J Dermatol* (2010) 163(6):1194–204. doi:10.1111/j.1365-2133.2010.10036.x
92. Johnston A, Fritz Y, Dawes SM, Diaconu D, Al-Attar PM, Guzman AM, et al. Keratinocyte overexpression of IL-17C promotes psoriasiform skin inflammation. *J Immunol* (2013) 190(5):2252–62. doi:10.4049/jimmunol.1201505
93. Vandeghinste N, Klattig J, Jagerschmidt C, Lavazais S, Marsais F, Haas JD, et al. Neutralization of IL-17C reduces skin inflammation in mouse models of psoriasis and atopic dermatitis. *J Invest Dermatol* (2018) 138(7):1555–63. doi:10.1016/j.jid.2018.01.036
94. Johansen C, Riis JL, Gedebjerg A, Kragballe K, Iversen L. Tumor necrosis factor alpha-mediated induction of interleukin 17C in human keratinocytes is controlled by nuclear factor kappaB. *J Biol Chem* (2011) 286(29):25487–94. doi:10.1074/jbc.M111.240671
95. Roth SA, Simanski M, Rademacher F, Schroder L, Harder J. The pattern recognition receptor NOD2 mediates *Staphylococcus aureus*-induced IL-17C expression in keratinocytes. *J Invest Dermatol* (2014) 134(2):374–80. doi:10.1038/jid.2013.313
96. Ramirez-Carrozzi V, Sambandam A, Luis E, Lin Z, Jeet S, Lesch J, et al. IL-17C regulates the innate immune function of epithelial cells in an autocrine manner. *Nat Immunol* (2011) 12(12):1159–66. doi:10.1038/ni.2156
97. Song X, Zhu S, Shi P, Liu Y, Shi Y, Levin SD, et al. IL-17RE is the functional receptor for IL-17C and mediates mucosal immunity to infection with intestinal pathogens. *Nat Immunol* (2011) 12(12):1151–8. doi:10.1038/ni.2155
98. Monin L, Gudjonsson JE, Childs EE, Amatya N, Xing X, Verma AH, et al. MCPIP1/regnase-1 restricts IL-17A- and IL-17C-dependent skin inflammation. *J Immunol* (2017) 198(2):767–75. doi:10.4049/jimmunol.1601551
99. Friedrich M, Tillack C, Wollenberg A, Schauber J, Brand S. IL-36gamma sustains a proinflammatory self-amplifying loop with IL-17C in anti-TNF-induced psoriasiform skin lesions of patients with Crohn's disease. *Inflamm Bowel Dis* (2014) 20(11):1891–901. doi:10.1097/MIB.0000000000000198
100. Fritz Y, Klenotic PA, Swindell WR, Yin ZQ, Groft SG, Zhang L, et al. Induction of alternative proinflammatory cytokines accounts for sustained psoriasiform skin inflammation in IL-17C+IL-6KO mice. *J Invest Dermatol* (2017) 137(3):696–705. doi:10.1016/j.jid.2016.10.021
101. Reynolds JM, Martinez GJ, Nallaparaju KC, Chang SH, Wang YH, Dong C. Cutting edge: regulation of intestinal inflammation and barrier function by IL-17C. *J Immunol* (2012) 189(9):4226–30. doi:10.4049/jimmunol.1103014
102. Im E, Jung J, Rhee SH. Toll-like receptor 5 engagement induces interleukin-17C expression in intestinal epithelial cells. *J Interferon Cytokine Res* (2012) 32(12):583–91. doi:10.1089/jir.2012.0053
103. Friedrich M, Diegelmann J, Schauber J, Auernhammer CJ, Brand S. Intestinal neuroendocrine cells and goblet cells are mediators of IL-17A-amplified epithelial IL-17C production in human inflammatory bowel disease. *Mucosal Immunol* (2015) 8(4):943–58. doi:10.1038/mi.2014.124
104. Hwang SY, Kim HY. Expression of IL-17 homologs and their receptors in the synovial cells of rheumatoid arthritis patients. *Mol Cells* (2005) 19(2):180–4.
105. Chang SH, Reynolds JM, Pappu BP, Chen G, Martinez GJ, Dong C. Interleukin-17C promotes Th17 cell responses and autoimmune disease via interleukin-17 receptor E. *Immunity* (2011) 35(4):611–21. doi:10.1016/j.immuni.2011.09.010
106. Butcher MJ, Waseem TC, Galkina EV. Smooth muscle cell-derived interleukin-17C plays an atherogenic role via the recruitment of proinflammatory interleukin-17A+ T cells to the aorta. *Arterioscler Thromb Vasc Biol* (2016) 36(8):1496–506. doi:10.1161/ATVBAHA.116.307892
107. Golden JB, Wang Y, Fritz Y, Diaconu D, Zhang X, Debanne SM, et al. Chronic, not acute, skin-specific inflammation promotes thrombosis in psoriasis murine models. *J Transl Med* (2015) 13:382. doi:10.1186/s12967-015-0738-z
108. Jungnickel C, Schmidt LH, Bittigkoffer L, Wolf L, Wolf A, Ritzmann F, et al. IL-17C mediates the recruitment of tumor-associated neutrophils and lung tumor growth. *Oncogene* (2017) 36(29):4182–90. doi:10.1038/onc.2017.28
109. Xu M, Dong C. IL-25 in allergic inflammation. *Immunol Rev* (2017) 278(1):185–91. doi:10.1111/imr.12558
110. Angkasekwinai P, Park H, Wang YH, Wang YH, Chang SH, Corry DB, et al. Interleukin 25 promotes the initiation of proallergic type 2 responses. *J Exp Med* (2007) 204(7):1509–17. doi:10.1084/jem.20061675
111. Hvid M, Vestergaard C, Kemp K, Christensen GB, Deleuran B, Deleuran M. IL-25 in atopic dermatitis: a possible link between inflammation and skin barrier dysfunction? *J Invest Dermatol* (2011) 131(1):150–7. doi:10.1038/jid.2010.277
112. Deleuran M, Hvid M, Kemp K, Christensen GB, Deleuran B, Vestergaard C. IL-25 induces both inflammation and skin barrier dysfunction in atopic dermatitis. *Chem Immunol Allergy* (2012) 96:45–9. doi:10.1159/000331871
113. Aktar MK, Kido-Nakahara M, Furue M, Nakahara T. Mutual upregulation of endothelin-1 and IL-25 in atopic dermatitis. *Allergy* (2015) 70(7):846–54. doi:10.1111/all.12633
114. Kim BE, Bin L, Ye YM, Ramamoorthy P, Leung DY. IL-25 enhances HSV-1 replication by inhibiting filaggrin expression, and acts synergistically with Th2 cytokines to enhance HSV-1 replication. *J Invest Dermatol* (2013) 133(12):2678–85. doi:10.1038/jid.2013.223
115. Suto H, Nambu A, Morita H, Yamaguchi S, Numata T, Yoshizaki T, et al. IL-25 enhances Th17 cell-mediated contact dermatitis by promoting IL-1beta production by dermal dendritic cells. *J Allergy Clin Immunol* (2018). doi:10.1016/j.jaci.2017.12.1007
116. Gumus P, Buduneli E, Biyikoglu B, Aksu K, Sarac F, Nile C, et al. Gingival crevicular fluid, serum levels of receptor activator of nuclear factor-kappaB ligand, osteoprotegerin, and interleukin-17 in patients with rheumatoid arthritis and osteoporosis and with periodontal disease. *J Periodontol* (2013) 84(11):1627–37. doi:10.1902/jop.2013.120595
117. Liu D, Cao T, Wang N, Liu C, Ma N, Tu R, et al. IL-25 attenuates rheumatoid arthritis through suppression of Th17 immune responses in an IL-13-dependent manner. *Sci Rep* (2016) 6:36002. doi:10.1038/srep36002
118. Caruso R, Sarra M, Stolfi C, Rizzo A, Fina D, Fantini MC, et al. Interleukin-25 inhibits interleukin-12 production and Th1 cell-driven inflammation in the gut. *Gastroenterology* (2009) 136(7):2270–9. doi:10.1053/j.gastro.2009.02.049
119. Reynolds JM, Lee YH, Shi Y, Wang X, Angkasekwinai P, Nallaparaju KC, et al. Interleukin-17B antagonizes interleukin-25-mediated mucosal inflammation. *Immunity* (2015) 42(4):692–703. doi:10.1016/j.immuni.2015.03.008
120. Kleinschek MA, Owyang AM, Joyce-Shaikh B, Langrish CL, Chen Y, Gorman DM, et al. IL-25 regulates Th17 function in autoimmune inflammation. *J Exp Med* (2007) 204(1):161–70. doi:10.1084/jem.20061738
121. Mantani P, Duner P Jr, Bengtsson E Sr, Ljungcrantz I, Sundius L, To F Jr, et al. Interleukin 25 (IL-25) has a protective role in atherosclerosis development in the aortic arch in mice. *J Biol Chem* (2018). doi:10.1074/jbc.RA117.000292

122. Mantani PT, Duner P, Bengtsson E, Alm R, Ljungcrantz I, Soderberg I, et al. IL-25 inhibits atherosclerosis development in apolipoprotein E deficient mice. *PLoS One* (2015) 10(1):e0117255. doi:10.1371/journal.pone.0117255
123. Salimi M, Barlow JL, Saunders SP, Xue L, Gutowska-Owsiak D, Wang X, et al. A role for IL-25 and IL-33-driven type-2 innate lymphoid cells in atopic dermatitis. *J Exp Med* (2013) 210(13):2939–50. doi:10.1084/jem.20130351
124. Lonati PA, Brembilla NC, Montanari E, Fontao L, Gabrielli A, Vettori S, et al. High IL-17E and low IL-17C dermal expression identifies a fibrosis-specific motif common to morphea and systemic sclerosis. *PLoS One* (2014) 9(8):e105008. doi:10.1371/journal.pone.0105008
125. Letuve S, Lajoie-Kadoch S, Audusseau S, Rothenberg ME, Fiset PO, Ludwig MS, et al. IL-17E upregulates the expression of proinflammatory cytokines in lung fibroblasts. *J Allergy Clin Immunol* (2006) 117(3):590–6. doi:10.1016/j.jaci.2005.10.025
126. Otsuka A, Miyachi Y, Kabashima K. Narrowband ultraviolet B phototherapy decreased the serum IL-17E level in a patient with psoriasis vulgaris. *J Eur Acad Dermatol Venereol* (2012) 26(11):1455–6. doi:10.1111/j.1468-3083.2011.04345.x
127. Fort MM, Cheung J, Yen D, Li J, Zurawski SM, Lo S, et al. IL-25 induces IL-4, IL-5, and IL-13 and Th2-associated pathologies in vivo. *Immunity* (2001) 15(6):985–95. doi:10.1016/S1074-7613(01)00243-6
128. Pan G, French D, Mao W, Maruoka M, Risser P, Lee J, et al. Forced expression of murine IL-17E induces growth retardation, jaundice, a Th2-biased response, and multiorgan inflammation in mice. *J Immunol* (2001) 167(11):6559–67. doi:10.4049/jimmunol.167.11.6559
129. Kim MR, Manoukian R, Yeh R, Silbiger SM, Danilenko DM, Scully S, et al. Transgenic overexpression of human IL-17E results in eosinophilia, B-lymphocyte hyperplasia, and altered antibody production. *Blood* (2002) 100(7):2330–40. doi:10.1182/blood-2002-01-0012
130. Fallon PG, Ballantyne SJ, Mangan NE, Barlow JL, Dasvarma A, Hewett DR, et al. Identification of an interleukin (IL)-25–dependent cell population that provides IL-4, IL-5, and IL-13 at the onset of helminth expulsion. *J Exp Med* (2006) 203(4):1105–16. doi:10.1084/jem.20051615
131. Ballantyne SJ, Barlow JL, Jolin HE, Nath P, Williams AS, Chung KF, et al. Blocking IL-25 prevents airway hyperresponsiveness in allergic asthma. *J Allergy Clin Immunol* (2007) 120(6):1324–31. doi:10.1016/j.jaci.2007.07.051
132. Lebwohl M, Strober B, Menter A, Gordon K, Weglowska J, Puig L, et al. Phase 3 studies comparing brodalumab with ustekinumab in psoriasis. *N Engl J Med* (2015) 373(14):1318–28. doi:10.1056/NEJMoa1503824
133. Conrad C, Gilliet M. Psoriasis: from pathogenesis to targeted therapies. *Clin Rev Allergy Immunol* (2018) 54(1):102–13. doi:10.1007/s12016-018-8668-1
134. Sawyer L, Fotheringham I, Gibbons C, Møller A. Brodalumab versus secukinumab in moderate-to-severe psoriasis: an indirect comparison of 52-week efficacy outcomes. *EADV (E-poster #1839)* (2017).
135. Angkasekwinai P, Srimanote P, Wang YH, Pootong A, Sakolvaree Y, Pattanapanyasat K, et al. Interleukin-25 (IL-25) promotes efficient protective immunity against *Trichinella spiralis* infection by enhancing the antigen-specific IL-9 response. *Infect Immun* (2013) 81(10):3731–41. doi:10.1128/IAI.00646-13
136. Owyang AM, Zaph C, Wilson EH, Guild KJ, McClanahan T, Miller HR, et al. Interleukin 25 regulates type 2 cytokine-dependent immunity and limits chronic inflammation in the gastrointestinal tract. *J Exp Med* (2006) 203(4):843–9. doi:10.1084/jem.20051496
137. Glatt S, Helmer E, Haier B, Strimenopoulou F, Price G, Vajjah P, et al. First-in-human randomized study of bimekizumab, a humanized monoclonal antibody and selective dual inhibitor of IL-17A and IL-17F, in mild psoriasis. *Br J Clin Pharmacol* (2017) 83(5):991–1001. doi:10.1111/bcp.13185
138. Iboshi Y, Nakamura K, Fukaura K, Iwasa T, Ogino H, Sumida Y, et al. Increased IL-17A/IL-17F expression ratio represents the key mucosal T helper/regulatory cell-related gene signature paralleling disease activity in ulcerative colitis. *J Gastroenterol* (2017) 52(3):315–26. doi:10.1007/s00535-016-1231-z

19

Systemic Inflammation and Cardiovascular Comorbidity in Psoriasis Patients: Causes and Consequences

Wolf-Henning Boehncke*[1,2]

[1] Department of Pathology and Immunology, Faculty of Medicine, University of Geneva, Geneva, Switzerland,
[2] Division of Dermatology and Venereology, Geneva University Hospitals, Geneva, Switzerland

***Correspondence:**
Wolf-Henning Boehncke
wolf-henning.boehncke@hcuge.ch

Psoriasis is a common inflammatory skin disease characterized by the appearance of red scaly plaques that can affect any part of the body. High prevalence, chronicity, disfiguration, disability, and associated comorbidity make it a challenge for clinicians of multiple specialties. Likewise, its complex pathogenesis, comprising inflammation, hyperproliferation, and angioneogenesis, intrigues numerous scientific disciplines, namely, immunology. From a clinical perspective, the severity of psoriasis is highlighted by its increased mortality, with cardiovascular diseases contributing the highest excess risk. From a scientific point of view, psoriasis has to be considered a systemic inflammatory condition, as blood biomarkers of inflammation are elevated and imaging techniques document sites of inflammation beyond the skin. While the association of psoriasis with cardiovascular diseases is now widely accepted, causes and consequences of this association are controversially discussed. This review comments on epidemiologic, genetic, and mechanistic studies that analyzed the relation between psoriasis and cardiovascular comorbidity. The hypothesis of psoriasis potentially being an independent cardiovascular risk factor, driving atherosclerosis *via* inflammation-induced endothelial dysfunction, will be discussed. Finally, consequences for the management of psoriasis with the objective to reduce the patients' excess cardiovascular risk will be pointed out.

Keywords: psoriasis, coronary heart disease, stroke, atherosclerosis, insulin resistance, endothelial dysfunction, mortality

INTRODUCTION

Psoriasis is among the few non-communicable diseases the World Health Organization identified as a major global health problem (1). It is a common inflammatory skin disease, affecting around 2% of the population in Western countries (2). Its clinical hallmark are red scaly plaques that can affect any part of the body, but preferentially appear over elbows and knees as well as on the scalp, the umbilical, and perianal region. These lesions reflect the principal pathogenetic mechanisms underlying psoriasis, namely, inflammation, hyperproliferation, and angioneogenesis. To date, psoriasis is considered an immune-mediated disease, exhibiting an intense cross talk between components of the innate and the adaptive immune system, which then trigger the epidermal changes (3). Psoriatic inflammation goes more than skin deep, as signs of inflammation can readily be detected at sites outside the skin (4).

Comorbidity is a common feature of many immune-mediated inflammatory diseases across different medical specialties, including model diseases such as rheumatoid arthritis (5), inflammatory bowel disease (6), or multiple sclerosis (7). A wealth of data documents the association of psoriasis with numerous comorbid diseases, including cardiometabolic, gastrointestinal, and kidney diseases as well as malignancies, infections, and mood disorders (8). To this end, it is still controversial whether psoriatic arthritis should be considered an extracutaneous manifestation of psoriasis or as a separate entity, and thus comorbidity (9). Among the comorbid conditions, cardiovascular diseases are of particular importance, as they often directly impact the patients' mortality (10).

In the case of rheumatoid arthritis, currently available evidence is strong enough to allow the issue of recommendations that substantially change prevention and treatment goals for cardiovascular risk factors in these patients (11). And while the association with cardiovascular diseases also among psoriasis patients is now widely accepted, causes and consequences of this association are controversially discussed (12–14). This review comments on epidemiologic, genetic, and mechanistic studies that analyzed the relation between psoriasis and cardiovascular comorbidity. The hypothesis of psoriasis potentially being an independent cardiovascular risk factor, driving atherosclerosis *via* inflammation-induced endothelial dysfunction, will be discussed. Finally, consequences for the management of psoriasis with the objective to reduce the patients' excess cardiovascular risk will be pointed out.

EPIDEMIOLOGY

One of the first systematic analyses on disease concomitance based on more than 40,000 cases identified an association of psoriasis not only with cardiovascular disease but also with diseases that represent risk factors for atherosclerosis, such as diabetes mellitus or obesity. The authors concluded that a distinct pattern of associated diseases exists in patients with psoriasis and suggest a genetically determined selection (15). Since then, multiple epidemiologic studies have addressed the issue of cardiovascular comorbidity in psoriasis patients. And while some groups concluded that such a link does not exist (16–18), many others were able to reproduce this association recently summarized elsewhere (8, 19) (**Table 1**). Based on the currently available evidence, most experts agree that the association of psoriasis with cardiovascular comorbidity is real (20). This is also reflected by and justifies the inclusion of advice on the management of psoriasis patients with such comorbidities in guidelines and treatment recommendations (21, 22).

The fact that cardiovascular diseases are associated with psoriasis leads to the question on why that might be so. A strong argument in favor of an indirect link comes from the observation that psoriasis is associated with numerous conditions representing major cardiovascular risk factors in their own right (**Table 2**). In fact, the very first publication on psoriasis comorbidity reported an association with diabetes mellitus as early as 1897 (31). Also, the study by Henseler and Christophers cited above documents diabetes mellitus and obesity as concomitant conditions (15). Finally, Takeshita et al. recently summarized the evidence for obesity, hypertension, diabetes mellitus, dyslipidemia, and the metabolic syndrome as comorbid diseases in psoriasis (8), with the metabolic syndrome essentially representing the combined appearance of obesity, hypertension, insulin resistance, and dyslipidemia (32). These conditions are not only well-established major cardiovascular risk factors and therefore incorporated in the Framingham's Cardiovascular Disease Risk Scores used to predict cardiovascular risk in the general population (33), some of them, namely, smoking (34) and obesity (35), are also risk factors for the development of psoriasis.

TABLE 1 | Summary of studies analyzing the association between psoriasis and major adverse cardiovascular events.

Reference	Study characteristics	Key finding
Dowlatshahi et al. (16)	Population-based study (262 patients with mostly mild psoriasis, and 8,009 controls)	No increased risk for cardiovascular events
Parisi et al. (17)	Cohort study (48,000 patients and 200,000 controls)	No association of psoriasis with cardiovascular disease
Egeberg et al. (18)	Nationwide cohort study (adult population of Denmark)	Slight increase of myocardial infarction in patients with severe psoriasis
Armstrong et al. (23)	Systematic review and meta-analysis (220,000 patients and 10 mio controls)	Increased risk for myocardial infarction, stroke, and cardiovascular mortality among psoriasis patients
Gaeta et al. (24)	Meta-analysis (1.8 mio patients and 43 mio controls)	Increased risk for myocardial infarction and cardiovascular mortality among psoriasis patients
Gu et al. (25)	Meta-analysis of cohort studies (6.2 mio individuals overall)	Increased risk for myocardial infarction, stroke, and cardiovascular mortality among psoriasis patients
Horreau et al. (26)	Systematic literature review (324,000 patients and 5.3 mio controls)	Increased risk for myocardial infarction and stroke among psoriasis patients
Miller et al. (27)	Meta-analysis (500,000 patients and 29 mio controls)	Increased risk for cardiovascular disease among psoriasis patients
Pietrzak et al. (28)	Review (360,000 patients and 9.2 mio controls)	Increased risk for cardiovascular events among psoriasis patients
Samarasekera et al. (29)	Systematic review and meta-analysis (480,000 patients and 10 mio controls)	Increased risk for myocardial infarction, stroke, and cardiovascular mortality among psoriasis patients
Xu et al. (30)	Meta-analysis of cohort studies (326,000 patients and 5.2 mio controls)	Increased risk for myocardial infarction and stroke among psoriasis patients

TABLE 2 | Synopsis of arguments in favor or against the hypothesis of psoriasis representing an independent cardiovascular risk factor.

Domain	Psoriasis may be an independent cardiovascular risk factor	Psoriasis may *not* be an independent cardiovascular risk factor
Epidemiology	Dose effect: Population-based studies document a higher cardiovascular risk among patients with severe compared to those with mild psoriasis. The risk is also higher in patients with longer disease duration. In case–control studies, surrogate markers for increased cardiovascular risk are associated with psoriasis after thorough control for confounding factors.	Conventional cardiovascular risk factors such as several or even all components of the metabolic syndrome are associated with psoriasis throughout all age groups
Genetics	A comprehensive assessment of the catalog of genome-wide association studies shows that the genetic control of psoriasis is almost completely independent from both the metabolic syndrome and coronary heart disease	There may be some shared susceptibility loci between psoriasis and its comorbidities A missense mutation in the insulin-responsive peptidase links psoriasis to hypertension and diabetes mellitus
Pathophysiology	Remarkable similarities exist between the inflammatory processes in psoriatic and atherosclerotic plaques: • insulin resistance • endothelial dysfunction • T-lymphocyte driven • neutrophils involved • monocytes/macrophages involved • platelets involved	The exact role of several potentially shared components has yet to be established: • macrophages • IL-17A

Evidence in favor of psoriasis as an independent cardiovascular risk factor comes from studies showing a "dose effect" of psoriasis on the patients' cardiovascular risk (**Table 2**). A landmark study in this regard was conducted by Gelfand et al. who used the General Practice Research Database from 1987 to 2002, comprising prospective data collected from general practitioners in Great Britain. After adjusting for major cardiovascular risk factors, such as hypertension, diabetes mellitus, and hyperlipidemia, they found a slightly elevated adjusted relative risk for myocardial infarction among patients with mild psoriasis, and a substantially elevated adjusted relative risk among patients with severe psoriasis (36). Two meta-analyses also came to the conclusion that the cardiovascular risk of psoriasis patients correlates with the severity of their disease (29, 23). In line with this hypothesis, longer duration of psoriasis has also been associated with increased cardiovascular risk for the patients (37, 38). Another landmark study was performed by Ludwig et al. who quantified coronary artery calcification *via* CT scans, using the well-established Agatston score, among hospitalized psoriasis patients, thus suffering from severe psoriasis (39). Their scores were compared to controls matched for all major cardiovascular risk factors. The study showed highly significantly elevated coronary artery calcification, so that the study had to be stopped before the originally calculated number of patients had been included. This observation is even more alarming, as only patients with a negative history for current or previous heart problems were included.

The clinical relevance of psoriasis as an independent cardiovascular risk factor was quantified by Mehta et al. in a cohort study of severe psoriasis patients. There, the attributable risk of severe psoriasis on major cardiovascular events, i.e., namely, myocardial infarction and stroke, over a 10-year period was found to be around 6% (40). Others found the increased risk of such events associated with psoriasis to be comparable with that conferred by diabetes mellitus alone (41) or by rheumatoid arthritis (42). This is remarkable as the former is a well-accepted major cardiovascular risk factor, and the association of the latter with an increased cardiovascular risk already led to specific recommendations on how to address this extra risk, as pointed out above.

Taken together, despite few studies that did not show statistically significant associations between psoriasis and major cardiovascular events, a majority of studies using different methodical approaches suggests not only an association of psoriasis with cardiovascular diseases but also provides evidence for psoriasis as an independent cardiovascular risk factor (**Table 2**).

Noteworthy, chronic skin inflammation as such is not sufficient to explain the role of psoriasis as an independent cardiovascular risk factor, as a recent systematic review and meta analysis failed to provide evidence for atopic dermatitis, another common chronic inflammatory skin disease, exhibiting comparable effects (43). A major epidemiologic study documented even the inverse phenomenon, namely, a rather significantly decreased risk for myocardial infarction, stroke, or cardiovascular death (44). Therefore, genetic and pathogenetic analyses are needed to understand this association.

GENETICS

One possibility to explain the association of psoriasis with its comorbid conditions in general and cardiovascular disease in particular is that these entities share common genetics. A genetic predisposition of psoriasis can already be postulated based on the facts that many patients have a positive family history and that the concordance rate among monozygotic twins is much higher compared to dizygotic twins (45). The first psoriasis susceptibility locus (PSORS-1) identified is located on the short arm of chromosome 6 in the region coding for major histocompatibility complex (MHC) molecules. It is still the most reproducible among all PSORS loci identified and may explain up to 50% of the heritability of psoriasis (46). Namely genome-wide association studies (GWASs) shed more light on the genetics of psoriasis and allowed to identify at least 50 regions on the human genome which harbor at least 1 and sometimes more than 1 potential candidate gene associated with psoriasis. This database allows to group the respective genes according to pathways, with antigen presentation, interleukin-23 (IL-23) signaling, T-lymphocyte development and polarization, innate immunity, and negative regulators of immune responses as the key axes (47).

Following up on the notion that chronic skin inflammation as such does not suffice to explain increased cardiovascular risk, a GWAS showed some overlap between susceptibility loci for psoriasis and atopic dermatitis. This association was mediated by a combination of shared and opposing alleles, with the most significant effects operating in opposing directions, thus arguing in favor of distinct pathogenetic pathways of these diseases (48). This notion is supported by a much smaller study from Japan that observed only marginal associations between atopic dermatitis and susceptibility single-nucleotide polymorphisms for psoriasis (49). By contrast, rheumatoid arthritis as another chronic inflammatory disease with known cardiovascular comorbidity does exhibit a genetic architecture not too different from psoriasis: genetic variants in the MHC region account for more than 60% of the known genetic heritability of rheumatoid arthritis. Other associated genes are involved in the function of T-lymphocytes and monocytes representing the adaptive and the innate immune system, respectively. 35 rheumatoid arthritis risk loci gene products can be mapped to signaling pathways in T-lymphocytes and antigen-presenting cells (50). These include components of the tumor necrosis factor alpha (TNF-α) signaling cascade, the potential relevance of this finding will be discussed below.

Genetic variation and pathways in atherosclerosis do not show obvious overlap with the genetic signature of psoriasis or rheumatoid arthritis. Kessler et al. recently assigned 30 of 65 loci associated with coronary artery disease to 6 pathways with known pathophysiological roles in this disease, the function of the other 35 candidate genes is not sufficiently known to allow allocation to a particular pathway. These six pathways comprise inflammation, triglycerides, LDL cholesterol, blood pressure, vascular remodeling, and nitric oxide signaling (51).

Several groups have further analyzed the hypothesis of psoriasis and its comorbidities being genetically linked, following up on the observation that GWASs have shown overlap in the genetic susceptibility to different pathologies, namely, immune-mediated diseases (52). Ellinghaus et al. identified seven shared susceptibility loci for psoriasis and Crohn's disease; they went on to demonstrate a genetic overlap between five seronegative inflammatory diseases, namely psoriasis, Crohn's disease, ankylosing spondylitis, primary sclerosing cholangitis, and ulcerative colitis (53, 54). An observation pointing toward a genetic link between psoriasis and cardiovascular comorbidity was made by Cheng et al. who interpreted a missense mutation in the insulin-responsive aminopeptidase LNPEP as a potential link, namely between psoriasis, hypertension, and diabetes mellitus (55) (**Table 2**). The importance of insulin resistance in this context will be discussed in detail below. On the other hand, a comprehensive assessment of the catalog of GWASs by Gupta et al. shows that the genetic control of psoriasis is almost completely independent from both the metabolic syndrome and coronary heart disease (**Table 2**). To prove reliability of this approach, the authors were able to identified 10 common loci for the metabolic syndrome and coronary heart disease, using exactly the same data set (56).

Taken together, although some genetic overlap between psoriasis and several of its comorbid conditions exists, the observed association of psoriasis with cardiovascular comorbidity cannot satisfyingly be explained by shared genetics (**Table 2**).

PATHOGENESIS

Common Pathways of Psoriatic and Atherosclerotic Plaque Formation

To this end, epidemiological evidence in favor of psoriasis being associated with cardiovascular comorbidity and potentially functioning as an independent cardiovascular risk factor has been summarized. As genetic overlap cannot satisfyingly explain the excess cardiovascular risk of patients with severe psoriasis, mechanistic studies are needed to further clarify the link.

Often, animal models are a good starting point to unravel pathogenetic mechanisms. With regard to psoriasis, older models often highlighted the role of the adaptive immune system (57), while novel approaches such as mannan-induced psoriasis shed more light on the crucial role of the innate immune system (58). Few studies have been performed to analyze the link between psoriasis and its cardiovascular comorbidity. One such approach takes advantage of the capacity of the TLR7 agonist imiquimod to induce a psoriasis-like inflammation in murine skin. Jin et al. succeeded in inducing a state of systemic inflammation through topical application of imiquimod onto interleukin-10-deficient mice, but noticed a decrease of body weight in these mice, while psoriasis patients show a trend toward obesity (59). Shibata et al. studied imiquimod-induced psoriasiform inflammation in mice deficient of adiponectin, an anti-inflammatory adipokine, and found a more severe phenotype in these knockout mice. Furthermore, intraperitoneal injections of adiponectin had a therapeutic effect in adiponectin knockout mice (60). While this study explored an indirect link between psoriasis and cardiovascular disease *via* metabolic factors, the only direct link the author is aware of comes from a study in the type-II collagen-specific antibody-induced psoriatic arthritis model. Using this model, Sherlock et al. demonstrated that IL-23 drives inflammation in the aortic root through activation of $CD3^{+}CD4^{-}CD8^{-}$ T-lymphocytes (61).

Atherosclerosis as a key process in cardiovascular diseases has long been recognized as an inflammation-driven phenomenon (62, 63). This is also true for psoriasis (64, 65). The cardiologist Späh was among the first who discussed a potentially common inflammatory pathway and the idea of an integrated treatment approach (66). He stressed altered endothelial function and subsequent recruitment of leukocytes, primarily T-lymphocytes, to developing lesions as a shared early step in the process of plaque formation in atherosclerosis and psoriasis. Lymphocyte extravasation has indeed been studied in detail with the intention to develop targeted therapies for psoriasis, but to date, none of the potential candidates was found to be sufficiently effective to validate development into a marketed drug (67, 68). Meanwhile, many more shared mechanisms of atherosclerosis and psoriasis have been studied in detail.

Elaborating on the observations described above, a role namely for T-helper-1 lymphocytes (TH1 lymphocytes) has been established in atherosclerosis as well as psoriasis (**Table 2**). Although TH1 as well as TH2 lymphocyte responses can contribute to atherosclerosis, several lines of evidence suggest a predominant role of TH1 lymphocytes. These include the TH1 phenotype and function of most T-cell clones derived from atherosclerotic plaques as well as immunohistochemical studies on such plaques (69–71). Subsequently, high circulating levels of TH17 lymphocytes and IL-17 in patients with acute coronary syndrome, a positive correlation of IL-17 with levels of high-sensitivity C-reactive protein and IL-6 (predicting an increased risk of myocardial infarction) in those patients, and the observation that IL-17 inhibition in mice significantly reduces the size of atherosclerotic plaques, were all interpreted as indicators for a role of TH17 lymphocytes in atherosclerosis (72–74). Similarly, psoriasis was initially thought to be a prototypical TH1 lymphocyte-mediated disease, with these cells activating macrophages, neutrophils and CD8$^+$ cytotoxic lymphocytes (75). Then, the role of TH17 lymphocytes was stressed in the light of clinical studies documenting the high clinical efficacy of therapies targeting the IL-17 pathway (76).

While the role of the adaptive immune system in the pathogenesis of psoriasis has been thoroughly investigated ever since the accidental observation of the therapeutic efficacy of cyclosporine A in 1979 (77), interest in the important role of the innate immune system has only recently experienced a renaissance (**Table 2**). Evidence for the contribution of neutrophils, which are predominant in pustular forms, but readily detectable also in chronic plaque type psoriasis, where they form the so-called Munro's abscesses within the epidermis, comes from *in vivo* studies as well as organotypic 3D models and has recently been reviewed elsewhere (78). Further supporting the role of neutrophils is the clinical observation by Reich et al., who reported that psoriasis treatment with the anti-IL17A antibody secukinumab resulted in the near total elimination of intraepidermal IL-17-positive neutrophils as an early therapeutic effect (79). Neutrophils are equally important in atherosclerosis, as they interact with damaged endothelium, augment leukocyte recruitment *via* secretion of chemotactic mediators, and promote the development of foam cells, a macrophage subset driving atherosclerosis (80). Neutrophil localization to developing atherosclerotic plaques has been demonstrated in mouse models (81, 82) and human atherosclerotic lesions (83); their presence in occlusive thrombi and culprit lesions of acute coronary syndrome patients suggests a role in atherosclerotic progression (84).

As for neutrophils, involvement of monocytes and macrophages has readily been demonstrated in both diseases (**Table 2**). These are regularly detectable in psoriatic lesions (85). Using a mouse model where the psoriatic phenotype is induced by topical application of the immunomodulator imiquimod, Costa et al. demonstrated that induction of the phenotype depends exclusively on hematopoietic cells. Using conditional knockout mouse strains, the active contribution of monocytes and macrophages on disease propagation and exacerbation was shown (86). With regard to atherosclerosis, Tabas and Lichtman recently reviewed how macrophages can be programmed for functions on a spectrum from inflammatory and host defense to resolution and repair in atherosclerotic plaques (87). In general, inflammatory macrophages carry out processes that promote atherosclerosis progression, including plaque necrosis and thinning of a protective fibrous cap. By contrast, resolving macrophages carry out functions that can suppress plaque progression and promote plaque regression, including clearing dead cells and secreting collagen that can form a protective scar over the lesion (88).

Besides these vigorously studied cells of the adaptive immune system, platelets seem to also actively contribute to atherosclerosis and psoriasis (**Table 2**). Platelets are widely known to have prominent functions in hemostasis and thrombosis, but their involvement in immune and inflammatory processes is now more and more recognized (89). Their potential to influence such process is not surprising, given their capacity to release a plethora of mediators and to interact with numerous cells and tissues through a variety of adhesion molecules. In psoriasis, platelet activation can be used to monitor disease activity through quantification of platelet activation markers in the patients' blood (90). Mechanistically, it is thought that activated platelets facilitate leukocyte extravasation (91). Similar effects link platelets to atherosclerosis (92, 93). The clinically relevant role of platelets in this context is underlined by the success of platelet inhibitory drugs in treating and preventing acute arterial thromboembolic events (94).

In recent years, a factor attracting particular attention in the context of psoriatic as well as atherosclerotic inflammation is IL-17A. Its role as a major driver of psoriatic inflammation is now well accepted and underlined by the numerous lines of evidence, including the development of a psoriatic phenotype in mice overexpressing IL-17A in the epidermis (95), or the high efficacy of IL-17A-blocking biologics in the treatment of psoriasis (96). By contrast, deciphering the exact role of IL-17A in atherosclerosis remains a challenging task (**Table 2**). Numerous studies documented pro-atherogenic effects. For example, in a hypercholesterolemic animal model, IL-17A inhibition reduced atheroma area and stenosis. At the molecular level, expression of the chemokine CCL5 (CC chemokine ligand 5), the cytokines IL-6 and TNF-α, several adhesion molecules including vascular cell adhesion molecule 1, and the pro-thrombotic molecule TF was reduced (74). Complementary experiments were conducted in murine models, where addition of exogenous IL-17A-stimulated pathological changes associated with increased plaque instability, while IL-17A inhibition resulted in regression of atherosclerosis (97–99). *Ex vivo* studies on human plaque fragments showed that exposure to IL-17A induced pro-inflammatory, pro-thrombotic, plaque destabilizing, and cell-attracting effects (100). On the other hand, there is also some evidence suggesting that IL-17A may have anti-atherosclerotic effects, as another mouse model characterized by increased IL-17A expression showed significantly smaller atherosclerotic lesions. In the same publication, an association between IL-17A expression and plaque stability in human carotid artery plaques was reported (101). Moreover, a study from Simon et al. on almost 1,000 patients with acute myocardial infarction demonstrated that low serum levels of IL-17A are associated with a higher risk for major cardiovascular events (102). Overall, many experts lean toward the concept of IL-17A being primarily pro-atherogenic, although some uncertainty persists.

Psoriatic Inflammation as a Driver for Atherosclerosis

Thus, over the last decade, multiple shared pathogenetic mechanisms have been identified in psoriatic and atherosclerotic plaque formation. These similarities do not, however, explain why psoriasis might actually represent an independent cardiovascular risk factor, as suggested by the majority of epidemiologic studies. Of major importance in this regard was the notion that psoriasis cannot be regarded as isolated cutaneous inflammation, but rather represents a chronic systemic inflammatory disease. To this end, several groups have identified biomarkers of inflammation in the blood of psoriasis patients which correlate with psoriasis severity, such as C-reactive protein (103), erythrocyte sedimentation rate (104), and the platelet activation marker P-selectin (90). Documentation of vascular inflammation through (18)F-fluorodeoxyglucose positron emission tomography computed tomography (PET-CT) in psoriasis patients, pioneered by Mehta and co-workers, points into the same direction (4). More recently, the group demonstrated that psoriasis severity associates with aortic vascular inflammation detected by that method (93), suggesting that psoriatic inflammation affects blood vessels and induces inflammation in the vessel walls. Studies in mouse models confirm that chronic skin-specific inflammation can indeed induce vascular inflammation (94).

The pathogenetic link between psoriasis and cardiovascular comorbidity is likely provided through insulin resistance and endothelial dysfunction, as these are known drivers for atherosclerosis (105). Insulin resistance is typically defined as decreased sensitivity to metabolic actions of insulin that promote glucose disposal. This is not only an important feature of diabetes mellitus but also a prominent component of cardiovascular disorders, which are characterized by endothelial dysfunction (106). Conversely, endothelial dysfunction is also present in diabetes mellitus (107). In addition to its essential metabolic actions, insulin has important vascular actions that involve stimulation of the production of nitric oxide from endothelium, leading to vasodilation (**Figure 1A**). This effect has metabolic consequences, too, as increased blood flow ultimately leads to augmented glucose disposal in skeletal muscle (108). On the other hand, insulin signaling in endothelial cells regulates secretion of the vasoconstricting factor endothelin-1. Inflammation shifts this equilibrium as it induces insulin resistance *via* cytokines, which alter insulin signaling in endothelial cells, ultimately reducing the production of vasodilating nitric oxide and inducing endothelial dysfunction (109) (**Figure 1B**).

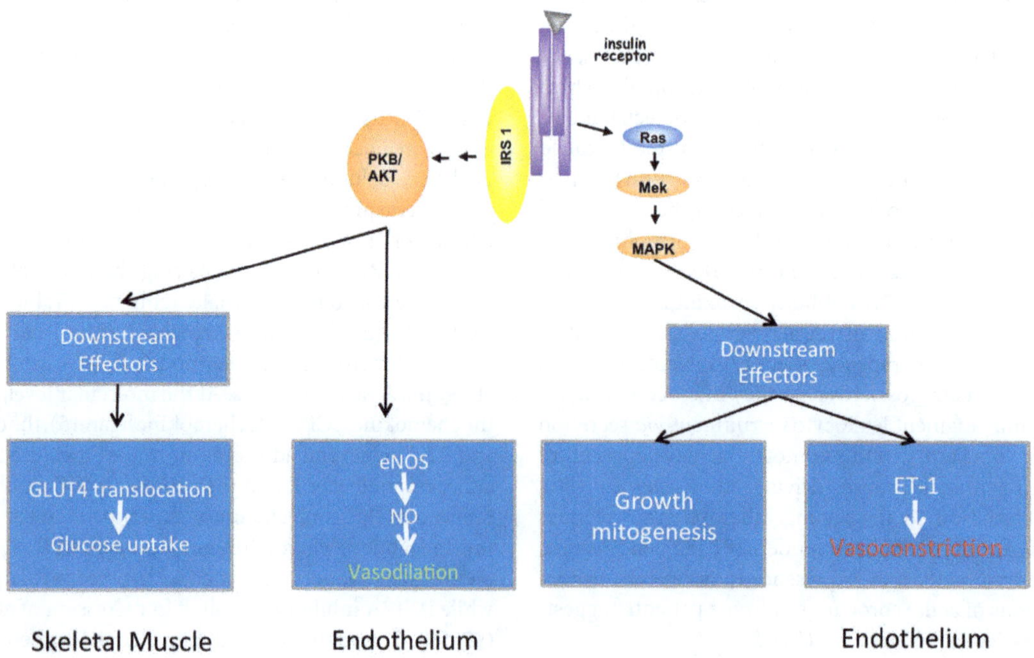

FIGURE 1 | Metabolic and vascular effects of insulin. Under physiologic conditions, the activated insulin receptor on endothelial cells leads to phosphorylation of endothelial nitric oxide synthase (eNOS) *via* activation of insulin receptor substrate (IRS) and phosphoinositide-3-kinase (a). This results in vasodilation *via* NO production. This branch also regulates GLUT4 translocation and glucose uptake in muscle cells. The mitogen-activated protein kinase (MAPK) pathway controls secretion of vasoconstrictive ET-1 in endothelial cells, and cell growth and mitogenesis in cells at large. Inflammation reduces NO production *via* blocking insulin receptor signaling at the level of the IRS-1 (b).

Noteworthy, TNF-α, a central cytokine in the pathogenesis of many chronic inflammatory diseases including psoriasis, is a major insulin antagonist (110).

The concept of the "psoriatic march" provides a framework to explain how psoriatic inflammation drives cardiovascular comorbidity *via* atherosclerosis independently from the presence of additional cardiovascular risk factors (111, 112) (**Figure 2**). According to this concept, psoriasis is a chronic systemic inflammatory disorder, as evidenced by elevated biomarkers of systemic inflammation. Noteworthy, not only classical markers for systemic inflammation have been shown to be elevated but also resistin and leptin (113, 114). These belong to a family of mediators secreted by adipocytes called adipokines. Resistin and leptin are insulin antagonizing adipokines. Collectively, the adipokine milieu in the blood of psoriasis patients is strikingly similar to that of prediabetic individuals and is a hint toward a state of insulin resistance. The diagnosis of insulin resistance is based on the so-called homeostasis model assessment of insulin resistance (HOMA-IR) index, calculated on the basis of a blood test, or an oral glucose tolerance test (115, 116). Using these approaches, two cross-sectional studies demonstrated that psoriasis patients exhibit insulin resistance at clinical levels (113, 117). Besides the insulin-antagonizing effects, numerous adipokines in general and leptin in particular may drive atherosclerosis through immunomodulation, including the upregulation of adhesion molecules on endothelial cells (118). At the level of endothelial cells, insulin resistance is thought to induce endothelial dysfunction *via* the pathway described above, resulting in vascular stiffness at the functional level. Indeed, several groups found evidence for endothelial dysfunction, using ultrasound methods. In particular, flow-mediated vascular dilation was impaired (119–122). In one of these studies, insulin resistance was assessed as well *via* the HOMA-IR and found to be significantly higher when compared to non-psoriatic controls, again stressing the link between insulin resistance and endothelial dysfunction in psoriasis (122). This cascade drives atherosclerosis, which ultimately causes cardiovascular diseases such as myocardial infarction and stroke.

Although not in the focus of this review, it is interesting to note that inflammation-induced insulin resistance may well help to explain the altered epidermal homeostasis observed in the epidermis of psoriatic plaques (123, 124), a phenomenon that might have implications beyond psoriasis (125).

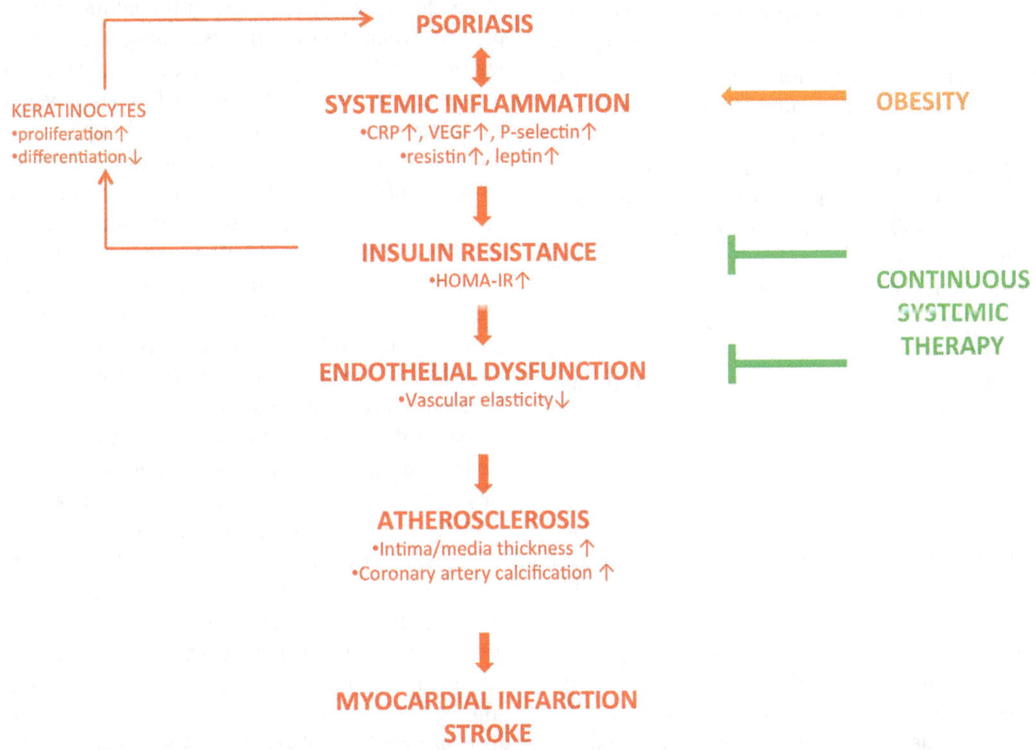

FIGURE 2 | The concept of the "psoriatic march." This hypothesis suggests that psoriasis is a systemic inflammatory condition, as numerous biomarkers of inflammation are elevated in the patients' blood compartment. Functional consequences are insulin resistance, evidenced by an increased HOMA-IR (homeostasis assessment of insulin resistance), and endothelial dysfunction, resulting in increased vascular stiffness. This provides the basis for atherosclerosis, observable through analysis of vessel wall composition *via* CTs or ultrasound. Depending on the sites of atherosclerosis, major cardiovascular events such as myocardial infarction and stroke result from this. This "backbone" (red, bold) may be developed further by adding additional "modules": insulin resistance has been shown to alter epidermal homeostasis (red, fine). Obesity, causing a state of systemic inflammation as well, is a known risk factor for psoriasis and may induce the phenotype (orange, bold). Whether systemic anti-inflammatory therapy is capable of reducing the patients' cardiovascular risk through reducing insulin resistance and endothelial dysfunction is still a matter of debate (green).

CONSEQUENCES FOR THE MANAGEMENT OF PSORIASIS

Monitoring

Most observations discussed so far support the notion that cardiovascular comorbidity is a clinically relevant problem for patients suffering from severe psoriasis. In spite of this, several studies document that these patients are not adequately monitored and treated for cardiovascular risk factors. A survey conducted between October 2010 and April 2011 among primary care physicians and cardiologists showed that most of the responding physicians (251 of 1,200 questionnaires sent out were returned) did not routinely screen psoriasis patients for cardiovascular risk factors (126). A cross-sectional study based on National Ambulatory Medical Care Survey data from 2005 to 2009 demonstrated that less than half of the psoriasis patients were screened for at least one cardiovascular risk factor (127). Finally, in a cross-sectional study of patients with hypertension in Great Britain, psoriasis patients were more likely to have uncontrolled hypertension compared with non-psoriatic individuals (128). This is in contrast to recommendations from numerous organizations and societies, who unanimously suggest such a screening (129–131). Takeshita et al. recently summarized what most experts currently agree upon, much of it being identical to what is comprised in current recommendations for the general adult population (132, 133): traditional cardiovascular risk factors should be evaluated. These include total and high-density lipoprotein cholesterol, systolic blood pressure, use of antihypertensive therapy, diabetes, and current smoking. In addition, lifestyle interventions, such as weight loss and smoking cessation, should be encouraged among patients who are obese and who are current smokers, respectively. A controlled clinical trial published a decade ago already showed the potential advantages of a more comprehensive approach to psoriasis treatment, as obese patients with moderate-to-severe psoriasis had a better response to low-dose cyclosporine A if a calorie-reduced diet was included in their treatment regimen (134).

Prevention

The state of chronic systemic inflammation in psoriasis may at least contribute to atherosclerosis *via* insulin resistance and endothelial dysfunction and therefore be partially responsible for the increased cardiovascular risk of patients with severe psoriasis. This raises the question whether continuous systemic anti-inflammatory treatments may help to reduce this excess risk. Recently, data from the CANTOS trial suggest that this is principally feasible. That trial evaluated the efficacy of the interleukin-1β-blocking antibody canakinumab in more than 10,000 patients with previous myocardial infarction and a high-sensitivity C-reactive protein level of 2 mg or more per liter on nonfatal myocardial infarction, nonfatal stroke, or cardiovascular death. At a median follow-up of 3.7 years, the incidence rate was 4.50 events per 100 patient-years in the placebo-group, and between 3.86 and 4.11 events per 100 patient-years in the different canakinumab dosing groups. Thus, the trial documented a small, but statistically significant reduction of recurrent cardiovascular events in a high-risk population (135).

An early hint that continuous systemic anti-inflammatory treatment might reduce the cardiovascular risk of psoriasis came from a retrospective study by Prodanovich et al. who analyzed the files of more than 7,000 American veterans who had been treated over extended periods of time with methotrexate for their psoriasis. They found a significantly reduced incidence of cardiovascular diseases in those patients (136). Since then, several observational studies analyzing the effects of methotrexate or TNF-α inhibitors came to similar conclusions (137, 138), while others failed to document such protective effects (139, 140). Complementary to these studies, small controlled trials were performed, evaluating changes of biomarkers for cardiovascular risk under systemic anti-psoriatic treatment. Indeed, several groups reported amelioration of such markers under successful therapy. These include cytokines, adipokines, endothelial dysfunction, and carotid intima-media thickness (141–145).

Based on some of these observations, more ambitious projects were launched, sponsored by pharmaceutical companies. A pilot study on 30 psoriasis patients looked at vascular inflammation in the ascending aorta and carotid arteries by means of PET-CTs. In this study, decreases in vascular inflammation were observed in patients treated with adalimumab compared with placebo when data for the ascending aorta and carotid arteries were analyzed separately at 15 weeks (146). A larger study including 107 patients showed no difference over 16 weeks in the adalimumab-treated group compared to placebo and a modest increase in vascular inflammation in the carotid arteries after 52 weeks of treatment with adalimumab (147). A commentary on that publication suggested that the study might have been too small or of insufficient duration to show an effect, and that it was the carotid arteries and ascending aorta that were studied, not the coronary arteries, which might explain the negative result (20). Another study using the IL-17A-blocking antibody secukinumab was performed in a multi-center setting in Germany. A recently presented abstract on the occasion of the congress of the European Academy for Dermatology and Venereology in Geneva in 2017 documented a trend toward improvement in vascular elasticity, but no date from that trial have so far been published in a peer-reviewed manner.

Taken together, there is some evidence in favor of the idea to reduce the excess cardiovascular risk of psoriasis patients through systemic anti-inflammatory therapy. TNF-α and IL-17A are interesting targets in this regard, as the former is an important insulin antagonist, and the latter seems to exhibit primarily pro-atherogenic effects, although some anti-atherogenic effects have also been reported (148). The CANTOS study can serve as proof of concept for the principal capacity of anti-inflammatory therapy to reduce the cardiovascular risk, but it also points out that even in a high-risk population the effect size might be relatively small. This may explain why much smaller and shorter studies can easily fail to show efficacy in this regard, even more so, if relatively health patients are enrolled, as has been the case in the German trial using secukinumab. Although this approach remains intellectually appealing, it may be more effective and efficient in a real-world scenario to address other major cardiovascular risk factors associated with psoriasis in order to reduce the patients' excess cardiovascular risk, e.g., through appropriate treatment of the metabolic syndrome or components thereof, or through lifestyle interventions (smoking!).

CONCLUSION

Psoriasis is currently regarded a chronic-recurrent, systemic inflammatory disease, driven by an intense cross talk between cells of the innate and adaptive immune system. It is associated with substantial cardiovascular comorbidity, which can only partially be explained through shared a genetic control. Evidence in favor of psoriasis as an independent cardiovascular risk factor comes from epidemiologic studies showing a "dose effect" of psoriasis on the patients' cardiovascular risk as well as from case–control studies looking at biomarkers for cardiovascular risk and specific manifestations of atherosclerosis. Inflammation-induced insulin resistance and endothelial dysfunction provide a pathogenetic link between psoriasis and atherosclerosis. Whether systemic anti-inflammatory therapy can reduce the patients' excess cardiovascular risk remains one of the hot research topics in the field. Independent of this discussion, a comprehensive approach to the management of psoriasis at least in patients with severe disease is mandatory based on current knowledge. This must include regular screening and monitoring of traditional cardiovascular risk factors as well as their guideline-oriented treatment.

AUTHOR CONTRIBUTIONS

W-HB is the sole author of this manuscript. He defined the content, performed the literature search, wrote the text, and created figures and the table.

REFERENCES

1. WHO. *Document EB133.R2, Agenda Item 6.2.* (2013).
2. Boehncke WH, Schön MP. Psoriasis. *Lancet* (2015) 386(9997):983–94. doi:10.1016/S0140-6736(14)61909-7
3. Capon F, Burden AD, Trembath RC, Barker JN. Psoriasis and other complex trait dermatoses: from Loci to functional pathways. *J Invest Dermatol* (2012) 132(3 Pt 2):915–22. doi:10.1038/jid.2011.395
4. Mehta NN, Yu Y, Saboury B, Foroughi N, Krishnamoorthy P, Raper A, et al. Systemic and vascular inflammation in patients with moderate to severe psoriasis as measured by [18F]-fluorodeoxyglucose positron emission tomography-computed tomography (FDG-PET/CT): a pilot study. *Arch Dermatol* (2011) 147(9):1031–9. doi:10.1001/archdermatol.2011.119
5. Dougados M. Comorbidities in rheumatoid arthritis. *Curr Opin Rheumatol* (2016) 28(3):282–8. doi:10.1097/BOR.0000000000000267
6. Román AL, Muñoz F. Comorbidity in inflammatory bowel disease. *World J Gastroenterol* (2011) 17(22):2723–33. doi:10.3748/wjg.v17.i22.2723
7. Wens I, Dalgas U, Stenager E, Eijnde BO. Risk factors related to cardiovascular diseases and the metabolic syndrome in multiple sclerosis – a systematic review. *Mult Scler* (2013) 19(12):1556–64. doi:10.1177/1352458513504252
8. Takeshita J, Grewal S, Langan SM, Mehta NN, Ogdie A, Van Voorhees AS, et al. Psoriasis and comorbid diseases: epidemiology. *J Am Acad Dermatol* (2017) 76(3):377–90. doi:10.1016/j.jaad.2016.07.064
9. Boehncke WH. Psoriasis and psoriatic arthritis: flip sides of the coin? *Acta Derm Venereol* (2016) 96(4):436–41. doi:10.2340/00015555-2385
10. Abuabara K, Azfar RS, Shin DB, Neimann AL, Troxel AB, Gelfand JM. Cause-specific mortality in patients with severe psoriasis: a population-based cohort study in the U.K. *Br J Dermatol* (2010) 163(3):586–92. doi:10.1111/j.1365-2133.2010.09941.x
11. Agca R, Heslinga SC, Rollefstad S, Heslinga M, McInnes IB, Peters MJ, et al. EULAR recommendations for cardiovascular disease risk management in patients with rheumatoid arthritis and other forms of inflammatory joint disorders: 2015/2016 update. *Ann Rheum Dis* (2017) 76(1):17–28. doi:10.1136/annrheumdis-2016-209775
12. Stern RS. Psoriasis is not a useful independent risk factor for cardiovascular disease. *J Invest Dermatol* (2010) 130(4):917–9. doi:10.1038/jid.2009.446
13. Lai YC, Yew YW. Psoriasis as an independent risk factor for cardiovascular disease: an epidemiologic analysis using a national database. *J Cutan Med Surg* (2016) 20(4):327–33. doi:10.1177/1203475415602842
14. Ogdie A, Troxel AB, Mehta NN, Gelfand JM. Psoriasis and cardiovascular risk: strength in numbers part 3. *J Invest Dermatol* (2015) 135(9):2148–50. doi:10.1038/jid.2015.218
15. Henseler T, Christophers E. Disease concomitance in psoriasis. *J Am Acad Dermatol* (1995) 32(6):982–6. doi:10.1016/0190-9622(95)91336-X
16. Dowlatshahi EA, Kavousi M, Nijsten T, Ikram MA, Hofman A, Franco OH, et al. Psoriasis is not associated with atherosclerosis and incident cardiovascular events: the Rotterdam Study. *J Invest Dermatol* (2013) 133(10):2347–54. doi:10.1038/jid.2013.131
17. Parisi R, Rutter MK, Lunt M, Young HS, Symmons DPM, Griffiths CEM, et al. Psoriasis and the risk of major cardiovascular events: cohort study using the clinical practice research datalink. *J Invest Dermatol* (2015) 135(9):2189–97. doi:10.1038/jid.2015.87
18. Egeberg A, Thyssen JP, Jensen P, Gislason GH, Skov L. Risk of myocardial infarction in patients with psoriasis and psoriatic arthritis: a nationwide cohort study. *Acta Derm Venereol* (2017) 97(7):819–24. doi:10.2340/00015555-2657
19. Raaby L, Ahlehoff O, de Thurah A. Psoriasis and cardiovascular events: updating the evidence. *Arch Dermatol Res* (2017) 309(3):225–8. doi:10.1007/s00403-016-1712-1
20. Lebwohl M. Does treatment of psoriasis reduce cardiovascular comorbidities? *J Invest Dermatol* (2017) 137(8):1612–3. doi:10.1016/j.jid.2017.06.001
21. Nast A, Gisondi P, Ormerod AD, Saiag P, Smith C, Spuls PI, et al. European S3-Guidelines on the systemic treatment of psoriasis vulgaris – Update 2015 – Short version – EDF in cooperation with EADV and IPC. *J Eur Acad Dermatol Venereol* (2015) 29(12):2277–94. doi:10.1111/jdv.13354
22. Coates LC, Kavanaugh A, Mease PJ, Soriano ER, Laura Acosta-Felquer M, Armstrong AW, et al. Group for research and assessment of psoriasis and psoriatic arthritis 2015 treatment recommendations for psoriatic arthritis. *Arthritis Rheumatol* (2016) 68(5):1060–71. doi:10.1002/art.39573
23. Armstrong EJ, Harskamp CT, Armstrong AW. Psoriasis and major adverse cardiovascular events: a systematic review and meta-analysis of observational studies. *J Am Heart Assoc* (2013) 2(2):e000062. doi:10.1161/JAHA.113.000062
24. Gaeta M, Castelvecchio S, Ricci C, Pigatto P, Pellissero G, Cappato R. Role of psoriasis as independent predictor of cardiovascular disease: a meta-regression analysis. *Int J Cardiol* (2013) 168(3):2282–8. doi:10.1016/j.ijcard.2013.01.197
25. Gu WJ, Weng CL, Zhao YT, Liu QH, Yin RX. Psoriasis and risk of cardiovascular disease: a meta-analysis of cohort studies. *Int J Cardiol* (2013) 168(5):4992–6. doi:10.1016/j.ijcard.2013.07.127
26. Horreau C, Pouplard C, Brenaut E, Barnetche T, Misery L, Cribier B, et al. Cardiovascular morbidity and mortality in psoriasis and psoriatic arthritis: a systematic literature review. *J Eur Acad Dermatol Venereol* (2013) 27(Suppl 3):12–29. doi:10.1111/jdv.12163
27. Miller IM, Ellervik C, Yazdanyar S, Jemec GB. Meta-analysis of psoriasis, cardiovascular disease, and associated risk factors. *J Am Acad Dermatol* (2013) 69(6):1014–24. doi:10.1016/j.jaad.2013.06.053

28. Pietrzak A, Bartosińska J, Chodorowska G, Szepietowski JC, Paluszkiewicz P, Schwartz RA. Cardiovascular aspects of psoriasis: an updated review. *Int J Dermatol* (2013) 52(2):153–62. doi:10.1111/j.1365-4632.2012.05584.x
29. Samarasekera EJ, Neilson JM, Warren RB, Parnham J, Smith CH. Incidence of cardiovascular disease in individuals with psoriasis: a systematic review and meta-analysis. *J Invest Dermatol* (2013) 133(10):2340–6. doi:10.1038/jid.2013.149
30. Xu T, Zhang YH. Association of psoriasis with stroke and myocardial infarction: meta-analysis of cohort studies. *Br J Dermatol* (2012) 167(6): 1345–50. doi:10.1111/bjd.12002
31. Strauss H. Zur Lehre von der neurogenen und der thyreogenen Glykosurie. *DtscMed Wochenschr* (1897) 20:309–12. doi:10.1055/s-0029-1204995
32. Kassi E, Pervanidou P, Kaltsas G, Chrousos G. Metabolic syndrome: definitions and controversies. *BMC Med* (2011) 9:48. doi:10.1186/1741-7015-9-48
33. D'Agostino RB Sr, Vasan RS, Pencina MJ, Wolf PA, Cobain M, Massaro JM, et al. General cardiovascular risk profile for use in primary care: the Framingham Heart Study. *Circulation* (2008) 117(6):743–53. doi:10.1161/CIRCULATIONAHA.107.699579
34. Lee EJ, Han KD, Han JH, Lee JH. Smoking and risk of psoriasis: a nationwide cohort study. *J Am Acad Dermatol* (2017) 77(3):573–5. doi:10.1016/j.jaad.2017.04.015
35. Danielsen K, Wilsgaard T, Olsen AO, Furberg AS. Overweight and weight gain predict psoriasis development in a population-based cohort. *Acta Derm Venereol* (2017) 97(3):332–9. doi:10.2340/00015555-2530
36. Gelfand JM, Neimann AL, Shin DB, Wang X, Margolis DJ, Troxel AB. Risk of myocardial infarction in patients with psoriasis. *JAMA* (2006) 296(14):1735–41. doi:10.1001/jama.296.14.1735
37. Armstrong AW, Harskamp CT, Ledo L, Rogers JH, Armstrong EJ. Coronary artery disease in patients with psoriasis referred for coronary angiography. *Am J Cardiol* (2012) 109(7):976–80. doi:10.1016/j.amjcard.2011.11.025
38. Li WQ, Han JL, Manson JE, Rimm EB, Rexrode KM, Curhan GC, et al. Psoriasis and risk of nonfatal cardiovascular disease in U.S. women: a cohort study. *Br J Dermatol* (2012) 166(4):811–8. doi:10.1111/j.1365-2133.2011.10774.x
39. Ludwig RJ, Herzog C, Rostock A, Ochsendorf FR, Zollner TM, Thaci D, et al. Psoriasis: a possible risk factor for development of coronary artery calcification. *Br J Dermatol* (2007) 156(2):271–6. doi:10.1111/j.1365-2133.2006.07562.x
40. Mehta NN, Yu Y, Pinnelas R, Krishnamoorthy P, Shin DB, Troxel AB, et al. Attributable risk estimate of severe psoriasis on major cardiovascular events. *Am J Med* (2011) 124(8):775.e1–6. doi:10.1016/j.amjmed.2011.03.028
41. Ahlehoff O, Gislason GH, Charlot M, Jørgensen CH, Lindhardsen J, Olesen JB, et al. Psoriasis is associated with clinically significant cardiovascular risk: a Danish nationwide cohort study. *J Intern Med* (2011) 270(2):147–57. doi:10.1111/j.1365-2796.2010.02310.x
42. Ogdie A, Yu Y, Haynes K, Love TJ, Maliha S, Jiang Y, et al. Risk of major cardiovascular events in patients with psoriatic arthritis, psoriasis and rheumatoid arthritis: a population-based cohort study. *Ann Rheum Dis* (2015) 74(2):326–32. doi:10.1136/annrheumdis-2014-205675
43. Thyssen JP, Halling-Overgaard AS, Andersen YMF, Gislason G, Skov L, Egeberg A. The association between cardiovascular disease and type 2 diabetes in adults with atopic dermatitis: a systematic review and meta-analysis. *Br J Dermatol* (2017). doi:10.1111/bjd.16215
44. Andersen YM, Egeberg A, Gislason GH, Hansen PR, Skov L, Thyssen JP. Risk of myocardial infarction, ischemic stroke, and cardiovascular death in patients with atopic dermatitis. *J Allergy Clin Immunol* (2016) 138(1):310–2.e3. doi:10.1016/j.jaci.2016.01.015
45. Elder JT, Nair RP, Guo SW, Henseler T, Christophers E, Voorhees JJ. The genetics of psoriasis. *Arch Dermatol* (1994) 130(2):216–24. doi:10.1001/archderm.1994.01690020082014
46. Nair RP, Stuart PE, Nistor I, Hiremagalore R, Chia NV, Jenisch S, et al. Sequence and haplotype analysis supports HLA-C as the psoriasis susceptibility 1 gene. *Am J Hum Genet* (2006) 78(5):827–51. doi:10.1086/503821
47. Harden JL, Krueger JG, Bowcock AM. The immunogenetics of psoriasis: a comprehensive review. *J Autoimmun* (2015) 64:66–73. doi:10.1016/j.jaut.2015.07.008
48. Weidinger S, Willis-Owen SA, Kamatani Y, Baurecht H, Morar N, Liang L, et al. A genome-wide association study of atopic dermatitis identifies loci with overlapping effects on asthma and psoriasis. *Hum Mol Genet* (2013) 22(23):4841–56. doi:10.1093/hmg/ddt317
49. Tamari M, Saeki H, Hayashi M, Umezawa Y, Ito T, Fukuchi O, et al. An association study of 36 psoriasis susceptibility loci for psoriasis vulgaris and atopic dermatitis in a Japanese population. *J Dermatol Sci* (2014) 76(2):156–7. doi:10.1016/j.jdermsci.2014.08.005
50. Kim K, Bang SY, Lee HS, Bae SC. Update on the genetic architecture of rheumatoid arthritis. *Nat Rev Rheumatol* (2017) 13(1):13–24. doi:10.1038/nrrheum.2016.176
51. Kessler T, Vilne B, Schunkert H. The impact of genome-wide association studies on the pathophysiology and therapy of cardiovascular disease. *EMBO Mol Med* (2016) 8(7):688–701. doi:10.15252/emmm.201506174
52. Parkes M, Cortes A, van Heel DA, Brown MA. Genetic insights into common pathways and complex relationships among immune-mediated diseases. *Nat Rev Genet* (2013) 14(9):661–73. doi:10.1038/nrg3502
53. Ellinghaus D, Ellinghaus E, Nair RP, Stuart PE, Esko T, Metspalu A, et al. Combined analysis of genome-wide association studies for Crohn disease and psoriasis identifies seven shared susceptibility loci. *Am J Hum Genet* (2012) 90(4):636–47. doi:10.1016/j.ajhg.2012.02.020
54. Ellinghaus D, Jostins L, Spain SL, Cortes A, Bethune J, Han B, et al. Analysis of five chronic inflammatory diseases identifies 27 new associations and highlights disease-specific patterns at shared loci. *Nat Genet* (2016) 48(5):510–8. doi:10.1038/ng.3528
55. Cheng H, Li Y, Zuo XB, Tang HY, Tang XF, Gao JP, et al. Identification of a missense variant in LNPEP that confers psoriasis risk. *J Invest Dermatol* (2014) 134(2):359–65. doi:10.1038/jid.2013.317
56. Gupta Y, Möller S, Zillikens D, Boehncke WH, Ibrahim SM, Ludwig RJ. Genetic control of psoriasis is relatively distinct from that of metabolic syndrome and coronary artery disease. *Exp Dermatol* (2013) 22(8):552–3. doi:10.1111/exd.12192
57. Boehncke WH, Schön MP. Animal models of psoriasis. *Clin Dermatol* (2007) 25(6):596–605. doi:10.1016/j.clindermatol.2007.08.014
58. Hagert C, Sareila O, Kelkka T, Jalkanen S, Holmdahl R. The macrophage mannose receptor regulate mannan-induced psoriasis, psoriatic arthritis, and rheumatoid arthritis-like disease models. *Front Immunol* (2018) 9:114. doi:10.3389/fimmu.2018.00114
59. Jin SP, Koh SJ, Yu DA, Kim MW, Yun HT, Lee DH, et al. Imiquimod-applied interleukin-10 deficient mice better reflects severe and persistent psoriasis with systemic inflammatory state. *Exp Dermatol* (2018) 27(1):43–9. doi:10.1111/exd.13403
60. Shibata S, Tada Y, Hau CS, Mitsui A, Kamata M, Asano Y, et al. Adiponectin regulates psoriasiform skin inflammation by suppressing IL-17 production from γδ-T cells. *Nat Commun* (2015) 6:7687. doi:10.1038/ncomms8687
61. Sherlock JP, Joyce-Shaikh B, Turner SP, Chao CC, Sathe M, Grein J, et al. IL-23 induces spondyloarthropathy by acting on ROR-γt+ CD3+CD4-CD8- entheseal resident T cells. *Nat Med* (2012) 18(7):1069–76. doi:10.1038/nm.2817
62. Hansson GK. Inflammation, atherosclerosis, and coronary artery disease. *N Engl J Med* (2005) 352(16):1685–95. doi:10.1056/NEJMra043430
63. Hansson GK. Inflammation and atherosclerosis: the end of a controversy. *Circulation* (2017) 136(20):1875–7. doi:10.1161/CIRCULATIONAHA.117.030484
64. Schön MP, Boehncke WH. Psoriasis. *N Engl J Med* (2005) 352(18):1899–912. doi:10.1056/NEJMra041320
65. Lowes MA, Suárez-Fariñas M, Krueger JG. Immunology of psoriasis. *Annu Rev Immunol* (2014) 32:227–55. doi:10.1146/annurev-immunol-032713-120225
66. Späh F. Inflammation in atherosclerosis and psoriasis: common pathogenic mechanisms and the potential for an integrated treatment approach. *Br J Dermatol* (2008) 159(Suppl 2):10–7. doi:10.1111/j.1365-2133.2008.08780.x
67. Boehncke WH, Schön MP. Interfering with leukocyte rolling – a promising therapeutic approach in inflammatory skin disorders? *Trends Pharmacol Sci* (2003) 24(2):49–52. doi:10.1016/S0165-6147(02)00039-1
68. Boehncke WH, Schön MP, Girolomoni G, Griffiths C, Bos JD, Thestrup-Pedersen K. Leukocyte extravasation as a target for anti-inflammatory therapy – which molecule to choose? *Exp Dermatol* (2005) 14(1):70–80. doi:10.1111/j.0906-6705.2005.290a.x

69. Stemme S, Faber B, Holm J, Wiklund O, Witztum JL, Hansson GK. T lymphocytes from human atherosclerotic plaques recognize oxidized low density lipoprotein. *Proc Natl Acad Sci U S A* (1995) 92(9):3893–7. doi:10.1073/pnas.92.9.3893
70. Frostegård J, Ulfgren AK, Nyberg P, Hedin U, Swedenborg J, Andersson U, et al. Cytokine expression in advanced human atherosclerotic plaques: dominance of pro-inflammatory (Th1) and macrophage-stimulating cytokines. *Atherosclerosis* (1999) 145(1):33–43. doi:10.1016/S0021-9150(99)00011-8
71. Methe H, Brunner S, Wiegand D, Nabauer M, Koglin J, Edelman ER. Enhanced T-helper-1 lymphocyte activation patterns in acute coronary syndromes. *J Am Coll Cardiol* (2005) 45(12):1939–45. doi:10.1016/j.jacc.2005.03.040
72. Cheng X, Yu X, Ding YJ, Fu QQ, Xie JJ, Tang TT, et al. The Th17/Treg imbalance in patients with acute coronary syndrome. *Clin Immunol* (2008) 127(1):89–97. doi:10.1016/j.clim.2008.01.009
73. Hashmi S, Zeng QT. Role of interleukin-17 and interleukin-17-induced cytokines interleukin-6 and interleukin-8 in unstable coronary artery disease. *Coron Artery Dis* (2006) 17(8):699–706. doi:10.1097/01.mca.0000236288.94553.b4
74. Erbel C, Chen L, Bea F, Wangler S, Celik S, Lasitschka F, et al. Inhibition of IL-17A attenuates atherosclerotic lesion development in apoE-deficient mice. *J Immunol* (2009) 183(12):8167–75. doi:10.4049/jimmunol.0901126
75. Nickoloff BJ. Skin innate immune system in psoriasis: friend or foe? *J Clin Invest* (1999) 104(9):1161–4. doi:10.1172/JCI8633
76. Girolomoni G, Strohal R, Puig L, Bachelez H, Barker J, Boehncke WH, et al. The role of IL-23 and the IL-23/T_H 17 immune axis in the pathogenesis and treatment of psoriasis. *J Eur Acad Dermatol Venereol* (2017) 31(10):1616–26. doi:10.1111/jdv.14433
77. Mueller W, Herrmann B. Cyclosporin A for psoriasis. *N Engl J Med* (1979) 301(10):555. doi:10.1056/NEJM197909063011015
78. Lorthois I, Asselineau D, Seyler N, Pouliot R. Contribution of in vivo and organotypic 3D models to understanding the role of macrophages and neutrophils in the pathogenesis of psoriasis. *Mediators Inflamm* (2017) 2017:7215072. doi:10.1155/2017/7215072
79. Reich K, Papp KA, Matheson RT, Tu JH, Bissonnette R, Bourcier M, et al. Evidence that a neutrophil-keratinocyte crosstalk is an early target of IL-17A inhibition in psoriasis. *Exp Dermatol* (2015) 24(7):529–35. doi:10.1111/exd.12710
80. Soehnlein O. Multiple roles for neutrophils in atherosclerosis. *Circ Res* (2012) 110(6):875–88. doi:10.1161/CIRCRESAHA.111.257535
81. van Leeuwen M, Gijbels MJ, Duijvestijn A, Smook M, van de Gaar MJ, Heeringa P, et al. Accumulation of myeloperoxidase-positive neutrophils in atherosclerotic lesions in LDLR-/- mice. *Arterioscler Thromb Vasc Biol* (2008) 28(1):84–9. doi:10.1161/ATVBAHA.107.154807
82. Rotzius P, Thams S, Soehnlein O, Kenne E, Tseng CN, Björkström NK, et al. Distinct infiltration of neutrophils in lesion shoulders in ApoE-/- mice. *Am J Pathol* (2010) 177(1):493–500. doi:10.2353/ajpath.2010.090480
83. Hosokawa T, Kumon Y, Kobayashi T, Enzan H, Nishioka Y, Yuri K, et al. Neutrophil infiltration and oxidant-production in human atherosclerotic carotid plaques. *Histol Histopathol* (2011) 26(1):1–11. doi:10.14670/HH-26.1
84. Kramer MC, Rittersma SZ, de Winter RJ, Ladich ER, Fowler DR, Liang YH, et al. Relationship of thrombus healing to underlying plaque morphology in sudden coronary death. *J Am Coll Cardiol* (2010) 55(2):122–32. doi:10.1016/j.jacc.2009.09.007
85. Deng Y, Chang C, Lu Q. The inflammatory response in psoriasis: a comprehensive review. *Clin Rev Allergy Immunol* (2016) 50(3):377–89. doi:10.1007/s12016-016-8535-x
86. Costa S, Marini O, Bevilacqua D, DeFranco AL, Hou B, Lonardi S, et al. Role of MyD88 signaling in the imiquimod-induced mouse model of psoriasis: focus on innate myeloid cells. *J Leukoc Biol* (2017) 102(3):791–803. doi:10.1189/jlb.3MA0217-054RR
87. Tabas I, Lichtman AH. Monocyte-macrophages and T cells in atherosclerosis. *Immunity* (2017) 47(4):621–34. doi:10.1016/j.immuni.2017.09.008
88. Peled M, Fisher EA. Dynamic aspects of macrophage polarization during atherosclerosis progression and regression. *Front Immunol* (2014) 5:579. doi:10.3389/fimmu.2014.00579
89. Tamagawa-Mineoka R. Important roles of platelets as immune cells in the skin. *J Dermatol Sci* (2015) 77(2):93–101. doi:10.1016/j.jdermsci.2014.10.003
90. Garbaraviciene J, Diehl S, Varwig D, Bylaite M, Ackermann H, Ludwig RJ, et al. Platelet P-selectin reflects a state of cutaneous inflammation: possible application to monitor treatment efficacy in psoriasis. *Exp Dermatol* (2010) 19(8):736–41. doi:10.1111/j.1600-0625.2010.01095.x
91. Ludwig RJ, Schultz JE, Boehncke WH, Podda M, Tandi C, Krombach F, et al. Activated, not resting, platelets increase leukocyte rolling in murine skin utilizing a distinct set of adhesion molecules. *J Invest Dermatol* (2004) 122(3):830–6. doi:10.1111/j.0022-202X.2004.22318.x
92. Gawaz M, Langer H, May AE. Platelets in inflammation and atherogenesis. *J Clin Invest* (2005) 115(12):3378–84. doi:10.1172/JCI27196
93. Gisterå A, Hansson GK. The immunology of atherosclerosis. *Nat Rev Nephrol* (2017) 13(6):368–80. doi:10.1038/nrneph.2017.51
94. Jamasbi J, Ayabe K, Goto S, Nieswandt B, Peter K, Siess W. Platelet receptors as therapeutic targets: past, present and future. *Thromb Haemost* (2017) 117(7):1249–57. doi:10.1160/TH16-12-0911
95. Croxford AL, Karbach S, Kurschus FC, Wörtge S, Nikolaev A, Yogev N, et al. IL-6 regulates neutrophil microabscess formation in IL-17A-driven psoriasiform lesions. *J Invest Dermatol* (2014) 134(3):728–35. doi:10.1038/jid.2013.404
96. Amin M, Darji K, No DJ, Bhutani T, Wu JJ. Review of IL-17 inhibitors for psoriasis. *J Dermatolog Treat* (2017) 10:1–6. doi:10.1080/09546634.2017.1395796
97. Gao Q, Jiang Y, Ma T, Zhu F, Gao F, Zhang P, et al. A critical function of Th17 proinflammatory cells in the development of atherosclerotic plaque in mice. *J Immunol* (2010) 185(10):5820–7. doi:10.4049/jimmunol.1000116
98. Smith E, Prasad KM, Butcher M, Dobrian A, Kolls JK, Ley K, et al. Blockade of interleukin-17A results in reduced atherosclerosis in apolipoprotein E-deficient mice. *Circulation* (2010) 121(15):1746–55. doi:10.1161/CIRCULATIONAHA.109.924886
99. Madhur MS, Funt SA, Li L, Vinh A, Chen W, Lob HE, et al. Role of interleukin 17 in inflammation, atherosclerosis, and vascular function in apolipoprotein e-deficient mice. *Arterioscler Thromb Vasc Biol* (2011) 31(7):1565–72. doi:10.1161/ATVBAHA.111.227629
100. Erbel C, Akhavanpoor M, Okuyucu D, Wangler S, Dietz A, Zhao L, et al. IL-17A influences essential functions of the monocyte/macrophage lineage and is involved in advanced murine and human atherosclerosis. *J Immunol* (2014) 193(9):4344–55. doi:10.4049/jimmunol.1400181
101. Taleb S, Romain M, Ramkhelawon B, Uyttenhove C, Pasterkamp G, Herbin O, et al. Loss of SOCS3 expression in T cells reveals a regulatory role for interleukin-17 in atherosclerosis. *J Exp Med* (2009) 206(10):2067–77. doi:10.1084/jem.20090545
102. Simon T, Taleb S, Danchin N, Laurans L, Rousseau B, Cattan S, et al. Circulating levels of interleukin-17 and cardiovascular outcomes in patients with acute myocardial infarction. *Eur Heart J* (2013) 34(8):570–7. doi:10.1093/eurheartj/ehs263
103. Strober B, Teller C, Yamauchi P, Miller JL, Hooper M, Yang YC, et al. Effects of etanercept on C-reactive protein levels in psoriasis and psoriatic arthritis. *Br J Dermatol* (2008) 159(2):322–30. doi:10.1111/j.1365-2133.2008.08628.x
104. Kanelleas A, Liapi C, Katoulis A, Stavropoulos P, Avgerinou G, Georgala S, et al. The role of inflammatory markers in assessing disease severity and response to treatment in patients with psoriasis treated with etanercept. *Clin Exp Dermatol* (2011) 36(8):845–50. doi:10.1111/j.1365-2230.2011.04131.x
105. Kim JA, Montagnani M, Koh KK, Quon MJ. Reciprocal relationships between insulin resistance and endothelial dysfunction: molecular and pathophysiological mechanisms. *Circulation* (2006) 113(15):1888–904. doi:10.1161/CIRCULATIONAHA.105.563213
106. Reaven GM. Role of insulin resistance in human disease (syndrome X): an expanded definition. *Annu Rev Med* (1993) 44:121–31. doi:10.1146/annurev.me.44.020193.001005
107. McVeigh GE, Cohn JN. Endothelial dysfunction and the metabolic syndrome. *Curr Diab Rep* (2003) 3(1):87–92. doi:10.1007/s11892-003-0059-0
108. Montagnani M, Quon MJ. Insulin action in vascular endothelium: potential mechanisms linking insulin resistance with hypertension. *Diabetes Obes Metab* (2000) 2(5):285–92. doi:10.1046/j.1463-1326.2000.00092.x
109. Kim JA, Koh KK, Quon MJ. The union of vascular and metabolic actions of insulin in sickness and in health. *Arterioscler Thromb Vasc Biol* (2005) 25(5):889–91. doi:10.1161/01.ATV.0000164044.42910.6b

110. Hotamisligil GS, Shargill NS, Spiegelman BM. Adipose expression of tumor necrosis factor-alpha: direct role in obesity-linked insulin resistance. *Science* (1993) 259(5091):87–91. doi:10.1126/science.7678183
111. Boehncke WH, Boehncke S, Schön MP. Managing comorbid disease in patients with psoriasis. *BMJ* (2010) 340:b5666. doi:10.1136/bmj.b5666
112. Boehncke WH, Boehncke S, Tobin AM, Kirby B. The 'psoriatic march': a concept of how severe psoriasis may drive cardiovascular comorbidity. *Exp Dermatol* (2011) 20(4):303–7. doi:10.1111/j.1600-0625.2011.01261.x
113. Boehncke S, Thaci D, Beschmann H, Ludwig RJ, Ackermann H, Badenhoop K, et al. Psoriasis patients show signs of insulin resistance. *Br J Dermatol* (2007) 157(6):1249–51. doi:10.1111/j.1365-2133.2007.08190.x
114. Cerman AA, Bozkurt S, Sav A, Tulunay A, Elbaşi MO, Ergun T. Serum leptin levels, skin leptin and leptin receptor expression in psoriasis. *Br J Dermatol* (2008) 159(4):820–6. doi:10.1111/j.1365-2133.2008.08742.x
115. Matthews DR, Hosker JP, Rudenski AS, Naylor BA, Treacher DF, Turner RC. Homeostasis model assessment: insulin resistance and beta-cell function from fasting plasma glucose and insulin concentrations in man. *Diabetologia* (1985) 28(7):412–9. doi:10.1007/BF00280883
116. National Diabetes Data Group. Classification and diagnosis of diabetes mellitus and other categories of glucose intolerance. National Diabetes Data Group. *Diabetes* (1979) 28(12):1039–57. doi:10.2337/diab.28.12.1039
117. Ucak S, Ekmekci TR, Basat O, Koslu A, Altuntas Y. Comparison of various insulin sensitivity indices in psoriatic patients and their relationship with type of psoriasis. *J Eur Acad Dermatol Venereol* (2006) 20(5):517–22. doi:10.1111/j.1468-3083.2006.01499.x
118. Lago R, Gómez R, Lago F, Gómez-Reino J, Gualillo O. Leptin beyond body weight regulation – current concepts concerning its role in immune function and inflammation. *Cell Immunol* (2008) 252(1–2):139–45. doi:10.1016/j.cellimm.2007.09.004
119. Gisondi P, Fantin F, Del Giglio M, Valbusa F, Marino F, Zamboni M, et al. Chronic plaque psoriasis is associated with increased arterial stiffness. *Dermatology* (2009) 218(2):110–3. doi:10.1159/000182256
120. Balci DD, Balci A, Karazincir S, Ucar E, Iyigun U, Yalcin F, et al. Increased carotid artery intima-media thickness and impaired endothelial function in psoriasis. *J Eur Acad Dermatol Venereol* (2009) 23(1):1–6. doi:10.1111/j.1468-3083.2008.02936.x
121. Ulusoy RE, Karabudak O, Yokusoglu M, Kilicaslan F, Kirilmaz A, Cebeci BS. Noninvasive assessment of impaired endothelial function in psoriasis. *Rheumatol Int* (2010) 30(4):479–83. doi:10.1007/s00296-009-0995-3
122. Karadag AS, Yavuz B, Ertugrul DT, Akin KO, Yalcin AA, Deveci OS, et al. Is psoriasis a pre-atherosclerotic disease? Increased insulin resistance and impaired endothelial function in patients with psoriasis. *Int J Dermatol* (2010) 49(6):642–6. doi:10.1111/j.1365-4632.2009.04358.x
123. Buerger C, Richter B, Woth K, Salgo R, Malisiewicz B, Diehl S, et al. Interleukin-1β interferes with epidermal homeostasis through induction of insulin resistance: implications for psoriasis pathogenesis. *J Invest Dermatol* (2012) 132(9):2206–14. doi:10.1038/jid.2012.123
124. Buerger C, Shirsath N, Lang V, Berard A, Diehl S, Kaufmann R, et al. Inflammation dependent mTORC1 signaling interferes with the switch from keratinocyte proliferation to differentiation. *PLoS One* (2017) 12(7):e0180853. doi:10.1371/journal.pone.0180853
125. Malisiewicz B, Boehncke S, Lang V, Boehncke WH, Buerger C. Epidermal insulin resistance as a therapeutic target in acanthosis nigricans? *Acta Derm Venereol* (2014) 94(5):607–8. doi:10.2340/00015555-1778
126. Parsi KK, Brezinski EA, Lin TC, Li CS, Armstrong AW. Are patients with psoriasis being screened for cardiovascular risk factors? A study of screening practices and awareness among primary care physicians and cardiologists. *J Am Acad Dermatol* (2012) 67(3):357–62. doi:10.1016/j.jaad.2011.09.006
127. Alamdari HS, Gustafson CJ, Davis SA, Huang W, Feldman SR. Psoriasis and cardiovascular screening rates in the United States. *J Drugs Dermatol* (2013) 12(1):e14–9.
128. Takeshita J, Wang S, Shin DB, Mehta NN, Kimmel SE, Margolis DJ, et al. Effect of psoriasis severity on hypertension control: a population-based study in the United Kingdom. *JAMA Dermatol* (2015) 151(2):161–9. doi:10.1001/jamadermatol.2014.2094
129. Kimball AB, Gladman D, Gelfand JM, Gordon K, Horn EJ, Korman NJ, et al. National Psoriasis Foundation clinical consensus on psoriasis comorbidities and recommendations for screening. *J Am Acad Dermatol* (2008) 58(6):1031–42. doi:10.1016/j.jaad.2008.01.006
130. Daudén E, Castañeda S, Suárez C, García-Campayo J, Blasco AJ, Aguilar MD, et al. Clinical practice guideline for an integrated approach to comorbidity in patients with psoriasis. *J Eur Acad Dermatol Venereol* (2013) 27(11):1387–404. doi:10.1111/jdv.12024
131. Radtke MA, Mrowietz U, Feuerhahn J, Härter M, von Kiedrowski R, Nast A, et al. Early detection of comorbidity in psoriasis: recommendations of the National Conference on Healthcare in Psoriasis. *J Dtsch Dermatol Ges* (2015) 13(7):674–90. doi:10.1111/ddg.12643
132. Takeshita J, Grewal S, Langan SM, Mehta NN, Ogdie A, Van Voorhees AS, et al. Psoriasis and comorbid diseases: implications for management. *J Am Acad Dermatol* (2017) 76(3):393–403. doi:10.1016/j.jaad.2016.07.065
133. Goff DC Jr, Lloyd-Jones DM, Bennett G, Coady S, D'Agostino RB Sr, Gibbons R, et al. 2013 ACC/AHA guideline on the assessment of cardiovascular risk: a report of the American College of Cardiology/American Heart Association Task Force on Practice Guidelines. *J Am Coll Cardiol* (2014) 63(25 Pt B):2935–59. doi:10.1016/j.jacc.2013.11.005
134. Gisondi P, Del Giglio M, Di Francesco V, Zamboni M, Girolomoni G. Weight loss improves the response of obese patients with moderate-to-severe chronic plaque psoriasis to low-dose cyclosporine therapy: a randomized, controlled, investigator-blinded clinical trial. *Am J Clin Nutr* (2008) 88(5):1242–7.
135. Ridker PM, Everett BM, Thuren T, MacFadyen JG, Chang WH, Ballantyne C, et al. Antiinflammatory therapy with canakinumab for atherosclerotic disease. *N Engl J Med* (2017) 377(12):1119–31. doi:10.1056/NEJMoa1707914
136. Prodanovich S, Ma F, Taylor JR, Pezon C, Fasihi T, Kirsner RS. Methotrexate reduces incidence of vascular diseases in veterans with psoriasis or rheumatoid arthritis. *J Am Acad Dermatol* (2005) 52(2):262–7. doi:10.1016/j.jaad.2004.06.017
137. Wu JJ, Poon KY, Channual JC, Shen AY. Association between tumor necrosis factor inhibitor therapy and myocardial infarction risk in patients with psoriasis. *Arch Dermatol* (2012) 148(11):1244–50. doi:10.1001/archdermatol.2012.2502
138. Ahlehoff O, Skov L, Gislason G, Lindhardsen J, Kristensen SL, Iversen L, et al. Cardiovascular disease event rates in patients with severe psoriasis treated with systemic anti-inflammatory drugs: a Danish real-world cohort study. *J Intern Med* (2013) 273(2):197–204. doi:10.1111/j.1365-2796.2012.02593.x
139. Abuabara K, Lee H, Kimball AB. The effect of systemic psoriasis therapies on the incidence of myocardial infarction: a cohort study. *Br J Dermatol* (2011) 165(5):1066–73. doi:10.1111/j.1365-2133.2011.10525.x
140. Chen YJ, Chang YT, Shen JL, Chen TT, Wang CB, Chen CM, et al. Association between systemic antipsoriatic drugs and cardiovascular risk in patients with psoriasis with or without psoriatic arthritis: a nationwide cohort study. *Arthritis Rheum* (2012) 64(6):1879–87. doi:10.1002/art.34335
141. Coimbra S, Oliveira H, Reis F, Belo L, Rocha S, Quintanilha A, et al. Circulating adipokine levels in Portuguese patients with psoriasis vulgaris according to body mass index, severity and therapy. *J Eur Acad Dermatol Venereol* (2010) 24(12):1386–94. doi:10.1111/j.1468-3083.2010.03647.x
142. Coimbra S, Oliveira H, Reis F, Belo L, Rocha S, Quintanilha A, et al. Interleukin (IL)-22, IL-17, IL-23, IL-8, vascular endothelial growth factor and tumour necrosis factor-α levels in patients with psoriasis before, during and after psoralen-ultraviolet A and narrowband ultraviolet B therapy. *Br J Dermatol* (2010) 163(6):1282–90. doi:10.1111/j.1365-2133.2010.09992.x
143. Boehncke S, Fichtlscherer S, Salgo R, Garbaraviciene J, Beschmann H, Diehl S, et al. Systemic therapy of plaque-type psoriasis ameliorates endothelial cell function: results of a prospective longitudinal pilot trial. *Arch Dermatol Res* (2011) 303(6):381–8. doi:10.1007/s00403-010-1108-6
144. Boehncke S, Salgo R, Garbaraviciene J, Beschmann H, Hardt K, Diehl S, et al. Effective continuous systemic therapy of severe plaque-type psoriasis is accompanied by amelioration of biomarkers of cardiovascular risk: results of a prospective longitudinal observational study. *J Eur Acad Dermatol Venereol* (2011) 25(10):1187–93. doi:10.1111/j.1468-3083.2010.03947.x
145. Martinez-Lopez A, Blasco-Morente G, Perez-Lopez I, Tercedor-Sanchez J, Arias-Santiago S. Studying the effect of systemic and biological drugs on intima-media thickness in patients suffering from moderate and severe psoriasis. *J Eur Acad Dermatol Venereol* (2018). doi:10.1111/jdv.14841

146. Bissonnette R, Tardif JC, Harel F, Pressacco J, Bolduc C, Guertin MC. Effects of the tumor necrosis factor-α antagonist adalimumab on arterial inflammation assessed by positron emission tomography in patients with psoriasis: results of a randomized controlled trial. *Circ Cardiovasc Imaging* (2013) 6(1):83–90. doi:10.1161/CIRCIMAGING.112.975730
147. Bissonnette R, Harel F, Krueger JG, Guertin MC, Chabot-Blanchet M, Gonzalez J, et al. TNF-α antagonist and vascular inflammation in patients with psoriasis vulgaris: a randomized placebo-controlled study. *J Invest Dermatol* (2017) 137(8):1638–45. doi:10.1016/j.jid.2017.02.977
148. Gong F, Liu Z, Liu J, Zhou P, Liu Y, Lu X. The paradoxical role of IL-17 in atherosclerosis. *Cell Immunol* (2015) 297(1):33–9. doi:10.1016/j.cellimm.2015.05.007

20

Neutrophils in Psoriasis

Chih-Chao Chiang[1,2,3†], Wei-Jen Cheng[1,4,5†], Michal Korinek[6,7,8], Cheng-Yu Lin[6] and Tsong-Long Hwang[4,6,7,9,10,11]*

[1] Graduate Institute of Clinical Medical Sciences, College of Medicine, Chang Gung University, Taoyuan, Taiwan, [2] Supervisor Board, Taoyuan Chinese Medicine Association, Taoyuan, Taiwan, [3] Puxin Fengze Chinese Medicine Clinic, Taoyuan, Taiwan, [4] School of Traditional Chinese Medicine, Chang Gung University, Taoyuan, Taiwan, [5] Center for Traditional Chinese Medicine, Chang Gung Memorial Hospital, Taoyuan, Taiwan, [6] Graduate Institute of Natural Products, College of Medicine, Chang Gung University, Taoyuan, Taiwan, [7] Research Center for Chinese Herbal Medicine, Research Center for Food and Cosmetic Safety, and Graduate Institute of Health Industry Technology, Chang Gung University of Science and Technology, Taoyuan, Taiwan, [8] Department of Biotechnology, College of Life Science, Kaohsiung Medical University, Kaohsiung, Taiwan, [9] Chinese Herbal Medicine Research Team, Healthy Aging Research Center, Chang Gung University, Taoyuan, Taiwan, [10] Department of Anesthesiology, Chang Gung Memorial Hospital, Taoyuan, Taiwan, [11] Department of Chemical Engineering, Ming Chi University of Technology, New Taipei City, Taiwan

***Correspondence:**
Tsong-Long Hwang
htl@mail.cgu.edu.tw

†These authors have contributed equally to this work

Neutrophils are the most abundant innate immune cells. The pathogenic roles of neutrophils are related to chronic inflammation and autoimmune diseases. Psoriasis is a chronic systemic inflammatory disease affecting ~2–3% of the world population. The abundant presence of neutrophils in the psoriatic skin lesions serves as a typical histopathologic hallmark of psoriasis. Recent reports indicated that oxidative stress, granular components, and neutrophil extracellular traps from psoriatic neutrophils are related to the initial and maintenance phases of psoriasis. This review provides an overview on the recent (up to 2019) advances in understanding the role of neutrophils in the pathophysiology of psoriasis, including the effects of respiratory burst, degranulation, and neutrophil extracellular trap formation on psoriatic immunity and the clinical relationships.

Keywords: neutrophils, psoriasis, immunity, respiratory burst, degranulation, neutrophil extracellular traps

INTRODUCTION

Neutrophils are the most abundant cells in innate immunity. The main offensive functions of neutrophils include respiratory burst accompanied by reactive oxygen species (ROS) generation, degranulation (release of granules), and the formation of neutrophil extracellular traps (NETs) (**Figure 1**) (1, 2). Neutrophils shape adaptive immunity because they communicate and interact with the antigen-presenting cells and lymphocytes at the sites of inflammation (3, 4). Recently great attention was brought to the role of neutrophils in the development and progression of autoimmune diseases such as psoriasis.

Psoriatic neutrophils produce augmented respiratory burst with an overt accumulation of oxidative stress involving complicated inflammatory pathways. Proteases released in the degranulation step by neutrophils, such as myeloperoxidase (MPO), neutrophil elastase (NE), proteinase 3, and cathepsin G, participate in the generation of ROS, proteolytical activation of inflammatory mediators, and formation of autoantigens in psoriasis. The complexity and prevalence of psoriasis among the population since antiquity encouraged scientists to study the etiology of the disease and its relation to the immune system and inflammatory responses. Elegant reviews described the role of inflammation and immune system in the development of psoriasis (5, 6), the importance of biologic therapies targeting systemic inflammation (7), the significance of utilizing specific antibodies (8), the contribution of platelets to regulation of NET formation (9), the antimicrobial and pathogenetic roles of neutrophils in autoimmune, autoinflammatory, metabolic (10) and cardiovascular diseases (11). Also, recent books summarized the causes, symptoms, and treatment options of psoriasis (12–15).

However, the role of neutrophils in psoriasis was not deeply analyzed and summarized based on recent literature. Thus, in this work, we focus on summarizing recent findings on the main offensive features of neutrophils including respiratory burst, degranulation and NETs and their direct connection with development and progression of psoriasis (**Figure 2**). We hope that our work would provide a foundation for further studies to attenuate overstimulation of neutrophils in psoriasis and aid patients with a debilitating disease.

PSORIASIS

Psoriasis affects ~2–3% of the world population (>125 million people). Psoriasis is a common, chronic, immune-mediated disease that is manifested mainly as skin lesions and extracutaneous comorbidities (16, 17). It is associated with systemic inflammation, similar to that observed in obesity, malignancy, psoriatic arthritis, cardiovascular disorders, chronic obstructive pulmonary diseases, type 2 diabetes mellitus, liver and renal diseases, and inflammatory bowel diseases (18–20). Psoriasis affects men and women equally and usually starts to be manifested at the age of 20 to 30, but children and teenagers can be also affected (21). Clinical types of psoriasis include psoriasis vulgaris, guttate psoriasis, inverse psoriasis, pustular psoriasis, and erythrodermic psoriasis (22). Typical skin manifestations of psoriasis include erythematous, indurated, and scaling plaques that are painful, itchy, and have a burning sensation (16, 23). Psoriasis decreases patients' quality of life due to unpleasant symptoms and related public stigma (24, 25). The unpleasant skin appearance contributes to reduced employment levels and thus, affects the financial status of patients (26). Depression and suicidal tendencies are also increased in patients with psoriasis (27, 28). Therefore, psoriasis results in long-term physical, psychological, and economic burden at both the individual and societal levels.

NEUTROPHILS IN PSORIASIS

Psoriasis is an immunogenetic disease that is associated with the interactions between the innate and adaptive immune systems (29). The immunology disturbance in psoriasis is related to overstimulation of neutrophils, dendritic cells, T cells, keratinocytes, fibroblasts (6, 30), mast cells (31), and melanocytes (30, 32). Munro's microabscesses filled with neutrophils, which were first described in 1898, are considered as one of the major histopathological hallmarks of psoriasis (33). Neutrophils are now thought to be regulators between the innate and adaptive immune systems (34, 35).

There is no cure for psoriasis, however the symptoms can be reduced either by avoiding triggers or by medications. Currently, the available treatments such as phototherapy, topical therapy (corticosteroids, vitamin D analogs), systemic therapy (methotrexate, apremilast, cyclosporin), and biological treatments offer a relieve for patients with different severity of psoriasis. However, the risk-benefit ratio must be well-considered on individual basis, particularly, considering the chronic course of the disease and limitations of the long-term use of certain drugs (16). Although T cell immunology-related treatments have emerged as attractive options for psoriasis, according to a systematic review of adherence and satisfaction to current treatment covering studies conducted in 2002 (36) or between beginning of 2009 and end of 2014 in European Union (37), psoriatic patients expressed only moderate satisfaction with the available treatments as evidenced by the poor adherence rates, in particular to topical treatments (36, 37). That might be the biggest motivating factor for the use of alternative treatment methods such as traditional Chinese medicine and herbs (*Scutellaria baicalensis*, *Zingiber officinale*, *Indigo naturalis*, *Mahonia aquifolium*, *Aloe vera*) (38), dietary supplements (fish oil, vitamin D) or other (39). Furthermore, the combination of certain alternative medicines with conventional drug therapies has been shown to improve the treatment efficacy, which points to the importance of evaluation of safety of combined treatments, education of doctors but also improvements in patient-doctor interactions (40). Indeed, modern biological therapies demonstrate improved safety and efficacy, as well as better satisfaction in patients, but belong to an expensive class of drugs, with limited availability (41). Biological therapies of psoriasis include monoclonal antibodies or inhibitors targeting tumor necrosis factor (TNF)α (infliximab, adalimumab; etanercept) (42–44), interleukin (IL)-23/IL-12 (ustekinumab) (42), IL-23 (guselkumab, tildrakizumab, risankizumab) (45, 46), or IL-17 (secukinumab, ixekizumab, brodalumab) (11, 47, 48). The available therapies indirectly affect the function and numbers of neutrophils. According to previous studies, the neutrophil-to-lymphocyte ratio (NLR) and platelet-to-lymphocyte ratio (PLR) are significantly increased in patients with psoriasis (49). While the elevated NLR and PLR values are particularly associated with psoriasis, they do not indicate the severity of the condition (50). The importance of NLR level in the progression of the disease was demonstrated by the reduction in NLR level following psoriasis treatment (51). That brings in question the effectiveness of certain treatments such as narrow-band ultraviolet B phototherapy which does not affect the increased level of NLR (52). Increased NLR and PLR levels emerged as unrecognized predictors of subclinical atherosclerosis in patients with psoriasis (53). The presence of excessive amount of neutrophils is characteristic for the generalized pustular psoriasis. Recent reports indicated that the depletion of neutrophils significantly relieves the symptoms of pustular psoriasis in patients that did not respond well to conventional treatments (54). Understanding the role of

Abbreviations: CCL, CC-chemokine ligand; CXCL, chemokine (C-X-C motif) ligand; IL, interleukin; IFN, interfenon; LPS, lipopolysaccharide; mDCs, myeloid dendritic cells; MPO, myeloperoxidase; NET, neutrophil extracellular trap; NOX, NADPH oxidase; NE, neutrophil elastase; NLR, neutrophil-to-lymphocyte ratio, pDCs, plasmacytoid dendritic cells; PLR, platelet-to-lymphocyte ratio; Th, T helper cell; TLR, Toll-like receptor; TNF, tumor necrosis factor.

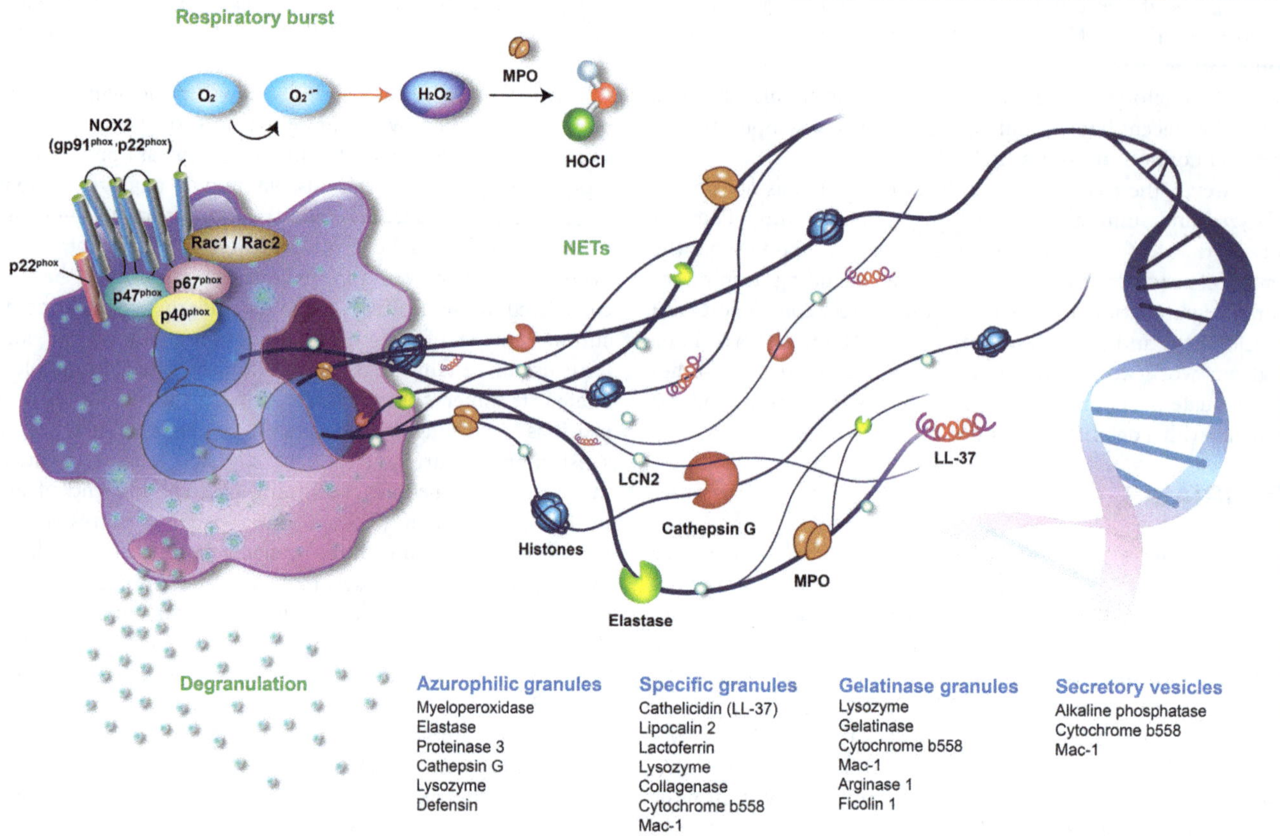

FIGURE 1 | The offensive mechanisms of neutrophils in inflammation. In the activated neutrophils, respiratory burst, degranulation, and the formation of neutrophil extracellular traps (NETs) are the main mechanisms responsible for inflammation. During the respiratory burst, neutrophils utilize oxygen to produce reactive oxygen species (ROS) such as superoxide (O_2^-), peroxide H_2O_2 or hypochlorous acid (HOCl) by activating NADPH oxidase (NOX2) and myeloperoxidase (MPO). As activation processes are triggered by diverse stimuli, neutrophils mobilize different granules including azurophilic granules, specific granules, gelatinase granules, and secretory vesicles. Subsequently, neutrophils degranulate and release various granular compounds of which neutrophil elastase (NE), MPO, proteinase 3, LL37, and lipocalin 2 play an important role in the pathogenesis of psoriasis. NETs are novel and pivotal components of neutrophils composed of extruded sticky and decondensed chromatin decorated with many antimicrobial compounds, such as histones, MPO, NE, and cathepsin G. The formation of NETs is involved in complicated inflammatory reactions and contributes to the pathogenesis of psoriasis. MPO, myeloperoxidase; NADPH, reduced nicotinamide adenine dinucleotide phosphate; NE, neutrophil elastase; NET, neutrophil extracellular trap; NOX2, NADPH oxidase.

neutrophils in psoriasis attracted the attention of scientific community aiming to develop treatment protocols focusing on attenuating neutrophil overstimulation in this disease (55).

RESPIRATORY BURST AND PSORIASIS

Circulating neutrophils are recruited to inflammatory sites following inflammatory signals. They are then activated to generate and release large amounts of ROS in a phenomenon known as respiratory burst. NADPH oxidase (NOX2) and MPO are two key enzymes that contribute to the respiratory burst (56, 57). NOX2 is composed of transmembrane cytochrome b558 ($p22^{phox}$ and $gp91^{phox}$) and cytosolic subunits ($p40^{phox}$, $p47^{phox}$, $p67^{phox}$, and Rac1/2). The assembled NOX2 complex, at the phagosomal and plasma membranes, is fully activated to generate superoxide anion ($O_2^{\bullet -}$), which is the origin of various ROS produced by neutrophils. Superoxide ($O_2^{\bullet -}$) is rapidly converted to hydrogen peroxide (H_2O_2) by superoxide dismutase (SOD). MPO, a heme peroxidase enzyme which is released in a process known as degranulation, utilizes H_2O_2 to produce many secondary reactive products. These products include hypochlorous acid (HOCl), chloramines (R-NHCl), and hypothiocyanite (OSCN−), as well as organic radicals such as products of lipid peroxidation (**Figure 1**) (58, 59).

ROS production is an integral part of the antimicrobial activity of neutrophils. However, the overproduction or inadequate clearance of ROS can cause various oxidative stress-related dysfunctions. These include cell and tissue damage; peroxidation and modification of DNA, lipids, and proteins; autoimmune NET formation; and autoantibody generation (58, 60). Neutrophils obtained from patients with psoriasis were shown to possess increased MPO and NOX2 activities, and release more ROS compared with neutrophils from healthy individuals (61, 62). Keratinocytes and T cells in psoriatic lesions produce priming agents of neutrophils, which results in an augmented respiratory burst by neutrophils with the overproduction of ROS (63–66). Accumulation of oxidative radicals also contributes to the pathogenesis of psoriasis. In response to the overproduction of

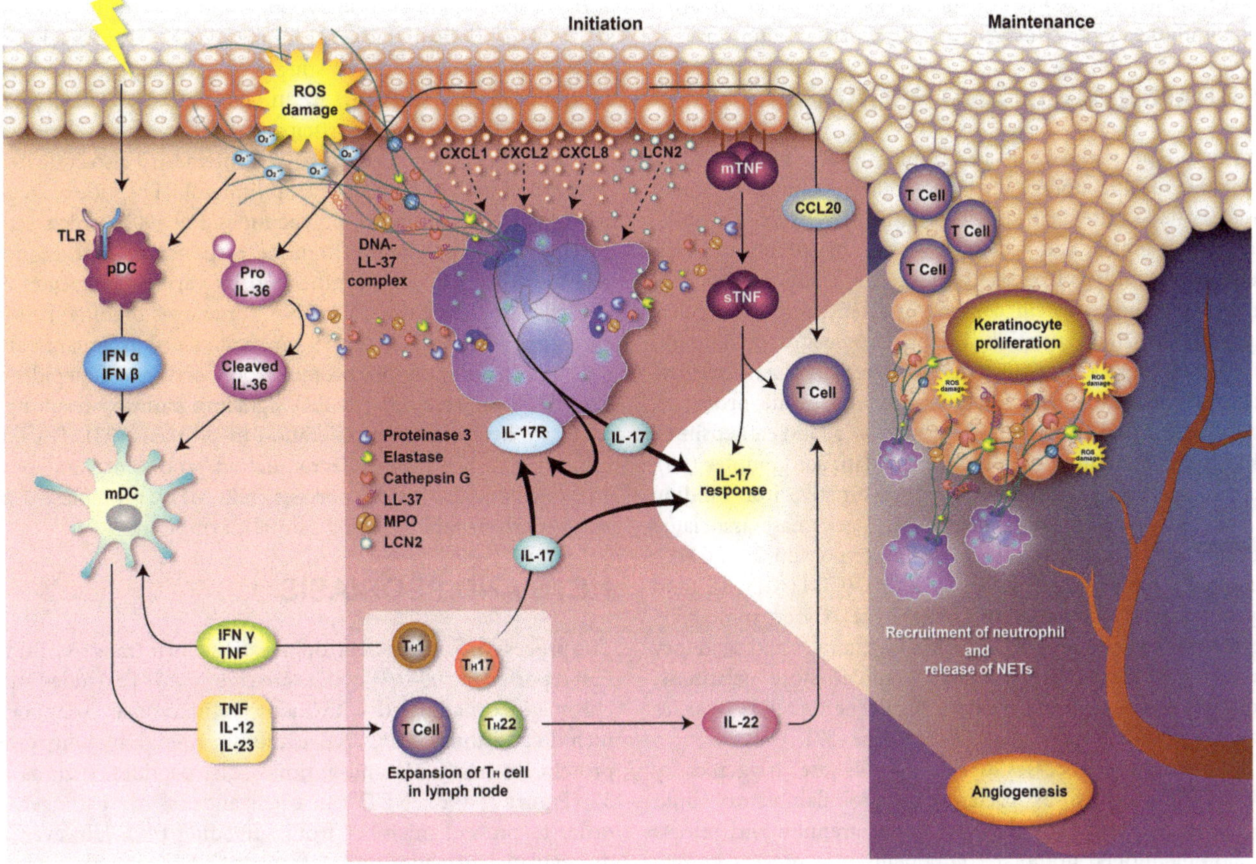

FIGURE 2 | Role of neutrophils in psoriasis. Various and diverse endogenous and exogenous impulses such as antigens, trauma, infection, or emotional stress can trigger the complex immune reactions leading to psoriasis. The interplay of neutrophils, dendritic cells, and T cells bridges the innate immune and adaptive immune systems. T cells and keratinocytes release chemokines, such as IL-17, CXCL1, CXCL2, and CXCL8, that mediate the recruitment of neutrophils. Circulating neutrophils migrate to the psoriatic lesions and induce respiratory burst, degranulation, and formation of NETs, thereby contributing to the immunopathogenesis of psoriasis which involves T cell imbalance, keratinocyte proliferation, angiogenesis, and auto-antigen formation. Neutrophils from patients with psoriasis have enhanced NOX2 and MPO activity and augmented respiratory burst. MPO also participates in generating oxidative stress and upregulating degranulation. The accumulated oxidative stress produced by neutrophils could stimulate the antigen-presenting cells pDCs via TLR receptors 7 and 9 which stimulate antigen-specific CD8+ T cells (memory T cells in dermis and naive T cells in lymph node) to release cytokines, chemokines, and other innate immune mediators. These T cells may also migrate to epidermis and trigger local inflammation and keratinocyte proliferation via MHC I receptor of keratinocytes. Production of IFN-α and IFN-β by pDCs then stimulates mDCs to secrete pro-inflammatory mediators such as TNF, IL-12 and IL-23. Proteinase 3 released from neutrophils cleaves pro-IL-36 to activated IL-36 cytokine amplifying the response of mDCs. TNF, IL-12, and IL-23 play an important role in the initiation of the Th1, Th17, and Th22 cells immune response in lymph node, leading to a secretion of various cytokines and chemokines. IL-1 is further amplifying Th17 response while TNF and IFN-γ is creating a back loop to mDCs activation. Th17 activation then leads to the production of IL-17 activating neutrophils and keratinocytes via IL-17 receptors which generates profound IL-17 response. Keratinocytes produce TNF and CCL20, a chemotactic for T cell and DCs. Neutrophils degranulate and release MPO, NE, proteinase 3, cathepsin G and lipocalin. Proteinase 3 cleaves and converts the resting TNFα located in membrane of epithelial cells (mTNFα) to an activated state called soluble TNFα (sTNFα). Proteinase 3 also contributes to the formation of the LL-37 which serves as autoantigen. The chromatin of NETs (DNA) combined with LL-37 have a profound role in the initiation and maintenance of immune response in psoriasis. NETs further supply IL-17 and induce Th17 cells to release more IL-17, which plays a decisive role in the maintenance of psoriasis. These processes participate in the psoriasis complex inflammatory reactions and lead to the escalation of local psoriatic tissue inflammation. IL-22 contributes to the formation of characteristic psoriatic skin lesions including epidermal hyperplasia and acanthosis (thickening of skin). The activation of the following transcription factors promote TNF and IL-17 production and formation of downstream amplification loops in psoriasis: the Janus kinase (JAK)–signal transducer and activator of transcription (STAT) family, nuclear factor-κB (NF-κB) and cyclic AMP. Furthermore, the activation of endothelial cells induces vascular proliferation, angiogenesis and the expression of adhesion molecules in the endothelium to recruit additional inflammatory cells into the skin such as mast cells and macrophages contributing to the pathogenesis of psoriasis. CCL, CC-chemokine ligand; CXCL, chemokine (C-X-C motif) ligand; IL, interleukin; IFN, interfenon; MHC I, major histocompatibility complex class I, MPO, myeloperoxidase; NET, neutrophil extracellular trap; NOX, NADPH oxidase; NE, neutrophil elastase; pDCs, plasmacytoid dendritic cells; mDCs, myeloid dendritic cells; TLR, Toll-like receptor; TNF, tumor necrosis factor.

ROS, dendritic cells are stimulated to present antigens to the T cells which results in an imbalance of T helper cell (Th)1 and Th2 cells, stimulation of keratinocytes proliferation, and promotion of angiogenesis (**Figure 2**). ROS then serve as the second messenger to activate mitogen-activated protein kinase (MAPK), nuclear factor-kappa B (NF-κB), or the Janus kinase-signal transducer and activator of transcription proteins (JAK-STAT)-related inflammatory pathways (67, 68). Suppression of respiratory burst of neutrophils emerged as a plausible pathway of attenuating overly immune response associated with psoriatic symptoms.

DEGRANULATION AND PSORIASIS

Neutrophils possess a multi-lobed nucleus, few mitochondria, and many specific storage organelles called granules. Granules are classified into azurophilic granules, specific granules, gelatinase granules, and secretory vesicles depending on their size, reaction with peroxidase-reactive dye, staining with 3,3'-diaminobenzidine, protein content, and tendency to mobilize (**Figure 1**) (69, 70). Azurophilic (peroxidase-positive or primary) granules are packed with MPO, bactericidal/permeability-increasing protein, defensins, lysozyme, and serine proteases, such as neutrophil elastase (NE), proteinase 3, and cathepsin G. Lysozyme is also found in specific and gelatinase granules (55). Specific (secondary) granules contain distinctive iron-binding glycoprotein lactoferrin, neutrophil gelatinase-associated lipocalin (NGAL, also called serum lipocalin-2, LCN2), collagenase, cytochrome b558, MAC-1 (CD11/CD18), and importantly, cathelicidins such as LL-37 (71). Cytochrome b558 and MAC-1 are also present in gelatinase granules and secretory vesicles (55). Gelatinase (tertiary) granules store gelatinase, lysozyme, arginase 1, and ficolin 1 (72). The secretory vesicles contain a characteristic alkaline phosphatase (57).

As activation processes of neutrophils are triggered by diverse stimuli such as bacterial or proinflammatory lipid mediators, neutrophils mobilize different granules and release the aforementioned granular components in a process known as degranulation or exocytosis (57). Degranulation is regulated by complicated control mechanisms, such as calcium signaling and actin remodeling (72–74). Azurophilic granules discharge toxic components into phagosomes and at inflammation sites. The secretion of specific and gelatinase granules promotes migration of neutrophils and the antimicrobial activity. The main purpose of releasing secretory vesicles is to facilitate neutrophils recruitment. Therefore, the degranulation process promotes firm adhesion, migration, respiratory burst, and successive NET formation of activated neutrophils (75). However, the dysregulation of neutrophil degranulation could damage tissues as observed in various diseases, such as hypoxia-related airway injury (76), severe pneumonia and chronic obstructive pulmonary diseases (77), atherosclerosis (78, 79), acute inflammatory liver injury (80), and rheumatoid arthritis (81, 82).

In psoriasis, MPO is significantly increased in skin plaques and is positively correlated with the severity of psoriasis (83). Serum MPO is also increased in patients with psoriasis, which may be related to recruited leukocytes in psoriatic skin lesions (84). MPO, the major enzymatic content of neutrophil granules, accounts for ~5% of the dry weight of the cell and represents the most toxic enzyme expressed by neutrophils (85). MPO is involved in the respiratory burst and can bind to CD11b/CD18 integrins, thereby contributing to the upregulation and augmentation of neutrophil degranulation in psoriasis (86). Furthermore, the neutrophil granule-derived serine proteinases, such as NE, proteinase 3, and cathepsin G, can activate interleukin (IL)-36 cytokine and lead to the escalation of local psoriatic tissue inflammation (87, 88). Proteinase 3 cleaves and converts the resting TNFα located in membrane of epithelial cells (mTNFα) to an activated state called soluble TNFα (sTNFα), which participates in the psoriasis complex inflammatory reactions (**Figure 2**). Proteinase 3 also contributes to the formation of the LL-37, an antimicrobial peptide belonging to cathelicidin family of polypeptides (89, 90), which serves as autoantigen mediating immune response in psoriasis (33). Antimicrobial peptides, synthesized by various leukocytes and epithelial cells, act via DNA/RNA complexes binding Toll-like receptors (TLR) 7, 8, and 9 to facilitate skin inflammation (91, 92). In addition, NE proteolytically activates the epidermal growth factor receptor (EGFR) signaling pathway resulting in excessive keratinocyte proliferation in psoriasis (93). Thus, the inhibition of neutrophils degranulation process or some of the enzymes contributing to psoriasis (NE, MPO, proteinase 3) are feasible targets for alleviating psoriatic symptoms.

NETS AND PSORIASIS

The process of forming neutrophil extracellular traps (NETs) was first reported in 2004 (94). NETs are composed of extruded sticky chromatin ornamented with many antimicrobial components including histones, MPO, NE, cathepsin G, high mobility group protein B1 (HMGB1) and antimicrobial peptides, such as LL-37 (**Figure 1**) (95). NETs can catch and destroy pathogens in order to prevent microbes from spreading (96). However, the dysregulated formation and clearance of NETs can result in many diseases. These include autoimmune diseases, such as systemic lupus erythematosus, anti-neutrophil cytoplasmic autoantibody (ANCA)-associated vasculitis, rheumatoid arthritis, gout (97), and autoimmune hepatitis (98); cardiovascular diseases, such as atherosclerosis, thrombosis, and abdominal aortic aneurysm (99–101); respiratory disorders inclusive of asthma, chronic obstructive pulmonary disease, cystic fibrosis, tuberculosis, bacterial and viral pneumonia, and transfusion-related acute lung injury (102, 103); digestive diseases, such as inflammatory bowel diseases, primary sclerosing cholangitis, primary biliary cholangitis (98); and cancer-related organ damage, metastasis, and thrombosis (9). Recently, a role of NETs in awakening of dormant cancer cells was discovered (104).

The process of NET formation is termed NETosis, which is subdivided into lytic NETosis and non-lytic NETosis. In lytic NETosis (also called suicidal NETosis), activated neutrophils generate NETs (it takes 2–4 h) and undergo a programmed cell death, which differs from necrosis, necroptosis, and apoptosis (105). Lytic NET formation is triggered by various stimuli undergoing different pathways. For instance, phorbol myristate acetate (PMA) increases cytosol calcium, activates protein kinase C (PKC)/Raf/MEK/ERK pathway, and induces NOX2 to generate ROS. ROS then acts as the second messenger to disintegrate the nuclear membrane and stimulate MPO to translocate NE to the nucleus where it causes proteolysis of histones and decondensation of chromatin. Afterward, peptidyl arginine deiminase 4 (PAD4)-mediated hypercitrullination of histones allows decondensed chromatin, the main component of NETs, to be readily expelled from the cell nucleus. Finally, as the plasma membrane dissolves, the chromatin decorated with granular components is released as extracellular traps (106). Other pathways of lytic NETosis include stimulation by fungi (such as *Aspergillus* spp.) through Dectin 2 and complement receptor 3 (CR3) (107), LPS (lipopolysaccharide) under special conditions described later in detail (108) or by monosodium urate crystals via receptor-interacting serine/threonine-protein kinase 1 (RIPK1) and RIPK3 pathway (109). All of these pathways involve NOX2, MPO, and NE activation (105). Nevertheless, there are other stimulators of NETosis acting independently of NOX2 such as ionomycin, or immune complexes (110). Ionomycin induces NETs via small conductance calcium-activated potassium channel protein 3 (SK3) and protein kinase C ζ (PKCζ), mitochondrial ROS (mitoROS), NE, and protein-arginine deiminase type 4 (PAD4) (111). Immune complexes related NETosis through FcγRIIIb are highly dependent on mitoROS (110, 112). The lytic-NETosis inducers such as PMA, ionomycin, or living bacteria were confirmed using a live imaging confocal microscopy, however, dead bacteria, LPS, glucose, or activated platelets alone failed to induce NETosis in the *in vitro* experiment (113). Such discrepancy might be due to variations in the experimental design of various studies.

On the other hand, non-lytic NETosis (also called vital NETosis) does not require neutrophils lysis or even the breach of the plasma membrane. Following the release of NETs, neutrophils are alive and keep their functions, such as chemotactic movement, phagocytotic ability, and respiratory burst power (98). This form of NETosis usually occurs early in infection by Gram-positive bacteria in human and mice. The process is very rapid (5–60 min to form NETs), requires both TLR 2 and complement-mediated opsonization, and is independent of NOX2 (114). Non-lytic NETosis can be induced by *Staphylococcus aureus* via a unique mechanism where the inner and outer nuclear membranes are separated, and the vesicles filled with nuclear DNA are extruded intact into the extracellular space where they rupture and release chromatins. Despite that this type of NETs keep a limited amount of proteolytic activity it is still able to kill *S. aureus* (115). Non-lytic NETosis can also be stimulated by *Candida albicans* via interaction with CR3 and fibronectin (116). Moreover, a special type of non-lytic NETosis, which releases mitochondrial DNA and is dependent on ROS, is stimulated by the granulocyte-macrophage colony-stimulating factor (GM-CSF) and LPS (10). Interestingly, Leishmania parasites induce both lytic and non-lytic NETosis (117). In that case, the chromatin decondensed by PAD4 is mixed with granular proteins and subsequently excreted with a minor nuclear envelope disruption and without cell membrane disorganization (10, 98). Delgado-Rizo et al. previously summarized the microbial inducers of NETs (10) but we would like to clarify the effect of LPS. Lipopolysaccharide (LPS) is an important component of the outer membrane of gram-negative bacteria known to trigger immune response (118). For a long time, it was unclear whether the direct interaction between LPS and neutrophils causes NETs release, because several reports showed LPS-induced lytic NET formation (94, 119) while other not (113, 120). Recently, it has been shown that only species- and serotype-specific LPS is able to induce NETs by direct interaction with neutrophils. It was demonstrated that LPS has to be derived from specific bacterial strain of *Escherichia coli* (O128:B12) and *Pseudomonas aeruginosa* (serotype 10) and must be present at sufficient concentration (8 pg per neutrophil). The neutrophils then undergo a lytic-NETosis independent of TLR4. However, non-lytic NETosis is triggered when sufficient amount of LPS regardless of bacterial origin interacts with TLR4 of platelets (108). The process is followed by binding of platelets to the P-selectin glycoprotein ligand-1 (PSGL-1) of neutrophils, and the release of HMGB1 by platelets (9, 95). Moreover, there is a growing evidence of crucial role of the other endogenous and immune factors in the process of NET formation, such as presence of platelets (95, 120), glucose (10), or other effectors (121). To orchestrate inflammatory response, NETs in combination with LPS were shown to induce the production of IL-1β by J774 macrophages via the caspase-1 and caspase-8 pathways (122).

In patients with psoriasis, neutrophils are pre-activated and form NETs in psoriatic skin lesions (55, 123). NETs are increased in blood samples and correlate with the severity of psoriasis (124, 125). They create an extremely immunogenic environment and participate in the initial and maintenance phases of psoriasis (126, 127). NETs stimulate epidermis to release inflammatory cytokines via TLR4 and IL-36 receptor crosstalk (123). Various exogenous and endogenous stimuli and ROS generated by neutrophils initiate immune reaction leading to psoriasis which involves T cell imbalance, keratinocyte proliferation, angiogenesis, and auto-antigen formation (**Figure 2**). The chromatin of NETs in psoriasis plaques is accompanied with antimicrobial peptide LL-37 released by keratinocytes to stimulate the synthesis of inflammatory mediators including IFN-α and IFN-β in plasmacytoid dendritic cells (pDCs) (16). Myeloid DCs (mDCs) are then activated to release many pro-inflammatory mediators, such as IL-6, IL-12, IL-23, and TNFα (91, 92), which play an important role in the initiation of the Th1, Th17, and Th22 cells immune response (16). Proteinase 3 released from neutrophils cleaves pro-IL-36 to activated IL-36 cytokine which is together with TNF and IFN-γ amplifying the response of mDCs. Th17 activation then leads to the production of IL-17 activating neutrophils and keratinocytes via IL-17 receptors which generates profound IL-17 response (16). Secretory leukocyte protease inhibitor (SLPI), a component of NETs with an inhibitory function on NET formation, may bind to DNA and NE in psoriatic skin lesions and activate the pDCs to produce type 1 interferons (IFN-α, IFN-β, etc.) which regulates autoimmunity in psoriasis (128–130). In addition, NETs allow the mDCs to readily sense the neutrophilic antigens and allow the T cells to be primed directly (45, 131, 132). Thus, NETs play an important role in the pathophysiology of psoriasis due to their link between the innate and adaptive immune systems. Psoriasis is accompanied with increased serum levels of TNF-α, interferon (IFN)-γ, IL-1, IL-2, IL-4, IL-6, IL-8, IL-10, IL-12, IL-17, IL-18 (133), IL-22 (134), chemerin, resistin (135), lipocalin-2 (LCN2) (123), soluble E-selectin (sE-selectin) (136), complement 3 (137), and decreased levels of transforming growth factor-beta (TGF-β) and adiponectin (133). These cytokines may therefore serve as potential biomarkers for psoriasis and treatment response in patients. According to a cross-sectional study, psoriasis patients had increased proinflammatory macrophage type 1 (IL-1, IL-6, TNF-α), Th1 (IL-2, IL-12, IFN-γ), Th17 (IL-6, IL-17) but also anti-inflammatory Th2/T regulatory (Treg) (IL-4, IL-10) profiles which may be correlated to the severity of psoriasis (133). Among the important mediators in psoriasis, LCN2 acts as an antimicrobial protein as well as adipokine associated with obesity, insulin resistance, and atherosclerotic disease, and is also responsible for the activation of the immune system in response to inflammatory and toxic stimuli. Importantly, serum LCN2 levels are elevated in psoriatic patients (138) and correlate with the severity of itching and thus might be used as a clinical marker for itching in psoriasis (139). Not only granulocytes but also keratinocytes of epidermis secrete LCN2, which drives the chemotaxis of neutrophils and sustains NET formation, and thereby in turn maintains the psoriatic inflammation (123). The increased LCN2 blood levels were observed in patients with palmoplantar pustular psoriasis (140) as well as other chronic inflammatory skin diseases such as acne inversa (141) or atopic dermatitis (142). Wolk et al. reported a positive correlation between the LCN2 production and IL-1β levels in the epidermis, which was further enhanced by IL-17 and TNF-α, but not by IL-22. The contribution of LCN2 on skin neutrophil infiltration is apparent (141). In the clinical setting, tissue LCN2 was found to be also significantly higher in psoriasis, regardless of dyslipidemia, or metabolic disturbance in patients. But the LCN2 levels together with psoriasis area and severity index (PASI) score significantly dropped after NBUVB treatment (143). The *in vivo* effects of LCN2 on topical imiquimod (IMQ)-induced psoriasis-like skin in BALB/c mice were evaluated by Hau group (138). In addition to markedly exacerbated erythema and scaling in IMQ-treated murine skin, LCN2 increased the mRNA expression of interleukin (IL)-17A, IL-17F, IL-22, IL-23, CC-chemokine ligand (CCL)20, TNF-α, chemokine (C-X-C motif) ligand (CXCL)1, CXCL2, LCN2, and S100A7 while it did not affect the mRNA levels of IFN-γ, or CXCL10 in the skin. Similar effects were observed *in vitro* on human keratinocytes (138). The data suggest a link between NETs-related cytokines and Th-17 activation in psoriasis.

NET-TH17 AXIS AND PSORIASIS

Psoriasis has been considered as a T-helper (Th)1/Th17-mediated, chronic inflammatory dermatosis with relation to metabolic syndromes (144). Apart from keratinocytes and T lymphocytes (145), neutrophils are one of the major cellular sources of IL-17 via NET formation in psoriasis (146), and also mast cells were reported to generate extracellular traps (147). NETs activation has been linked with Th17 responses in psoriasis and has drawn particular attention recently (148). In an experimental model, NETs induced the generation of $CD3^{+}CD4^{+}IL\text{-}17^{+}$ (Th17) cells from peripheral blood mononuclear cells, which requires monocyte and cell-to-cell contact. Th17 induction was enhanced by a psoriasis risk-associated variant in the TRAF3IP2 gene encoding the D10N variant of Act1 which serves as a key mediator of IL-17 signal transduction. That provides an evidence of genetic basis for the enhanced IL-17 expression in psoriasis. IL-17-expressing T cells and neutrophils were suggested to have a cross-talk because IL-17-expressing T cells produce cytokines which promote the development, recruitment, and lifespan of neutrophils (149).

Although many immune diseases including psoriasis or atopic dermatitis have been traditionally classified as Th1/Th2 biphasic disorders, there is a growing evidence supporting a rather systemic activation of other multiple Th-cell subsets, such as Th17 cells producing IL-17 and IL-22 (**Figure 2**). Interestingly, in comparison with psoriasis, atopic dermatitis showed reduced genomic expression of IL-23, IL-17, IFN-γ, and other innate defense genes (hBD2, elafin, LL-37) (150). Elevated IL-17 is detected in psoriatic skin lesions and in the blood (151). IL-17 mainly stimulates keratinocytes to produce neutrophil-tropic chemokines CXCL-1, CXCL-2, CXCL-8 (IL-8), and antimicrobial peptides, such as LL-37. IL-17 serves as an autocrine-amplifying mediator that is simultaneously involved in the recruitment, activation, and survival of neutrophils (6). There are several subtypes of IL-17 family cytokines binding to IL-17 receptors, namely IL-17A, IL-17B, IL-17C, IL-17D, IL-17E (also known as IL-25) and IL-17F (145). IL-17A from neutrophils stimulates keratinocytes to express CCL20, attracting Th17 cells with CCR6 expression to release IL-17A, and finally resulting in positive feedback and the development of the psoriatic lesions (8). IL-17C is a unique cytokine that is produced by keratinocytes and that is involved in such synergistic loops that may be responsible for amplifying the inflammation in both psoriasis and atopic dermatitis. This may ultimately lead to induction of S100As and other molecules that accompany epidermal hyperplasia. Thus, antagonism of IL-17C may be beneficial for psoriasis and atopic dermatitis treatment (152). IL-17E then recruits neutrophils by activating macrophages and contributes to the infiltration of psoriatic neutrophils (153). Besides other innate immune cells, neutrophils significantly contribute to IL-17-related immune regulations in psoriasis by employing several mechanisms including the formation of NETs (45). Moreover, IL-17 released by NETs leads to endothelial dysfunction in atherosclerosis and keratinocyte proliferation in psoriasis, which may explain why patients with psoriasis also suffer from increased risk of atherosclerosis (11). Anti-IL-17 drugs, such as secukinumab, clear the neutrophils in the epidermis and can be used to effectively treat psoriasis (48). The targeted biologic therapies are of great importance with regards to an increasing number of comorbidities associated with psoriasis together with its systemic inflammation nature indicating that these diseases are sharing some common pathological mechanisms (7). In summary, NETs were demonstrated as potential upstream drug targets for the treatment of psoriasis.

CONCLUSION

Neutrophils in psoriasis are of interest, particularly, because of their crucial roles in the innate and adaptive immune system. The respiratory burst with ROS generation, degranulation, and formation of NETs are the main offensive functions of neutrophils and contribute to the immunopathogenesis of psoriasis. Recently, great attention was brought to the role of NETs in psoriasis because activated neutrophils producing NETs are abundant in psoriatic skin plaques and pustules, as well as in the serum of patients with psoriasis. Overexpression of NETs leads to the activation of other cells releasing IL-17, which stimulates the synthesis of inflammatory mediators and in turn leads to auto-amplification of neutrophils. Therefore, further development of inhibitors and biologic drugs targeting overexpressed offensive features of neutrophils, i.e., respiratory burst, degranulation, and NET formation, is of great importance. We believe that the consideration of the role of neutrophil defense mechanisms in the pathogenesis of psoriasis offered in this review highlights the need to further investigate neutrophils for possible improvements of available treatments in the future.

AUTHOR CONTRIBUTIONS

C-CC and W-JC wrote and revised the manuscript. MK consulted and revised the manuscript. C-YL drew the figures. T-LH initiated the concept and supervised the writing. All authors read and approved the final manuscript.

ACKNOWLEDGMENTS

We are grateful to Assoc. Prof. Mohamed El-Shazly for valuable comments and revision of the manuscript. Special thanks to Editage English Editorial Office, Taiwan for English editing. The authors wish to thank Miss Ingrid Kuo and the Center for Big Data Analytics and Statistics (Grant CLRPG 3D0045) at Chang Gung Memorial Hospital for creating the illustrations used herein.

REFERENCES

1. Tecchio C, Cassatella MA. Neutrophil-derived chemokines on the road to immunity. *Semin Immunol.* (2016) 28:119–28. doi: 10.1016/j.smim.2016.04.003
2. Nauseef WM, Borregaard N. Neutrophils at work. *Nat Immunol.* (2014) 15:602–11. doi: 10.1038/ni.2921
3. Leliefeld PH, Koenderman L, Pillay J. How Neutrophils Shape Adaptive Immune Responses. *Front Immunol.* (2015) 6:471. doi: 10.3389/fimmu.2015.00471
4. Rosales C, Lowell CA, Schnoor M, Uribe-Querol E. Neutrophils: Their Role in Innate and Adaptive Immunity 2017. *J Immunol Res.* (2017) 2017:9748345. doi: 10.1155/2017/9748345
5. Georgescu SR, Tampa M, Caruntu C, Sarbu MI, Mitran CI, Mitran MI, et al. Advances in understanding the immunological pathways in psoriasis. *Int J Mol Sci.* (2019) 20:739. doi: 10.3390/ijms20030739
6. Chiricozzi A, Romanelli P, Volpe E, Borsellino G, Romanelli M. Scanning the Immunopathogenesis of Psoriasis. *Int J Mol Sci.* (2018) 19:E179. doi: 10.3390/ijms19010179
7. Korman NJ. Management of psoriasis as a systemic disease: What is the evidence? *Br J Dermatol.* (2019). doi: 10.1111/bjd.18245. [Epub ahead of print].
8. Katayama H. Development of psoriasis by continuous neutrophil infiltration into the epidermis. *Exp Dermatol.* (2018) 27:1084–91. doi: 10.1111/exd.13746
9. Cedervall J, Hamidi A, Olsson AK. Platelets, NETs and cancer. *Thromb Res.* (2018) 164(Suppl 1):S148–52. doi: 10.1016/j.thromres.2018.01.049
10. Delgado-Rizo V, Martínez-Guzmán MA, Iñiguez-Gutierrez L, García-Orozco A, Alvarado-Navarro A, Fafutis-Morris M. Neutrophil extracellular traps and its implications in inflammation: an overview. *Front Immunol.* (2017) 8:81. doi: 10.3389/fimmu.2017.00081
11. Sanda GE, Belur AD, Teague HL, Mehta NN. Emerging Associations Between Neutrophils, Atherosclerosis, and Psoriasis. *Curr Atheroscler Rep.* (2017) 19:53. doi: 10.1007/s11883-017-0692-8
12. Bagchi D, Kundu-Raychaudhuri SK, Raychaudhuri SP. *Psoriasis and Psoriatic Arthritis: Pathophysiology, Therapeutic Intervention, and Complementary Medicine.* Portland, OR: CRC Press/Taylor & Francis Group (2018) p. 413.
13. Menter A. RC. *Psoriasis.* 2nd ed. Portland, OR: CRC Press/Taylor & Francis Group (2017). p. 268
14. Warren R. MA. *Handbook of Psoriasis and Psoriatic Arthritis.* Springer International Publishing (2016). p. 116.
15. Adebajo A, Gladman DD, Mease PJ. *Psoriatic Arthritis and Psoriasis: Pathology and Clinical Aspects.* Springer International Publishing (2016). p. 316.
16. Greb JE, Goldminz AM, Elder JT, Lebwohl MG, Gladman DD, Wu JJ, et al. Psoriasis. *Nat Rev Dis Primers.* (2016) 2:16082. doi: 10.1038/nrdp.2016.83
17. Sticherling M. Psoriasis and autoimmunity. *Autoimmun Rev.* (2016) 15:1167–70. doi: 10.1016/j.autrev.2016.09.004
18. Kaushik SB, Lebwohl MG. CME Part I Psoriasis: which therapy for which patient psoriasis comorbidities and preferred systemic agents. *J Am Acad Dermatol.* (2019) 80:27–40. doi: 10.1016/j.jaad.2018.06.057
19. Geller S, Xu H, Lebwohl M, Nardone B, Lacouture ME, Kheterpal M. Malignancy risk and recurrence with psoriasis and its treatments: a concise update. *Am J Clin Dermatol.* (2018) 19:363–75. doi: 10.1007/s40257-017-0337-2
20. Gelfand JM. Psoriasis, type 2 diabetes mellitus, and obesity: weighing the evidence. *JAMA Dermatol.* (2016) 152:753–4 doi: 10.1001/jamadermatol.2016.0670
21. Armstrong AW. Psoriasis. *JAMA Dermatol.* (2017) 153:956. doi: 10.1001/jamadermatol.2017.2103
22. Raychaudhuri SK, Maverakis E, Raychaudhuri SP. Diagnosis and classification of psoriasis. *Autoimmun Rev.* (2014) 13:490–5. doi: 10.1016/j.autrev.2014.01.008
23. Nestle FO, Kaplan DH, Barker J. Psoriasis. *N Engl J Med.* (2009) 361:496–509. doi: 10.1056/NEJMra0804595
24. Vanderpuye-Orgle J, Zhao Y, Lu J, Shrestha A, Sexton A, Seabury S, et al. Evaluating the economic burden of psoriasis in the United States. *J Am Acad Dermatol.* (2015) 72:961–7.e5. doi: 10.1016/j.jaad.2015.02.1099
25. Brezinski EA, Dhillon JS, Armstrong AW. Economic burden of psoriasis in the United States: a systematic review. *JAMA Dermatol.* (2015) 151:651–8. doi: 10.1001/jamadermatol.2014.3593
26. Hawro T, Zalewska A, Hawro M, Kaszuba A, Krolikowska M, Maurer M. Impact of psoriasis severity on family income and quality of life. *J Eur Acad Dermatol Venereol.* (2015) 29:438–43. doi: 10.1111/jdv.12572
27. Singh S, Taylor C, Kornmehl H, Armstrong AW. Psoriasis and suicidality: a systematic review and meta-analysis. *J Am Acad Dermatol.* (2017) 77:425–40.e2. doi: 10.1016/j.jaad.2017.05.019
28. Dowlatshahi EA, Wakkee M, Arends LR, Nijsten T. The prevalence and odds of depressive symptoms and clinical depression in psoriasis patients: a systematic review and meta-analysis. *J Invest Dermatol.* (2014) 134:1542–51. doi: 10.1038/jid.2013.508

29. Prinz JC. Autoimmune aspects of psoriasis: heritability and autoantigens. *Autoimmun Rev.* (2017) 16:970–9. doi: 10.1016/j.autrev.2017.07.011
30. Hwang ST, Nijsten T, Elder JT. Recent highlights in psoriasis research. *J Invest Dermatol.* (2017) 137:550–6. doi: 10.1016/j.jid.2016.11.007
31. Harvima IT, Nilsson G, Suttle MM, Naukkarinen A. Is there a role for mast cells in psoriasis? *Arch Dermatol Res.* (2008) 300:461–78. doi: 10.1007/s00403-008-0874-x
32. Prinz JC. Melanocytes: target cells of an HLA-C*06:02-restricted autoimmune response in psoriasis. *J Invest Dermatol.* (2017) 137:2053–8. doi: 10.1016/j.jid.2017.05.023
33. Mrowietz U. Neutrophils' sexiness is independent of trendy fashion. *Exp Dermatol.* (2017) 26:312–3. doi: 10.1111/exd.13102
34. Mantovani A, Cassatella MA, Costantini C, Jaillon S. Neutrophils in the activation and regulation of innate and adaptive immunity. *Nat Rev Immunol.* (2011) 11:519–31. doi: 10.1038/nri3024
35. Jaillon S, Galdiero MR, Del Prete D, Cassatella MA, Garlanda C, Mantovani A. Neutrophils in innate and adaptive immunity. *Semin Immunopathol.* (2013) 35:377–94. doi: 10.1007/s00281-013-0374-8
36. Dubertret L, Mrowietz U, Ranki A, van de Kerkhof PC, Chimenti S, Lotti T, et al. European patient perspectives on the impact of psoriasis: the EUROPSO patient membership survey. *Br J Dermatol.* (2006) 155:729–36. doi: 10.1111/j.1365-2133.2006.07405.x
37. Belinchón I, Rivera R, Blanch C, Comellas M, Lizán L. Adherence, satisfaction and preferences for treatment in patients with psoriasis in the European Union: a systematic review of the literature. *Patient Prefer Adherence.* (2016) 10:2357–67. doi: 10.2147/PPA.S117006
38. Meng S, Lin Z, Wang Y, Wang Z, Li P, Zheng Y. Psoriasis therapy by Chinese medicine and modern agents. *Chin Med.* (2018) 13:16. doi: 10.1186/s13020-018-0174-0
39. Damevska K, Franca K, Lotti T, Nikolovska S, Pollozhani N. Complementary and integrative therapies for psoriasis: looking forward. *Dermatol Ther.* (2018) 31:e12627. doi: 10.1111/dth.12627
40. Talbott W, Duffy N. Complementary and alternative medicine for psoriasis: what the dermatologist needs to know. *Am J Clin Dermatol.* (2015) 16:147–65. doi: 10.1007/s40257-015-0128-6
41. Costanzo A, Malara G, Pelucchi C, Fatiga F, Barbera G, Franchi A, et al. Effectiveness end points in real-world studies on biological therapies in psoriasis: systematic review with focus on drug survival. *Dermatology.* (2018) 234:1–12. doi: 10.1159/000488586
42. Yamanaka K, Umezawa Y, Yamagiwa A, Saeki H, Kondo M, Gabazza EC, et al. Biologic therapy improves psoriasis by decreasing the activity of monocytes and neutrophils. *J Dermatol.* (2014) 41:679–85. doi: 10.1111/1346-8138.12560
43. de Groot M, Picavet DI, van Kuijk AW, Tak PP, Bos JD, de Rie MA, et al. A prospective, randomized, placebo-controlled study to identify biomarkers associated with active treatment in psoriatic arthritis: effects of adalimumab treatment on lesional and nonlesional skin. *Dermatology.* (2012) 225:298–303. doi: 10.1159/000343290
44. Tan JK, Aphale A, Malaviya R, Sun Y, Gottlieb AB. Mechanisms of action of etanercept in psoriasis. *J Investig Dermatol Symp Proc.* (2007) 12:38–45. doi: 10.1038/sj.jidsymp.5650037
45. Schon MP, Erpenbeck L. The Interleukin-23/Interleukin-17 Axis Links Adaptive and Innate Immunity in Psoriasis. *Front Immunol.* (2018) 9:1323. doi: 10.3389/fimmu.2018.01323
46. Chen F, Cao A, Yao S, Evans-Marin HL, Liu H, Wu W, et al. mTOR Mediates IL-23 Induction of Neutrophil IL-17 and IL-22 Production. *J Immunol.* (2016) 196:4390–9. doi: 10.1097/01.ccm.0000508877.60312.7c
47. Liu L, Lu J, Allan BW, Tang Y, Tetreault J, Chow CK, et al. Generation and characterization of ixekizumab, a humanized monoclonal antibody that neutralizes interleukin-17A. *J Inflamm Res.* (2016) 9:39–50. doi: 10.2147/JIR.S100940
48. Reich K, Papp KA, Matheson RT, Tu JH, Bissonnette R, Bourcier M, et al. Evidence that a neutrophil-keratinocyte crosstalk is an early target of IL-17A inhibition in psoriasis. *Exp Dermatol.* (2015) 24:529–35. doi: 10.1111/exd.12710
49. Polat M, Bugdayci G, Kaya H, Oguzman H. Evaluation of neutrophil-to-lymphocyte ratio and platelet-to-lymphocyte ratio in Turkish patients with chronic plaque psoriasis. *Acta Dermatovenerol Alp Pannonica Adriat.* (2017) 26:97–100. doi: 10.15570/actaapa.2017.28
50. Paliogiannis P, Satta R, Deligia G, Farina G, Bassu S, Mangoni AA, et al. Associations between the neutrophil-to-lymphocyte and the platelet-to-lymphocyte ratios and the presence and severity of psoriasis: a systematic review and meta-analysis. *Clin Exp Med.* (2019) 19:37–45. doi: 10.1007/s10238-018-0538-x
51. Balevi A, Olmuscelik O, Ustuner P, Ozdemir M. Is there any correlation between red cell distribution width, mean platelet volume neutrophil count, lymphocyte count, and psoriasis area severity index in patients under treatment for psoriasis? *Acta Dermatovenerol Croat.* (2018) 26:199–205.
52. Erek Toprak A, Ozlu E, Uzuncakmak TK, Yalcinkaya E, Sogut S, Karadag AS. Neutrophil/lymphocyte ratio, serum endocan, and nesfatin-1 levels in patients with psoriasis vulgaris undergoing phototherapy treatment. *Med Sci Monit.* (2016) 22:1232–7. doi: 10.12659/MSM.898240
53. Yurtdas M, Yaylali YT, Kaya Y, Ozdemir M, Ozkan I, Aladag N. Neutrophil-to-lymphocyte ratio may predict subclinical atherosclerosis in patients with psoriasis. *Echocardiography.* (2014) 31:1095–104. doi: 10.1111/echo.12511
54. Ikeda S, Takahashi H, Suga Y, Eto H, Etoh T, Okuma K, et al. Therapeutic depletion of myeloid lineage leukocytes in patients with generalized pustular psoriasis indicates a major role for neutrophils in the immunopathogenesis of psoriasis. *J Am Acad Dermatol.* (2013) 68:609–17. doi: 10.1016/j.jaad.2012.09.037
55. Schon MP, Broekaert SM, Erpenbeck L. Sexy again: the renaissance of neutrophils in psoriasis. *Exp Dermatol.* (2017) 26:305–11. doi: 10.1111/exd.13067
56. Belambri SA, Rolas L, Raad H, Hurtado-Nedelec M, Dang PM, El-Benna J. NADPH oxidase activation in neutrophils: role of the phosphorylation of its subunits. *Eur J Clin Invest.* (2018) 2:e12951. doi: 10.1111/eci.12951
57. Amulic B, Cazalet C, Hayes GL, Metzler KD, Zychlinsky A. Neutrophil function: from mechanisms to disease. *Annu Rev Immunol.* (2012) 30:459–89. doi: 10.1146/annurev-immunol-020711-074942
58. Glennon-Alty L, Hackett AP, Chapman EA, Wright HL. Neutrophils and redox stress in the pathogenesis of autoimmune disease. *Free Radic Biol Med.* (2018) 125:25–35. doi: 10.1016/j.freeradbiomed.2018.03.049
59. Winterbourn CC, Kettle AJ, Hampton MB. Reactive oxygen species and neutrophil function. *Annu Rev Biochem.* (2016) 85:765–92. doi: 10.1146/annurev-biochem-060815-014442
60. Hoffmann MH, Griffiths HR. The dual role of ROS in autoimmune and inflammatory diseases: Evidence from preclinical models. *Free Radic Biol Med.* (2018) 125:62–71. doi: 10.1016/j.freeradbiomed.2018.03.016
61. Bloomfield FJ, Young MM. Enhanced release of inflammatory mediators from lithium-stimulated neutrophils in psoriasis. *Br J Dermatol.* (1983) 109:9–13. doi: 10.1111/j.1365-2133.1983.tb03985.x
62. Bloomfield FJ, Young MM. Enhanced chemiluminescence production by phagocytosing neutrophils in psoriasis. *Inflammation.* (1988) 12:153–9. doi: 10.1007/BF00916398
63. Martin G, Guerard S, Fortin MM, Rusu D, Soucy J, Poubelle PE, et al. Pathological crosstalk *in vitro* between T lymphocytes and lesional keratinocytes in psoriasis: necessity of direct cell-to-cell contact. *Lab Invest.* (2012) 92:1058–70. doi: 10.1038/labinvest.2012.69
64. Vogt KL, Summers C, Chilvers ER, Condliffe AM. Priming and de-priming of neutrophil responses *in vitro* and *in vivo*. *Eur J Clin Invest.* (2018) 47:e12967. doi: 10.1111/eci.12967
65. Boehncke WH, Schon MP. Psoriasis. *Lancet.* (2015) 386:983–94. doi: 10.1016/S0140-6736(14)61909-7
66. Guerard S, Allaeys I, Martin G, Pouliot R, Poubelle PE. Psoriatic keratinocytes prime neutrophils for an overproduction of superoxide anions. *Arch Dermatol Res.* (2013) 305:879–89. doi: 10.1007/s00403-013-1404-z
67. Lin X, Huang T. Oxidative stress in psoriasis and potential therapeutic use of antioxidants. *Free Radic Res.* (2016) 50:585–95. doi: 10.3109/10715762.2016.1162301
68. Lai R, Xian D, Xiong X, Yang L, Song J, Zhong J. Proanthocyanidins: novel treatment for psoriasis that reduces oxidative stress and modulates Th17 and Treg cells. *Redox Rep.* (2018) 23:130–5. doi: 10.1080/13510002.2018.1462027
69. Lacy P. Mechanisms of degranulation in neutrophils. *Allergy Asthma Clin Immunol.* (2006) 2:98–108. doi: 10.1186/1710-1492-2-3-98

70. Sheshachalam A, Srivastava N, Mitchell T, Lacy P, Eitzen G. Granule protein processing and regulated secretion in neutrophils. *Front Immunol.* (2014) 5:448. doi: 10.3389/fimmu.2014.00448
71. Kahlenberg JM, Kaplan MJ. Little peptide, big effects: the role of LL-37 in inflammation and autoimmune disease. *J Immunol.* (2013) 191:4895–901. doi: 10.4049/jimmunol.1302005
72. Cowland JB, Borregaard N. Granulopoiesis and granules of human neutrophils. *Immunol Rev.* (2016) 273:11–28. doi: 10.1111/imr.12440
73. Mitchell T, Lo A, Logan MR, Lacy P, Eitzen G. Primary granule exocytosis in human neutrophils is regulated by Rac-dependent actin remodeling. *Am J Physiol Cell Physiol.* (2008) 295:C1354–65. doi: 10.1152/ajpcell.00239.2008
74. Jog NR, Rane MJ, Lominadze G, Luerman GC, Ward RA, McLeish KR. The actin cytoskeleton regulates exocytosis of all neutrophil granule subsets. *Am J Physiol Cell Physiol.* (2007) 292:C1690–700. doi: 10.1152/ajpcell.00384.2006
75. Yin C, Heit B. Armed for destruction: formation, function and trafficking of neutrophil granules. *Cell Tissue Res.* (2018) 371:455–71. doi: 10.1007/s00441-017-2731-8
76. Hoenderdos K, Lodge KM, Hirst RA, Chen C, Palazzo SG, Emerenciana A, et al. Hypoxia upregulates neutrophil degranulation and potential for tissue injury. *Thorax.* (2016) 71:1030–8. doi: 10.1136/thoraxjnl-2015-207604
77. Polverino E, Rosales-Mayor E, Dale GE, Dembowsky K, Torres A. The role of neutrophil elastase inhibitors in lung diseases. *Chest.* (2017) 152:249–62. doi: 10.1016/j.chest.2017.03.056
78. Chistiakov DA, Bobryshev YV, Orekhov AN. Neutrophil's weapons in atherosclerosis. *Exp Mol Pathol.* (2015) 99:663–71. doi: 10.1016/j.yexmp.2015.11.011
79. Sivalingam Z, Larsen SB, Grove EL, Hvas AM, Kristensen SD, Magnusson NE. Neutrophil gelatinase-associated lipocalin as a risk marker in cardiovascular disease. *Clin Chem Lab Med.* (2017) 56:5–18. doi: 10.1515/cclm-2017-0120
80. Ramaiah SK, Jaeschke H. Role of neutrophils in the pathogenesis of acute inflammatory liver injury. *Toxicol Pathol.* (2007) 35:757–66. doi: 10.1080/01926230701584163
81. Wright HL, Moots RJ, Bucknall RC, Edwards SW. Neutrophil function in inflammation and inflammatory diseases. *Rheumatology.* (2010) 49:1618–31. doi: 10.1093/rheumatology/keq045
82. Wright HL, Moots RJ, Edwards SW. The multifactorial role of neutrophils in rheumatoid arthritis. *Nat Rev Rheumatol.* (2014) 10:593–601. doi: 10.1038/nrrheum.2014.80
83. Dilek N, Dilek AR, Taskin Y, Erkinuresin T, Yalcin O, Saral Y. Contribution of myeloperoxidase and inducible nitric oxide synthase to pathogenesis of psoriasis. *Postepy Dermatol Alergol.* (2016) 33:435–9. doi: 10.5114/ada.2016.63882
84. Cao LY, Soler DC, Debanne SM, Grozdev I, Rodriguez ME, Feig RL, et al. Psoriasis and cardiovascular risk factors: increased serum myeloperoxidase and corresponding immunocellular overexpression by Cd11b. (+) CD68. (+) macrophages in skin lesions. *Am J Transl Res.* (2013) 6:16–27.
85. Strzepa A, Pritchard KA, Dittel BN. Myeloperoxidase: a new player in autoimmunity. *Cell Immunol.* (2017) 317:1–8. doi: 10.1016/j.cellimm.2017.05.002
86. Lau D, Mollnau H, Eiserich JP, Freeman BA, Daiber A, Gehling UM, et al. Myeloperoxidase mediates neutrophil activation by association with CD11b/CD18 integrins. *Proc Natl Acad Sci USA.* (2005) 102:431–6. doi: 10.1073/pnas.0405193102
87. Guo J, Tu J, Hu Y, Song G, Yin Z. Cathepsin G cleaves and activates IL-36γ and promotes the inflammation of psoriasis. *Drug Des Devel Ther.* (2019) 13:581–8. doi: 10.2147/DDDT.S194765
88. Henry CM, Sullivan GP, Clancy DM, Afonina IS, Kulms D, Martin SJ. Neutrophil-derived proteases escalate inflammation through activation of IL-36 family cytokines. *Cell Rep.* (2016) 14:708–22. doi: 10.1016/j.celrep.2015.12.072
89. Xhindoli D, Pacor S, Benincasa M, Scocchi M, Gennaro R, Tossi A. The human cathelicidin LL-37–A pore-forming antibacterial peptide and host-cell modulator. *Biochim Biophys Acta.* (2016) 1858:546–66. doi: 10.1016/j.bbamem.2015.11.003
90. Durr UH, Sudheendra US, Ramamoorthy A. LL-37, the only human member of the cathelicidin family of antimicrobial peptides. *Biochim Biophys Acta.* (2006) 1758:1408–25. doi: 10.1016/j.bbamem.2006.03.030
91. Ganguly D, Chamilos G, Lande R, Gregorio J, Meller S, Facchinetti V, et al. Self-RNA-antimicrobial peptide complexes activate human dendritic cells through TLR7 and TLR8. *J Exp Med.* (2009) 206:1983–94. doi: 10.1084/jem.20090480
92. Lande R, Gregorio J, Facchinetti V, Chatterjee B, Wang YH, Homey B, et al. Plasmacytoid dendritic cells sense self-DNA coupled with antimicrobial peptide. *Nature.* (2007) 449:564–9. doi: 10.1038/nature06116
93. Meyer-Hoffert U, Wingertszahn J, Wiedow O. Human leukocyte elastase induces keratinocyte proliferation by epidermal growth factor receptor activation. *J Invest Dermatol.* (2004) 123:338–45. doi: 10.1111/j.0022-202X.2004.23202.x
94. Brinkmann V, Reichard U, Goosmann C, Fauler B, Uhlemann Y, Weiss DS, et al. Neutrophil extracellular traps kill bacteria. *Science.* (2004) 303:1532–5. doi: 10.1126/science.1092385
95. Kim SJ, Jenne CN. Role of platelets in neutrophil extracellular trap. (NET) production and tissue injury. *Semin Immunol.* (2016) 28:546–54. doi: 10.1016/j.smim.2016.10.013
96. Branzk N, Lubojemska A, Hardison SE, Wang Q, Gutierrez MG, Brown GD, et al. Neutrophils sense microbe size and selectively release neutrophil extracellular traps in response to large pathogens. *Nat Immunol.* (2014) 15:1017–25. doi: 10.1038/ni.2987
97. Apel F, Zychlinsky A, Kenny EF. The role of neutrophil extracellular traps in rheumatic diseases. *Nat Rev Rheumatol.* (2018) 14:467–75. doi: 10.1038/s41584-018-0039-z
98. Honda M, Kubes P. Neutrophils and neutrophil extracellular traps in the liver and gastrointestinal system. *Nat Rev Gastroenterol Hepatol.* (2018) 15:206–21. doi: 10.1038/nrgastro.2017.183
99. Fernandez-Ruiz I. Inflammation: NETs are involved in AAA. *Nat Rev Cardiol.* (2018) 15:257. doi: 10.1038/nrcardio.2018.28
100. Doring Y, Soehnlein O, Weber C. Neutrophil extracellular traps in atherosclerosis and atherothrombosis. *Circ Res.* (2017) 120:736–43. doi: 10.1161/CIRCRESAHA.116.309692
101. Dabrowska D, Jablonska E, Garley M, Sawicka-Powierza J, Nowak K. The Phenomenon of Neutrophil Extracellular Traps in Vascular Diseases. *Arch Immunol Ther Exp.* (2018) 66:273–81. doi: 10.1007/s00005-018-0505-y
102. Porto BN, Stein RT. Neutrophil extracellular traps in pulmonary diseases: too much of a good thing? *Front Immunol.* (2016) 7:311. doi: 10.3389/fimmu.2016.00311
103. Liu T, Wang FP, Wang G, Mao H. Role of neutrophil extracellular traps in asthma and chronic obstructive pulmonary disease. *Chin Med J.* (2017) 130:730–6. doi: 10.4103/0366-6999.201608
104. Albrengues J, Shields MA, Ng D, Park CG, Ambrico A, Poindexter ME, et al. Neutrophil extracellular traps produced during inflammation awaken dormant cancer cells in mice. *Science.* (2018) 361:eaao4227. doi: 10.1126/science.aao4227
105. Kenny EF, Herzig A, Kruger R, Muth A, Mondal S, Thompson PR, et al. Diverse stimuli engage different neutrophil extracellular trap pathways. *Elife.* (2017) 6:e24437. doi: 10.7554/eLife.24437
106. Papayannopoulos V, Metzler KD, Hakkim A, Zychlinsky A. Neutrophil elastase and myeloperoxidase regulate the formation of neutrophil extracellular traps. *J Cell Biol.* (2010) 191:677–91. doi: 10.1083/jcb.201006052
107. Loures FV, Rohm M, Lee CK, Santos E, Wang JP, Specht CA, et al. Recognition of Aspergillus fumigatus hyphae by human plasmacytoid dendritic cells is mediated by dectin-2 and results in formation of extracellular traps. *PLoS Pathog.* (2015) 11:e1004643. doi: 10.1371/journal.ppat.1004643
108. Pieterse E, Rother N, Yanginlar C, Hilbrands LB, van der Vlag J. Neutrophils discriminate between lipopolysaccharides of different bacterial sources and selectively release neutrophil extracellular traps. *Front Immunol.* (2016) 7:484. doi: 10.3389/fimmu.2016.00484
109. Desai J, Kumar SV, Mulay SR, Konrad L, Romoli S, Schauer C, et al. PMA and crystal-induced neutrophil extracellular trap formation involves RIPK1-RIPK3-MLKL signaling. *Eur J Immunol.* (2016) 46:223–9. doi: 10.1002/eji.201545605
110. Papayannopoulos V. Neutrophil extracellular traps in immunity and disease. *Nat Rev Immunol.* (2018) 18:134–47. doi: 10.1038/nri.2017.105
111. Douda DN, Khan MA, Grasemann H, Palaniyar N. SK3 channel and mitochondrial ROS mediate NADPH oxidase-independent NETosis

induced by calcium influx. *Proc Natl Acad Sci USA.* (2015) 112:2817–22. doi: 10.1073/pnas.1414055112

112. Behnen M, Leschczyk C, Moller S, Batel T, Klinger M, Solbach W, et al. Immobilized immune complexes induce neutrophil extracellular trap release by human neutrophil granulocytes via FcgammaRIIIB and Mac-1. *J Immunol.* (2014) 193:1954–65. doi: 10.4049/jimmunol.1400478
113. Hoppenbrouwers T, Autar ASA, Sultan AR, Abraham TE, van Cappellen WA, Houtsmuller AB, et al. *In vitro* induction of NETosis: Comprehensive live imaging comparison and systematic review. *PLoS ONE.* (2017) 12:e0176472. doi: 10.1371/journal.pone.0176472
114. Yipp BG, Petri B, Salina D, Jenne CN, Scott BN, Zbytnuik LD, et al. Infection-induced NETosis is a dynamic process involving neutrophil multitasking *in vivo*. *Nat Med.* (2012) 18:1386–93. doi: 10.1038/nm.2847
115. Pilsczek FH, Salina D, Poon KK, Fahey C, Yipp BG, Sibley CD, et al. A novel mechanism of rapid nuclear neutrophil extracellular trap formation in response to *Staphylococcus aureus*. *J Immunol.* (2010) 185:7413–25. doi: 10.4049/jimmunol.1000675
116. Byrd AS, O'Brien XM, Johnson CM, Lavigne LM, Reichner JS. An extracellular matrix-based mechanism of rapid neutrophil extracellular trap formation in response to Candida albicans. *J Immunol.* (2013) 190:4136–48. doi: 10.4049/jimmunol.1202671
117. Rochael NC, Guimaraes-Costa AB, Nascimento MT, DeSouza-Vieira TS, Oliveira MP, Garcia e Souza LF, et al. Classical ROS-dependent and early/rapid ROS-independent release of neutrophil extracellular traps triggered by Leishmania parasites. *Sci Rep.* (2015) 5:18302. doi: 10.1038/srep18302
118. Chandler CE, Ernst RK. Bacterial lipids: powerful modifiers of the innate immune response. *F1000Res.* (2017) 6:F1000. doi: 10.12688/f1000research.11388.1
119. Petretto A, Bruschi M, Pratesi F, Croia C, Candiano G, Ghiggeri G, et al. Neutrophil extracellular traps. (NET) induced by different stimuli: a comparative proteomic analysis. *PLoS ONE.* (2019) 14:e0218946. doi: 10.1371/journal.pone.0218946
120. Clark SR, Ma AC, Tavener SA, McDonald B, Goodarzi Z, Kelly MM, et al. Platelet TLR4 activates neutrophil extracellular traps to ensnare bacteria in septic blood. *Nat Med.* (2007) 13:463–9. doi: 10.1038/nm1565
121. Liu S, Su X, Pan P, Zhang L, Hu Y, Tan H, et al. Neutrophil extracellular traps are indirectly triggered by lipopolysaccharide and contribute to acute lung injury. *Sci Rep.* (2016) 6:37252. doi: 10.1038/srep37252
122. Hu Z, Murakami T, Tamura H, Reich J, Kuwahara-Arai K, Iba T, et al. Neutrophil extracellular traps induce IL-1β production by macrophages in combination with lipopolysaccharide. *Int J Mol Med.* (2017) 39:549–58. doi: 10.3892/ijmm.2017.2870
123. Shao S, Fang H, Dang E, Xue K, Zhang J, Li B, et al. Neutrophil extracellular traps promote inflammatory responses in psoriasis via activating epidermal TLR4/IL-36R crosstalk. *Front Immunol.* (2019) 10:746. doi: 10.3389/fimmu.2019.00746
124. Hu SC, Yu HS, Yen FL, Lin CL, Chen GS, Lan CC. Neutrophil extracellular trap formation is increased in psoriasis and induces human β-defensin-2 production in epidermal keratinocytes. *Sci Rep.* (2016) 6:31119. doi: 10.1038/srep31119
125. Lee KH, Kronbichler A, Park DD, Park Y, Moon H, Kim H, et al. Neutrophil extracellular traps (NETs) in autoimmune diseases: a comprehensive review. *Autoimmun Rev.* (2017) 16:1160–73. doi: 10.1016/j.autrev.2017.09.012
126. Lowes MA, Suárez-Fariñas M, Krueger JG. Immunology of psoriasis. *Annu Rev Immunol.* (2014) 32:227–55. doi: 10.1146/annurev-immunol-032713-120225
127. Pinegin B, Vorobjeva N, Pinegin V. Neutrophil extracellular traps and their role in the development of chronic inflammation and autoimmunity. *Autoimmun Rev.* (2015) 14:633–40. doi: 10.1016/j.autrev.2015.03.002
128. Skrzeczynska-Moncznik J, Wlodarczyk A, Zabieglo K, Kapinska-Mrowiecka M, Marewicz E, Dubin A, et al. Secretory leukocyte proteinase inhibitor-competent DNA deposits are potent stimulators of plasmacytoid dendritic cells: implication for psoriasis. *J Immunol.* (2012) 189:1611–7. doi: 10.4049/jimmunol.1103293
129. Zabieglo K, Majewski P, Majchrzak-Gorecka M, Wlodarczyk A, Grygier B, Zegar A, et al. The inhibitory effect of secretory leukocyte protease inhibitor. (SLPI) on formation of neutrophil extracellular traps. *J Leukoc Biol.* (2015) 98:99–106. doi: 10.1189/jlb.4AB1114-543R
130. Majewski P, Majchrzak-Gorecka M, Grygier B, Skrzeczynska-Moncznik J, Osiecka O, Cichy J. Inhibitors of serine proteases in regulating the production and function of neutrophil extracellular traps. *Front Immunol.* (2016) 7:261. doi: 10.3389/fimmu.2016.00261
131. Tillack K, Breiden P, Martin R, Sospedra M. T lymphocyte priming by neutrophil extracellular traps links innate and adaptive immune responses. *J Immunol.* (2012) 188:3150–9. doi: 10.4049/jimmunol.1103414
132. Sangaletti S, Tripodo C, Chiodoni C, Guarnotta C, Cappetti B, Casalini P, et al. Neutrophil extracellular traps mediate transfer of cytoplasmic neutrophil antigens to myeloid dendritic cells toward ANCA induction and associated autoimmunity. *Blood.* (2012) 120:3007–18. doi: 10.1182/blood-2012-03-416156
133. Cataldi C, Mari NL, Lozovoy MAB, Martins LMM, Reiche EMV, Maes M, et al. Proinflammatory and anti-inflammatory cytokine profiles in psoriasis: use as laboratory biomarkers and disease predictors. *Inflamm Res.* (2019) 68:557–67. doi: 10.1007/s00011-019-01238-8
134. Murakami M, Hagforsen E, Morhenn V, Ishida-Yamamoto A, Iizuka H. Patients with palmoplantar pustulosis have increased IL-17 and IL-22 levels both in the lesion and serum. *Exp Dermatol.* (2011) 20:845–7. doi: 10.1111/j.1600-0625.2011.01325.x
135. Gisondi P, Lora V, Bonauguri C, Russo A, Lippi G, Girolomoni G. Serum chemerin is increased in patients with chronic plaque psoriasis and normalizes following treatment with infliximab. *Br J Dermatol.* (2013) 168:749–55. doi: 10.1111/bjd.12118
136. Shveta, Agarwal K, Ranchander, Agarwal S. Serum sE-selectin levels in newly diagnosed psoriasis patients and correlation with psoriasis area and severity index score. *J Clin Diagnost Res.* (2017) 11:EC09–12. doi: 10.7860/JCDR/2017/29957.10831
137. Torres T, Bettencourt N, Mendonca D, Vasconcelos C, Silva BM, Selores M. Complement C3 as a marker of cardiometabolic risk in psoriasis. *Arch Dermatol Res.* (2014) 306:653–60. doi: 10.1007/s00403-014-1467-5
138. Hau CS, Kanda N, Tada Y, Shibata S, Uozaki H, Fukusato T, et al. Lipocalin-2 exacerbates psoriasiform skin inflammation by augmenting T-helper 17 response. *J Dermatol.* (2016) 43:785–94. doi: 10.1111/1346-8138.13227
139. Aizawa N, Ishiuji Y, Tominaga M, Sakata S, Takahashi N, Yanaba K, et al. Relationship between the degrees of itch and serum lipocalin-2 levels in patients with psoriasis. *J Immunol Res.* (2019) 2019:8171373. doi: 10.1155/2019/8171373
140. Wolk K, Frambach Y, Jacobi A, Wilsmann-Theis D, Phillipp S, Witte-Handel E, et al. Increased levels of lipocalin 2 in palmoplantar pustular psoriasis. *J Dermatol Sci.* (2018) 90:68–74. doi: 10.1016/j.jdermsci.2017.12.018
141. Wolk K, Wenzel J, Tsaousi A, Witte-Handel E, Babel N, Zelenak C, et al. Lipocalin-2 is expressed by activated granulocytes and keratinocytes in affected skin and reflects disease activity in acne inversa/hidradenitis suppurativa. *Br J Dermatol.* (2017) 177:1385–93. doi: 10.1111/bjd.15424
142. Esaki H, Brunner PM, Renert-Yuval Y, Czarnowicki T, Huynh T, Tran G, et al. Early-onset pediatric atopic dermatitis is TH2 but also TH17 polarized in skin. *J Allergy Clin Immunol.* (2016) 138:1639–51. doi: 10.1016/j.jid.2016.02.064
143. Abdel Hay R, Samir N, Safwat M, Rashed L, Soliman M. Tissue lipocalin-2 in psoriasis: is it a marker of metabolic disturbance or a possible marker of therapeutic efficacy after narrow band ultraviolet B? *J Dermatolog Treat.* (2019) 17:1–5. doi: 10.1080/09546634.2019.1605141
144. Cai Y, Fleming C, Yan J. New insights of T cells in the pathogenesis of psoriasis. *Cell Mol Immunol.* (2012) 9:302–9. doi: 10.1038/cmi.2012.15
145. Brembilla NC, Senra L, Boehncke WH. The IL-17 family of cytokines in psoriasis: IL-17A and beyond. *Front Immunol.* (2018) 9:1682. doi: 10.3389/fimmu.2018.01682
146. Blauvelt A, Chiricozzi A. The immunologic role of IL-17 in psoriasis and psoriatic arthritis pathogenesis. *Clin Rev Allergy Immunol.* (2018) 55:379–90. doi: 10.1007/s12016-018-8702-3

147. Lin AM. Mast cells and neutrophils release IL-17 through extracellular trap formation in psoriasis. *J Immunol.* (2011) 187:490–500. doi: 10.4049/jimmunol.1100123
148. Di Domizio J, Gilliet M. Psoriasis caught in the NET. *J Invest Dermatol.* (2019) 139:1426–9. doi: 10.1016/j.jid.2019.04.020
149. Lambert S, Hambro CA, Johnston A, Stuart PE, Tsoi LC, Nair RP, et al. Neutrophil extracellular traps induce human Th17 cells: effect of psoriasis-associated TRAF3IP2 genotype. *J Invest Dermatol.* (2019) 139:1245–53. doi: 10.1016/j.jid.2018.11.021
150. Guttman-Yassky E, Lowes MA, Fuentes-Duculan J, Zaba LC, Cardinale I, Nograles KE, et al. Low expression of the IL-23/Th17 pathway in atopic dermatitis compared to psoriasis. *J Immunol.* (2008) 181:7420–7. doi: 10.4049/jimmunol.181.10.7420
151. Chen K, Kolls JK. Interluekin-17A (IL17A). *Gene.* (2017) 614:8–14. doi: 10.1016/j.gene.2017.01.016
152. Guttman-Yassky E, Krueger JG. IL-17C: a unique epithelial cytokine with potential for targeting across the spectrum of atopic dermatitis and psoriasis. *J Invest Dermatol.* (2018) 138:1467–9. doi: 10.1016/j.jid.2018.02.037
153. Senra L, Mylonas A, Kavanagh RD, Fallon PG, Conrad C, Borowczyk-Michalowska J, et al. IL-17E (IL-25) Enhances innate immune responses during skin inflammation. *J Invest Dermatol.* (2019) 139:1732–42.e17. doi: 10.1016/j.jid.2019.01.021

21

T Cell Hierarchy in the Pathogenesis of Psoriasis and Associated Cardiovascular Comorbidities

Fabio Casciano[1], Paolo D. Pigatto[2], Paola Secchiero[1], Roberto Gambari[3] and Eva Reali[3,4]*

[1] Department of Morphology, Surgery and Experimental Medicine and LTTA Centre, University of Ferrara, Ferrara, Italy, [2] Department of Dermatology and Venereology, I.R.C.C.S. Istituto Ortopedico Galeazzi, University of Milan, Milan, Italy, [3] Department of Life Sciences and Biotechnology, University of Ferrara, Ferrara, Italy, [4] Laboratory of Translational Immunology, I.R.C.C.S. Istituto Ortopedico Galeazzi, Milan, Italy

***Correspondence:**
Eva Reali
eva.reali@unife.it,
eva.reali@grupposandonato.it

The key role of T cells in the pathogenesis of cutaneous psoriasis has been well described in the last decade and the knowledge of the relative role of the different subsets of T cells in psoriasis pathogenesis has considerably evolved. Now, it is clear that IL-17A-producing T cells, including Th17/Tc17, have a central role in the pathogenesis of cutaneous psoriasis and therapies blocking the IL-17A pathway show high clinical efficacy. By contrast, the contribution of IFNγ-producing T cells has progressively become less clear because of the lack of efficacy of anti-IFNγ antibodies in clinical studies. In parallel, the role of $CD8^+$ T cells specific for self-antigens has been revived and increasing evidence now indicates that in psoriatic skin the majority $CD8^+$ T cells are present in the form of epidermal tissue-resident memory T cells. In the last years it also emerged the possibility of a contribution of T cell recirculation in the pathogenesis of psoriasis and its systemic manifestations. The aim of this review is to define a hierarchy for the different subsets of T cells in the T cell-mediated inflammatory cascade in psoriatic skin. This analysis will possibly help to distinguish the subsets that initiate the disease, those involved in the establishment of the self-sustaining amplification loop that leads to the cutaneous clinical manifestations and finally the subsets that act as downstream players in established lesions. Specific T cell subpopulations finally will be considered for their possible role in propagating inflammation at distant sites and for representing a link with systemic inflammation and cardiovascular comorbidities.

Keywords: psoriasis, skin, inflammation, psoriatic arthritis, TCR repertoire, comorbidities

INTRODUCTION

Psoriasis is a chronically relapsing inflammatory disease of the skin affecting about 2% of the population worldwide.

Histologically, psoriasis is characterized by three principal features: epidermal hyperplasia, leukocyte infiltrate, and an increased number of tortuous and leaky vessels in the dermis (1–3). In recent studies, the presence of lymphoid aggregates/memory T cell clusters in the dermis of psoriatic plaques has been reported (4, 5).

20–30% of patients with psoriasis also develops psoriatic arthritis (PsA) and there is evidence that psoriasis is associated with systemic inflammation and with comorbidities, such as cardiovascular disease (6–12).

With regards to the pathogenesis, it is now emerging that psoriasis is an immune-mediated disease with a central autoimmune component mediated by T cells. Specifically, the disease pathogenesis involves a dynamic interplay between dermal dendritic cells, T cells ($CD8^+$ autoreactive T cells, Th1, and Th17) and keratinocytes giving rise to a self-sustaining inflammatory cycle that develops around the TNF/IL-23/IL-17A axis (13–17). Despite this evidence, the hierarchical sequence of T cell-mediated events in the psoriatic inflammatory cascade is not completely defined. On the basis of the current literature and results of cytokine-blocking therapies it is possible to distinguish, in the T cell-mediated psoriatic inflammatory cascade, (i) an initial skin T cell activation phase, (ii) the establishment of chronic inflammation, (iii) the maintenance of clinically established lesions, and (iv) the egress from the skin of specific subsets of T cells that could possibly take part in the development of extra-cutaneous manifestations of psoriasis, including joint inflammation and cardiovascular comorbidities (18, 19).

T CELL HIERARCHY IN THE FORMATION OF PSORIATIC PLAQUES

T cell responses against self-antigens in psoriasis are initiated by dendritic cells in the dermis of pre-psoriatic skin (20). Mature dermal dendritic cells can produce TNFα and IL-23, present self-antigens, and stimulate the activation of autoreactive $CD8^+$ T cells together with a fraction of $CD4^+$ T cells polarized toward Th17 phenotype or the $IL\text{-}17^+IFN\gamma^+$ pathogenic Th1/Th17 as described by Annunziato and co-workers and Eisdmo and co-workers (20–23).

Activated T cells can migrate to the epidermis and recognize epidermal autoantigens and possibly progress toward differentiation to tissue-resident memory T cells (T_{RM}) characterized by $CD69^+CD103^+CCR7^-CD45RA^-CD62L^-$ phenotype (24, 25). Recognition of epidermal autoantigens by Tc1/Tc17 induces the secretion of cytokines, including IL-22, that mediate the initial phase of epidermal hyperproliferation and activation of keratinocytes (**Figure 1A**). These will produce chemokines and antimicrobial peptides, which lead to the progression of the inflammatory process (26–29).

Epidermal autoantigens include LL-37 antimicrobial peptide expressed by keratinocytes, keratin 17, and melanocyte-derived antigen ADAMTS-like protein 5 (ADAMTSL5) recognized by IL-17A-producing $CD8^+$ T cells, restricted by HLA-C*06:02 (26, 30–35).

This evidence together with early studies strongly supports that $CD8^+$ T cells represent the autoimmune core of the disease. In psoriatic skin lesions, $CD8^+$ T cells accumulate in the form of T_{RM} with a pathogenic IFNγ–IL-17A cytokine profile that were detected also in resolved psoriatic lesions and identified as potential mechanisms of site-specific disease memory (20, 25, 36–42).

The major role of $CD8^+$ T cells is also strongly supported by the fact that the main psoriasis risk gene is the HLA-class I allele HLA-C*06:02 on psoriasis susceptibility locus 1 on chromosome 6 and additional HLA-class I alleles are associated with psoriasis (43, 44).

Among tissue-resident T cells in human psoriatic skin, Clark and co-workers have recently shown that the vast majority has an αβ TCR (42), despite γδ T cells have been reported to play a role in the production of IL-17A and maintenance of inflammation (45, 46).

As regards to the TCR repertoire, studies of TCRBV chain sequencing showed mono or oligoclonal expansions of T cells mainly of $CD8^+$ lineage in psoriatic skin (47–49). TCRBV expansion indicates antigen-driven $CD8^+$ T cell responses, whereas the $CD4^+$ T cell fraction was reported to be polyclonal (50). In patients with cutaneous psoriasis, however, the presence of oligoclonal TCRBV expansion in peripheral blood is debated (51, 52). Two different studies of high-throughput sequencing of the entire TCR repertoire have shown that alongside with a limited oligoclonally expanded T cell subpopulation in psoriatic skin that was in part retained in resolved lesions, there was a vast majority of polyclonal T cells (42, 53). This data suggests that similarly to what has been described in PsA by Winchester and co-workers, antigen-driven mono and oligoclonally expanded T cell populations represent a limited component of the T cell reactions in psoriatic skin, whereas the vast majority is represented by polyclonal $CD4^+$ T cells that are not present in resolved lesions (54).

This evidence together confers to autoreactive $CD8^+$ T cells a dominant role in the plaque formation and in psoriasis recurrence and possibly a common role in psoriasis and PsA. It also underlines the importance of mechanisms of T cell plasticity and polarization toward pathogenic phenotypes.

With respect to CD8 T cell targetability, a recent study on a AGR mouse model of psoriasis has reported the accumulation of epidermal $CD8^+$ T cells during psoriasis development which was associated with IL-17A production and increased keratinocyte proliferation. Importantly, in this study injection of anti-CD8 antibody completely prevented psoriasis development (29).

Nevertheless, it is likely that Tc1/Tc17 autoreactive $CD8^+$ T_{RM} cells overlap their features and functions with the cells that under physiological conditions work as immune sentinels at barrier tissue. For this reason in a clinical setting, it could be difficult to target epidermal $CD8^+$ T_{RM} cells by the available immunotherapeutic tools without incurring in major adverse effects (20, 28, 29, 37).

As regards T helper cells, they have been reported to be more abundant in psoriatic skin lesions. While initially they were described mainly as Th1 cells, more recently the attention has been focused on IL-17-producing cells and the IL-23/Th17 axis clearly emerged as central in the control of the pro-inflammatory cycle in psoriatic plaques (14, 15). The high efficacy and fast outcome of IL-17A blocking therapies in resolving cutaneous clinical symptoms has strongly supported this concept (28, 55, 56). In addition, at skin level an expanded subset of T cells that produces IL-22 but not IL-17A (Th22) with a main role in the induction of acanthosis was identified. Importantly, these cells were found to be present also in resolved psoriatic lesions (57, 58).

In line with the key role of IL-17A, the main gene variants associated with psoriasis outside the MHC locus are single nucleotide polymorphisms, belonging to the IL-23/IL-17A axis (*IL23R*, *IL12B*, and *IL23A*) and the NF-κB pathway (*TNFAIP3*) (44, 59). It is, however, possible to hypothesize that Th17 or pathogenic Th1/Th17 cells could be expanded in the dermis as an event downstream of the epidermal autoimmune T_{RM} and occurs through bystander activation mechanisms like the one described by Winchester and co-workers in psoriatic synovial tissues (54).

In this view, the cycle that develops around the IL-23/IL-17A axis could involve some antigen-driven populations and a

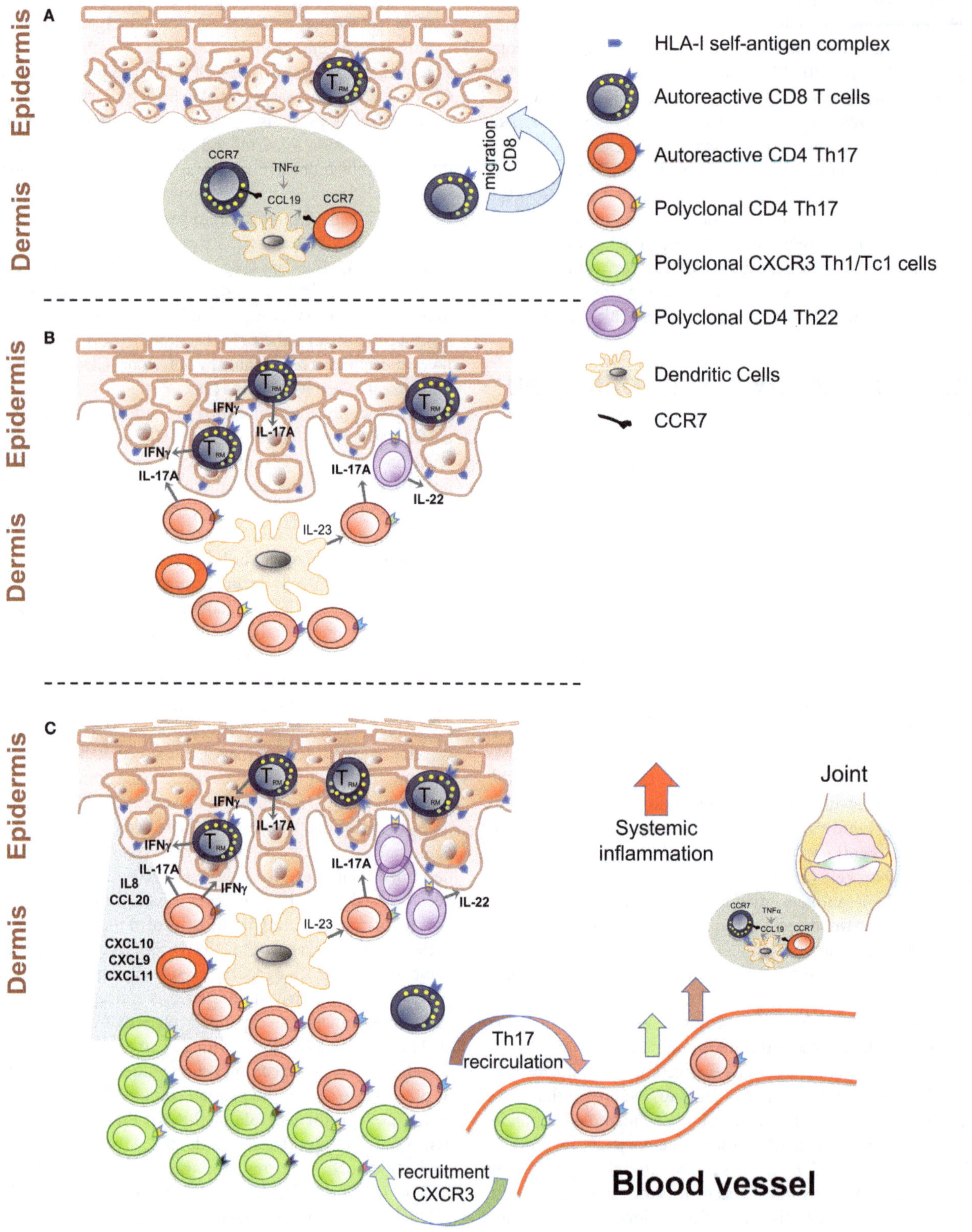

FIGURE 1 | T cell mediated events in the psoriatic inflammatory cascade. **(A)** Activation of autoreactive T cells by self-antigens presented in the dermal lymphoid aggregates. Establishment of CD8+ T_{RM} cells as central autoimmune component of disease pathogenesis and potential mechanisms of site-specific disease memory. **(B)** Polyclonal T cells proliferation and Th17/Tc17-mediated inflammation around the IL-23/IL-17A axis. **(C)** Recruitment of Th1/Tc1 cells, with multiple specificities, from the blood stream, induced by CXCL10 chemokines. Recirculation of T cells from the skin to the blood can spread inflammation at systemic level and at distant sites.

considerable fraction of polyclonally expanded T cells that can represent the second step of the pro-inflammatory cascade, responsible for the amplification of inflammation and for the exacerbation of clinical symptoms (**Figure 1B**).

As a consequence of the strong evidence of the central role of IL-17A-producing cells, the relevance of Th1 cells and IFNγ has become less clear. In lesional skin of psoriasis patients, Th1 cells and IFNγ levels are clearly increased (60, 61). However, in a small pilot study in patients with psoriasis, treatment with a humanized anti-IFNγ antibody induced improvement of histological and some clinical parameters but only minor therapeutic effects (62).

These controversial findings focus on the complexity of the interplay between the Th1/Tc1 and Th17/Tc17 cells in the pathogenesis of psoriasis and it is not clear how the marked increase of IFNγ and IFNγ-producing cells in psoriatic skin can actually link with the failure of IFNγ-blockade to show therapeutic efficacy.

Results from a study by Kryczek et al. have suggested that IFNγ exerts one of its effects by programming myeloid dendritic cells to produce CCL20, ligand of CCR6, and to secrete IL-23. This in turn would favor the recruitment and expansion of IL-17A-producing cells (63, 64). On the other hand, IFNγ mRNA is markedly upregulated in psoriatic plaques and noticeably IFNγ-induced genes, such as *CXCL9*, *CXCL10*, and *CXCL11* are strongly increased in psoriatic lesions (65).

In line with this evidence, we have previously reported gene expression data in psoriatic skin showing significant enhancement of *CXCR3* and *CXCL10* expression with an inverse correlation between the circulating fraction of CXCR3$^+$ CD4$^+$ effector memory T cells and the severity of cutaneous psoriasis (66, 67). Therefore, we can postulate an ultimate downstream phase in the psoriatic cascade, driven by the CXCL10/CXCR3 axis which induces the recruitment of Th1/Tc1 from the blood stream (**Figure 1C**).

T CELLS IN THE PATHOGENESIS OF PsA

Psoriatic arthritis develops in a fraction of patients with psoriasis and in the majority of cases it follows the development of the cutaneous disease by a mean of 10 years (68).

In addition to the skin, PsA targets the attachment sites of ligament to bone (entheses), the peripheral joints, and the spine (12, 69).

Enthesitis is indeed a distinctive feature of PsA and it has been hypothesized that, in PsA joints, inflammation can start from the entheses. The disease progression, in patients with PsA, can finally lead to destructive bone loss and 67% of patients exhibit signs of erosive bone disease (70).

Similarly to psoriasis, T cells are involved in the pathogenesis of PsA and reduction of CD3$^+$ cells in PsA synovium correlated with the clinical response to biological therapies (71).

In PsA patients, Canete and co-workers have evidenced the presence of lymphoid aggregates in synovial tissues that was significantly reduced by TNF-blocking agents. This result could be paralleled by the observation of lymphoid aggregates in psoriatic skin and the role of CCR7/CCL19 axis, modulated by TNF in the initial clustering of dendritic cells and T cells in the dermis (4, 5, 72–75).

In line with the concept of shared pathogenic mechanisms between psoriasis and PsA, Belasco and colleagues provided the evidence that gene expression in PsA synovium was more closely related to gene expression in the PsA patient skin than to gene expression in the synovium of patients with other forms of arthritis. *IL17* gene, however, was upregulated more in skin than in the synovium, whereas *TNF* and *IFNγ* were similarly upregulated in both tissues (76).

As regards the TCR repertoire analysis in PsA joints, Tassiulas et al. (47) showed oligoclonal and monoclonal T cell expansions in the synovial tissue, some of which were shared with the skin. In a subsequent study, Curran et al. performed TCR β-chain nucleotide sequencing in peripheral blood and synovial tissues/fluid showing that 76% of the clones in inflamed tissues were polyclonal, whereas 12% of the expanded clones had structurally homologous CDR3 β-chain sequence and were only CD8$^+$ in lineage (54). Interestingly, some of the expanded CD8$^+$ clones identified in the synovial tissue were present also in peripheral blood and joint fluid.

A second population of moderately expanded inflammation-related clones, that were either of CD4$^+$ or CD8$^+$ lineage, was identified only in inflamed synovial tissue and joint fluid. These cells could represent a secondary consequence of the inflammation induced by other proliferating clones.

Finally, one major population consisted of unexpanded polyclonal CD4$^+$ T cells that did not persist in the tissue during methotrexate treatment, were most likely effector memory CD4$^+$ T cells recruited by inflammatory chemokines released by other cell populations. The lack of clonal expansion in CD4$^+$ T cells suggests a lower hierarchical role in driving inflammation.

These findings together suggest a role for cognate T cell responses in the pathogenesis of PsA and further suggest that T cell clones specific for identical or homologous antigens in skin and synovium may represent central elements in promoting inflammation in both tissues (47).

It remains to be established how self-reactive T cell responses in the skin, can be mechanistically linked to the one found in the synovial fluid and how these events can occur with years of time-lapse.

To this end, genetic association studies can provide some interpretation keys. In addition to the HLA-C*06:02 which is common with psoriatic plaque, additional HLA-alleles are associated with PsA. These HLA-alleles include B*08:01:01, B*27:05:02, B*38:01:01, and B*39:01:01 (77).

This underlines the importance of CD8$^+$ T cells recognizing HLA-class I associated self-antigens in the pathogenesis of PsA and suggests that the autoimmune basis of PsA may be even broader than the one of cutaneous psoriasis. In this view, enthesis that anatomically links mechanical stress to immunologically active tissue (synovium), could be central for the pathogenesis (78).

Entheses are commonly subject to microdamage associated with local cytokine release, which may evolve into subsequent inflammation (79, 80). Inflammation in turn can favor cross-presentation of self-antigens.

It is, therefore, possible that recirculation of pathogenic skin T cells recognizing common self-antigens can start subclinical inflammation by localizing to the synovioenthesial complex (**Figure 1C**).

Patients with psoriatic disease have shown an increased level of circulating CCR6$^+$ CD4$^+$ T_{EM} and T_{EFF} cells that correlated positively with systemic inflammation (66). Therefore, it is possible to hypothesize that a fraction of IL-17-producing T cells recirculates from the skin and relocalize to the entheses.

This is reinforced by the findings of Sherlock et al. reporting that IL-17A$^+$ cells locate mainly at the entheses and synovial tissues and by the evidence that among the genetic risk factors outside the MHC locus there are gene variants falling into the IL-23/IL-17A axis (77, 80–85). Importantly, it has been reported that IL-23 is expressed in synovial membrane with ectopic lymphoid tissue (78).

The fraction of IL-17A-producing cells recirculating from the skin could, therefore, determines subclinical inflammation and favor, in the long-term, cross-presentation of self-antigens and epitope spreading phenomena (73, 78).

In established PsA, it has also been reported an increased percentage of IL-17A-producing CD8$^+$ T cells in synovial fluid which correlate with bone erosion and disease severity (86–88).

In the light of a hierarchical T cell clonality in psoriatic tissue and the evidence of the multiple-specific clones, including EBV-specific clones, observed in synovial fluid, we can postulate that massive recruitment of T cells with Th1/Tc1 phenotype from peripheral blood occurs as a consequences of inflammatory chemokine release (54). By analogy with the observation in psoriatic skin and by evidence from the data provided by Gladman and co-workers it is possible that CXCL10/CXCR3 axis can act as a downstream cell recruitment mechanism of tissue inflammation common to cutaneous psoriasis and PsA (89–91).

T CELLS IN PSORIASIS-ASSOCIATED CARDIOVASCULAR COMORBIDITIES

Increasing epidemiological and clinical evidence indicates that psoriasis is an independent risk factor for cardiovascular disease (92, 93).

As a consequence of poorly controlled tissue inflammation, psoriasis patients can develop systemic inflammation and atherosclerosis. In this process, it has been postulated that inflamed tissue-derived factors or cells may directly affect distant vessels for the development of athero-thrombosis (7, 94, 95). Nevertheless, the cellular mechanisms that link the cutaneous manifestations of plaque psoriasis with the initiation and progression of atherosclerosis in psoriasis patients are largely unknown.

A recent study on human tissues showed that psoriasis and atherosclerosis exhibit significant overlap of their transcriptomes and in particular that *TNF*, *IFNg*, and IFNγ-induced genes, which are common between psoriasis and atherosclerosis may provide the link between the two diseases (96). By contrast, *IL-17A* and *CCL20* were higher in psoriasis than in atherosclerotic tissue, whereas *IL17R* gene was expressed at similar levels.

Because of the link between IL-17A and neutrophil infiltration in atherosclerotic plaques and its key role in the pathogenesis of psoriasis it has been suggested that the IL-17A/neutrophil axis could take part to atherogenesis associated with psoriatic disease (97). Nevertheless, the role of IL-17A in psoriasis-associated atherosclerosis is still controversial. Indeed, Usui et al. reported that IL-17A deficiency protected against atherosclerosis in apoE$^{-/-}$ mice due to reduced macrophage infiltration and inflammatory cytokine secretion in the lesions (98).

Other mouse studies have indicated that IL-17A may promote plaque stability by contributing to fibrous cap formation (99). Collectively, the results indicate that IL-17A may exert both anti- and pro-atherogenic effects, depending on the inflammatory context. However, further studies will be necessary to clarify the contribution of T cells recirculating from the psoriatic plaque in the development of atherosclerosis.

IMPLICATIONS FOR THE DEVELOPMENT OF THERAPEUTIC PROTOCOLS

From this analysis it emerges a differential contribution of the individual subsets of T cells in the pathogenesis of psoriasis, PsA, and associated cardiovascular comorbidities namely, atherosclerosis. In particular, TNFα has a relevant role in inducing the CCL19/CCR7-mediated formation of clusters of dendritic cells and T cells in both psoriasis and PsA. It also emphasizes the role of IL-23/IL-17 axis in the amplification loop critical for the clinical manifestations of cutaneous psoriasis and possibly in the initial phase of join inflammation.

On the other hand, the possibility of a third step of CXCL10/CXCR3-mediated recruitment of Th1/Tc1 cells from the blood stream may explain the apparent controversy between the high amount of IFNγ-producing cells and the low therapeutic efficacy of anti-IFNγ antibody treatment.

CONCLUSION

By defining the hierarchy of the T cell-mediated events of the psoriatic cascade in psoriatic plaques it is possible to distinguish a core antigen-driven oligo or monoclonally expanded autoreactive CD8$^+$ T cell component, a secondary self-reactive CD4$^+$ T cell component, a polyclonal CD4$^+$ Th17 and pathogenic Th1/Th17 population amplified by the IL-23/IL-17A axis, and a downstream recruitment of CXCR3$^+$ T cells with different specificities induced by the upregulation of CXCL10 chemokine. Similarly in PsA the analysis of the TCR repertoire has evidenced central antigen-driven expansion of mainly CD8$^+$ T cells and broad polyclonal CD4$^+$ T cells expansion. In addition, a group of common clones were also expanded in peripheral blood of patients with PsA and T cell clones specific for identical or homologous antigens were present in both skin and in synovial tissues. These may represent central elements in promoting inflammation in both tissues. In addition, oligoclonally expanded clones in peripheral blood of patients with PsA may also suggest that T cell recirculation can represent a mechanistic link between skin and joints inflammation.

AUTHOR CONTRIBUTIONS

FC wrote parts of the manuscript and prepared the figures. PP collaborated to the writing. PS and RG discussed the content and critically revised the manuscript. ER supervised the work and wrote the final version of the manuscript.

REFERENCES

1. Boehncke WH, Brembilla NC. Unmet needs in the field of psoriasis: pathogenesis and treatment. *Clin Rev Allergy Immunol* (2017). doi:10.1007/s12016-017-8634-3
2. Boehncke WH, Schon MP. Psoriasis. *Lancet* (2015) 386(9997):983–94. doi:10.1016/S0140-6736(14)61909-7
3. Raychaudhuri SK, Maverakis E, Raychaudhuri SP. Diagnosis and classification of psoriasis. *Autoimmun Rev* (2014) 13(4–5):490–5. doi:10.1016/j.autrev.2014.01.008
4. Mitsui H, Suarez-Farinas M, Belkin DA, Levenkova N, Fuentes-Duculan J, Coats I, et al. Combined use of laser capture microdissection and cDNA microarray analysis identifies locally expressed disease-related genes in focal regions of psoriasis vulgaris skin lesions. *J Invest Dermatol* (2012) 132(6):1615–26. doi:10.1038/jid.2012.33
5. Bose F, Petti L, Diani M, Moscheni C, Molteni S, Altomare A, et al. Inhibition of CCR7/CCL19 axis in lesional skin is a critical event for clinical remission induced by TNF blockade in patients with psoriasis. *Am J Pathol* (2013) 183(2):413–21. doi:10.1016/j.ajpath.2013.04.021
6. Golden JB, McCormick TS, Ward NL. IL-17 in psoriasis: implications for therapy and cardiovascular co-morbidities. *Cytokine* (2013) 62(2):195–201. doi:10.1016/j.cyto.2013.03.013
7. Boehncke WH, Gladman DD, Chandran V. Cardiovascular comorbidities in psoriasis and psoriatic arthritis: pathogenesis, consequences for patient management, and future research agenda: a report from the GRAPPA 2009 annual meeting. *J Rheumatol* (2011) 38(3):567–71. doi:10.3899/jrheum.101124
8. Siegel D, Devaraj S, Mitra A, Raychaudhuri SP, Raychaudhuri SK, Jialal I. Inflammation, atherosclerosis, and psoriasis. *Clin Rev Allergy Immunol* (2013) 44(2):194–204. doi:10.1007/s12016-012-8308-0
9. Boehncke WH, Kirby B, Fitzgerald O, van de Kerkhof PC. New developments in our understanding of psoriatic arthritis and their impact on the diagnosis and clinical management of the disease. *J Eur Acad Dermatol Venereol* (2014) 28(3):264–70. doi:10.1111/jdv.12222
10. Boehncke WH, Menter A. Burden of disease: psoriasis and psoriatic arthritis. *Am J Clin Dermatol* (2013) 14(5):377–88. doi:10.1007/s40257-013-0032-x
11. Coates LC, FitzGerald O, Helliwell PS, Paul C. Psoriasis, psoriatic arthritis, and rheumatoid arthritis: is all inflammation the same? *Semin Arthritis Rheum* (2016) 46(3):291–304. doi:10.1016/j.semarthrit.2016.05.012
12. Wittkowski KM, Leonardi C, Gottlieb A, Menter A, Krueger GG, Tebbey PW, et al. Clinical symptoms of skin, nails, and joints manifest independently in patients with concomitant psoriasis and psoriatic arthritis. *PLoS One* (2011) 6(6):e20279. doi:10.1371/journal.pone.0020279
13. Di Cesare A, Di Meglio P, Nestle FO. The IL-23/Th17 axis in the immunopathogenesis of psoriasis. *J Invest Dermatol* (2009) 129(6):1339–50. doi:10.1038/jid.2009.59
14. Lowes MA, Russell CB, Martin DA, Towne JE, Krueger JG. The IL-23/T17 pathogenic axis in psoriasis is amplified by keratinocyte responses. *Trends Immunol* (2013) 34(4):174–81. doi:10.1016/j.it.2012.11.005
15. Gaffen SL, Jain R, Garg AV, Cua DJ. The IL-23-IL-17 immune axis: from mechanisms to therapeutic testing. *Nat Rev Immunol* (2014) 14(9):585–600. doi:10.1038/nri3707
16. Chiricozzi A, Krueger JG. IL-17 targeted therapies for psoriasis. *Expert Opin Investig Drugs* (2013) 22(8):993–1005. doi:10.1517/13543784.2013.806483
17. Girolomoni G, Strohal R, Puig L, Bachelez H, Barker J, Boehncke WH, et al. The role of IL-23 and the IL-23/TH 17 immune axis in the pathogenesis and treatment of psoriasis. *J Eur Acad Dermatol Venereol* (2017) 31(10):1616–26. doi:10.1111/jdv.14433
18. Diani M, Altomare G, Reali E. T cell responses in psoriasis and psoriatic arthritis. *Autoimmun Rev* (2015) 14(4):286–92. doi:10.1016/j.autrev.2014.11.012
19. Lowes MA, Suarez-Farinas M, Krueger JG. Immunology of psoriasis. *Annu Rev Immunol* (2014) 32:227–55. doi:10.1146/annurev-immunol-032713-120225
20. Gallais Serezal I, Classon C, Cheuk S, Barrientos-Somarribas M, Wadman E, Martini E, et al. Resident T cells in resolved psoriasis steer tissue responses that stratify clinical outcome. *J Invest Dermatol* (2018). doi:10.1016/j.jid.2018.02.030
21. Cosmi L, Liotta F, Maggi E, Romagnani S, Annunziato F. Th17 and non-classic Th1 cells in chronic inflammatory disorders: two sides of the same coin. *Int Arch Allergy Immunol* (2014) 164(3):171–7. doi:10.1159/000363502
22. Zaba LC, Fuentes-Duculan J, Eungdamrong NJ, Abello MV, Novitskaya I, Pierson KC, et al. Psoriasis is characterized by accumulation of immunostimulatory and Th1/Th17 cell-polarizing myeloid dendritic cells. *J Invest Dermatol* (2009) 129(1):79–88. doi:10.1038/jid.2008.194
23. Zaba LC, Krueger JG, Lowes MA. Resident and "inflammatory" dendritic cells in human skin. *J Invest Dermatol* (2009) 129(2):302–8. doi:10.1038/jid.2008.225
24. Mackay LK, Kallies A. Transcriptional regulation of tissue-resident lymphocytes. *Trends Immunol* (2017) 38(2):94–103. doi:10.1016/j.it.2016.11.004
25. Cheuk S, Wiken M, Blomqvist L, Nylen S, Talme T, Stahle M, et al. Epidermal Th22 and Tc17 cells form a localized disease memory in clinically healed psoriasis. *J Immunol* (2014) 192(7):3111–20. doi:10.4049/jimmunol.1302313
26. Lande R, Botti E, Jandus C, Dojcinovic D, Fanelli G, Conrad C, et al. The antimicrobial peptide LL37 is a T-cell autoantigen in psoriasis. *Nat Commun* (2014) 5:5621. doi:10.1038/ncomms6621
27. Lande R, Chamilos G, Ganguly D, Demaria O, Frasca L, Durr S, et al. Cationic antimicrobial peptides in psoriatic skin cooperate to break innate tolerance to self-DNA. *Eur J Immunol* (2014) 45(1):203–13. doi:10.1002/eji.201344277
28. Conrad C, Gilliet M. Psoriasis: from pathogenesis to targeted therapies. *Clin Rev Allergy Immunol* (2018) 54(1):102–13. doi:10.1007/s12016-018-8668-1
29. Di Meglio P, Villanova F, Navarini AA, Mylonas A, Tosi I, Nestle FO, et al. Targeting CD8(+) T cells prevents psoriasis development. *J Allergy Clin Immunol* (2016) 138(1):274–6.e6. doi:10.1016/j.jaci.2015.10.046
30. Arakawa A, Siewert K, Stohr J, Besgen P, Kim SM, Ruhl G, et al. Melanocyte antigen triggers autoimmunity in human psoriasis. *J Exp Med* (2015) 212(13):2203–12. doi:10.1084/jem.20151093
31. Gudmundsdottir AS, Sigmundsdottir H, Sigurgeirsson B, Good MF, Valdimarsson H, Jonsdottir I. Is an epitope on keratin 17 a major target for autoreactive T lymphocytes in psoriasis? *Clin Exp Immunol* (1999) 117(3):580–6. doi:10.1046/j.1365-2249.1999.01013.x
32. Johnston A, Gudjonsson JE, Sigmundsdottir H, Love TJ, Valdimarsson H. Peripheral blood T cell responses to keratin peptides that share sequences with streptococcal M proteins are largely restricted to skin-homing CD8(+) T cells. *Clin Exp Immunol* (2004) 138(1):83–93. doi:10.1111/j.1365-2249.2004.00600.x
33. McFadden J, Valdimarsson H, Fry L. Cross-reactivity between streptococcal M surface antigen and human skin. *Br J Dermatol* (1991) 125(5):443–7. doi:10.1111/j.1365-2133.1991.tb14769.x
34. Valdimarsson H, Sigmundsdottir H, Jonsdottir I. Is psoriasis induced by streptococcal superantigens and maintained by M-protein-specific T cells that cross-react with keratin? *Clin Exp Immunol* (1997) 107(Suppl 1):21–4.
35. Valdimarsson H, Thorleifsdottir RH, Sigurdardottir SL, Gudjonsson JE, Johnston A. Psoriasis as an autoimmune disease caused by molecular mimicry. *Trends Immunol* (2009) 30(10):494–501. doi:10.1016/j.it.2009.07.008
36. Cheuk S, Schlums H, Gallais Serezal I, Martini E, Chiang SC, Marquardt N, et al. CD49a expression defines tissue-resident CD8(+) T cells poised for cytotoxic function in human skin. *Immunity* (2017) 46(2):287–300. doi:10.1016/j.immuni.2017.01.009
37. Boyman O, Conrad C, Tonel G, Gilliet M, Nestle FO. The pathogenic role of tissue-resident immune cells in psoriasis. *Trends Immunol* (2007) 28(2):51–7. doi:10.1016/j.it.2006.12.005
38. Conrad C, Boyman O, Tonel G, Tun-Kyi A, Laggner U, de Fougerolles A, et al. Alpha1beta1 integrin is crucial for accumulation of epidermal T cells and the development of psoriasis. *Nat Med* (2007) 13(7):836–42. doi:10.1038/nm1605
39. Hijnen D, Knol EF, Gent YY, Giovannone B, Beijn SJ, Kupper TS, et al. CD8(+) T cells in the lesional skin of atopic dermatitis and psoriasis patients are an important source of IFN-gamma, IL-13, IL-17, and IL-22. *J Invest Dermatol* (2013) 133(4):973–9. doi:10.1038/jid.2012.456
40. Ortega C, Fernandez AS, Carrillo JM, Romero P, Molina IJ, Moreno JC, et al. IL-17-producing CD8+ T lymphocytes from psoriasis skin plaques are cytotoxic effector cells that secrete Th17-related cytokines. *J Leukoc Biol* (2009) 86(2):435–43. doi:10.1189/JLB.0109046
41. Res PC, Piskin G, de Boer OJ, van der Loos CM, Teeling P, Bos JD, et al. Overrepresentation of IL-17A and IL-22 producing CD8 T cells in lesional skin suggests their involvement in the pathogenesis of psoriasis. *PLoS One* (2010) 5(11):e14108. doi:10.1371/journal.pone.0014108
42. Matos TR, O'Malley JT, Lowry EL, Hamm D, Kirsch IR, Robins HS, et al. Clinically resolved psoriatic lesions contain psoriasis-specific IL-17-producing alphabeta T cell clones. *J Clin Invest* (2017) 127(11):4031–41. doi:10.1172/JCI93396

43. Gudjonsson JE, Karason A, Antonsdottir A, Runarsdottir EH, Hauksson VB, Upmanyu R, et al. Psoriasis patients who are homozygous for the HLA-Cw*0602 allele have a 2.5-fold increased risk of developing psoriasis compared with Cw6 heterozygotes. *Br J Dermatol* (2003) 148(2):233–5. doi:10.1046/j.1365-2133.2003.05115.x
44. Harden JL, Krueger JG, Bowcock AM. The immunogenetics of psoriasis: a comprehensive review. *J Autoimmun* (2015) 64:66–73. doi:10.1016/j.jaut.2015.07.008
45. Cai Y, Shen X, Ding C, Qi C, Li K, Li X, et al. Pivotal role of dermal IL-17-producing gammadelta T cells in skin inflammation. *Immunity* (2011) 35(4):596–610. doi:10.1016/j.immuni.2011.08.001
46. Laggner U, Di Meglio P, Perera GK, Hundhausen C, Lacy KE, Ali N, et al. Identification of a novel proinflammatory human skin-homing Vgamma9Vdelta2 T cell subset with a potential role in psoriasis. *J Immunol* (2011) 187(5):2783–93. doi:10.4049/jimmunol.1100804
47. Tassiulas I, Duncan SR, Centola M, Theofilopoulos AN, Boumpas DT. Clonal characteristics of T cell infiltrates in skin and synovium of patients with psoriatic arthritis. *Hum Immunol* (1999) 60(6):479–91. doi:10.1016/S0198-8859(99)00034-8
48. Lin WJ, Norris DA, Achziger M, Kotzin BL, Tomkinson B. Oligoclonal expansion of intraepidermal T cells in psoriasis skin lesions. *J Invest Dermatol* (2001) 117(6):1546–53. doi:10.1046/j.0022-202x.2001.01548.x
49. Bour H, Puisieux I, Even J, Kourilsky P, Favrot M, Musette P, et al. T-cell repertoire analysis in chronic plaque psoriasis suggests an antigen-specific immune response. *Hum Immunol* (1999) 60(8):665–76. doi:10.1016/S0198-8859(99)00027-0
50. Norris DA, Travers JB, Leung DY. Lymphocyte activation in the pathogenesis of psoriasis. *J Invest Dermatol* (1997) 109(1):1–4. doi:10.1111/1523-1747.ep12276285
51. Cao X, Wa Q, Wang Q, Li L, Liu X, An L, et al. High throughput sequencing reveals the diversity of TRB-CDR3 repertoire in patients with psoriasis vulgaris. *Int Immunopharmacol* (2016) 40:487–91. doi:10.1016/j.intimp.2016.10.004
52. Borgato L, Puccetti A, Beri R, Codella O, Frigo A, Simeoni S, et al. The T cell receptor repertoire in psoriatic synovitis is restricted and T lymphocytes expressing the same TCR are present in joint and skin lesions. *J Rheumatol* (2002) 29(9):1914–9.
53. Harden JL, Hamm D, Gulati N, Lowes MA, Krueger JG. Deep sequencing of the T-cell receptor repertoire demonstrates polyclonal T-cell infiltrates in psoriasis. *F1000Res* (2015) 4:460. doi:10.12688/f1000research.6756.1
54. Curran SA, FitzGerald OM, Costello PJ, Selby JM, Kane DJ, Bresnihan B, et al. Nucleotide sequencing of psoriatic arthritis tissue before and during methotrexate administration reveals a complex inflammatory T cell infiltrate with very few clones exhibiting features that suggest they drive the inflammatory process by recognizing autoantigens. *J Immunol* (2004) 172(3):1935–44.
55. Cho JH, Feldman M. Heterogeneity of autoimmune diseases: pathophysiologic insights from genetics and implications for new therapies. *Nat Med* (2015) 21(7):730–8. doi:10.1038/nm.3897
56. Canavan TN, Elmets CA, Cantrell WL, Evans JM, Elewski BE. Anti-IL-17 medications used in the treatment of plaque psoriasis and psoriatic arthritis: a comprehensive review. *Am J Clin Dermatol* (2016) 17(1):33–47. doi:10.1007/s40257-015-0162-4
57. Eyerich S, Eyerich K, Pennino D, Carbone T, Nasorri F, Pallotta S, et al. Th22 cells represent a distinct human T cell subset involved in epidermal immunity and remodeling. *J Clin Invest* (2009) 119(12):3573–85. doi:10.1172/JCI40202
58. Diani M, Altomare G, Reali E. T helper cell subsets in clinical manifestations of psoriasis. *J Immunol Res* (2016) 2016:7692024. doi:10.1155/2016/7692024
59. Cargill M, Schrodi SJ, Chang M, Garcia VE, Brandon R, Callis KP, et al. A large-scale genetic association study confirms IL12B and leads to the identification of IL23R as psoriasis-risk genes. *Am J Hum Genet* (2007) 80(2):273–90. doi:10.1086/511051
60. Uyemura K, Yamamura M, Fivenson DF, Modlin RL, Nickoloff BJ. The cytokine network in lesional and lesion-free psoriatic skin is characterized by a T-helper type 1 cell-mediated response. *J Invest Dermatol* (1993) 101(5):701–5. doi:10.1111/1523-1747.ep12371679
61. Zaba LC, Suarez-Farinas M, Fuentes-Duculan J, Nograles KE, Guttman-Yassky E, Cardinale I, et al. Effective treatment of psoriasis with etanercept is linked to suppression of IL-17 signaling, not immediate response TNF genes. *J Allergy Clin Immunol* (2009) 124(5):1022–10.e1–395. doi:10.1016/j.jaci.2009.08.046
62. Harden JL, Johnson-Huang LM, Chamian MF, Lee E, Pearce T, Leonardi CL, et al. Humanized anti-IFN-gamma (HuZAF) in the treatment of psoriasis. *J Allergy Clin Immunol* (2015) 135(2):553–6. doi:10.1016/j.jaci.2014.05.046
63. Kryczek I, Bruce AT, Gudjonsson JE, Johnston A, Aphale A, Vatan L, et al. Induction of IL-17+ T cell trafficking and development by IFN-gamma: mechanism and pathological relevance in psoriasis. *J Immunol* (2008) 181(7):4733–41. doi:10.4049/jimmunol.181.7.4733
64. Kryczek I, Wei S, Gong W, Shu X, Szeliga W, Vatan L, et al. Cutting edge: IFN-gamma enables APC to promote memory Th17 and abate Th1 cell development. *J Immunol* (2008) 181(9):5842–6. doi:10.4049/jimmunol.181.9.5842
65. Gottlieb AB, Chamian F, Masud S, Cardinale I, Abello MV, Lowes MA, et al. TNF inhibition rapidly down-regulates multiple proinflammatory pathways in psoriasis plaques. *J Immunol* (2005) 175(4):2721–9. doi:10.4049/jimmunol.175.4.2721
66. Diani M, Galasso M, Cozzi C, Sgambelluri F, Altomare A, Cigni C, et al. Blood to skin recirculation of CD4+ memory T cells associates with cutaneous and systemic manifestations of psoriatic disease. *Clin Immunol* (2017) 180:84–94. doi:10.1016/j.clim.2017.04.001
67. Sgambelluri F, Diani M, Altomare A, Frigerio E, Drago L, Granucci F, et al. A role for CCR5(+)CD4 T cells in cutaneous psoriasis and for CD103(+) CCR4(+) CD8 Teff cells in the associated systemic inflammation. *J Autoimmun* (2016) 70:80–90. doi:10.1016/j.jaut.2016.03.019
68. Dhir V, Aggarwal A. Psoriatic arthritis: a critical review. *Clin Rev Allergy Immunol* (2013) 44(2):141–8. doi:10.1007/s12016-012-8302-6
69. Anandarajah AP, Ritchlin CT. Pathogenesis of psoriatic arthritis. *Curr Opin Rheumatol* (2004) 16(4):338–43.
70. van Kuijk AW, Tak PP. Synovitis in psoriatic arthritis: immunohistochemistry, comparisons with rheumatoid arthritis, and effects of therapy. *Curr Rheumatol Rep* (2011) 13(4):353–9. doi:10.1007/s11926-011-0181-y
71. Pontifex EK, Gerlag DM, Gogarty M, Vinkenoog M, Gibbs A, Burgman I, et al. Change in CD3 positive T-cell expression in psoriatic arthritis synovium correlates with change in DAS28 and magnetic resonance imaging synovitis scores following initiation of biologic therapy – a single centre, open-label study. *Arthritis Res Ther* (2011) 13(1):R7. doi:10.1186/ar3228
72. Kim TG, Jee H, Fuentes-Duculan J, Wu WH, Byamba D, Kim DS, et al. Dermal clusters of mature dendritic cells and T cells are associated with the CCL20/CCR6 chemokine system in chronic psoriasis. *J Invest Dermatol* (2014) 134(5):1462–5. doi:10.1038/jid.2013.534
73. Canete JD, Santiago B, Cantaert T, Sanmarti R, Palacin A, Celis R, et al. Ectopic lymphoid neogenesis in psoriatic arthritis. *Ann Rheum Dis* (2007) 66(6):720–6. doi:10.1136/ard.2006.062042
74. Celis R, Planell N, Fernandez-Sueiro JL, Sanmarti R, Ramirez J, Gonzalez-Alvaro I, et al. Synovial cytokine expression in psoriatic arthritis and associations with lymphoid neogenesis and clinical features. *Arthritis Res Ther* (2012) 14(2):R93. doi:10.1186/ar3817
75. Chimenti MS, Triggianese P, Nuccetelli M, Terracciano C, Crisanti A, Guarino MD, et al. Auto-reactions, autoimmunity and psoriatic arthritis. *Autoimmun Rev* (2015) 14(12):1142–6. doi:10.1016/j.autrev.2015.08.003
76. Belasco J, Louie JS, Gulati N, Wei N, Nograles K, Fuentes-Duculan J, et al. Comparative genomic profiling of synovium versus skin lesions in psoriatic arthritis. *Arthritis Rheumatol* (2015) 67(4):934–44. doi:10.1002/art.38995
77. Winchester R, Giles J, Jadon D, Haroon M, McHugh N, FitzGerald O. Implications of the diversity of class I HLA associations in psoriatic arthritis. *Clin Immunol* (2016) 172:29–33. doi:10.1016/j.clim.2016.07.019
78. Lories RJ, McInnes IB. Primed for inflammation: enthesis-resident T cells. *Nat Med* (2012) 18(7):1018–9. doi:10.1038/nm.2854
79. Novelli L, Chimenti MS, Chiricozzi A, Perricone R. The new era for the treatment of psoriasis and psoriatic arthritis: perspectives and validated strategies. *Autoimmun Rev* (2014) 13(1):64–9. doi:10.1016/j.autrev.2013.08.006
80. Sherlock JP, Buckley CD, Cua DJ. The critical role of interleukin-23 in spondyloarthropathy. *Mol Immunol* (2014) 57(1):38–43. doi:10.1016/j.molimm.2013.06.010
81. Benham H, Norris P, Goodall J, Wechalekar MD, FitzGerald O, Szentpetery A, et al. Th17 and Th22 cells in psoriatic arthritis and psoriasis. *Arthritis Res Ther* (2013) 15(5):R136. doi:10.1186/ar4317
82. Suzuki E, Mellins ED, Gershwin ME, Nestle FO, Adamopoulos IE. The IL-23/IL-17 axis in psoriatic arthritis. *Autoimmun Rev* (2014) 13(4–5):496–502. doi:10.1016/j.autrev.2014.01.050

83. Sherlock JP, Joyce-Shaikh B, Turner SP, Chao CC, Sathe M, Grein J, et al. IL-23 induces spondyloarthropathy by acting on ROR-gammat+ CD3+CD4-CD8- entheseal resident T cells. *Nat Med* (2012) 18(7):1069–76. doi:10.1038/nm.2817
84. Nograles KE, Brasington RD, Bowcock AM. New insights into the pathogenesis and genetics of psoriatic arthritis. *Nat Clin Pract Rheumatol* (2009) 5(2):83–91. doi:10.1038/ncprheum0987
85. Apel M, Uebe S, Bowes J, Giardina E, Korendowych E, Juneblad K, et al. Variants in RUNX3 contribute to susceptibility to psoriatic arthritis, exhibiting further common ground with ankylosing spondylitis. *Arthritis Rheum* (2013) 65(5):1224–31. doi:10.1002/art.37885
86. Menon B, Gullick NJ, Walter GJ, Rajasekhar M, Garrood T, Evans HG, et al. Interleukin-17+CD8+ T cells are enriched in the joints of patients with psoriatic arthritis and correlate with disease activity and joint damage progression. *Arthritis Rheumatol* (2014) 66(5):1272–81. doi:10.1002/art.38376
87. Adamopoulos IE, Bowman EP. Immune regulation of bone loss by Th17 cells. *Arthritis Res Ther* (2008) 10(5):225. doi:10.1186/ar2502
88. Adamopoulos IE, Chao CC, Geissler R, Laface D, Blumenschein W, Iwakura Y, et al. Interleukin-17A upregulates receptor activator of NF-kappaB on osteoclast precursors. *Arthritis Res Ther* (2010) 12(1):R29. doi:10.1186/ar2936
89. Chandran V, Gladman DD. Update on biomarkers in psoriatic arthritis. *Curr Rheumatol Rep* (2010) 12(4):288–94. doi:10.1007/s11926-010-0107-0
90. Muntyanu A, Abji F, Liang K, Pollock RA, Chandran V, Gladman DD. Differential gene and protein expression of chemokines and cytokines in synovial fluid of patients with arthritis. *Arthritis Res Ther* (2016) 18(1):296. doi:10.1186/s13075-016-1196-6
91. Abji F, Pollock RA, Liang K, Chandran V, Gladman DD. Brief report: CXCL10 is a possible biomarker for the development of psoriatic arthritis among patients with psoriasis. *Arthritis Rheumatol* (2016) 68(12):2911–6. doi:10.1002/art.39800
92. Eder L, Gladman DD. Atherosclerosis in psoriatic disease: latest evidence and clinical implications. *Ther Adv Musculoskelet Dis* (2015) 7(5):187–95. doi:10.1177/1759720X15591801
93. Eder L, Joshi AA, Dey AK, Cook R, Siegel EL, Gladman DD, et al. TNF-alpha inhibitors are associated with reduced indices of subclinical atherosclerosis in patients with psoriatic disease. *Arthritis Rheumatol* (2017) 70(3):408–16. doi:10.1002/art.40366
94. Wang Y, Gao H, Loyd CM, Fu W, Diaconu D, Liu S, et al. Chronic skin-specific inflammation promotes vascular inflammation and thrombosis. *J Invest Dermatol* (2012) 132(8):2067–75. doi:10.1038/jid.2012.112
95. Szentpetery A, Healy GM, Brady D, Haroon M, Gallagher P, Redmond CE, et al. Higher coronary plaque burden in psoriatic arthritis is independent of metabolic syndrome and associated with underlying disease severity. *Arthritis Rheumatol* (2018) 70(3):396–407. doi:10.1002/art.40389
96. Mehta NN, Teague HL, Swindell WR, Baumer Y, Ward NL, Xing X, et al. IFN-gamma and TNF-alpha synergism may provide a link between psoriasis and inflammatory atherogenesis. *Sci Rep* (2017) 7(1):13831. doi:10.1038/s41598-017-14365-1
97. Sanda GE, Belur AD, Teague HL, Mehta NN. Emerging associations between neutrophils, atherosclerosis, and psoriasis. *Curr Atheroscler Rep* (2017) 19(12):53. doi:10.1007/s11883-017-0692-8
98. Usui F, Kimura H, Ohshiro T, Tatsumi K, Kawashima A, Nishiyama A, et al. Interleukin-17 deficiency reduced vascular inflammation and development of atherosclerosis in Western diet-induced apoE-deficient mice. *Biochem Biophys Res Commun* (2012) 420(1):72–7. doi:10.1016/j.bbrc.2012.02.117
99. Taleb S, Tedgui A, Mallat Z. IL-17 and Th17 cells in atherosclerosis: subtle and contextual roles. *Arterioscler Thromb Vasc Biol* (2015) 35(2):258–64. doi:10.1161/ATVBAHA.114.303567

Permissions

All chapters in this book were first published by Frontiers; hereby published with permission under the Creative Commons Attribution License or equivalent. Every chapter published in this book has been scrutinized by our experts. Their significance has been extensively debated. The topics covered herein carry significant findings which will fuel the growth of the discipline. They may even be implemented as practical applications or may be referred to as a beginning point for another development.

The contributors of this book come from diverse backgrounds, making this book a truly international effort. This book will bring forth new frontiers with its revolutionizing research information and detailed analysis of the nascent developments around the world.

We would like to thank all the contributing authors for lending their expertise to make the book truly unique. They have played a crucial role in the development of this book. Without their invaluable contributions this book wouldn't have been possible. They have made vital efforts to compile up to date information on the varied aspects of this subject to make this book a valuable addition to the collection of many professionals and students.

This book was conceptualized with the vision of imparting up-to-date information and advanced data in this field. To ensure the same, a matchless editorial board was set up. Every individual on the board went through rigorous rounds of assessment to prove their worth. After which they invested a large part of their time researching and compiling the most relevant data for our readers.

The editorial board has been involved in producing this book since its inception. They have spent rigorous hours researching and exploring the diverse topics which have resulted in the successful publishing of this book. They have passed on their knowledge of decades through this book. To expedite this challenging task, the publisher supported the team at every step. A small team of assistant editors was also appointed to further simplify the editing procedure and attain best results for the readers.

Apart from the editorial board, the designing team has also invested a significant amount of their time in understanding the subject and creating the most relevant covers. They scrutinized every image to scout for the most suitable representation of the subject and create an appropriate cover for the book.

The publishing team has been an ardent support to the editorial, designing and production team. Their endless efforts to recruit the best for this project, has resulted in the accomplishment of this book. They are a veteran in the field of academics and their pool of knowledge is as vast as their experience in printing. Their expertise and guidance has proved useful at every step. Their uncompromising quality standards have made this book an exceptional effort. Their encouragement from time to time has been an inspiration for everyone.

The publisher and the editorial board hope that this book will prove to be a valuable piece of knowledge for researchers, students, practitioners and scholars across the globe.

List of Contributors

Maria Sole Chimenti, Flavia Sunzini, Giulia Lavinia Fonti, Paola Conigliaro, Paola Triggianese and Roberto Perricone
Rheumatology, Allergology and Clinical Immunology, University of Rome Tor Vergata, Rome, Italy

Laura Fiorucci and Roberto Santucci
Department of Clinical Sciences and Translational Medicine, University of Rome Tor Vergata, Rome, Italy

Elisabetta Botti, Luca Bianchi and Maria Esposito
Dermatology, University of Rome Tor Vergata, Rome, Italy

Luisa Costa and Francesco Caso
Rheumatology Unit, Department of Clinical Medicine and Surgery, University of Naples Federico II, Naples, Italy

Alessandro Giunta
Dermatology Unit, Department of Systems Medicine, University of Rome Tor Vergata, Rome, Italy

Charlie Bridgewood
Centre of Skin Sciences, School of Chemistry and Biosciences, University of Bradford, Bradford, United Kingdom

Gareth W. Fearnley and Sreenivasan Ponnambalam
Endothelial Cell Biology Unit, School of Molecular and Cellular Biology, University of Leeds, Leeds, United Kingdom

Anna Berekmeri
Department of Dermatology, Chapel Allerton Hospital, Leeds, United Kingdom
Faculty of Biological Sciences, School of Molecular and Cellular Biology, University of Leeds, Leeds, United Kingdom

Philip Laws
Department of Dermatology, Chapel Allerton Hospital, Leeds, United Kingdom
National Institute of Health Research (NIHR), Leeds Biomedical Research Centre (BRC), Chapel Allerton Hospital, Leeds, United Kingdom

Tom Macleod and Martin Stacey
Faculty of Biological Sciences, School of Molecular and Cellular Biology, University of Leeds, Leeds, United Kingdom

Anne Graham
Biomedical Sciences, School of Chemistry and Biosciences, University of Bradford, Bradford, United Kingdom

Miriam Wittmann
Centre of Skin Sciences, School of Chemistry and Biosciences, University of Bradford, Bradford, United Kingdom
National Institute of Health Research (NIHR), Leeds Biomedical Research Centre (BRC), Chapel Allerton Hospital, Leeds, United Kingdom
Leeds Institute of Rheumatic and Musculoskeletal Medicine (LIRMM), University of Leeds, Leeds, United Kingdom

Peng Hu, Jinhui Li and Dezhi Mu
West China Second University Hospital, Sichuan University, Chengdu, China
Department of Pediatrics, West China Second University Hospital, Sichuan University, Chengdu, China
Key Laboratory of Obstetrics & Gynecologic and Pediatric Diseases and Birth Defects of the Ministry of Education, Sichuan University, Chengdu, China

Mengyao Wang and Ai Zheng
West China Second University Hospital, Sichuan University, Chengdu, China
Key Laboratory of Birth Defects and Related Diseases of Women and Children, Sichuan University, Ministry of Education, Chengdu, China

Hu Gao
West China Second University Hospital, Sichuan University, Chengdu, China
Key Laboratory of Birth Defects and Related Diseases of Women and Children, Sichuan University, Ministry of Education, Chengdu, China
Department of Emergency, West China Second University Hospital, Sichuan University, Chengdu, China

Jiyu Tong
West China Second University Hospital, Sichuan University, Chengdu, China
Key Laboratory of Birth Defects and Related Diseases of Women and Children, Sichuan University, Ministry of Education, Chengdu, China
Department of Immunology, West China School of Basic Medical Sciences and Forensic Medicine, Sichuan University, Chengdu, China

Alessio Mylonas and Curdin Conrad
Department of Dermatology, University Hospital CHUV, Lausanne, Switzerland

Aparna P. Sajja, Aditya A. Joshi, Heather L. Teague, Amit K. Dey and Nehal N. Mehta
National Heart, Lung, and Blood Institute, National Institutes of Health, Bethesda, MD, United States

Marzia Dolcino, Giuseppe Patuzzo, Elisa Tinazzi and Claudio Lunardi
Department of Medicine, University of Verona, Verona, Italy

Andrea Pelosi and Piera Filomena Fiore
Immunology Area, Pediatric Hospital Bambino Gesù, Rome, Italy

Antonio Puccetti
Department of Experimental Medicine - Section of Histology, University of Genova, Genova, Italy

Claudia Buerger
Department of Dermatology, Venerology and Allergology, Clinic of the Goethe University, Frankfurt

Jörg Christoph Prinz
Department of Dermatology, University Clinics, Ludwig-Maximilian-University of Munich, Munich, Germany

Giuseppina Caiazzo, Gabriella Fabbrocini, Roberta Di Caprio, Annunziata Raimondo, Emanuele Scala and Nicola Balato
Department of Clinical Medicine and Surgery, University of Naples Federico II, Napoli, Italy

Anna Balato
Department of Advanced Biomedical Sciences, University of Naples Federico II, Napoli, Italy

Cristina Albanesi and Stefania Madonna
Laboratory of Experimental Immunology, Istituto Dermopatico dell'Immacolata (IDI), IRCCS, Rome, Italy

Paolo Gisondi and Giampiero Girolomoni
Section of Dermatology, Department of Medicine, University of Verona, Verona, Italy

Haiming Chen
The Second Affiliated Hospital, Guangzhou University of Chinese Medicine, Guangzhou, China
Postdoctoral Programme, Guangzhou University of Chinese Medicine, Guangzhou, China
Guangdong Provincial Hospital of Chinese Medicine, Guangzhou, China
Guangdong Provincial Academy of Chinese Medical Sciences, Guangzhou, China

Huazhen Liu, Maojie Wang, Xiong Li, Wanling Yu and Zhenhua Dai
The Second Affiliated Hospital, Guangzhou University of Chinese Medicine, Guangzhou, China
Guangdong Provincial Hospital of Chinese Medicine, Guangzhou, China
Guangdong Provincial Academy of Chinese Medical Sciences, Guangzhou, China

Chuanjian Lu and Ling Han
The Second Affiliated Hospital, Guangzhou University of Chinese Medicine, Guangzhou, China
Guangdong Provincial Hospital of Chinese Medicine, Guangzhou, China
Guangdong Provincial Academy of Chinese Medical Sciences, Guangzhou, China
Guangdong Provincial Key Laboratory of Clinical Research on Traditional Chinese Medicine Syndrome, Guangzhou, China

Hui Zhao
Key Laboratory for Regenerative Medicine, Ministry of Education, Faculty of Medicine, School of Biomedical Sciences, The Chinese University of Hong Kong, Hong Kong, China
Kunming Institute of Zoology Chinese Academy of Sciences-The Chinese University of Hong Kong Joint Laboratory of Bioresources and Molecular Research of Common Diseases, Hong Kong, China

Yuhong Yan
The Second Affiliated Hospital, Guangzhou University of Chinese Medicine, Guangzhou, China
Guangdong Provincial Hospital of Chinese Medicine, Guangzhou, China

Michael P. Schön
Department of Dermatology, Venereology and Allergology, University Medical Center Göttingen, Göttingen, Germany
Lower Saxony Institute of Occupational Dermatology, University Medical Center Göttingen, University of Osnabrück, Osnabrück, Germany

Luise Erpenbeck
Department of Dermatology, Venereology and Allergology, University Medical Center Göttingen, Göttingen, Germany

Maria J. E. Visser and Etheresia Pretorius
Department of Physiological Sciences, Faculty of Science, Stellenbosch University, Stellenbosch, South Africa

Gareth Tarr
Department of Physiological Sciences, Faculty of Science, Stellenbosch University, Stellenbosch, South Africa
Division of Rheumatology, Institute of Orthopaedics and Rheumatology, Winelands Mediclinic Orthopaedic Hospital, Stellenbosch, South Africa

Lipeng Tang
Department of Pharmacology of Traditional Chinese Medicine, The Second Affiliated Hospital of Guangzhou University of Chinese Medicine, Guangzhou, Guangdong, China

Xiaozhi Yang, Yongxin Liang and Hesong Xie
School of Bioscience and Bio-Pharmaceutics, Guangdong Pharmaceutical University, Guangzhou, Guangdong, China

Guangjuan Zheng
Department of Pharmacology of Traditional Chinese Medicine, The Second Affiliated Hospital of Guangzhou University of Chinese Medicine, Guangzhou, Guangdong, China
Department of Pathology, The Second Affiliated Hospital of Guangzhou University of Chinese Medicine, Guangzhou, Guangdong, China

Loredana Frasca, Raffaella Palazzo and Roberto Lande
Istituto Superiore di Sanità, National Center for Drug Research and Evaluation, Rome, Italy

Stefano Alivernini and Elisa Gremese
Division of Rheumatology, Fondazione Policlinico Universitario A. Gemelli, IRCCS, Rome, Italy
Division of Rheumatology, Università Cattolica del Sacro Cuore, Rome, Italy

Barbara Tolusso and Luca Petricca
Division of Rheumatology, Fondazione Policlinico Universitario A. Gemelli, IRCCS, Rome, Italy

Laura Bui and Antonella Evangelista
Institute of Pathology, Fondazione Policlinico Universitario A. Gemelli, Rome, Italy

Barbara Marinari
Dermatology Unit, Department of Systems Medicine, University of Rome Tor Vergata, Rome, Italy

Simone E. Auteri, Francesca R. Spinelli, Tania Colasanti, Cristiano Alessandri, Fabrizio Conti and Guido Valesini
Rheumatology Unit, Department of Internal Medicine and Medical Specialties, Sapienza University of Rome, Rome, Italy

Francesca Spadaro
Confocal Microscopy Unit, Core Facilities, Istituto Superiore di Sanità, Rome, Italy

Mario Falchi
National AIDS Center, Istituto Superiore di Sanità, Rome, Italy

Immacolata Pietraforte
Department of Oncology and Molecular Medicine, Istituto Superiore di Sanità, Rome, Italy

Antonio Costanzo
Skin Pathology Lab, Humanitas Clinical and Research Center, Milan, Italy

Maria S. Chimenti and Giulia L. Fonti
Rheumatology, Allergology and Clinical Immunology, University of Rome Tor Vergata, Rome, Italy

Cong Qi, Yazhuo Wang, Ping Li and Jingxia Zhao
Beijing Hospital of Traditional Chinese Medicine, Capital Medical University, Beijing, China
Beijing Key Laboratory of Clinic and Basic Research with Traditional Chinese Medicine on Psoriasis, Beijing Institute of Traditional Chinese Medicine, Beijing, China

Carmen De Jesús-Gil, Ester Ruiz-Romeu and Luis F. Santamaria-Babí
Translational Immunology, Department of Cellular Biology, Physiology and Immunology, Faculty of Biology, Universitat de Barcelona, Barcelona, Spain

Marta Ferran, Gustavo Deza and Ramon M. Pujol
Department of Dermatology, Hospital del Mar. Barcelona, Barcelona, Spain
IMIM (Hospital del Mar Medical Research Institute), Barcelona, Spain

Anca Chiriac
Nicolina Medical Center, Department of Dermatology, Iasi, Romania
Apollonia University, Iasi, Romania "P.Poni" Institute of Macromolecular Chemistry, Romanian Academy, Iasi, Romania

Péter Hóllo
Department of Dermatovenerology and Oncodermatology, Semmelweis Egyetem, Budapest, Hungary

Antonio Celada
Macrophage Biology, Department of Cellular Biology, Physiology and Immunology, Faculty of Biology, Universitat de Barcelona, Barcelona, Spain

Nicolo Costantino Brembilla and Luisa Senra
Department of Pathology and Immunology, Faculty of Medicine, University of Geneva, Geneva, Switzerland

Wolf-Henning Boehncke
Department of Pathology and Immunology, Faculty of Medicine, University of Geneva, Geneva, Switzerland
Division of Dermatology and Venereology, Geneva University Hospitals, Geneva, Switzerland

Chih-Chao Chiang
Graduate Institute of Clinical Medical Sciences, College of Medicine, Chang Gung University, Taoyuan, Taiwan
Supervisor Board, Taoyuan Chinese Medicine Association, Taoyuan, Taiwan
Puxin Fengze Chinese Medicine Clinic, Taoyuan, Taiwan

Wei-Jen Cheng
Graduate Institute of Clinical Medical Sciences, College of Medicine, Chang Gung University, Taoyuan, Taiwan
School of Traditional Chinese Medicine, Chang Gung University, Taoyuan, Taiwan
Center for Traditional Chinese Medicine, Chang Gung Memorial Hospital, Taoyuan, Taiwan

Michal Korinek
Graduate Institute of Natural Products, College of Medicine, Chang Gung University, Taoyuan, Taiwan
Research Center for Chinese Herbal Medicine, Research Center for Food and Cosmetic Safety, and Graduate Institute of Health Industry Technology, Chang Gung University of Science and Technology, Taoyuan, Taiwan
Department of Biotechnology, College of Life Science, Kaohsiung Medical University, Kaohsiung, Taiwan

Cheng-Yu Lin
Graduate Institute of Natural Products, College of Medicine, Chang Gung University, Taoyuan, Taiwan

Tsong-Long Hwang
School of Traditional Chinese Medicine, Chang Gung University, Taoyuan, Taiwan
Graduate Institute of Natural Products, College of Medicine, Chang Gung University, Taoyuan, Taiwan
Research Center for Chinese Herbal Medicine, Research Center for Food and Cosmetic Safety, and Graduate Institute of Health Industry Technology, Chang Gung University of Science and Technology, Taoyuan, Taiwan
Chinese Herbal Medicine Research Team, Healthy Aging Research Center, Chang Gung University, Taoyuan, Taiwan
Department of Anesthesiology, Chang Gung Memorial Hospital, Taoyuan, Taiwan
Department of Chemical Engineering, Ming Chi University of Technology, New Taipei City, Taiwan

Fabio Casciano and Paola Secchiero
Department of Morphology, Surgery and Experimental Medicine and LTTA Centre, University of Ferrara, Ferrara, Italy

Paolo D. Pigatto
Department of Dermatology and Venereology, I.R.C.C.S. Istituto Ortopedico Galeazzi, University of Milan, Milan, Italy

Roberto Gambari and Eva Reali
Department of Life Sciences and Biotechnology, University of Ferrara, Ferrara, Italy
Laboratory of Translational Immunology, I.R.C.C.S. Istituto Ortopedico Galeazzi, Milan, Italy

Index

A

Acanthosis, 27-28, 32, 36, 40, 44, 72, 102, 104, 109, 132, 142, 153, 212, 217, 227

Adaptive Immunity, 5, 40, 47, 98, 100, 117, 119, 143, 214, 222

Angiogenesis, 2-3, 5, 7-8, 11-13, 15-17, 19, 21-25, 54, 57, 92, 115, 129, 143, 148, 156, 187-188, 217, 219

Apoptosis, 1-3, 5-10, 53-54, 63, 71, 73, 76-77, 101, 114-115, 123, 137, 145, 154, 177, 218

Atherosclerosis, 7, 10-11, 19, 24, 46-54, 86-89, 92-94, 96, 121, 144, 146, 195-196, 199-202, 204-211, 213, 215, 218, 220-223, 230-231, 233

Atopic Dermatitis, 10, 43-44, 140-141, 143, 184, 187, 190, 192-193, 195, 198-200, 203-204, 210, 220, 224-225, 231

Autoantigens, 3-4, 6, 10, 26-27, 32, 36-37, 49, 56, 79-83, 85, 98, 101, 103, 119, 156, 163, 165, 168-170, 185-186, 214, 222, 227, 232

Autoimmune Disorder, 147

B

Biological Function, 171-172

C

Candida Albicans, 183, 186-187, 219, 224

Carbamylation, 6, 10, 155-156, 160, 164-166, 168

Cardiovascular Comorbidities, 12, 71, 94, 226-227, 229-231, 233

Cardiovascular Disease, 26, 46-47, 49-55, 67, 70-71, 86-87, 93-95, 130-131, 134, 139, 141, 144, 172, 189-190, 193-195, 202-203, 209-210, 212, 223, 226, 230

Cardiovascular Risk, 7, 47, 50-52, 86, 94-95, 130, 140, 201-204, 207-210, 212, 223

Cathelicidin, 4, 23, 26, 44, 82, 99-100, 103, 123, 128, 132, 155-156, 168-169, 218, 223

Cell Death, 1-3, 7-9, 11, 77, 104, 128-129, 170, 178

Cell Development, 29, 43, 148, 172, 178-179

Cell Proliferation, 9, 27-28, 32, 43-44, 62, 77, 100, 105-108, 111-114, 148, 154, 159, 163, 174-176

Chemokine, 29, 37-38, 43-44, 50, 70, 100, 114, 132-133, 143, 145, 169, 174-177, 181, 184, 198, 205, 215, 217, 220, 230, 232

Chromatin, 8, 56, 67, 123-124, 129, 198, 216-219

Chronic Inflammatory Disease, 47, 50, 119, 204

Citrullination, 129, 155-156, 159-160, 164-165

Comorbid Diseases, 119, 121-122, 140, 202, 209, 212

Confocal Microscopy, 155-158, 160-163, 165-168, 219

Coronary Heart Disease, 46, 50-51, 201, 203-204

Cytokines, 2-7, 12-13, 20, 31-33, 36, 42-50, 53-55, 57, 67, 79, 82, 92, 998-107, 110-111, 119-126, 128-129, 134-137, 140, 147, 149-150, 152-153, 156, 166, 171, 181, 184-185, 188-200, 208, 211, 217, 223-224, 227, 231, 233

Cytoplasm, 2, 7, 81

D

Degranulation, 159, 163, 214-218, 220-223

Depression, 26, 131, 134, 140, 143, 150, 152, 154, 188, 215, 221

Diabetes Mellitus, 26, 106, 143, 172, 202-203, 206, 215, 221

Disease Recurrence, 172

Dyslipidemia, 46-47, 67, 87, 92, 202, 220

E

Endothelial Dysfunction, 47-50, 94, 135, 139-140, 201-203, 206-209, 211, 220

Endothelium, 12, 21-22, 49, 130-131, 135-136, 139, 141, 146, 205-206, 211, 217

Epidermal Autoantigens, 37, 227

Epitope, 32, 83, 85, 167, 187, 230-231

G

Gene Expression, 56-58, 67, 70, 94, 101, 132, 136, 143, 145, 153-154, 169, 179-180, 193, 198, 229

Gene Module, 56

H

Human Leukocyte Antigen, 27, 79-81, 83, 85, 131, 133

Hypercitrullination, 123, 164, 169, 219

Hypercoagulability, 130-131, 135, 139

Hyperkeratosis, 27, 36, 72, 109, 148

Hypertension, 26, 46, 54, 87, 92, 94, 134-135, 148, 202-204, 208, 211-212

I

Immune Cells, 1-2, 5-6, 9, 26-28, 31, 38, 46-47, 50-51, 56, 75, 77, 89, 98-99, 101, 103, 112, 114, 117, 121-122, 125, 132, 135, 148-149, 152, 177-178, 188, 190, 194-195, 211, 214, 220, 231

Immune Complexes, 128, 158, 160, 219, 224

Innate Immunity, 5-7, 33, 40, 42, 44, 47, 52, 69, 98-99, 101-103, 117, 119, 121, 123, 125-129, 141-142, 145, 204, 214, 222

Insulin Resistance, 47, 50, 54, 67, 70-71, 77, 87, 134, 201-204, 206-208, 211-212, 220

K

Keratinocyte Hyperproliferation, 36-39, 42

Keratinocytes, 1-6, 8-10, 13, 20, 22-24, 26-28, 31-32, 37-41, 44, 47, 53-54, 72-77, 80, 82, 89, 98-104, 106, 112-114, 116, 118-121, 123, 125-126, 128-129, 132, 134, 142-143, 145, 148-150, 153, 156, 174-177, 188-190, 193, 195, 197, 199, 215-217, 219-220, 222, 224, 227

L

Ligand, 3, 43, 73, 103, 132-133, 137, 139, 146, 150-151, 154, 172, 175-177, 191, 197, 199, 205, 215, 217, 219-220, 229

Lipid, 4-5, 7, 10, 27, 48-50, 63, 67, 73, 98-99, 101, 106, 113, 216, 218

Liver Disease, 134, 144

Lymph Nodes, 43-44, 105, 111, 113-114, 174, 176-177, 180, 182

M

Macrophages, 3, 5-6, 10, 12-16, 20-22, 24-25, 38, 47-48, 50, 54, 70, 87, 92, 99, 113, 118, 121-123, 128, 132, 143-144, 146, 148, 153-154, 158, 175, 195, 203, 205, 211, 217, 219-220, 223-224

Metabolic Syndrome, 51, 56, 67, 69-72, 87, 93, 106, 134, 144, 188, 202-204, 209-210, 233

Monocytes, 7, 12-15, 19-22, 24-25, 42, 44-45, 48, 53-54, 87, 92, 101, 132, 135, 143, 145, 169, 175, 194, 203-205, 222

Myeloid Cells, 12, 20, 24, 120, 122-123, 190, 195, 211

N

Neutrophil Extracellular Traps, 48, 54, 117, 124, 128-129, 170, 214, 216, 218, 223-225

Neutrophils, 5-6, 9, 27, 32, 36, 38-40, 44, 47-50, 54, 99-102, 123-129, 132, 142, 146, 149, 153, 155-156, 158-161, 163-165, 169, 174-177, 180, 189-190, 194-197, 199, 203, 205, 211, 214-223, 225, 233

Nuclear Receptor, 147, 149-150, 153-154

O

Obesity, 26, 46, 50-51, 54, 67, 70, 84, 87, 106, 131-132, 134, 141, 172, 202, 204, 207, 212, 215, 220-221

Oxidative Stress, 1-2, 4-11, 115, 132, 139, 214, 216-217, 222

P

Palmoplantar Pustulosis, 84, 119, 127, 147, 224

Paradoxical Psoriasis, 36-37, 39-42, 194

Parakeratosis, 27, 36, 40, 72, 74, 106, 109

Pathogenesis, 1-7, 9-11, 27-29, 36-39, 41-43, 45, 50, 56-59, 61, 63, 69-77, 79-81, 89, 94, 96, 101-104, 113-114, 125-128, 130-132, 141-142, 147-148, 156, 162-163, 171-172, 181, 183, 194, 200-201, 204, 207, 216-217, 226-233

Peptide, 4-6, 9, 23, 27, 32, 37, 42, 44, 47, 57, 76, 79-85, 100, 103, 119, 123, 126, 128-129, 132, 142, 148, 153, 156-157, 162, 164, 166-169, 177, 190, 197, 218-219, 223, 227, 231

Peripheral Blood, 6-7, 9-10, 24-25, 28, 32, 43, 57-58, 70, 74, 77, 89, 130, 153, 165, 168, 172-175, 179, 181, 190, 220, 227, 229-231

Plaque Psoriasis, 14, 24, 29, 32-36, 39, 41-44, 52, 94-97, 103, 126, 128, 141, 144-145, 148, 152-153, 166, 171, 181, 183-184, 187, 197, 212, 222, 224, 230, 232

Polymorphisms, 24-25, 36, 41, 45, 81, 102, 119, 182, 192, 197, 204, 227

Protein-protein Interaction, 56, 58, 63-64

Psoriasis, 1-16, 18-58, 60, 62, 64, 66-68, 70-160, 162, 164, 166-233

Psoriatic Arthritis, 1-11, 14, 16, 18, 24, 28, 30, 32, 38, 40, 42, 44, 56-71, 78, 80-84, 94, 96, 100, 102, 110, 114, 118-120, 122, 124, 126, 128, 134, 136, 138, 144, 146, 150, 172, 174, 180, 182, 184, 186, 192, 194, 200, 202, 204, 206, 212, 218, 224, 226, 228-233

Psoriatic Disease, 1-2, 5, 22, 46, 52, 89-90, 93, 168, 229-230, 232-233

Psoriatic Lesions, 12, 20, 23, 27, 29, 31, 40, 42-43, 48, 71, 73, 84, 87, 100-101, 119, 131-132, 142, 149, 176, 185, 187, 205, 216-217, 220, 227, 229, 231

Psoriatic Phenotype, 22, 27, 36-40, 42, 102, 205

Psoriatic Skin, 4-6, 10, 25, 27, 29, 32, 37-38, 44, 54, 73, 76-77, 81, 87, 89, 94, 99-103, 105, 109, 113, 116, 118, 120, 122-124, 127, 132, 134, 136, 145, 152, 156, 166, 175-176, 181, 185, 187, 190-192, 195-199, 214, 217-221, 226-227, 229, 231-232

Pustular Psoriasis, 13-14, 23-24, 119, 126, 129, 147, 189, 197, 215, 220, 222

R

Rapamycin, 67, 72-75, 77-78, 108, 175

Respiratory Burst, 214, 216-218, 220

S

Skin Disease, 2, 36, 48, 72, 79, 94, 98, 103, 126, 140, 142, 147-148, 152, 166, 171, 188, 201, 203

Skin Inflammation, 2, 5-6, 9-10, 22, 24-25, 27, 32-33, 38, 43-44, 48, 53, 93, 98, 103-104, 115-116, 119, 125, 129, 142, 147, 171, 176-178, 181-182, 188, 190, 193-195, 198-199, 203-204, 210, 218, 224-225, 232

Skin Lesions, 2, 5-6, 23, 36-37, 39-41, 48, 75, 79, 81, 84, 98, 101-103, 109-110, 115, 123, 129, 134, 136, 149, 156, 162, 178, 181-182, 199, 214-215, 217, 219-220, 223, 227, 231-232

Spleens, 105, 111, 113-114

Streptococcus Pyogenes, 132, 183-184, 186-187

Systemic Inflammation, 5, 70, 76, 89, 93-94, 105, 125, 130, 134-135, 139-140, 166, 190, 197, 201, 203-205, 207-209, 211, 213-215, 226, 229-230, 232

T

Tissue Inflammation, 13, 153, 217-218, 230

Topical Treatment, 75, 166

Tumor Necrosis Factor, 2, 10, 24, 27, 30, 42-43, 45-46, 49-50, 54, 56-57, 86, 88, 91, 94-95, 127, 141-142, 145-146, 148-150, 153-154, 175, 198, 204, 213, 215, 217

V

Vascular Inflammation, 46-47, 52-53, 55, 94, 143, 206, 208-209, 213, 233

www.ingramcontent.com/pod-product-compliance
Lightning Source LLC
LaVergne TN
LVHW082138200926
848484LV00008B/2070
* 9 7 9 8 8 8 7 4 0 4 0 3 5 *